Cardiovascular Problems in Emergency Medicine

Current Topics in Emergency Medicine

Series editor-in-chief, Peter Rosen
Associate series editor-in-chief, Shamai A. Grossman

Cardiovascular Problems in Emergency Medicine

A discussion-based review

Editor-in-chief

Shamai A. Grossman, MD, MS, FACEP

Director, Cardiac Emergency Center and Clinical Decision Unit
Beth Israel Deaconess Medical Center
Assistant Professor of Medicine
Harvard Medical School
Boston, Massachusetts, USA

Senior editor

Peter Rosen, MD, FACS, FACEP

Director of Education
Beth Israel Deaconess Medical Center
Senior Lecturer in Medicine
Harvard Medical School
Boston, Massachusetts, USA

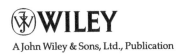

A John Wiley & Sons, Ltd., Publication

Library of Congress Cataloging-in-Publication Data
Cardiovascular problems in emergency medicine : a discussion-based review /edited by Shamai Grossman ; associate editor-in-chief, Peter Rosen.
       p. ; cm. – (Current topics in emergency medicine)
    Includes bibliographical references and index.
    ISBN-13: 978-0-470-67067-5 (pbk. : alk. paper)
    ISBN-10: 978-0-470-67067-3 (pbk. : alk. paper)
    ISBN-13: 978-1-119-95977-9 (ePDF)
    ISBN-13: 978-1-119-95980-9 (Wiley Online Library)
    [etc.]
  1. Cardiovascular emergencies--Case studies. 2. Evidence-based medicine–Case studies. I. Grossman, Shamai A. II. Rosen, Peter III. Series: Current topics in emergency medicine.
    [DNLM: 1. Cardiovascular Diseases–Case Reports. 2. Emergency Treatment–Case Reports. 3. Critical Care–Case Reports. 4. Emergency Medical Services–methods–Case Reports. 5. Evidence-Based Medicine–Case Reports. WG 205]
   RC675.C39 2011
   616.1'025--dc23
                                                                                2011024785
A catalogue record for this book is available from the British Library.

This book is published in the following electronic formats: ePDF 9781119959779; Wiley Online Library 9781119959809; ePub 9781119959786; Mobi 9781119959793

Set in 9/11.5pt Sabon by Thomson Digital, Noida, India

1   2011

Contents

List of Contributors

Editor-in-chief

Shamai A. Grossman, M.D., M.S. FACEP
Director, Cardiac Emergency Center and Clinical
 Decision Unit
Beth Israel Deaconess Medical Center
Assistant Professor of Medicine
Harvard Medical School
Boston, Massachusetts, USA

Senior editor

Peter Rosen, M.D., FACS, FACEP
Director of Education
Beth Israel Deaconess Medical Center
Senior Lecturer in Medicine
Harvard Medical School
Boston, Massachusetts, USA

Editors

William J Brady, MD
Vice Chair
Department of Emergency Medicine
Professor of Emergency Medicine and Medicine
University of Virginia Health System
Charlottesville, VA, USA

David F M Brown, MD
Vice Chair
Department of Emergency Medicine
Massachusetts General Hospital
Associate Professor
Harvard Medical School
Boston, Massachusetts, USA

Theodore C. Chan, MD
Medical Director
Department of Emergency Medicine
University of California, San Diego Medical Center
Professor of Clinical Medicine
University of California, San Diego
San Diego, California, USA

Richard Harrigan, M.D.
Professor of Emergency Medicine
Temple University School of Medicine
Philadelphia, PA, USA

Amal Mattu, MD, FAAEM, FACEP
Professor and Residency Director
Department of Emergency Medicine
University of Maryland School
 of Medicine
Baltimore, Maryland, USA

Edward Ullman, MD
Assistant Professor of Medicine
Harvard Medical School
Director of Medical Student Education
Division of Emergency Medicine
Beth Israel Deaconess Medical Center
Boston, Massachusetts, USA

Contributing authors

Jonathan Anderson, MD
Instructor of Medicine
Harvard Medical School
Beth Israel Deaconess Medical Center
Boston, Massachusetts, USA

Russell Berger, MD
Children's Hospital Boston
Junior Toxicology Fellow
Harvard Medical Toxicology Fellowship
Children's Hospital Boston,
 Massachusetts, USA

J. Stephen Bohan, MD, MS
Executive Vice Chair
Department of Emergency Medicine
Brigham and Women's Hospital
Assistant Professor of Medicine
Harvard Medical School
Boston, Massachusetts, USA

Michael A. Bohrn, MD, FAAEM, FACEP
Clinical Associate Professor of
  Emergency Medicine
Penn State University College of Medicine
Hershey, PA, USA

Kenneth J. Bramwell, MD
Academic: Director
Pediatric Emergency Medicine
Emergency Medicine of Idaho
St. Luke's Regional Medical Center
Boise, Idaho, USA

Brian J. Browne, MD, FAAEM, FACEP
Professor and Chairman
Department of Emergency Medicine
University of Maryland School of Medicine
Baltimore, Maryland, USA

Nathan Charlton, MD
Assistant Professor of Emergency Medicine
Department of Emergency Medicine
Consultant in Toxicology
Division of Medical Toxicology, Department of
  Emergency Medicine
Medical Director, Blueridge Poison Center
University of Virginia Health System
Charlottesville, VA, USA

Catherine Cleaveland, M.D.
Fellow, Division of EMS
Attending Physician, Department of
  Emergency Medicine
University of Virginia Health System
Charlottesville, VA, USA

Kristen Cochran, MD
Instructor in Medicine
Harvard Medical School
Beth Israel Deaconess Medical Center
Boston, Massachusetts, USA

Jeffrey Green, M.D.
Associate Professor of Emergency Medicine
U.C. Davis School of Medicine
Sacramento, CA, USA

Alden Landry, MD
Instructor in Medicine
Harvard Medical School
Beth Israel Deaconess Medical Center
Fellow
Commonwealth Fund/ Harvard University
  Minority Health Policy Fellowship
Boston, Massachusetts, USA

Benjamin J. Lawner, DO, EMT-P
Clinical Assistant Professor
Department of Emergency Medicine
University of Maryland School of Medicine
Deputy EMS Medical Director
Baltimore City Fire Department
Baltimore, Maryland, USA

Keith A. Marill, MD
Assistant Professor, Division of
  Emergency Medicine,
Harvard Medical School
Attending Physician, Department of
  Emergency Medicine,
Massachusetts General Hospital.
Boston Massachusetts, USA

Jehangir Meer, MD, FACEP, FRCPC, RDMS
Director of Emergency Ultrasound
St Agnes Hospital Center
Baltimore, Maryland

Laura Oh, MD
Department of Emergency Medicine
University of Virginia
  School of Medicine
Charlottesville, VA, USA

John T Nagurney, MD MPH
Assistant Professor of Surgery, Division of
  Emergency Medicine,
Harvard Medical School
Attending Physician and
  Director of Research,
Department of Emergency Medicine,
Massachusetts General Hospital
Boston, Massachusetts, USA

Robin Naples, M.D.
Assistant Professor of Emergency Medicine
Temple University School of Medicine
Philadelphia, Pennsylvania, USA

David A. Peak, MD
Assistant Professor, Division of Emergency Medicine,
Harvard Medical School
Attending Physician and Assistant
    Residency Director,
Department of Emergency Medicine,
Massachusetts General Hospital
Boston, Massachusetts, USA

David Plitt, MD
Department of Medicine
University of Virginia School of Medicine
Charlottesville, VA, USA

Kevin C. Reed, MD, FACEP, FAAEM
Assistant Professor of Clinical
    Emergency Medicine
Georgetown University School of Medicine
Department of Emergency Medicine,
Washington, USA

Jeffrey Soderman, MD
Attending Physician
Department of Emergency Medicine
Beverly Hospital
Beverly, MA, USA

Shannon Straszewski, MD
Chief Resident
Harvard Affiliated Residency in Emergency Medicine
Beth Israel Deaconess Medical Center
Boston, Massachusetts, USA

Jefferson G. Williams, MD, MPH
EMS Fellow and Clinical Instructor
University of North Carolina Department of
    Emergency Medicine
Chapel Hill, North Carolina, USA

Carrie D Tibbles, MD
Associate Director, Graduate Medical Education
Beth Israel Deaconess Medical Center
Associate Residency Director Harvard Affiliated
    Emergency Medicine Residency
Assistant Professor of Medicine
Harvard Medical School

Transcription editors

Colleen Birmingham, MD
Fellow in Medical Toxicology
New York University Medical Center/
    New York City Poison Center
New York, New York, USA

Jessica Klausmeier, MD
Division of Emergency Medicine
Beth Israel Deaconess Medical Center
Boston, Massachusetts, USA

Ashleigh Hegedus, MD
Instructor in medicine
Harvard Medical School
Division of Emergency Medicine
Beth Israel Deaconess Medical Center
Boston, Massachusetts, USA

Acknowledgements

Meaningful endeavors are seldom created in a vacuum. The authors would like to acknowledge a number of people who have enabled this book to come to fruition. Firstly, I would like to thank my mentor par excellence and chair, Dr Rich Wolfe, without whose creativity, few of my dreams would have been achieved. To Dr Peter Rosen, whose wisdom and leadership is apparent in every page of this book, I am forever indebted. To Maureen Blicker, your uncanny organizational skill made 27 weekly case discussions a reality. To my colleagues and residents in emergency medicine at Beth Israel Deaconess Medical Center, it is you who portray excellence in health care on a daily basis and motivate this text. I thank my beloved parents, Rabbi Rafael and Shirley Grossman, who have taught me well the words of Herzl, "if you will it, it shall not be a dream". My remarkable children, Naamah, Ezra, Atira, Meira, Tehila, Elianna and Netanel, you continue to inspire and teach me new ideas daily. To my wife Sharon, your partnership is equal in all of life's accomplishments; this book is a product of your endeavors as much as mine, ". . . and you have exceeded them all" (Proverbs 31:29). Lastly, I thank G-d for all his wisdom and kindness bestowed upon me. Ultimately, it is "the Lord who is thy healer" (Exodus 15:26).

Shamai A. Grossman

To Drs. Tim Marshall and Wayne Pinto. Without your expertise, I could not have worked on this book.

Peter Rosen

I would like to thank my wife, King, for everything that she does; without her, none of this work would be possible. I would also like to thank my children, Lauren, Anne, Chip, and Katherine, for being both wonderful and my inspiration. Lastly, I must also thank my emergency medicine colleagues, both at the University of Virginia and elsewhere, for their "most excellent" care of the patient, at times under less than optimal conditions in today's healthcare world.

William J Brady

Dedicated to past, present, and future Harvard Affiliated EM residents - thank you for inspiring me every day.

David FM Brown

Thanks to my wife, Diana, and children, Lauren and Taylor, for their love and support.

Theodore C. Chan

Thank you to my children, Quinn and Kelly, for continuing to open my eyes to what life is and what it should be, and showing me how to make those two things one.

Richard A. Harrigan

Dedicated to the "big rocks" in my life: my wife, Sejal, and my children Nikhil, Eleena, and Kamran, for their support and continued reminders of the priorities of life; and to the students, residents, and faculty of the Department of Emergency Medicine at the University of Maryland School of Medicine for their commitment to education.

Amal Mattu

To my parents, for their continuous support; to my beautiful daughters Maya and Sienna, who brighten and bring such joy to my day; to my wife Sonal, who makes me a better person and doctor, and to the patients who put their trust in me.

Edward Ullman

Preface

The hardest part of practicing medicine is knowing what questions must be answered. In discussions about our field, it quickly becomes apparent that many of the critical questions involve cardiac emergencies. We therefore decided to dedicate a monogram to the focused discussion of cardiac problems. For many decades, the right cardiac question was: "Is this patient having an acute myocardial infarction?" Yet, as we have become more sophisticated in being able to care for this disease process, it has become apparent that this is no longer the right question. Now we must struggle with: "Is this patient having an acute ischemic coronary syndrome?"

As we all struggle to answer the correct question and deal with it in an efficient, safe and practical fashion, we decided that it would be useful to query some of our colleagues about which questions to ask, and how they answer them.

With the emphasis today on making medical decisions based upon evidence, we wished to not only provide examples of that evidence at work, but to show how it is expressed through the experience and expertise of practicing Emergency Physicians.

We hope that this book will not only be of interest, but of some utility for those young physicians who are in the process of becoming fluent in the language of Emergency Medicine, as well as those students who are considering the field as a career. We also hope that those physicians who are already practicing Emergency Medicine will find these discussions not only interesting, but helpful to their daily management decisions as well.

We also remembered that we ourselves learned best from relevant clinical cases. We therefore decided to have each topic introduced by a clinical case, chosen from our actual practice, with a discussion of the case by our editorial board, sometimes supplemented by the chapter author.

Each chapter is divided into four sections: a relevant case, a discussion, a concept section, and a management section. Each chapter concludes with a management section that summarizes care of each disease in an algorithm or chart format. This final section is intended to serve as both a review and ultimately as an easily used reference guide while caring for patients.

While the cases represent our own styles and those of the institutions within which we practice, we hope that these examples will help instruct those who are struggling to formulate their own safe approaches to clinical management and provide a safe background upon which to build clinical confidence and expertise. Clearly these practices will continue to evolve as we acquire more evidence to solve some of the ongoing dilemmas that still exist about management. Precisely for that reason, we offer this book as a safe place from which to start, to improvise and to modify, so as to achieve the best outcomes for the patients with these complex and critical problems.

Shamai A. Grossman
Peter Rosen
October 2011

Cardiac Ischemia

SECTION ONE

Cardiac Ischemia

Chapter 1

Chest pain

Michael Bohrn[1], Amal Mattu[2] & Brian Browne[3]

[1] *Clinical Associate Professor of Emergency Medicine, Penn State University College of Medicine, Hershey, PA, USA*
[2] *Professor and Residency Director, Department of Emergency Medicine, University of Maryland School of Medicine, Baltimore, Maryland, USA*
[3] *Professor and Chairman, Department of Emergency Medicine, University of Maryland School of Medicine, Baltimore, Maryland, USA*

Section I: Case presentation

A 46-year-old man presented to the emergency department (ED) complaining of chest pain. The pain had begun while he was carrying some heavy boxes at home four hours prior, and had persisted since. He described the pain as a severe ache in the midsternal area, but there were superimposed sharp pains that radiated to the left shoulder when he took a deep breath. It did not appear to change with body or arm position, with walking, or with swallowing. He felt dyspneic and nauseated, and he also reported that he was diaphoretic during the first 20 minutes of the pain. The pain did not improve with ibuprofen, so he decided to come to the ED.

The past medical history was notable for HIV and hypertension. The patient had stated that he had been noncompliant with medications and primary care follow-up during the prior year. The last CD4 count one year ago was approximately 500. He had smoked one pack of cigarettes per day for more than 20 years, and had used crack cocaine regularly for 10 years, although he had not used cocaine for a week. He was uncertain if there was a family history of early cardiac disease or sudden death. He had been admitted for chest pain approximately six months earlier at a nearby hospital, and had a "negative" stress test at that time.

The vital signs were: temperature 37°C, pulse 90 beats/min, respirations 20 breaths/min, blood pressure 180/110 mmHg, pulse oximetry 98%. The cardiac and pulmonary examinations were normal with the exception of mild, sharp, left-sided chest pain with deep inspiration. The chest wall was mildly tender. The pulses and jugular venous pulsations were normal. There was no peripheral edema. The rest of the physical examination was normal. An electrocardiogram (EKG) was obtained, and demonstrated sinus rhythm with voltage criteria for left ventricular hypertrophy and diffuse T-wave flattening across the precordium. The chest X-ray study was normal.

Section II: Case discussion

Dr Peter Rosen: We are always taught that the most important part of the evaluation of ischemic chest pain is the history. Yet, for 30 years I have been trying to find a description of ischemic chest pain that enables me to say, "this chest pain is ischemic, and that is musculoskeletal, and that is gastrointestinal." Do you have any clues for us, or is that just one of the legends of clinical medicine?

Dr David Brown: I don't think there is an answer to your question that is clinically useful. Each of us could probably describe classic chest pain and classic findings for all of the conditions you just mentioned, but there is considerable overlap between these disease presentations such that I don't think the emergency

Cardiovascular Problems in Emergency Medicine: A discussion-based review, First Edition.
Edited by Shamai A. Grossman and Peter Rosen.
© 2011 John Wiley & Sons, Ltd. Published 2011 by John Wiley & Sons, Ltd.

physician can use the history alone to reliably exclude an acute coronary syndrome in a patient like this one.

PR: Do you think there is any benefit to the patient describing isometric exercise such as shoveling snow or, as in this history, less isometric exercise in that he was carrying boxes? Would a more isometric history, such as if he had said that the pain came on while he was lifting the boxes up onto a shelf, be more useful?

DB: If you have additional history from him regarding whether or not any use of the muscles or movement of his arm might have precipitated the pain, and can fully reproduce it now while he is in the ED, this may be useful. But I don't think there is a lot of utility in differentiating whether this exercise was isometric because one could say that he was walking at the same time, and that there was an aerobic component that precipitated the pain.

PR: The drug abuse history in this case makes me far less suspicious that this is ischemic pain. Once I get a history of cocaine use in a patient who says he hasn't used it in the past week, although time is relative for users, I find it is more likely to be nonspecific chest wall pain rather than ischemia. Is there any way you can distinguish these patients from history alone, or does it require a full workup?

Dr Shamai Grossman: Patients with cocaine chest pain always worry me because I find that they have more atypical presentations. These patients seem to present often, as this one has, with chest pain that can be from multiple different etiologies. Once they tell me that they use cocaine, I tend to not trust them to be telling me the truth when they say they haven't used cocaine in the last week. I would simply assume that the patient has actually used cocaine very recently, likely within the last 24 hours. Once I assume this, I also have to assume that the chest pain is cardiac in etiology until it has been fully proven otherwise.

PR: This patient also has a past history of HIV. I'm not aware of HIV causing ischemic cardiac disease. I have seen cardiac ischemia with pulmonic, oncologic, and gastrointestinal problems, but I don't believe I've ever seen a patient with HIV present with an ischemic coronary syndrome. Is this true?

SG: HIV can cause a dilated cardiomyopathy, although not an ischemic cardiomyopathy. In addition, recent data seem to suggest an increased incidence of coronary

artery disease with protease inhibitors, and HIV patients appear to be more likely to have traditional cardiac risk factors then the general population.[1–9] All of this requires one to truly think broadly when trying to sort out a diagnosis in this patient.

PR: What is the utility of that CD4 count that's a year old?

Dr Ted Chan: It suggests that, a year ago, he was not significantly immunosuppressed, and not at risk for many of the atypical infections associated with HIV. It's difficult to say what it might be now, particularly if he has been non-compliant with his medications over the past year.

PR: Would you say the same thing about his "negative" stress test from six months earlier?

SG: The same suspicions that I had about this patient's report that he hadn't used cocaine in a week would make me skeptical about his report of a negative stress test, and I wouldn't accept this at face value. The value of any stress test that is six months old is controversial, although some studies suggest that there is utility in a negative stress test anywhere from one and one-half to three years later.[10–13] However, the utility of a stress test is related to the pre- and post-test probability that this patient's symptoms are ischemic in etiology.

PR: This is the kind of patient who is going to be a significant management problem in the ED because no cardiologist is going to be excited about working him up, and he may be very hard to admit. We become very cynical about these patients because of their social circumstances, and they may have to prove to us that they are experiencing something nefarious before we will listen to their story. What should the extent of his workup in the ED be before you would push for a cardiology consult?

DB: Given an EKG that is nonspecific, a history that is suggestive but nondiagnostic, and no cardiac markers, we have little compelling data to prompt a cardiology consultation at this point. What he does need now is a first set of cardiac markers and a careful look at his electrocardiogram, perhaps obtaining an old EKG if one's available. There are some data to suggest that a rapid rule-out over 6 to 8 hours, including two sets of negative markers followed by some sort of provocative testing, is sufficient to evaluate patients with cocaine-related chest pain.[14]

SG: There are a couple of studies looking at the utility of stress testing in patients with cocaine chest pain, which suggest that they are not useful in the first few weeks following cocaine use.[15-18] In our institution, we tend not to obtain stress tests on these patients while they are in the observation unit or in the hospital. In patients at high risk based on their histories and EKGs suggestive of ischemia, we would likely take them for a cardiac catheterization. If they were a little lower risk, in this day and age, I might consider a cardiac computed tomography (CT) angiogram.

PR: I presume you would get a chest X-ray study to see if there is a noncardiac disease declaring itself as the source of the pleuritic pain. Would you get a repeat CD4 count?

TC: I would most likely not check a CD4 count, as we would probably not get it back in a timely manner. Furthermore, unless he is manifesting some other symptoms suggestive of an opportunistic infection, it probably would not be that helpful in terms of the emergency care.

PR: Since there is a pleuritic component to the history, would you evaluate him up for a pulmonary embolism (PE)?

TC: True, there is a pleuritic component to his pain, but he has minimal respiratory complaints, and the oxygenation is normal. Unless there is additional history of some immobilization, prior trauma, or something similar, I would put him in a low-risk category for PE, and perhaps screen him with a D-dimer.

PR: I was told by one of the county hospital faculty in a high cocaine use neighborhood that, one Saturday night, they did a toxicologic screen on all of the patients in the ED, and 100% of them tested positive for cocaine. Obviously you can't admit 100% of your patients to the observation unit, so can you limit utilizing the unit for the high-risk cocaine user only? I've been perhaps too cavalier in my own practice, because unless they have an enzyme elevation or a significant EKG change, I have not been doing further work-up on them, but maybe I should be treating them more diligently?

SG: Again, in a low-risk patient who had used cocaine (unclear if it was during the previous 24 hours, but within the last week), we would probably do serial enzymes 6 hours apart, and if they were negative, and if the patient were pain free with an unchanged follow-up EKG, we would probably discharge him home. We would arrange a follow-up, and possibly a stress test in the next 1 to 2 weeks. The patient with other risk factors, or a more worrisome story, is more likely to get a stress test as an outpatient 2 weeks later, or a coronary CT while in the ED.

PR: I've read some literature that says that while these patients seem to have an increased incidence of coronary artery disease over the general population, they do not respond to reperfusion when they appear to be having a myocardial infarction (MI) that is induced by cocaine. This leaves me puzzled as to what should the approach be for these patients? Do they require a stent, or are they better off treated with vasodilators like calcium channel blockade?

SG: Even though cocaine accelerates atherosclerosis, if these patients are having infarctions, it is more likely from coronary vasospasm than thrombosis. When the etiology is vasospasm, a stent is not going to be useful. In the acute setting, we generally use benzodiazepines as a first line treatment. Nevertheless, if the patient presents with an EKG suggestive of an acute MI, he would still be a candidate for thrombolytic therapy and coronary intervention, simply because you can't tell definitively, without visualizing the vessels, whether the etiology is vasospasm or atherosclerotic in etiology. For that reason, given a choice between thrombolytic therapy and taking the patient to the catheterization laboratory, I would certainly favor taking them to the catheterization laboratory; if you take them to the catheterization laboratory and it turns out that they have coronary vasospasm, then you could treat the vasospasm without subjecting the patient to the dangers of thrombolytic therapy.

PR: Do you have any different experiences in your institution?

TC: Our cardiologists may be more reticent to go to the catheterization laboratory right away, but I think that's just a function of their own practice.

PR: What about a nonspecific EKG change? It's easy to recognize an abnormality if it is new, but this case is a classic example of a patient who may have had EKG changes for a long time, and we may not be able to prove it because we won't be able to obtain a prior tracing. He also has a history of hypertension, so left ventricular hypertrophy with these changes wouldn't be unusual. Is this EKG reassuring if his enzymes are not elevated?

SG: In a patient with a nonspecific story, a nonspecific EKG that doesn't evolve when you do serial EKGs concurrent with serial cardiac enzymes tends to be much more useful. If the repeat EKG has changed, which I find is more often the case than that the enzymes have changed, then I become more concerned that this is cardiac ischemia. On the other hand, if the EKG is unchanged, I find myself more reassured that this is likely to be the baseline EKG, and that the presentation less likely to be cardiac ischemia in etiology.

PR: As many of these patients are often not just smoking cocaine but also abusing drugs intravenously, do you think there is any utility here for obtaining an echocardiogram to make sure you are not missing an endocarditis?

SG: Endocarditis should always be in your differential diagnosis, particularly in patients who are likely to engage in intravenous drug abuse. Unless there were other pieces of information suggestive of endocarditis, such as a concomitant fever, a murmur, splinter hemorrhages, or telangiectasias that would point towards endocarditis, I probably wouldn't pursue this diagnosis. Nevertheless, an echocardiogram is not an unreasonable test to do to help differentiate the etiologies of chest pain. One might be able to evaluate the valves and regional wall motion at the same time, and this might make it a very useful test.

PR: Over the years I've been confused about what pharmacotherapy to utilize in a cocaine user. Are aspirin, beta-blockers or anti-coagulants useful?

TC: Aspirin is inexpensive and rarely harmful in any patient, and that would include those with cocaine chest pain. Beta-blockers, depending on whether this patient had just ingested cocaine, might be problematic because of unrestricted alpha agonism. With anticoagulation, it depends on how you categorize this patient in terms of the likelihood of having an acute coronary syndrome (ACS) event. The higher the probability, the more anticoagulation is reasonable. With low-risk patients, cocaine by itself would not push me to start a glycoprotein 2b/3a inhibitor or heparin.

DB: I want to reiterate that cocaine chest pain patients should be approached the same way as other patients who present with chest pain, and should be evaluated like non-cocaine using patients. Their workup and treatment are dictated by the history, EKG and cardiac marker findings, and the persistence of symptoms.

Case resolution

The patient was admitted to a chest pain observation unit adjacent to the ED and ruled out for myocardial infarction based on negative troponin values. The EKG demonstrated no changes. The patient underwent an exercise stress test during which he developed recurrence of the chest tightness, accompanied by frank T-wave inversions in the lateral leads. The patient was then sent for cardiac catheterization that demonstrated mild diffuse atherosclerotic disease and a critical occlusion in the left circumflex artery. He was treated with a stent, and was discharged 2 days later in good condition.

Section III: Concepts

Background

Chest pain is one of the four most-common chief complaints for adult patients presenting to EDs in the United States.[19] While medical professionals and the lay public alike typically associate chest pain with a cardiac source (i.e., cardiac ischemia or infarction), a significant portion of patients with chest pain will have other etiologies of their pain. One study finds that nearly 21% of patients with chest pain have a noncardiac cause of their symptoms.[20] Chest pain may be caused by a variety of serious and life-threatening illnesses. Emergency department evaluation of the patient with chest pain therefore must focus on excluding the most dangerous conditions first. To accomplish this, care should be taken to employ a systematic approach to avoid missing one of these key diagnoses. Dangerous diagnoses associated with chest pain may be distilled down to a few easy to remember diagnoses. Acute coronary syndromes (acute myocardial infarction and unstable angina), aortic dissection, pulmonary embolism, tension pneumothorax, cardiac tamponade, and esophageal rupture are the most rapidly life-threatening diagnoses associated with chest pain symptoms. Evaluation of each chest pain patient should include consideration of each of these diagnoses. A careful clinical history and physical examination and consideration of individual risks versus benefits are important in determining the ultimate evaluation and treatment course for a specific patient.

Initial chest pain workup

Physicians evaluating a patient with chest pain should have a systematic approach to these patients, and the resulting workup should be based on the etiologies of chest pain, history, and physical examination findings.

Acute coronary syndrome (ACS)

An ACS is a frequent concern for emergency healthcare providers when evaluating patients with chest pain. The prospect of missing the diagnosis of acute myocardial infarction in the ED has been the topic of several papers. The commonly quoted "miss rate" for MI stands at 2.1%, and the consequences are significant, both for patient care and from a medico-legal perspective.[21] Missed MI accounts for 10% of malpractice claims against emergency physicians, but comprise 25% of the total cost of these malpractice claims.[22] Thus, consideration of cardiac ischemia or infarction should always occur when evaluating patients with chest pain.

A careful history and physical examination are the starting points for evaluating patients with possible ACS. Chest pain radiating to the left arm, right shoulder, or both arms is associated with a progressively higher likelihood of MI.[23] A history of a previous MI, diaphoresis, an S3 heart sound on auscultation, nausea and vomiting, hypotension, and pulmonary rales are also factors that increase the likelihood of MI.[23] Chest pain worsened by changes in position or described as sharp or stabbing has been associated with a lower likelihood of an acute MI, as has chest pain of very short duration.[24,25] In previous studies, chest pain of very short or very long duration is associated with a very low risk of acute cardiac events.[26] In addition, reproducible chest wall pain does not exclude a cardiac cause, including acute MI; in one study, up to 7% of patients with acute MI present with fully reproducible chest wall pain.[27]

Coronary artery disease risk factors are often used to help differentiate high- and low-risk patient groups in the ED. While the classic risk factors of diabetes mellitus, hypertension, older age, male gender, hyperlipidemia, smoking, and premature family history of coronary artery disease are useful in determining long-term risk of a patient developing coronary artery disease, the use of risk factors has very limited utility in the ED when trying to determine the *acute* risk of ACS.[28–30] The 2007 American College of Cardiology (ACC)/American Heart Association (AHA) Guidelines have affirmed that the most important factor associated with predicting ACS in a patient presenting with chest pain is the history of the present illness, clearly exceeding the predictive value of cardiac risk factors.[31,32]

Physical examination findings noted above, including diaphoresis, an S3 heart sound, and pulmonary rales, are all nonspecific and, in isolation, not overly helpful for pointing the overall diagnosis to acute MI. However, in conjunction with other historical findings, these may lead to an increased likelihood of MI.[24] The main benefit of the physical examination in patients with an acute MI is to exclude the acute complications of MI (e.g. valvular rupture, acute congestive heart failure), or other non-ACS diagnostic possibilities. Esophageal rupture, cardiac tamponade, tension pneumothorax, and aortic dissection may all have physical examination findings that suggest these entities instead of an acute MI.[33–36]

Aortic dissection

Aortic dissection is much less common than an acute MI or unstable angina, but the emergency physician must still be alert to the possibility of this entity. There is some overlap of clinical findings with those seen with myocardial ischemia, but several factors are helpful in determining the presence of acute aortic dissection. Chest pain is the most common symptom of acute aortic dissection, and though a description of "ripping" or "tearing" pain has been shown to have a significantly increased likelihood of aortic dissection, more recent registry data shows that sharp pain may be even more common.[37] Pain that is sudden in onset and pain which reaches maximal intensity at onset is also associated with aortic dissection. Several factors relating to the location of pain may be helpful. Tearing-type pain in the posterior thoracic or interscapular area may signify dissection involving the descending aorta, while pain in the neck or jaw may mean that the dissection affects the brachiocephalic or common carotid arteries and the aortic arch.[36,37] Typically, anterior chest pain may signify a dissection site at the root or ascending portion of the aorta.[37]

Several other presenting symptoms are well reported and varied, often depending on the location and extension of the dissection, including: neurologic deficits or stroke-like symptoms, flank pain, syncope, and altered mental status.[36] Other historical components include an increased incidence in men compared with women, as well as increased incidence with hypertension, especially following cocaine use. Finally, there are associations of aortic dissection with genetic connective tissue disease such as Marfan syndrome and Ehlers-Danlos syndrome, which may be found in nearly 5% of patients with acute aortic dissection. Pregnancy, syphilis, and bicuspid aortic valves have also been associated with aortic dissection.[37] Physical examination occasionally reveals pulse inequities between the upper and lower extremities. A blood pressure difference of 20 mmHg or more between the upper extremities has been associated specifically with aortic dissection.[38] Hypertension is the classic blood pressure finding with aortic dissection, and is seen in nearly half of all cases (although hypotension may be seen as well).[37,38] Hypotension associated with aortic dissection suggests a poor prognosis, as this typically signifies other complications, such as inferior wall MI, cardiac tamponade, or volume loss/bleeding.[37] Other common findings include neurologic deficits, which can be present in up to 20% of patients, and include stroke-like syndromes with extremity weakness or paresthesias or altered mental status.[37] A variety of other findings including shortness of breath, new diastolic murmur from acute aortic insufficiency, and dysphagia or hoarseness may be seen.[37]

Pulmonary embolism

Because of the difficulties in diagnosing pulmonary embolism (PE), a large body of medical literature exists on this topic, but it is still a most challenging condition to assess. The most commonly seen symptoms of PE include shortness of breath (60–79% of patients) and chest pain (17–64%).[39,40] The classic symptom triad of dyspnea, chest pain, and hemoptysis has been found to have poor sensitivity and specificity. Pleuritic chest pain is found in a significant proportion of patients with PE, though this complaint also has poor specificity for PE.[39,40] Several other symptoms may be seen, but none are very specific for PE; these include: syncope, palpitations, tachycardia, wheezing, cough, seizure, fever, lower extremity edema, diaphoresis, and cyanosis.[40] Unfortunately, no specific symptom is sufficient to diagnose PE. Physical findings with PE are similarly nonspecific and include fever, tachycardia, accentuated second heart sound, rales, tachypnea, and new cardiac murmurs or S3/S4 cardiac gallop. Additionally, cardiac dysrhythmias, especially atrial dysrhythmias such as atrial fibrillation, atrial flutter, and atrial premature contractions, may be present.[41] Given the difficulties in finding specific historical or physical findings for PE, assessment for risk factors for venous thromboembolism should be considered next. There are a wide variety of risks for venous thromboembolism, but a few important risks include: a history of previous deep venous thrombosis (DVT) or PE; hematologic factors such as protein C, protein S, antithrombin III deficiencies, or Factor V Leiden; prothrombin 2010 gene mutation; and a host of miscellaneous less common factors.[42] Additional recognized complications include recent travel or immobilization, history of cancer, recent trauma or surgery, estrogen hormone use, pregnancy, and the post-partum period.[43]

Using risk assessment in conjunction with standard history and physical examination findings, a variety of clinical prediction rules have been developed. While no rule is perfect, these tools may aid initial decision-making. The most well-known scoring system is the Well's score, which assigns points for any of the following findings: clinical signs/symptoms of DVT, heart rate over 100 beats per minute, immobilization, previous history of DVT/PE, hemoptysis, malignancy, and a determination of the likelihood of PE as compared with that of alternative diagnoses.[43] Another popular scoring system is the revised Geneva score (RGS).[44] The RGS is also a point-scoring system, and assigns points for any of the following: age >65, previous DVT or PE, major surgery or lower limb fracture within one month, malignancy within the past year, unilateral lower-limb pain, hemoptysis, rapid heart rate, and pain on lower-limb deep venous palpation or unilateral edema. Both the Well's score and the RGS assign low, intermediate, and high clinical probabilities of thromboembolism based on the point total. The use of these clinical probabilities can be combined with certain testing (e.g. D-dimer assay) to determine how far to progress with the workup.

For very low-risk patients in whom additional testing is being debated, use of the Pulmonary Embolism Rule-out Criteria (PERC) rule may be useful. This rule utilizes eight criteria: age <50 years, pulse <100 bpm,

$SaO_2 > 94\%$, no unilateral leg swelling, no hemoptysis, no recent trauma or surgery, no previous DVT or PE, and no hormone use.[45] In a more recent prospective multicenter evaluation, the PERC rule (PERC negative) in conjunction with a low clinical probability of PE reduced the probability of venous thromboembolism to $<2\%$.[46]

Tension pneumothorax
Tension pneumothorax is a life-threatening cause of chest pain. Clinical history is key with any history of trauma or associated respiratory issues. A recent military-based study shows a prevalence of tension pneumothorax in 3–4% of battlefield casualties.[47] A history of an obstructive airway process (e.g., asthma, chronic obstructive pulmonary disease) or of positive pressure ventilation (e.g., recent intubation, recent surgery, etc.) is very important in determining whether to pursue this diagnosis. A chest X-ray study or other imaging modality should be not be sought until the tension has been relieved, as the time spent in proving the diagnosis with an imaging study may prevent a successful relief of the tension pressures. Clinical findings are often present in support of this, with abnormal breath sounds—decreased breath sounds on the affected side or hyperresonance to percussion over the affected side—and deviation of the trachea away from the affected side representing the most common findings. Rapid imaging is indicated in patients with a suspected pneumothorax, with bedside ultrasound showing excellent sensitivity and specificity.[48] A chest X-ray study is the most common imaging modality utilized, although as stated, it is more prudent to relieve the tension than to prove its presence. In the setting of suspected tension pneumothorax, other imaging is also reserved for evaluation post-intervention, but CT scanning is more sensitive than chest X-ray for finding a small pneumothorax in general.

Cardiac tamponade
Cardiac tamponade is another condition with key historical and physical examination features. General history taking should include consideration of typical causes of pericardial effusion, including uremia, malignancy, HIV, tuberculosis, and other previous medical conditions and surgical procedures.[49,50] Recent pacemaker placement, central venous catheter insertion, cardiac catheterization, trauma, or other thoracic surgical procedures can lead to a very rapid development of pericardial fluid

and tamponade physiology.[50] A careful history including anticoagulant and antiplatelet use is also important, particularly if the presumed pericardial effusion is felt to be hemorrhagic in nature. Additional historical findings include weight loss, fatigue, night sweats, or symptoms suggestive of underlying rheumatologic or connective tissue disorders.[49] Specific symptoms to suggest current or impending cardiac tamponade include shortness of breath, dyspnea on exertion, tachypnea, air hunger, and tachycardia.[51]

The physical examination may demonstrate diaphoresis, tachycardia, and tachypnea, typically with clear lung fields.[49] The classic Beck's Triad consists of increased jugular venous pressure (JVP), hypotension, and diminished heart tones. This triad is typically seen with a significant pericardial effusion, and is more often seen with medical than traumatic etiologies.[49,52] Pulsus paradoxus is often described with cardiac tamponade. In severe tamponade, the pulses may disappear with inspiration. On auscultation, the difference between the first appearance of the first Korotkoff sound while obtaining the systolic blood pressure, and where it becomes steady, is the pulsus paradoxus. Greater than 10 mmHg is usually abnormal.[49] Transthoracic echocardiography at the bedside is probably the quickest way to confirm the presence of an effusion, and tamponade. The normal pathophysiologic response to tamponade is a tachycardia, but immediately prior to arrest, the patient will develop a bradycardia. The intrapericardial pressure must be relieved immediately when this is seen.

Esophageal rupture
The most common cause of esophageal rupture is iatrogenic, due to endoscopic or other procedures. The classic Boerhaave's syndrome, caused by repeated retching or vomiting, is seen in about 15% of cases of esophageal rupture, followed in incidence by toxic ingestions and penetrating trauma.[53] Other historical findings for classic esophageal rupture include a sudden onset of severe epigastric or chest pain following forceful vomiting or retching. Other potential causes include recent childbirth, heavy lifting or straining, blunt trauma, or bouts of severe coughing.[52-55] Some patients will complain of fever or of radiation of pain to the back, shoulder, or neck. Some patients will have difficulty with speech, or trouble swallowing. Previous esophageal conditions, cancer, or radiation treatment may also predispose patients to esophageal rupture.

Physical findings are varied with esophageal rupture, and many are nonspecific. Fever, tachypnea, tachycardia, and subcutaneous emphysema are important considerations. Subcutaneous emphysema is the most specific of these findings, but may take several hours to develop.[53–56] Hypotension may be a sign of septic shock from mediastinitis, and carries a grave prognosis. Hamman's crunch, a friction rub of the pericardium heard when auscultating the heart and occurring with each heart beat, is another useful finding that is fairly specific for mediastinal emphysema.[57] Esophageal rupture is best repaired early after the rupture surgically.

Testing for patients with chest pain

Once an initial differential diagnosis has been created, the next steps in the ED typically involve diagnostic testing. While each of the serious conditions outlined previously generate different workups, the workup for most ED patients with chest pain should start with an EKG and a chest X-ray study.

Electrocardiogram

The EKG is critically important in diagnosing ST-segment elevation MI (STEMI) and acute coronary syndromes, and also has benefit for non-ST-segment elevation MI (NSTEMI) and high-risk unstable angina patients. EKGs showing a STEMI will dictate rapid medical management, with either fibrinolytic therapy or percutaneous coronary intervention (PCI). For this reason, the initial EKG should be obtained and reviewed by the emergency physician within 10 minutes of the patient's arrival in the ED. The EKG can also help steer management toward other key diagnoses during the critical first few minutes of evaluation.

The EKG can be used to localize an acute STEMI to a specific wall or anatomic territory; commonly involved areas include the anterior, anterolateral, inferior, lateral, and septal territories.[58] Additionally, ST depressions in the right precordial leads (leads V1-V3) or ST elevation in specially placed posterior leads may signify an acute posterior wall STEMI.[59–61] Right-sided EKG leads should be obtained in patients with acute inferior STEMI.[62] This special placement of EKG leads can identify concurrent right ventricular infarction, which increases the possibility of complications, including hypotension (especially if nitroglycerin is utilized during treatment).[63–65]

EKGs demonstrating acute ST-segment deviation—ST depression or transient ST elevation—signify the need for rapid, aggressive medical management, or consideration of early invasive (PCI) therapy.[66] T-wave inversions can also be indicative of cardiac ischemia or non-ST-elevation MI, and a need for more aggressive medical management.[66] In addition, several specific findings on EKG may be suggestive of specific acute coronary syndromes or MI. ST elevation in lead aVR in patients with other findings suggestive of an acute coronary syndrome may be indicative of left main coronary artery occlusion.[67] The terminal T inversion and biphasic T wave pattern in precordial leads V2-V4 is sometimes known as Wellens' sign or Wellens' syndrome, indicating proximal occlusion of the left anterior descending coronary artery.[68,69]

Serial EKGs or continuous ST-segment monitoring are often useful in diagnosing an evolving ACS, and increase the sensitivity of the diagnostic process in these patients.[70] These options are especially important when managing ill-appearing patients with an initially unclear diagnostic evaluation, or those with persistent chest pain or other ischemic symptoms.

The EKG can also be a key diagnostic tool for other non-ACS conditions. The classic changes of diffuse ST elevation with PR depression suggest acute pericarditis, while low voltage and electrical alternans should raise suspicion for pericardial effusion and possible cardiac tamponade.[71,72,73] Aortic dissection may be associated with an acute STEMI when the coronary arteries are affected. A STEMI in conjunction with aortic dissection can involve the right coronary artery, and thus presents as an inferior wall STEMI.[74] Pulmonary embolism is associated with a wide variety of EKG changes, although none of these changes are specific enough to enable a diagnosis of PE from the EKG alone. In patients who might have a PE, the S1Q3T3 pattern has been seen with equal rates in patients with and without confirmed PE following testing.[75] Other EKG findings such as sinus tachycardia, nonspecific ST-T changes, right bundle branch block, atrial fibrillation or flutter may occur in the presence of acute PE as well.[76]

Chest X-ray study

The chest X-ray study represents the second test commonly obtained for ED patients presenting with chest pain. This study is useful in determining the presence or absence of a variety of pulmonary conditions, including pneumothorax, pneumonia, and pleural effusions, or obtaining information about other mediastinal structures. Supine chest X-ray sensitivity and specificity is lower than an upright chest X-ray study, with sensitivity typically listed in the 37–52% range even for those primary pulmonary disorders just mentioned, so reasonable attempts should be made to acquire upright rather than supine X-rays.[77–80]

Esophageal rupture may demonstrate a pleural effusion (usually on the left), pneumomediastinum, and subcutaneous emphysema.[81–83] Cardiac tamponade itself cannot be diagnosed by chest X-ray study, although the presence of a large, globular heart may suggest an underlying pericardial effusion.[84]

The most common manifestation of aortic dissection on chest X-ray (69% in one registry report) is a widened mediastinum, although the classic finding of aortic diameter of >5.5 cm for ascending (Type A) dissections has recently been questioned.[85] Several other chest X-ray findings may be seen with aortic dissection, including abnormal cardiac contour (51%), displacement or calcification of the aorta (7%), and pleural effusion (15%).[85] Most of these findings are seen with ascending aortic dissection, and not with descending aortic dissection. Aortic changes on the chest X-ray study may also be seen with traumatic aortic injury. Several findings may be seen, including left apical pleural cap, irregularity or loss of the aortic knob, tracheal shift to the right, depression of the left main bronchus, opacification of the aorticopulmonary window, and deviation of a nasogastric tube to the right or left as well as widening of the mediastinum.[86,87]

Finally, the chest X-ray study is probably of the lowest utility in evaluation of patients with presumed cardiac ischemia from acute MI or other acute coronary syndromes. In these patients, the primary benefit of a chest X-ray study is to differentiate alternative conditions that might be the cause of a patient's symptoms, or to identify concurrent heart failure.

Other diagnostic imaging studies

Following initial evaluation with EKG and the chest X-ray study, many patients require additional imaging to further delineate their clinical conditions. The mainstays of this imaging are CT scans and ultrasound-based studies (bedside ultrasound, echocardiography, etc.). For those patients with concerns regarding aortic dissection or pulmonary embolism, CT scanning with IV contrast is typically the next diagnostic study to be obtained, and "triple rule out" or other scanning techniques simultaneously evaluate for coronary artery disease, pulmonary embolism, and aortic dissection. These studies are currently being performed with low frequency, but may be more prevalent in the future as technology advances.[88] CT scanning has been shown to be very sensitive for determining the presence and location of acute aortic dissection, and EKG-gated protocols allow more reliable imaging.[89] This can be very helpful for determining the specific location of the dissection and its relation to the renal arteries— important information for surgical colleagues as they plan their management. As noted above, CT imaging can also be of assistance in diagnosing other potential intra-thoracic causes of chest pain, and can be used to assess for pulmonary embolism and coronary atherosclerotic disease.

CT scanning with IV contrast is very useful for diagnosing pulmonary embolism. The sensitivity and specificity for these scans is high, with one systematic review noting an overall negative predictive value following a negative CT scan for PE of 99.1%.[90] CT scans provide a high diagnostic yield, but do not come without potential pitfalls. The most common of these problems include IV contrast reactions and higher radiation exposure, although EKG-gating and reduced CT tube voltage may help to limit increases in radiation dose.[91]

Ultrasound-based studies may be obtained directly at the bedside by the emergency physician, or via colleagues in radiology or cardiology. Most patients requiring urgent ultrasonography for chest pain have time-sensitive clinical presentations or are considerably ill, and studies outside the ED are often not possible to obtain safely. A wide range of studies illustrates the utility of emergency ultrasound for these chest pain-related conditions, and a recent policy statement by the American College of Emergency Physicians emphasizes the increasing role ultrasound has in daily clinical practice.[92] Probably the easiest to perform and most-studied use of ultrasound is in determining the presence of a pericardial effusion. Additionally, more detail can be obtained by evaluating for right ventricular collapse, which is another finding readily seen on bedside ultrasound.[93] Right ventricular collapse points toward tamponade physiology. Several studies have looked at the utility of ultrasound in making the diagnosis of pneumothorax. A variety of signs can help the emergency physician identify pneumothorax via ultrasound, including the comet tail sign, sliding sign, etc.[48,94,95] While the ultrasonic image can demonstrate the pneumothorax, it cannot tell you the size, or whether there is tension pathophysiology. Ultrasonographic diagnosis of pneumothorax may be most useful in trauma, in the intensive care unit, or in other supine patients where initial chest X-ray imaging may not be sensitive enough to exclude a pneumothorax.[94,95] In addition, ultrasound use allows visualization of an associated hemothorax or pleural effusion.

Bedside echocardiography can be very helpful with diagnosing aortic dissection. For unstable patients who are unable to leave the ED for imaging, bedside echocardiography is the study of choice.[96] If available, transesophageal echocardiography is preferred. In addition, echocardiography can evaluate for associated valvular dysfunction, especially aortic insufficiency, which sometimes accompanies aortic dissection, as well as regional wall motion abnormalities and overall systolic function in patients with concurrent acute MI.

Esophageal rupture may be diagnosed by contrast-enhanced X-ray studies utilizing water-soluble contrast, or via direct endoscopy. Additional imaging may be needed via CT scanning or other studies in order to fully evaluate this condition.

Various other imaging modalities have currently or may have in the future a role in evaluating selected patients with acute chest pain. Chief among these tests, magnetic resonance imaging can be used for aortic dissection and other aortic injuries, formal aortography can also be obtained in appropriate patients, and ventilation-perfusion scans can be useful in specific patients being evaluated for pulmonary embolism. A wide variety of cardiac perfusion and other imaging can be utilized for patients with chest pain suggestive of an ACS.

Laboratory studies

Laboratory studies are not overly helpful for a number of chest pain syndromes. However, the diagnosis of ACS, including acute STEMI and non-STEMI ACS, is largely based on the use of cardiac biomarkers, primarily troponin. There is much in the medical literature regarding the use of cardiac markers in the evaluation of patients with chest pain. Various protocols involving myoglobin, creatine kinase-MB fraction (CK-MB) and troponins are currently in use. The diagnostic benefit of myoglobin involves a trade-off: very high sensitivity balanced by a relatively low specificity for acute MI. Most protocols utilizing myoglobin seek to exploit the high sensitivity in order to perform a rapid "rule-out" of MI.[97] CK-MB was the previously preferred test for evaluating for myocardial necrosis from MI. Troponins (troponin I or troponin T) are now being used as the primary markers for myocardial necrosis and MI, particularly when attempting to "rule in" a diagnosis of acute MI, and the American College of Cardiology and European Society of Cardiology embraced troponins in their 2000 joint statement on the definition of myocardial infarction.[62,97-99] All of these biomarkers are indicative of myocardial necrosis, and therefore they are only reliably elevated in MI, but the failure to detect a rise does not eliminate the presence of cardiac ischemia. Furthermore, because there is a delay in detectable serum levels of these biomarkers after MI, a single laboratory result does not reliably rule out MI if the level is obtained within the first few hours of the MI.[62,97] Serial cardiac markers, especially when obtained 6 hours or more following symptom onset, demonstrate a much improved sensitivity, nearing 98–100%.[100] Even when only one of the markers is elevated (e.g., elevated CK-MB in conjunction with a normal troponin value), patients are still at higher risk for adverse events. Troponin elevation, however, tends to be more reliably predictive of adverse events.[101,102]

Cardiac markers, especially troponin, are also being evaluated for their role in diagnosing aortic dissection and pulmonary embolism. Troponin levels may be elevated above the threshold defining acute myocardial infarction in close to 10–11% of patients with acute aortic dissection, especially with a type A or ascending dissection, but the specificity of troponin testing for aortic dissection is not adequate to differentiate this condition from an acute MI.[103-104] Several studies have examined the role of troponin T or troponin I testing for pulmonary embolism and, while some studies show elevated troponin levels with massive PE/right ventricular dysfunction, the overall specificity of troponin testing in differentiating a primary myocardial infarction remains unclear. Some suggest combined approaches that utilize troponin testing followed by acute echocardiography in appropriate patients.[105]

The other major laboratory test that has utility in the diagnosis of chest pain syndromes is the D-dimer. In one large, prospective observational study, the rate of developing venous thromboembolism at three months after the onset of symptoms in patients with a low clinical probability and negative D-dimer result is only 0.5%.[106] Obtaining D-dimer testing in very low-risk, or in moderate-to-high-risk patients, will result in significant numbers of false positive or false negative tests, respectively. The PIOPED II investigators also recommend clinical evaluation, followed by D-dimer testing in appropriate patients, with CT pulmonary angiography and CT venography for patients in whom further testing is needed.[107]

Other laboratory tests may have roles once a critical chest pain diagnosis is confirmed (e.g., correctable anemia in a patient with cardiac ischemia or acute MI), but there is little diagnostic benefit to most other laboratory tests for acute chest pain syndromes.

Disposition of emergency department patients with chest pain

Most of the critical diagnoses associated with chest pain represent serious conditions where admission to the hospital or directly to the operating room is indicated. This seems straightforward with patients diagnosed with acute MI, acute aortic dissection, pulmonary embolism, esophageal rupture, cardiac tamponade, or tension pneumothorax. Admission of patients with pericarditis is less clear, and often depends upon other co-morbid conditions and current clinical findings, as well as the underlying etiology of the pericarditis. Pneumothorax without tension presents similar challenges. While a large pneumothorax that requires a tube thoracostomy warrants an admission, it is less true for patients with a small pneumothorax. These patients often may be managed with a short-term (i.e., 6 hour) observation and repeat chest X-ray study, followed by discharge with close follow-up; needle aspiration of the pneumothorax in the ED followed by discharge home; or simple outpatient observation with close follow-up and repeat chest X-ray studies.[108] A variety of scoring systems have been used to assist with disposition decisions regarding patients with pneumonia, including the PORT score/pneumonia severity index and the CURB-65 score.[109-111] Some patients with chest pain may have musculoskeletal pain, and may be safely discharged to home, as can the majority of patients with acute herpes zoster-related pain. Patients may also have gastrointestinal-related symptoms such as esophageal spasm, gastroesophageal reflux disease, or other syndromes, and these patients usually can be discharged to home, if the diagnosis can be clearly established.

Unfortunately, there is considerable overlap in the clinical findings for these various conditions, and admission or further testing is warranted to exclude a serious potential cause of the chest pain. In all of these cases, clinical judgment supersedes all testing and guidelines.

Section IV: Decision making

- Careful consideration must be made of the critical chest pain differential diagnoses including:
  acute coronary syndrome
  aortic dissection
  pulmonary embolism
  esophageal rupture
  pericarditis/cardiac tamponade
  tension pneumothorax
- Less critical diagnoses include non-tension pneumothorax, pneumonia, musculoskeletal problems, and herpes zoster.
- Evaluation for all of these entities starts with a focused history and physical examination.
- EKG and chest X-ray study are indicated in most patients with chest pain.
- Further testing and consultations are guided by clinical presentation.
- Cardiac biomarkers and D-dimer testing should be considered.
- Chest pain attributable to one of the critical diagnoses above warrants admission.
- Use of clinical judgment is paramount.

References

1 Mary-Krause M, Cotte L, Simon A, Partisani M, Costagliola D. Increased risk of myocardial infarction with duration of protease inhibitor therapy in HIV-infected men. *Aids*. 2003;17:2479–2486.

2 Jutte A, Schwenk A, Franzen C, et al. Increasing morbidity from myocardial infarction during HIV protease inhibitor treatment? *Aids*. 1999;13:1796–1797.

3 Bozzette SA, Ake CF, Tam HK, Chang SW, Louis TA. Cardiovascular and cerebrovascular events in patients treated for human immunodeficiency virus infection. *N Engl J Med.* 2003;348:702–710.

4 Friis-Moller N, Sabin CA, Weber R, et al. Combination antiretroviral therapy and the risk of myocardial infarction. *N Engl J Med.* 2003;349:1993–2003.

5 Hsue PY, Giri K, Erickson S, et al. Clinical features of acute coronary syndromes in patients with human immunodeficiency virus infection. *Circulation.* 2004; 109:316–319.

6 Bergersen BM, Sandvik L, Dunlop O, Birkeland K, Bruun JN. Prevalence of hypertension in HIV-positive patients on highly active retroviral therapy (HAART) compared with HAART-naive and HIV-negative controls: results from a Norwegian study of 721 patients. *Eur J Clin Microbiol Infect Dis.* 2003;22:731–736.

7 Smith CJ, Levy I, Sabin CA, et al. Cardiovascular disease risk factors and antiretroviral therapy in an HIV-positive UK population. *HIV Med.* 2004;5:88–92.

8 Hadigan C, Meigs JB, Wilson PW, et al. Prediction of coronary heart disease risk in HIV-infected patients with fat redistribution. *Clin Infect Dis.* 2003;36:909–916.

9 Grunfeld C, Pang M, Doerrler W, et al. Lipids, lipoproteins, triglyceride clearance, and cytokines in human immunodeficiency virus infection and the acquired immunodeficiency syndrome. *J Clin Endocrinol Metab.* 1992;74:1045–1052.

10 Bangalore S, Yao S, Puthumana J, et al. Incremental prognostic value of stress echocardiography over clinical and stress electrocardiographic variables in patients with prior myocardial infarction: "warranty time" of a normal stress echocardiogram. *Echocardiography.* 2006;23(6):455–464.

11 Hachamovitch R, Hayes S, Friedman J, et al. Determinants of risk and its temporal variation in patients with normal stress myocardial perfusion scans: what is the warranty period of a normal scan? *J Am Coll Cardiol.* 2003; 41:1329–1340.

12 Mahenthiran J, Bangalore S, Yao S, et al. Comparison of prognostic value of stress echocardiography versus stress electrocardiography in patients with suspected coronary artery disease. *Am J Cardiol.* 2005;96:628–634.

13 Metz LD, Beattie M, Hom R, et al. The prognostic value of normal exercise myocardial perfusion imaging and exercise echocardiography: a meta analysis. *J Am Coll Cardiol.* 2007;49:227–237.

14 Weber JE, Shofer FS, Larkin GL, et al. Validation of a brief observation period for patients with cocaine-associated chest pain. *N Engl J Med.* 2003;348:510–517.

15 Littmann L, Miller RF, Monroe MH. Stress testing in patients with cocaine-associated chest pain. *J Emerg Med.* 2004;27:417–418.

16 Weber JE, Bonzheim SC, Boczar ME, et al. The uncertain benefit of immediate stress testing (ETT) for low-intermediate-risk patients with cocaine-associated chest pain in the ed-cardiac decision unit (CDU). *Acad Emerg Med.* 2001;8:553.

17 Kanneganti P, Nelson RA, Boyd SJ, et al. Exercise stress testing in recently abstinent chronic cocaine abusers. *Am J Drug Alcohol Abuse.* 2008;34:489–498.

18 McCord J, Jneid H, Hollander JE, et al. Management of cocaine-associated chest pain and myocardial infarction: a scientific statement from the American Heart Association Acute Cardiac Care Committee of the Council on Clinical Cardiology. *Circulation.* 2008;117:1897–1907.

19 Merrill CT, Owens PL, Stock CS. Emergency Department Visits for Adults in Community Hospitals from Selected States, 2005. Statistical Brief #47. Rockville, MD. Agency for Healthcare Research and Quality (AHRQ).

20 Miller CD, Lindsell CJ, Khandelwal S, et al. Is the initial diagnostic impression of "noncardiac" chest pain adequate to exclude cardiac disease? *Ann Emerg Med.* 2004;44:565–574.

21 Pope JH, Aufderheide TP, Ruthazer R, et al. Missed diagnoses of acute cardiac ischemia in the emergency department. *N Engl J Med.* 2000;342:1163–1170.

22 Karcz A, Korn R, Burke M, et al. Malpractice claims against emergency physicians in Massachusetts 1975-1993. Am J Emerg Med. 1996;14(4):341–345.

23 Panju AA, Hemmelgarn BR, Guyatt GH, et al. It this patient having a myocardial infarction? *JAMA.* 1998;280(14):1256–1263.

24 Lee TH, Cook EF, Weisberg M, et al. Acute chest pain in the emergency room. *Arch Intern Med.* 1985;145:65–69.

25 Solomon CG, Lee TH, Cook EF, et al. Comparison of clinical presentation of acute myocardial infarction in patients older than 65 years of age to younger patients: the Multicenter Chest Pain Study experience. *Am J Cardiol.* 1989;63:772–776.

26 Tatum JL, Jesse RL, Kontos MC, et al. Comprehensive strategy for the evaluation and triage of the chest pain patient. *Ann Emerg Med.* 1997;29(1):116–125.

27 Swap CJ, Nagurney JT. Value and limitations of chest pain history in evaluation of patients with suspected acute coronary syndromes. *JAMA.* 2005;294:2623–2629.

28 Han JH, Lindsell CJ, Storrow AB, et al. The role of cardiac risk factor burden in diagnosing acute coronary syndromes in the emergency department setting. *Ann Emerg Med.* 2007;49(2):145–152.

29 Jayes RL, Beshansky JR, D'Agostino RB, et al. Do patients' coronary risk factor reports predict acute cardiac ischemia in the emergency department? A multicenter study. *J Clin Epidemiol.* 1992;45(6):621–626.

30 Body R, McDowell G, Carley S, et al. Do risk factors for chronic coronary heart disease help diagnose acute myocardial infarction in the emergency department? *Resuscitation*. 2008;79:41–45.

31 Anderson JL, Adams CD, Antman EM, et al. ACC/AHA 2007 guidelines for the management of patients with unstable angina/non-ST-elevation myocardial infarction: executive summary. *Circulation*. 2007;116: 803–877.

32 Antman EM, Hand M, Armstrong PW, et al. 2007 focused update of the ACC/AHA 2004 guidelines for the management of patients with ST-elevation myocardial infarction: a report of the American College of Cardiology/American Heart Association Task Force on Practice Guidelines. *J Am Coll Cardiol*. 2008;51:210–247.

33 Eroglu A, Can Kurkcuoglu I, Karaoglanglu N, et al. Esophageal perforation: the importance of early diagnosis and primary repair. *Dis Esophagus*. 2004;17(1):91–94.

34 Aikat S, Ghaffari S. A review of pericardial diseases: clinical, ECG and hemodynamic features and management. *Cleve Clin J Med*. 2000;67(12):903–914.

35 Leigh-Smith S, Harris T. Tension pneumothorax: time for a re-think? *Emerg Med J*. 2005;22:8–16.

36 Chen K, Varon J, Wenker OC, et al. Acute thoracic aortic dissection: the basics. *J Emerg Med*. 1997;15(6): 859–867.

37 Hagan PG, Nienber CA, Isselbacher EM, et al. The international registry of acute aortic dissection (IRAD): new insights into an old disease. *JAMA*. 2000; 283(7):897–903.

38 Klompas M. Does this patient have an acute thoracic aortic dissection? *JAMA*. 2002;287(17):2262–2272.

39 Stein PD, Terrin ML, Hales CA, et al. Clinical, laboratory, roentgenographic, and electrocardiographic findings in patients with acute pulmonary embolism and no pre-existing cardiac or pulmonary disease. *Chest*. 1991;100:598–603.

40 Stein PD, Beemath A, Matta F, et al. Clinical characteristics of patient with acute pulmonary embolism: data from PIOPED II. *Am J Med*. 2007;120:871–879.

41 Ullman E, Brady WJ, Perron AD, et al. Electrocardiographic manifestations of pulmonary embolism. *Am J Emerg Med*. 2001;19(6):514–519.

42 Tapson VF. Acute pulmonary embolism. *N Engl J Med*. 2008;358:1037–1052.

43 Wells PS, Anderson DR, Rodger M, et al. Excluding pulmonary embolism at the bedside without diagnostic imaging: management of patients with suspected pulmonary embolism presenting to the emergency department by using a simple clinical model and D-dimer. *Ann Intern Med*. 2001;135:98–107.

44 LeGal G, Righini M, Roy P-M, et al. Prediction of pulmonary embolism in the emergency department: the revised Geneva score. *Ann Intern Med*. 2006;144: 165–171.

45 Kline JA, Mitchell AM, Kabrhel C, et al. Clinical criteria to prevent unnecessary diagnostic testing in emergency department patients with suspected pulmonary embolism. *J Thromb Haemost*. 2004;2:1247–1255.

46 Kline JA, Courtney DM, Kabrhel C, et al. Prospective multicenter evaluation of the pulmonary embolism rule-out criteria. *J Thromb Haemost*. 2008;6:772–780.

47 McPherson JJ, Feigin DS, Bellamy RF. Prevalence of tension pneumothorax in fatally wounded combat casualties. *J Trauma*. 2006;60(3):573–578.

48 Lichtenstein DA, Meziere G, Lascols N, et al. Ultrasound diagnosis of occult pneumothorax. *Crit Care Med*. 2005;33(6):1231–1238.

49 Roy CL, Minor MA, Brookhart A, et al. Does this patient with pericardial effusion have cardiac tamponade? *JAMA*. 2007;297(16):1810–1818.

50 Atar S, Chiu J, Forrester J, et al. Bloody pericardial effusion in patients with cardiac tamponade: Is the cause cancerous, tuberculous, or iatrogenic in the 1990s? *Chest*. 1999;116(6):1564–1569.

51 Spodick DH. Acute cardiac tamponade. *N Engl J Med*. 2003;349:684-690.

52 Guberman BA, Fowler NO, Engel PJ, et al. Cardiac tamponade in medical patients. *Circulation*. 1981;64: 633–640.

53 Vial CM, Whyte RI. Boerhaave's syndrome: diagnosis and management. *Surg Clin North Am*. 2005; 85(3):515–524.

54 Flynn AE, Verrier ED, Way LW, et al. Esophageal perforation. *Arch Surg*. 1989;124(10):1211–1215.

55 Gemer O, Popescu M, Lebowits O, et al. Pneumomediastinum in labor. *Arch Gynecol Obstet*. 1994; 255(1):47–49.

56 Bernard AW, Ben-David K, Pritts T. Delayed presentation of thoracic esophageal perforation after blunt trauma. *J Emerg Med*. 2008;34(1):49–53.

57 Ringstorm E, Freedman J. Approach to undifferentiated chest pain in the emergency department. *Mt Sinai J Med*. 2006;73(2):499–505.

58 Fuchs RM, Achuff SC, Grunwald L, et al. Electrocardiographic localization of coronary artery narrowing: studies during myocardial ischemia and infarction in patients with one vessel disease. *Circulation*. 1982;66: 1168–1176.

59 Gibson RS, Crampton RS, Watson DD, et al. Precordial ST segment depression during acute inferior myocardial infarction: clinical, scintigraphic, and angiographic correlations. *Circulation*. 1982;86:732–741.

60 Matetzky S, Freimark D, Feinberg M, et al. Acute myocardial infarction with isolated ST segment elevation in posterior chest leads V7-V9: "hidden" ST segment

elevations revealing posterior infarction. *J Am Coll Cardiol.* 1999;34(3):748–753.

61 Matetzky S, Freimark D, Chouraqui P, et al. Significance of ST segment elevations in posterior chest leads V7-V9 in patients with acute inferior myocardial infarction: application for thrombolytic therapy. *J Am Coll Cardiol.* 1998;31(3):506–511.

62 Antman EM, Ande DT, Armstrong PW, et al. ACC/AHA guidelines for the management of patients with ST elevation myocardial infarction—executive summary. *J Am Coll Cardiol.* 2004;44:671–719.

63 Moye S, Carney MF, Holstege C, et al. The ECG in right ventricular myocardial infarction. *Am J Emerg Med.* 2005;23(6):793–799.

64 Come PC, Pitt B. Nitroglycerin-induced severe hypotension and bradycardia in patients with acute myocardial infarction. *Circulation.* 1976;54(4):624–628.

65 Assali AR, Teplisky I, Ben-Dor I, et al. Prognostic importance of right ventricular infarction in an acute myocardial infarction cohort referred for comtemporary percutaneous reperfusion therapy. *Am Heart J.* 2007;153:231–237.

66 Cannon CP, McCabe CH, Stone PH. The electrocardiogram predicts one-year outcome of patients with unstable angina and non-Q-wave myocardial infarction: results of the TIMI-III registry ECG ancillary study. *J Am Coll Cardiol.* 1997;30(1):133–140.

67 Williamson K, Mattu A, Plautz CU, et al. Electrocardiographic applications of lead aVR. *Am J Emerg Med.* 2006;24:864–874.

68 deZwaan, Bar FW, Janssen JH, et al. Angiographic and clinical characteristics of patients showing an ECG pattern indicating critical narrowing of the proximal LAD coronary artery. *Am Heart J.* 1989;117(3):657–665.

69 Rhinehardt J, Brady WJ, Perron AD, et al. Electrocardiographic manifestations of Wellens' syndrome. *Am J Emerg Med.* 2002;20:638–643.

70 Jernberg T, Lindahl B, Wallentin L. Continuous multilead ST-segment monitoring should be part of the clinical routine [letter]. *Eur Heart J.* 2002;23(12):918–921.

71 Imazio M, Trinchero R. Triage and management of acute pericarditis. *Int J Cardiol.* 2007;118:286–294.

72 Demangone D. ECG manifestations: noncoronary heart disease. *Emerg Med Clin North Am.* 2006;24(1):113–131.

73 Little WC, Freeman GL. Pericardial disease. *Circulation.* 2006;113(12):1622–1632.

74 Dorman SH, Barry J. Acute aortic dissection mimicking an acute coronary syndrome through occlusion of the right coronary artery. *Emerg Med J.* 2008;25:462–463.

75 Rodger M, Makropoulos D, Turek M, et al. Diagnostic value of the electrocardiogram in suspected pulmonary embolism. *Am J Cardiol.* 2000;86:807–809.

76 Chan TC, Vike GM, Pollack ML, Brady WJ. Electrocardiographic manifestations: pulmonary embolism. *J Emerg Med.* 2001;21:263–270.

77 Tocino IM, Miller MH, Fairfax WR. Distribution of pneumothorax in the supine and semirecumbent critically ill adult. *Amer J Radiol.* 1985;144:901–905.

78 Carr JJ, Reed JC, Choplin RH, et al. Plain and computed radiology for detecting experimentally induced pneumothorax in cadavers: implications for detection in patients. *Radiology.* 1992;183:193–199.

79 Soldati G, Testa A, Sher S, et al. Occult traumatic pneumothorax: diagnostic accuracy of lung ultrasonography in the emergency department. *Chest.* 2008;133:204–211.

80 Spizarny DL, Goodman LR. Air in the minor fissure: A sign of right-sided pneumothorax. *Radiology.* 1986;160:329–331.

81 Ball C, Kirkpatrick AW, Fox DL, et al. Are occult pneumothoraces truly occult or simply missed? *J Trauma.* 2006;60(2):294–299.

82 Lemke T, Jagminas L. Spontaneous esophageal rupture: a frequently missed diagnosis. *Am Surg.* 1999;65(5):449–452.

83 Forshaw MJ, Khan AZ, Strauss DC, et al. Vomiting-induced pneumomediastinum and subcutaneous emphysema does not always indicate Boerhaave's syndrome: report of six cases. *Surg Today.* 2007;37:888–892.

84 Khan AN, Al-Jahdali H, Al-Ghanem S, Gouda A. Reading chest radiographs in the critically ill (Part I): Normal chest radiographic appearance, instrumentation and complications from instrumentation. *Ann Thorac Med.* 2009;4:75–87.

85 Pape LA, Tsai TT, Isselbacher EM, et al. Aortic diameter > 5.5 cm is not a good predictor of type A aortic dissection. *Circulation.* 2007;116:1120–1127.

86 Gundry SR, Burney RE, Mackenzie JR, et al. Assessment of mediastinal widening associated with traumatic rupture of the aorta. *J Trauma.* 1983;23(4):293–299.

87 Ekeh AP, Peterson W, Woods RJ, et al. Is chest x-ray an adequate screening tool for the diagnosis of blunt thoracic aortic injury? *J Trauma.* 2008;65(5):1088–1092.

88 Rogg JG, De Neve J-W, Huang C, et al. The triple work-up for emergency department patients with acute chest pain: how often does it occur? *J Emerg Med.* 2008 [E-pub ahead of print].

89 Johnson RTC, Nikolaou K, Wintersperger BJ, et al. ECG-gated 64-MDCT angiography in the differential diagnosis of acute chest pain. *Amer J Radiol.* 2007;188:76–82.

90 Quiroz R, Kucher N, Zou KH, et al. Clinical validity of a negative computed tomography scan in patients with

suspected pulmonary embolism. *JAMA*. 2005;293(16): 2012–2017.

91 Hausleiter J, Meyer T, Hadamitzky M, et al. Radiation dose estimates from cardiac multislice computed tomography in daily practice. Impact of different scanning protocols on effective dose estimates. *Circulation*. 2006;113:1305–1310.

92 Policy Statement—American College of Emergency Physicians. Emergency ultrasound guidelines. *Ann Emerg Med*. 2009;53:550–570.

93 Tekwani K, Girzadas DV, Lambert ML. Emergency department diagnosis of pericardial tamponade aided by goal-directed bedside echocardiography. *Acad Emerg Med*. 2008;15(9):872.

94 Blaivas M, Lyon M, Duggal S. A prospective comparison of supine chest radiography and bedside ultrasound for the diagnosis of traumatic pneumothorax. *Acad Emerg Med*. 2005;12:844–849.

95 Bouhemad B, Zhang M, Lu Q, et al. Clinical review: bedside lung ultrasound in critical care practice. *Crit Care*. 2007;11:205.

96 Perkins A, Liteplo A, Noble VE. Ultrasound diagnosis of type A aortic dissection. *J Emerg Med*. 2010;38: 490–493.

97 Anderson JL, Adams CD, Antman E. ACC/AHA 2007 guidelines for the management of patients with unstable angina/non-ST-elevation myocardial infarction—executive summary. *J Am Coll Cardiol*. 2007;50:652–726.

98 Jaffery Z, Nowak R, Khoury N, et al. Myoglobin and troponin I predict 5-year mortality in patients with undifferentiated chest pain in the emergency department. *Am Heart J*. 2008;156:939–945.

99 Joint European Society of Cardiology/American College of Cardiology Committee. Myocardial infarction redefined—a consensus document of the joint European Society of Cardiology/American College of Cardiology Committee for the Redefinition of Myocardial Infarction. *Eur Heart J*. 2000;21:1502–1513.

100 Eggers KM, Oldgren J, Nordenskjold A, et al. Diagnostic value of serial measurement of cardiac markers in patients with chest pain: limited value of adding myoglobin to troponin I for exclusion of myocardial infarction. *Am Heart J*. 2004;148:574–581.

101 Newby LK, Roe MT, Chen AY, et al. Frequency and clinical implications of discordant creatine kinase-MB and troponin measurements in acute coronary syndromes. *J Am Coll Cardiol*. 2006;47:312–318.

102 Storrow AB, Lindsell CJ, Han JH, et al. Discordant cardiac markers: frequency and outcomes in emergency department patients with chest pain. *Ann Emerg Med*. 2006;48(6):660–665.

103 Giannitsis E, Muller-Bardorff M, Kurowski V, et al. Independent prognostic value of cardiac troponin T in patients with confirmed pulmonary embolism. *Circulation*. 2000;102:211–217.

104 Meyer T, Binder L, Hruska N, et al. Cardiac troponin I elevation in acute pulmonary embolism is associated with right ventricular dysfunction. *J Am Coll Cardiol*. 2000;36(5):1632–1636.

105 Binder L, Pieske B, Olschewski M, et al. N-terminal pro-brain natriuretic peptide or troponin testing followed by echocardiography for risk stratification of acute pulmonary embolism. *Circulation*. 2005;112:1573–1579.

106 van Belle A, Buller HR, Huisman MV, et al. Effectiveness of managing suspected pulmonary embolism using an algorithm combining clinical probability, D-dimer testing, and computed tomography. *JAMA*. 2006;295(2):172–179.

107 Stein PD, Woodard PK, Weg JG, et al. Diagnostic pathways in acute pulmonary embolism: recommendations of the PIOPED II investigators. *Am J Med*. 2006;119:1048–1055.

108 Zehtabchi S, Rios CL. Management of emergency department patients with primary spontaneous pneumothorax: needle aspiration or tube thoracostomy. *Ann Emerg Med*. 2008;51(1):91–100.

109 Fine MJ, Auble TE, Yealy DM, et al. A prediction rule to identify low risk patients with community-acquired pneumonia. *N Engl J Med*. 1997;336:243–250.

110 Lim WS, van der Eerden MM, Laing R, et al. Defining community acquired pneumonia severity on presentation to hospital: an international derivation and validation study. *Thorax*. 2003;58:377–382.

111 Aujesky D, Auble TE, Yealy DM, et al. Prospective comparison of three validated prediction rules for prognosis in community-acquired pneumonia. *Am J Med*. 2005;118:384–392.

2

Non-ST segment elevation myocardial infarction

David Plitt[1] & William J. Brady[2]

[1] Department of Medicine, University of Virginia School of Medicine, Charlottesville, VA, USA
[2] Vice Chair, Department of Emergency Medicine, Professor of Emergency Medicine and Medicine, University of Virginia Health System, Charlottesville, VA, USA

Section I: Case presentation

A 58-year-old woman presented to the emergency department (ED) with chest pain. The patient had a history of myocardial infarction, hypertension, and diabetes mellitus. The chest pain had its onset 12 hours prior to presentation while the patient was at rest; the patient noted that the discomfort was similar to her past cardiac pains. The physical examination was notable for marked hypertension and mild diaphoresis; her vital signs were otherwise unremarkable. The 12-lead electrocardiogram (EKG) demonstrated nonspecific ST-segment and T wave abnormalities. While awaiting laboratory results, the patient received aspirin and nitrates. The chest radiograph demonstrated mild pulmonary congestion. The serum troponin value was 0.09 mg/dl (normal <0.02 mg/dl).

An acute coronary syndrome (ACS) was diagnosed. Plans were made for hospital admission while serial troponin testing was performed; the second value was 1.9 mg/dl. Heparin was added along with clopidogrel. A repeat 12-lead EKG demonstrated progressive ST-segment depression in the inferior leads. Mild pulmonary congestion was considered a relative contraindication to intravenous beta-blockade.

The patient was admitted to the hospital for serial troponin testing. Approximately 18 hours after presentation, the serum troponin value was 11.1 mg/dl; continued ST depression was noted in the right precordial leads. The patient was taken to the cardiac catheterization laboratory for coronary angiography. While on-call to the laboratory, the patient received a glycoprotein inhibitor. At catheterization, right and circumflex coronary arterial occlusions were noted, and both were successfully stented; inferior and posterior hypokinesis were noted as well. The patient was ultimately diagnosed with a non-ST-segment elevation myocardial infarction with congestive heart failure; the serum troponin peaked at 19.6 mg/dl.

Section II: Case discussion

Dr Peter Rosen: This is not a subtle case in terms of the problems that physicians often have in recognizing coronary ischemic syndromes in women, but the real question is: What are your triggers for management and admission? When would you be comfortable defining a patient like this as stable angina for whom not much has to be done, as opposed to unstable angina where a different strategy has to be undertaken?

Dr David Brown: To start, we should consider the differential diagnosis, with an acute coronary syndrome being the first, but not the only, item on the list. Could this also be an aortic dissection, as this is someone with a history of hypertension? We would also consider some other cause of chest pain, such as

Cardiovascular Problems in Emergency Medicine: A discussion-based review, First Edition.
Edited by Shamai A. Grossman and Peter Rosen.
© 2011 John Wiley & Sons, Ltd. Published 2011 by John Wiley & Sons, Ltd.

pericarditis, myocarditis, pneumothorax, or pneumonia. Then, we would obtain, in addition to the EKG, a chest X-ray study and cardiac markers, whichever type are done in this particular ED, including a troponin level. Assuming we reasonably exclude the diagnoses I mentioned, we would not need to do more in finding an alternative diagnosis. Nevertheless, in a patient who presents like this with typical ischemic chest pain that occurred at rest, as well as with a history of myocardial infarction, there is a need to have, at the very least, even with negative initial markers, some sort of risk stratification and a period of monitoring.

Dr William Brady: The use of biomarkers is not indicated in all adult chest pain patients. This testing modality should only be used in patients where the clinical suspicion includes ACS.

DB: If we are 12 hours out from the onset of the symptoms, a single set of markers might be reasonable. We still will require some sort of risk stratification to see whether this pain represents a provocable ischemia. I can't imagine a scenario in which this particular patient will be sent directly home from the ED.

WB: The patient under discussion clearly needs admission to the hospital. Recurrent chest discomfort with progressively rising biomarkers identifies this patient at high risk, requiring additional therapy and further diagnostic evaluation.

Dr Shamai Grossman: You have several options as far as admission. At some institutions, this patient might require a full admission, while in others an observation unit stay might be available; regardless, she will need serial testing and probably some form of stress imaging.

DB: Much will depend on the results of the first set of markers in the ED. If she has a normal EKG and a normal troponin, along with being 12 hours out from the onset of symptoms that sound like ischemic chest pain, then an observation admission and provocative testing would be reasonable. This testing, depending on the institution, might be an exercise tolerance test with or without nuclear imaging or stress echo. On the other hand, if the troponin level is positive, then she should not go to an observation unit. She would, by definition, have met criteria for a non-ST elevated myocardial infarction (NSTEMI or non-STEMI) and should be admitted, at least, to a cardiac step-down

unit. The next step, for a patient with an elevation of troponin, probably wouldn't be provocative testing; it would be cardiac catheterization in a non-emergent but urgent fashion, such as the next morning, assuming she remained in stable condition over night.

WB: To reiterate, this patient has elevated biomarkers with an early rising pattern concerning for ACS with myocardial injury. Such patients, as identified with positive biomarkers, are at high risk for acute and subacute cardiovascular complications, including death. These patients always should be admitted to the hospital.

PR: What would you do with this patient with an elevated troponin level if you were in an institution that didn't have a catheterization laboratory, or did not have someone doing angioplasty?

Dr Amal Mattu: Traditionally, these patients would be managed conservatively. Assuming they continued to be pain and symptom free, they tended to do pretty well with conservative management and medical treatment, and did not need an immediate trip to the catheterization laboratory unless there were complications or recurrent pain. This strategy is referred to as a "selective invasive approach."

DB: The TACTICS trial looked at this, although it's a few years old now. In 2001, this study looked at conservative versus aggressive management, in a time frame similar to the current era, with the significant addition of the use of antiplatelet therapy. The authors conclude that conservative management is inferior to more aggressive management. This conclusion means that in non-STEMIs, the group of patients managed with urgent but not emergent catheterization, followed by revascularization, does better. This strategy was proven by performing cardiac catheterization on all the non-STEMI patients, not just those with an abnormal post-MI stress test.

WB: If you are working in the ED of an institution without coronary angiography, you should consider transfer of such patients, assuming that logistical issues are acceptable, including a safe, appropriate EMS transport staff and vehicle; a reasonable distance to a receiving hospital; and favorable weather, to name only a few issues. In a patient who is stable, it is not unreasonable to consider admission to the noninvasive hospital with transfer the next day. In the more acute patient with progressive pathophysiology, earlier transfer should be considered, assuming it is possible in a practical sense.

SG: Based on this data, someone who comes to a community hospital and rules in for a non-STEMI ought to have cardiac catheterization over the next day or so to define their anatomy, and revascularize whatever is thought to be the culprit lesion or lesions.

PR: Assuming that you were going to transfer the patient for that to be done, what would you use, medically, to cover the patient while you're arranging the transfer?

DB: This decision depends on the patient. The patient we are discussing has been pain free for 12 hours. I think a patient like this can receive aspirin, nitrates, and anti-coagulation; whether that's low molecular weight heparin or unfractionated heparin is still debatable, and probably not relevant. Whether the patient should receive additional antiplatelet therapy beyond aspirin is controversial. Some believe that anyone with a positive troponin should receive a glycoprotein inhibitor until such time as they undergo revascularization, either in the catheterization laboratory or at coronary artery bypass graft surgery (CABG). This strategy is more compelling when a patient is showing signs of progressive ACS or instability.

AM: If someone is having a non-STEMI, and the decision has been made for urgent cardiac catheterization, I would place them on a glycoprotein inhibitor even if they've been relatively asymptomatic for the past nine to twelve hours. I think there's good evidence to indicate that these patients do better if they're on the glycoprotein inhibitor heading into the laboratory. There is still debate about how long the glycoprotein inhibitor needs to be on board prior to catheterization, but I think they do better if it's given when the catheterization procedure begins.

WB: I agree. The ACS patients who are mechanically managed (i.e., in the catheterization laboratory) likely benefit from glycoprotein inhibition. Other patient groups that can benefit are the ACS patients with ongoing ischemia with positive biomarkers, an evolving EKG, or instability.

SG: Part of the question here is whether or not the patient should actually have the glycoprotein inhibitor started in the community hospital when they're going to be transferred to a tertiary care center. The issues with starting someone in the community hospital on a glycoprotein inhibitor concern a possible prolongation of stay in the transferring department, as well as possibly having more complications if the transferring physician is unfamiliar with the use of platelet inhibitors. One must consider very carefully when you're in the community whether you want to be the person to start the glycoprotein inhibitor, or whether that should be started in the tertiary care facility where the procedure will be performed, and whether the incremental benefit of having a glycoprotein inhibitor on board for a brief period of time—for the 30 minutes to an hour of transport time—will allow this agent to actually help preserve the person's myocardium or put that patient at greater risk for an adverse outcome.

DB: I think we're combining several issues. The first is: can the drug be safely given in the community by doctors and nurses who are going to be relatively unfamiliar with this drug? The second question is: will the patient will be going directly for catheterization? I don't think that's likely to happen for patients with a non-STEMI. They are more likely to be transferred to a facility where they could be catheterized, but it's usually the next business day. Then the question becomes: does 12 or even 24 hours of coverage with a glycoprotein inhibitor while someone's evolving a non-STEMI before revascularization make a difference or not? These patients are not comparable to STEMI patients being transferred directly to the catheterization laboratory, for whom you can strongly argue that it doesn't make much difference whether the glycoprotein inhibitor is given in the ED or in the catheter laboratory. But this is a different group of patients. These patients evolving a non-STEMI are going to wait for 12 hours or more, in a coronary care unit (CCU) or perhaps even in an ED observation unit, and will not have an immediate revascularization procedure. There is no evidence to help answer that question right now.

PR: I believe that one of your obligations required in arranging a transfer is to find out what your accepting physician wants done. There is great virtue in sharing responsibility in these cases. I worry less about the ability to give a bolus or to run an infusion by both emergency physicians and transferring EMTs or flight nurses because I think that we now have enough experience in the United States to show that it can be done safely. To summarize, we have a patient with an ischemic coronary syndrome who has an abnormal set of biomarkers and who is pain free a number of hours after the onset of pain. It sounds like there is a controversy between routinely starting platelet inhibition and waiting to have the cardiologist do so. Where there is controversy, I think it becomes even more important to find out what the receiving cardiologist wants done.

Let me ask a permutation of the question; let's assume now that the patient has a slight elevation of the first troponin and a normal or a nonspecific abnormal EKG, but is having stuttering chest pain. Would that alter your decision making about starting platelet inhibition before transfer?

AM: I would still talk to the receiving cardiologist. The practice patterns of cardiologists vary markedly, even within a single institution, as to who likes glycoprotein inhibitor and who doesn't. Even within the group that likes the glycoprotein inhibitor, some want eptifibatide while others want abciximab, some of them don't want either of these, and want clopidogrel instead.

PR: I personally would rather start platelet inhibition in somebody who is having stuttering symptoms than in somebody who is pain free.

SG: Would you have used clopidogrel in this patient?

AM: This again would depend on what the specific cardiologist wanted. In the ED, we may not be aggressive in using clopidogrel largely because cardiac surgeons are highly concerned about perioperative bleeding, should these patients ultimately require operative revascularization. Nevertheless, some surgeons do not voice these concerns, and I would just base my utilization of clopidogrel on the preferences of the accepting cardiologist.

WB: With respect to clopidogrel, its use in the ACS patient is most appropriate in those individuals who will be managed conservatively (i.e., no percutaneous coronary intervention [PCI]), and those persons who will likely undergo PCI at least 6 hours beyond the administration time of this platelet inhibitor. In other words, clopidogrel most often benefits patients who are managed medically for at least the initial phase of their care. Using clopidogrel urgently and early in a patient who is undergoing urgent PCI for STEMI is likely of little benefit.

PR: Let's assume that this is a patient who has a normal first set of biomarkers and either a normal EKG or one with nonspecific changes. When would you try to do a precatheterization laboratory stress test with such a patient, knowing that this still is a patient who had an ischemic coronary syndrome, perhaps a myocardial infarction (MI) 2 years previously, and has had some cardiac symptoms intermittently since?

SG: If the patient has a positive biomarker, and you're not going to take the patient to the catheterization laboratory, you probably should wait about 5 days before you put that patient back on a treadmill. Even then, it's controversial concerning how far you should work the patient on the treadmill (whether you should do a full Bruce Protocol, or some modification), but I don't think anyone would immediately put a patient who has positive biomarkers on a treadmill.

PR: What if the biomarkers are normal?

DB: Someone whose biomarkers are negative falls into the moderate risk category, similar to patients with a history of MI, a history of risk factors, and an ischemic sounding event. At 12 hours with cardiac markers that are negative, it's a pretty good bet that he or she didn't have an MI. The decision to obtain a stress test might depend somewhat on what was known about the patient's coronary artery disease, and whether or not he or she had been having symptoms over the past year that seemed to be accelerating. If this was the first episode since the MI, whenever that was, it was 12 hours since the onset of symptoms, the patient had a negative biomarker and a nonspecific EKG, and continued to clinically look well, then that's a patient who I think benefits from a stress imaging test to try to determine whether that chest pain from yesterday was really angina or whether it was from something else.

PR: How long is information that's negative from a stress test useful? For example, what if we have a patient with a normal set of biomarkers and a normal or nonspecific EKG but had an episode that sounds clearly anginal? The patient had a stress test a year ago that was negative. Does that make you want to repeat the stress test, or is there a length of time during which you feel that provides adequate negative information?

AM: Anecdotally, I would say that a negative stress test is probably useful for about an hour. I've seen

21

people with a negative stress test and then a week, or even 3 days, later have a STEMI. In one case, a patient went into ventricular tachycardia (VT) 3 days after a completely negative stress test, and then ruled in. I don't think there's reliable evidence that says that if you get a stress test then you don't need to worry about cardiac ischemia for 3 months, 6 months, or a year. To be reasonable, you are not going to keep stressing a patient over and over. So generally we assume that if a patient had a negative stress test within the past few months, and they're returning with the exact same symptoms that led to the first stress test, the exact intensity, radiation, associated symptoms, then we would feel a lot more comfortable, though perhaps still not 100%, that the stress test is reliable. In almost all the cases where I've seen patients have MIs after a recent stress test, they experienced some change in their symptoms. Thus, if a patient returns with a change in symptoms, this change, I believe, excludes the utility of the prior stress test. Anecdotally, we've seen at least a dozen cases in the past five years where patients coming back with a change in symptoms have ended up ruling in, even though they've had negative stress tests, again, anywhere from 3 days out to within the prior 6 months.

WB: Although simple exercise stress testing is of limited value in ruling out significant coronary obstructive lesions, the addition of a nuclear scan to this testing modality markedly increases its ability to identify patients who would benefit from a more aggressive diagnostic evaluation.

PR: My personal prejudice is that stress tests only have utility when they're positive, and that negative stress tests have no meaning whatsoever. A common practice in the United States is to observe patients overnight, perform a stress test in the morning, and if it is negative, discharge the patient home. However, if they have symptoms suggesting accelerating angina, I personally wouldn't be comfortable with anything but a coronary angiogram.

SG: In truth, a test's results are only as good as the test itself. When Diamond first published data in the 1970s on stress testing, it was predicated on pretest and posttest probabilities, so that even a completely normal stress test, in a patient with a high pretest probability, did not rule out ischemic heart disease.

That patient will remain with a relatively high post-test probability of cardiac ischemia. One approach suggests that if a patient has a negative stress test, and has another presentation with chest discomfort that is either the same or different, one might try to use a different imaging modality. Such a situation is where a coronary computed tomography angiogram (CTA) in a younger patient with no history of coronary disease, or adding imaging to a stress test that was previously done without imaging, might be particularly useful.

DB: I don't imagine that anyone would risk-stratify a patient with known coronary disease and accelerating symptoms with just a plain treadmill stress test. If the pretest probability is so high that the current event represents coronary ischemia, in my institution we would obtain a stress test with sestamibi imaging. In some institutions, one might obtain a stress echocardiogram. The patient today would not be a candidate for a coronary CT because she has known coronary artery disease (CAD). The CT scan is an anatomic study that isn't going to show whether the known CAD seen on the scan is related to the symptoms of this particular event. I think nonimaging treadmill testing has a role in patients in whom the pretest probability is low, and who have a normal EKG. In that situation, we have to be careful to tell the patients that we're not excluding coronary artery disease, we're just doing a functional test to evaluate whether walking on a treadmill provokes symptoms or findings on the EKG that suggest coronary artery disease. If it does not, then the patient is generally safe to be discharged, with further work-up as an outpatient dictated by whoever manages the ongoing care. Where we can run into trouble, is if we unthinkingly and uniformly tell these patients, "You're fine. Your stress test was negative. You don't have coronary artery disease." This is overstating and overestimating the ability of the test.

On the other hand, I don't believe that someone who has been pain free for 12 hours and has a negative set of biomarkers should automatically be taken for cardiac catheterization, even if the presenting history is suggestive of cardiac ischemia. In this patient today, we don't really know what the etiology of yesterday's chest pain was. She has a worrisome history from an ischemic standpoint, but the markers are negative and the EKG is unchanged or nonspecific in its findings. If she has a cardiac catheterization, you will find CAD, of course, because we already know she has it; however, you will not know whether, in someone who has been pain free for 12 hours and has a negative set of biomarkers, that it is this disease that is causing her symptoms. I would favor a treadmill test with imaging to see whether symptoms and perfusion correlate with each other on the treadmill. If they do, then proceed with an angiogram.

SG: Thus, the stress test would be particularly useful if there were multiple lesions found on diagnostic catheterization.

PR: Let me change directions for a minute to management of two of her other medical problems. It sounds like she was not being well controlled in terms of her hypertension. I did not hear what antihypertensive medication she was taking but, clearly, her blood pressure was not in a desirable range during this visit. What would you do in terms of management of her hypertension in terms of hoping to end her coronary ischemia? Secondly, how would you manage her diabetes during this phase? Many of these patients are type II diabetics. There's been some argument in the literature about whether it's safe to continue managing them as a type II, or whether they should be placed on insulin while they're having their acute ischemic coronary syndrome.

AM: In terms of the hyperglycemia, let's assume that she was hyperglycemic from the start. Hyperglycemia at the time of admission or poorly controlled hyperglycemia during the in-hospital stay is associated with a marked increase in hospital mortality and short-term mortality and morbidity. No one has definitely shown that hyperglycemia per se is causing the morbidity; it may just be an association rather than causal, but more and more of these studies are suggesting that tight glucose control can improve morbidity and mortality. I would be inclined to use insulin in a patient who is hyperglycemic in the ED with an acute coronary syndrome. The parameter that they define in these studies for hyperglycemia is a glucose level of about 140 mg/dl—fairly tight glucose control. I would make an effort to control the glucose level early on, and expect that the admitting physicians will use insulin as well to get improved glucose control. Of note, hyperglycemia has been associated with worse outcomes in sepsis, stroke, and postcardiac arrest syndrome, so I think it's reasonable to assume

that hyperglycemia may have some causal association with increased morbidity and mortality in this form of ischemic cardiac disease.

WB: Regarding the hyperglycemia, while it is a potential marker of a less-than-optimal outcome, extremely tight control in the ED is not recommended. This control can be achieved during inpatient hospitalization.

AM: In terms of the hypertension, if she's having pain, my first choice would be to go with nitrates. It is probable that nitrates as well as pain control will bring down the blood pressure. If she's pain free and still hypertensive, then I'd initially give her either her regular blood pressure medication, or perhaps a small dose of a beta-blocker; however, I tend to use early beta-blockers less in ACS unless they have intractable hypertension.

WB: Elevated blood pressures must be watched closely. Yet, the mere presence of an elevated blood pressure itself does not require immediate antihypertensive therapy. Rather, the clinician must consider the presence or absence of acute end-organ dysfunction among other issues; if present, antihypertensive therapy is warranted. In fact, the patient with an elevated blood pressure and no acute end-organ malfunction should be observed. The use of antihypertensive agents can cause morbidity, particularly in the elderly patient with long-term blood pressure elevations and less ability to auto-regulate organ perfusion. The use of beta-blockers in suspected ACS patients early in their course is now in question. Earlier research had suggested that the MI patient demonstrates benefit when beta-blockers are given early in their course resulting in smaller infarctions, improved ejection fractions, and fewer acute cardiovascular complications (particularly malignant ventricular dysrhythmias). In the contemporary setting, we have many more options to offer the ACS patient, including antiplatelet and anticoagulant therapies, as well as more aggressive revascularization tools. More recent research indicates that certain ACS patients may not benefit from early, intravenous beta-blocker administration. In fact, certain patients experience higher rates of symptomatic bradycardia, hypotension, and pulmonary congestion while only demonstrating a marginal benefit in reduced occurrence of primary ventricular fibrillation. Thus, widespread use of beta-blockers in the suspected ACS patient early in their care should be reconsidered. These patients can receive oral beta-blockers within the initial 24 hours of hospitalization; this "delayed" management still provides physiologic benefit, and meets regulatory requirement to the appropriate ACS candidate as well.

SG: Any patient whose chest examination has rales or rhonchi, and on chest X-ray study there is mild pulmonary congestion, should not receive a beta-blocker in the ED, and should probably not receive a beta-blocker until they no longer have any evidence of congestive heart failure. However, if one excludes all diabetics from beta blockade, one would preclude a very large segment of the coronary artery disease population from receiving beta-blockers that, as therapy for cardiac ischemia, has a well established benefit in mortality reduction.

AM: The traditional relative contraindication for beta-blockers and diabetes is that diabetics usually recognize that they are becoming hypoglycemic because they get a catecholamine surge, and then develop symptoms such as diaphoresis, or lightheadedness. If they are taking a beta-blocker, they may not get this surge, and therefore may not feel themselves becoming hypoglycemic. It has also been suggested that the beta blockade has a direct lowering effect on the blood sugar.

SG: As beta-blockers remain one of the few agents that truly have long-term mortality benefit, it may be worth the risk of hypoglycemia to obtain their protection. Close monitoring of the blood glucose levels may enable one to obtain the benefits of the beta-blockers without the negative effects of hypoglycemia.

WB: The EKG must also be discussed in this case. As seen in our patient today, the EKG can be normal or minimally abnormal in the setting of an ACS presentation. In a simple majority of acute myocardial infarction patients, the EKG will be diagnostically abnormal at presentation, with obvious ST-segment changes and T wave abnormalities. In the remainder of patients, the presenting EKG can be nonspecifically abnormal or even normal. Also, patients can demonstrate confounding EKG patterns such as left bundle branch block, left ventricular hypertrophy, or a ventricular paced rhythm. Thus, while the EKG is a powerful tool used in the chest pain patient suspected of ACS, it cannot be relied upon solely to include

or exclude a diagnosis. The clinician must understand its limitations and make treatment decisions accordingly.

Section III: Concepts

Background

Chest pain accounts for 6 to 8 million ED visits in the United States each year,[1,2] and is the second most common presenting complaint accounting for 5% of all ED visits.[2,3] Approximately two-thirds of these patients are felt to have a presentation consistent with an acute coronary syndrome, and are admitted to the hospital, but only one-half of these admitted patients (one-third of all who present) receive a discharge diagnosis of unstable coronary artery disease.[2,4,5] This diagnostic discrepancy amounts to an annual estimated cost of 6 billion dollars for false-positive admissions.[2] However, approximately 2–8% of patients who present to the ED with an ACS are inadvertently or incorrectly sent home.[2,6–8] Factors associated with such discharges include younger age, female gender, non-Caucasian ethnicity, atypical symptoms, lack of a prior coronary history, and nonspecific EKG findings. Furthermore, these patients have significant short-term morbidity and mortality that is equivalent to or higher than those patients with an ACS who are admitted.[7,8] Given the highly effective short- and long-term therapies for unstable coronary artery disease, the tremendous costs associated with inappropriate hospital admissions, and the increased morbidity and mortality associated with a missed diagnosis, acute coronary syndromes remain a difficult problem to efficiently triage, diagnose, and treat.

The presenting symptoms of an ACS are well known, and have been extensively studied in both prospective and retrospective analyses. Chest pain is the prototypical chief complaint, but up to 25% of patients present atypically without significant chest discomfort.[3,9] Studies of patients presenting with nontraumatic chest pain suggestive of an ACS find that such descriptive terms as "burning" and "indigestion" are equally as predictive as the terms "pressure" and "suffocating," while the terms "sharp" and "stabbing" or pain that is positional, reproducible, or pleuritic make an ACS significantly less likely.[4,10,11] New chest pain that is exertional, or radiates to one or both arms, is a helpful predictor of an unstable coronary syndrome, with reported positive likelihood ratios greater than two.[6,9,11] The severity, duration, and size distribution of the chest pain are not helpful predictors, nor is the patient's response to nitroglycerin or a "GI cocktail."[6,11-13] Other elements of the history, such as nausea, diaphoresis, and dyspnea, do occur frequently in patients with acute coronary syndromes, but they generally play little role in differentiating such syndromes from other common causes of chest pain.[6,9-11]

Traditional risk factors are important long-term predictors for CAD, but their value in diagnosing acute ischemic syndromes in an ED setting is less certain if of any value at all.[14] One retrospective study finds that, for patients younger than age 40, the presence of traditional risk factors for CAD is additive and quite helpful, with positive likelihood ratios of approximately 3 and 7 for the presence of 2–3 and 3–5 risk factors, respectively. However, the presence of such risk factors are only modestly helpful in patients age 40–65, and not helpful at all in patients older than 65.[15] One study evaluating the predictive value of various combinations of elements of the history in patients with suspected ACS finds that of those patients who do not have a known history of CAD, and present with sharp or stabbing pain that is pleuritic, positional, or reproducible in nature, none are diagnosed with ischemic heart disease.[4] Thus, certain elements of the history are only minimally helpful in diagnosing an ACS, and while the combination of pertinent features is more helpful, history alone does not allow for safe triage of such patients.

The physical examination of patients presenting with a suspected ACS should focus initially on stability of the patient. Pertinent vital signs, such as heart rate, blood pressure, and oxygenation status should be closely monitored and corrected accordingly. Features of potential decompensation, such as elevated jugular venous pressure and auscultation of mitral regurgitation, rales, or an S3, are noteworthy when present, but the ability of clinicians to reliably and accurately ascertain these items is variable and not always possible during a rapid assessment in a noisy ED.[9] Pulmonary and abdominal examinations may provide clues to an alternative diagnosis. Largely, the physical examination of the ACS patient is either normal or nonspecifically abnormal; obvious abnormalities, if present, most often result from complications of ACS, rather than the event itself—e.g., hypotension

Table 2-1. Differential diagnosis for nontraumatic chest pain.

Life Threatening	Non-life Threatening
Cardiac	*Cardiac*
Acute coronary syndrome	Pericarditis
Aortic dissection	Stable angina
Noncardiac	*Noncardiac*
Pulmonary embolism	GERD
Pneumothorax	Peptic ulcer disease
Esophageal rupture	Pancreatitis
Pneumonia	Cholecystitis
	Esophageal spasm
	Costochondritis
	Cervical/thoracic spine disease
	Shingles
	Anxiety

and pulmonary congestion resulting from a large anterior wall infarction.

The differential diagnosis for patients presenting with a suspected ACS encompasses the spectrum of cardiovascular, pulmonary, gastrointestinal, and musculoskeletal disorders, among many others (see Table 2-1). The most important goal of an emergency physician is to consider those causes that are acutely life threatening. This consideration is most commonly accomplished through interventions such as the history of the event, physical examination, 12-lead electrocardiography, chest roentgenography, and routine blood tests. There are several etiologies of coronary ischemia, which represent a perfusion imbalance between myocardial oxygen supply and demand.[16] The AHA/ACC recognizes five types of myocardial ischemia or infarction (see Table 2-2 on page 26). Acute coronary syndromes are the most common cause of life-threatening myocardial ischemia, and encompass several disorders that represent a common pathology. The primary event in these disorders is the acute rupture of an intra-coronary atherosclerotic plaque resulting in platelet aggregation and subsequent thrombus formation.[17] The subtypes of an ACS exist on a continuum of severity and include: unstable angina (UA), non-ST-elevation myocardial infarction (NSTEMI), and ST-elevation myocardial infarction (STEMI). The first two subtypes result from the subtotal occlusion of a coronary artery; the only difference is positive

Table 2-2. Clinical classification of myocardial infarction.[14]

Type 1
Spontaneous myocardial infarction related to ischemia due to a primary coronary event such as plaque rupture (ACS) or dissection

Type 2
Myocardial infarction secondary to ischemia due to either increased oxygen demand or decreased supply; examples include coronary artery spasm, coronary embolism, severe anemia, tachydysrhythmias, hypertension, and hypotension (demand ischemia)

Type 3
Sudden unexpected cardiac death, including cardiac arrest, due to a primary coronary event but before routine diagnostic tests can be obtained

Type 4a
Myocardial infarction associated with PCI

Type 4b
Myocardial infarction associated with stent thrombosis

Type 5
Myocardial infarction associated with CABG

---

evidence of myocardial necrosis in NSTEMI, while STEMI results from the total occlusion of a coronary artery and produces transmural infarction with ST-segment elevation on the standard 12-lead EKG.[17] Because both UA and NSTEMI result from identical coronary pathophysiology, they are thus assessed and managed in similar fashion.

Beyond the focused history and physical examination, the 12-lead EKG is the most important bedside test in the initial evaluation of patient with a suspected ACS, and it should be performed without delay upon patient arrival. When possible, this EKG should be compared to a prior EKG to assess for ischemic changes. An observational study of 63,478 patients with a suspected ACS finds a median time of 15 minutes from arrival to initial EKG, but the delay is greater than 10 minutes in 65% of patients. Risk factors for such a delay are female gender, non-Caucasian ethnicity, active tobacco use, prior percutaneous transluminal coronary angioplasty, lack of medical insurance, and an off-hour presentation to a teaching hospital. Although there was also an associated delay in therapy in these patients, there was no difference in mortality or infarction rate.[18]

The diagnostic value of the initial EKG in patients presenting with a suspected ACS has been the subject of numerous studies. Unfortunately, these studies differ with respect to the patient population, the method for diagnosing an ACS, the definition of an abnormal EKG, and the experience of the interpreting physician. Commonly reported sensitivities range from 40–81% yet may be as low as 20%.[19–22,6] However, the sensitivity is proportional to the degree of ischemia, and is thus much higher for STEMI than it is for UA/NSTEMI,[23] and is also higher when performed during an episode of chest pain.[24] The specificity also ranges widely, but it is much higher for more definitive findings such as ST-elevation (as high as 95%) than for ST-depression or nonspecific T wave changes (as low as 35%).[2,20]

While the presence of ischemic changes on the EKG is certainly helpful in diagnosis, the absence of such changes does not safely rule out ACS as the cause of chest pain. The number of patients with a final diagnosis of an ACS whose initial EKG is read as normal ranges from 1–37%, while those with only nonspecific EKG changes upon presentation range from 3–46%.[1,4,20,25–28] Confounding this problem is the fact that 24–63% of patients who do not receive a final diagnosis of an ACS will have an initial EKG that is not completely normal.[4,10]

While a single EKG is rarely diagnostic, the value of electrocardiography is directly proportional to the number of EKGs performed.[2,26] Obtaining both prehospital and in-hospital EKGs has been shown to improve sensitivity, with a slight drop in specificity.[22] Furthermore, the use of continuous EKG monitoring with serial 12-lead EKGs has been shown to significantly improve sensitivity for the diagnosis of both an ACS and a myocardial infarction with little reduction in specificity.[29]

The prognostic value of the initial EKG in patients with an ACS has also been extensively studied. Severe outcomes are fortunately quite low in patients whose initial EKG is read as normal or nonspecific: 0–1% and 0.6–6% for death and life-threatening complications, respectively.[23,25–27] Not surprisingly, the outcomes for those patients whose initial EKGs show changes suspicious for ischemia are worse.[23,27] Furthermore, these risks appear to correlate with the type of ischemic changes present. One study reveals that the risk of death or MI at 30 days is 5.5%, 10.5%, 9.4%, and 12.5% for patients whose initial EKGs revealed isolated T-wave inversions, isolated ST-depressions, isolated ST-elevations, and both ST-depressions and elevations, respectively. A similar trend is seen at 6 months.[30]

In addition to an appropriate symptom and EKG abnormality, the diagnosis of myocardial infarction requires the elevation of one or more cardiac-specific biomarkers.[16] The most commonly used indicators are the cardiac-specific troponins I and T (TnI and TnT). Troponin molecules associate with tropomyosin within muscle fibers and thus regulate myocardial contraction via their interaction with the actin/myosin complex.[17] The cardiac-specific troponins have near 100% specificity for myocardial events, and are thus preferred over CK-MB for the diagnosis of myocardial infarction.[16] Elevated cardiac troponins imply myocardial necrosis, and thus will be present in STEMI and NSTEMI, but not in UA or stable angina. The sensitivities of TnT and TnI for NSTEMI have been reported at 94% and 100%, respectively.[21] Because such elevations can take 4–6 hours after an event to show, all patients with a suspected ACS should have serial troponins checked with at least one level collected 6 hours after the onset of symptoms.[2,21] Elevated cardiac-specific troponins indicate myocardial necrosis, which is not limited to primary coronary ischemia. Alternative causes range from non-urgent causes, including demand ischemia, extreme exertion, renal failure, pericarditis, and infiltrative or inflammatory myocardial processes, to potentially life-threatening etiologies, such as severe congestive heart failure, pulmonary embolism, sepsis, cardiac contusion, Takotsubo cardiomyopathy, and subarachnoid hemorrhage.[16,31,32]

Perhaps an equally important quality of cardiac-specific troponins is their prognostic value. Elevated levels are associated with a higher risk of death or MI at 48 hours, 14 days, and 30 days.[33] In one trial, the 42-day mortality of patients with UA/NSTEMI is directly related to the initial TnI value: 1%, 3.7%, and 7.5% for TnI <0.4 ng/ml, >0.4 ng/ml, and >9 ng/ml, respectively.[34] Furthermore, the 72-hour troponin value directly correlates to the extent of myocardial necrosis.[35] Thus, cardiac-specific troponins are an important diagnostic and prognostic tool.

While the diagnostic evaluation is ongoing, the clinician must determine the appropriate level of care for the patient. Unstable patients obviously require ICU admission, while those who are clinically stable, but have a definite or probable ACS, can be transferred to a floor bed with continuous telemetry monitoring. Patients in whom an ACS is considered unlikely can safely be discharged for outpatient noninvasive testing after ED evaluation. For patients whose diagnoses remain uncertain, chest pain centers have been shown to decrease hospital costs and lengths of stay, as opposed to inpatient evaluations, when further investigation is required.[2] Regardless of the disposition, patients with an ACS often receive initial therapy while in the ED. As opposed to patients with STEMI, where the goal is to open the occluded artery either medically with fibrinolysis or mechanically with PCI, those with UA/NSTEMI are usually treated medically, at least initially; fibrinolytic therapy is contraindicated and is of no benefit or even harmful in this patient population.[36–38] Thus, the goal is to restore a proper perfusion balance by decreasing oxygen demand through a reduction in myocardial workload, and increasing oxygen supply by halting ongoing thrombus formation (see Table 2-3). As discussed in detail below, all patients with suspected ACS should receive continuous oxygen therapy via nasal cannula, chewable aspirin, and nitroglycerin unless contraindicated, with further therapy once a definitive diagnosis is obtained.

Medical therapies that decrease myocardial oxygen demand include nitroglycerin, beta-blockers, and morphine. Nitroglycerin primarily works through decreasing venous return and thus cardiac preload, and to a lesser extent through coronary artery vasodilatation.[39] It is most commonly given in a dissolving sublingual form, but can also be given topically or intravenously. Nitroglycerin has been shown to significantly decrease the severity and number of chest pain episodes.[39,40] A

Table 2-3. Therapy for UA/NSTEMI.

Anti-Anginal	Anti-Ischemic	
	Antiplatelet	Antithrombotic
Oxygen	Aspirin	Unfractionated heparin
Nitrates	Clopidogrel	Low molecular weight heparins
Beta-blockers	Glycoprotein IIb/IIIa inhibitors	Direct thrombin inhibitors
Morphine sulfate		Fondaparinux

pooled analysis of more than 2000 patients with acute MI who were given nitrates (either nitroglycerin or nitroprusside) reveals a significant decrease in mortality versus placebo, with the benefit occurring early during hospitalization.[41] Long-term studies evaluating the use of intravenous, followed by oral, nitrates fails to show a long-term mortality benefit, but they verify that nitrates are safe to use in the initial phases of an ACS.[42,43] However, nitrate use requires caution in certain conditions, such as right ventricular infarction, cardiogenic shock, or co-existent aortic stenosis.

Beta-blockers are another cornerstone of ACS therapy. By reducing heart rate, blood pressure, and contractility through interfering with adrenergic stimulation, they reduce cardiac oxygen demand.[44] Many studies have evaluated their early (within 12 hours) use in an ACS with overall favorable results. The short-term benefits of early beta-blocker use include a reduction in chest pain, infarct size, re-infarction rate, cardiogenic shock, life-threatening dysrhythmias, and cardiac free-wall rupture.[44–51] There also seems to be a short-term mortality benefit to the early administration of beta-blockers, although there are mixed results from several studies, many of them were pre-1990 and were conducted on a heterogeneous patient population with mixed coronary syndromes.[44,48,49,51,52] Long-term follow-up confirms a mortality benefit of early beta-blocker administration after an ACS, and is primarily due to a reduction in cardiovascular death.[51,53–56] There are obvious safety concerns to administering beta-blockers to certain patient populations. It is best to avoid beta-blocker therapy in patients with bradycardia, hypotension, or signs of acute heart failure.[48,51,56] Studies show that beta-blockers are safe to administer to patients with a history of chronic obstructive pulmonary disease, even if it is severe, although one should only use cardioselective beta-blockers, and their use should be avoided in patients who may be having an acute exacerbation of the lung disease.[57,58] Should beta-blockers be contraindicated for pulmonary reasons, non-dihydropyridine calcium-channel blockers may be used instead.[5] Morphine sulfate is recommended for patients with persistent chest pain despite nitroglycerin and beta-blocker therapy because of its anxiolytic and mild venodilatatory properties.[5]

In 2005, the ClOpidogrel and Metoprolol in Myocardial Infarction Trial (COMMIT) was published, and casts serious doubt on whether early intravenous beta-blocker therapy has merit. No mortality benefit exists, yet the beta-blocker group noted a small reduction in infarct size and a slight decrease in the incidence of ventricular fibrillation. Unfortunately, this group also had a higher rate of cardiogenic shock, particularly in elderly patients as well as those with borderline perfusion; tachycardia; and mild acute pulmonary congestion. These same patients also developed bradycardia, hypotension, and pulmonary congestion more frequently than the non-beta-blocker treatment group. Thus, this study suggests that the use of intravenous beta-blockers early in the patient's ACS is potentially problematic.[48] We must also realize that the potential physiologic benefits of beta-blocker therapy can be achieved with oral administration within the first 24 hours of presentation. As such, the best course of treatment is to evaluate the patient, determine the physiologic status over a period of observation, and then offer the appropriate beta-blocker therapy.

Antiplatelet therapy is a key feature in the management of UA/NSTEMI. For more than 25 years, aspirin, an irreversible inhibitor of intracellular thromboxane A2 production, has been the antiplatelet drug of choice.[59] Numerous studies demonstrate benefits of early aspirin administration for UA/NSTEMI, in doses ranging from 75 mg once daily to 324 mg four times daily, which include both short- and long-term significant reductions in myocardial infarction and death.[60–66] The thienopyridines, clopidogrel and ticlopidine, antagonize the cell surface ADP-receptors that contribute to platelet aggregation.[59] Clopidogrel is generally preferred over ticlopidine because of its more favorable side effect profile, and early administration has been shown to improve short-term and long-term outcomes in patients with UA/NSTEMI.[66–71] Clopidogrel's benefit has been observed versus placebo, as well as in combination with aspirin versus aspirin alone and its beneficial qualities have been demonstrated in patients treated with both primary medical and interventional strategies.[66,67,69-73] For patients undergoing early PCI, studies evaluating the optimal dose and timing of clopidogrel administration report that a high loading dose of 600 mg requires only 2 hours to attain an adequate platelet inhibitory effect, while a lower loading dose of 300 mg may require up to 15 hours for maximal efficacy.[72,74,75] Because bleeding, including CABG-related bleeding (but not non-CABG-related life-threatening bleeding) is significantly increased by co-administration of aspirin and clopidogrel, it is recommended that clopidogrel be withheld if urgent CABG is considered likely.[68,69,72,73,76] The issue of clopidogrel therapy in the ED is unresolved with regards to the most appropriate patient for such therapy, as well as the time and location of administration.

Glycoprotein IIb/IIIa inhibitors, the third class of antiplatelet medications, work by inhibiting the glycoprotein IIb/IIIa receptor found on platelet cell membranes.[59] The benefits of abciximab and eptifibatide were initially observed in patients undergoing either urgent or elective PCI, including patients with UA/NSTEMI, where they significantly decrease important short-term cardiac outcomes.[77–85] Abciximab has since shown a long-term mortality benefit for this indication, but no advantage is seen when it is used as primary medical treatment for patients with UA/NSTEMI who are not undergoing revascularization.[86,87] Tirofiban and eptifibatide provide significant benefit in patients with UA/NSTEMI, either prior to PCI or as part of a noninvasive approach.[88–92] Lamifiban has more mixed results in this patient population.[93,94] A meta-analysis of all patients with UA/NSTEMI reveals significantly improved outcomes with glycoprotein inhibition, and particular benefit has been demonstrated in certain high-risk patients, such as those with elevated troponins, diabetes, and a TIMI score greater than three (Table 2-4).[59,73,95–99] In patients managed invasively, the benefit occurs both prior to and after PCI.[100] Trials investigating the optimal timing of glycoprotein inhibitor administration have shown possible superiority

Table 2-4. TIMI risk score for UA/NSTEMI.

Age ≥ 65
Known coronary stenosis ≥ 50%
ST-segment depression on initial ECG
≥ 2 episodes of angina in the past 24 hours
Use of aspirin in the past 7 days
Elevated cardiac biomarkers
≥ 3 risk factors for CAD*

*Family history of CAD, hypertension, hypercholesterolemia, diabetes, current smoking
Adapted from: Sabatine MS, Antman EM. The thrombolysis in myocardial infarction risk score in unstable angina/non-ST-segment elevation myocardial infarction. *J Am Coll Cardiol.* 2003;41:89S–95S.

to a routine upstream versus deferred selective (at the time of PCI) approach, but this subject has not been intensively investigated.[101,102] Despite the proven benefit of these agents, retrospective data suggest that they are underused, which may be due to the fact that most trials have invariably demonstrated an increase in bleeding complications, mostly minor but in some cases major.[95,103] Thus, the ideal form of anti-platelet therapy must weigh individual risks and benefits, but the fact that a small percentage of patients are resistant to the effects of one class of antiplatelet medication underscores the importance of having multiple available options.

Antithrombotic therapy is an important adjunct to antiplatelet therapy in patients with UA/NSTEMI, as the downstream effect of platelet aggregation is activation of the coagulation cascade. Unfractionated heparin (UFH) inhibits factor Xa and soluble factor IIa via antithrombin III activation in an approximately equal ratio.[104] Although individual trials have slight differences with regards to the timing, dosing, and route of administration of UFH, standard bolus and pTT-guided continuous infusion therapy are of overall short-term benefit in patients with UA/NSTEMI.[62,64,105–107] Although significantly improved outcomes have been demonstrated with isolation therapy, the largest benefit is seen in those patients treated with concomitant aspirin, as they act via complimentary mechanisms, and there seems to be some risk of rebound ischemia after the discontinuation of UFH in patients without aspirin protection.[105,108–110] The low molecular weight heparins (LMWH) selectively inhibit factor Xa to a greater extent than factor IIa, and have the advantage of more reliable pharmacokinetics, which eliminates the need for pTT-guided dose adjustments.[104] Three LMWH, nadroparin, dalteparin, and enoxaparin, have been studied as alternatives to UFH, and there are pharmacological and clinical differences between these three agents.[111] Enoxaparin has demonstrated superiority to standard UFH therapy with regards to efficacy, while *dalteparin* and nadroparin have shown more mixed results, but are acceptable alternatives.[104,111–119] Furthermore, only enoxaparin has a sustained benefit at long-term follow-up.[120] However, most trials revealing the superiority of enoxaparin were performed in the era prior to the routine use of stents and glycoprotein inhibitors. Later trials comparing UFH versus enoxaparin in the presence of glycoprotein inhibitors show less clear benefit, but have maintained its status as superior to UFH.[121-126] There is no benefit to long-term administration of any heparin agent, and one should not switch between individual heparins during acute treatment due to dosing differences that compromise efficacy or safety.[104,107,121] Minor bleeding is significantly increased with all LMWH versus UFH, with a possibility of increased major bleeding, but this risk must be balanced against the ease of administration of LMWH and the proven superior efficacy of enoxaparin.[104,111,127] LMWH are contraindicated in patients with renal failure or body weight extremes.

Direct thrombin inhibitors (DTI) act independently of antithrombin III to inactivate both soluble and fibrin-bound factor IIa.[128] The two most studied DTI, hirudin and bivalirudin, have equivalence or slight benefit with regards to efficacy versus UFH in patients with UA/NSTEMI, but most of these trials were performed prior to the routine use of stents and glycoprotein IIb/IIIa inhibitors, and primarily involved patients undergoing an early invasive strategy.[128-141] Furthermore, heterogeneity exists with regards to safety, as hirudin is associated with a significantly higher rate of major bleeding, while bivalirudin is associated with a significantly lower rate.[138] The addition of either upstream or downstream glycoprotein IIb/IIIa inhibitors to bivalirudin does increase the bleeding rate to approximate that of patients treated similarly with UFH, and while less bleeding has been observed with bivalirudin alone, there may be a loss of efficacy with bivalirudin in the absence of a glycoprotein inhibitor.[139,140,142-144] Fondaparinux, a direct factor Xa inhibitor, has recently been shown to have equivalent efficacy versus enoxaparin with a significant reduction in major bleeding for UA/NSTEMI patients.[145,146] As more therapies become available, the potential number of combinations of antiplatelet and antithrombotic agents is multiplying. Although this will hopefully improve anti-ischemic management, the potential for bleeding complications must always be carefully assessed, as supratherapeutic dosing does occur in the nonclinical trial-based world of everyday practice, and is associated with increased mortality and lengths of hospital stay.[147]

Section IV: Decision making

Please refer to Tables 2-1 through 2-4.

References

1 Pope JH, Ruthazer R, Beshansky JR, et al. Clinical features of emergency department patients presenting with symptoms suggestive of acute cardiac ischemia: A multicenter study. *J Thromb Thrombolysis.* 1998;6(1):63–74.

2 Storrow AB, Gibler WB. Chest pain centers: diagnosis of acute coronary syndromes. *Ann Emerg Med.* 2000;35:449–461.

3 Ringstrom E, Freedman J. Approach to undifferentiated chest pain in the emergency department: a review of recent medical literature and published practice guidelines. *Mt Sinai J Med.* 2006;73(2):499–505.

4 Lee TH, Cook EF, Weisberg M, et al. Acute chest pain in the emergency room. Identification and examination of low-risk patients. *Arch Intern Med.* 1985;145(1):65–69.

5 Gibler WB, Cannon CP, Blomkalns AL, et al. American Heart Association Council on Clinical Cardiology; American Heart Association Council on Cardiovascular Nursing; Quality of Care and Outcomes Research Interdisciplinary Working Group; Society of Chest Pain Centers. Practical implementation of the guidelines for unstable angina/non-ST-segment elevation myocardial infarction in the emergency department. *Ann Emerg Med.* 2005;46(2):185–197.

6 Goodacre S, Locker T, Morris F, et al. How useful are clinical features in the diagnosis of acute, undifferentiated chest pain? *Acad Emerg Med.* 2002;9(3):203–208.

7 Lee TH, Rouan GW, Weisberg MC, et al. Clinical characteristics and natural history of patients with acute myocardial infarction sent home from the emergency room. *Am J Cardiol.* 1987;60:219–224.

8 Pope JH, Aufderheide TP, Ruthazer R, et al. Missed diagnoses of acute cardiac ischemia in the emergency department. *N Engl J Med.* 2000;342:1163–1170.

9 Panju AA, Hemmelgarn BR, Guyatt GH, et al. The rational clinical examination. Is this patient having a myocardial infarction? *JAMA.* 1998;280(14):1256-1263.

10 Tierney WM, Roth BJ, Psaty B, et al. Predictors of myocardial infarction in emergency room patients. *Crit Care Med.* 1985;13(7):526–531.

11 Swap CJ, Nagurney JT. Value and limitations of chest pain history in the evaluation of patients with suspected acute coronary syndromes. *JAMA.* 2005;294(20):2623–2629.

12 Henrikson CA, Howell EE, Bush DE, et al. Chest pain relief by nitroglycerin does not predict active coronary artery disease. *Ann Intern Med.* 2003;139:979–986.

13 Shry EA, Dacus J, Van De Graaff E, et al. Usefulness of the response to sublingual GTN as a predictor of

ischemic chest pain in the emergency department. *Am J Cardiol.* 2002;90:1264–1266.

14 Jayes RL Jr, Beshansky JR, D'Agostino RB, et al. Do patients' coronary risk factor reports predict acute cardiac ischemia in the emergency department? A multicenter study. *J Clin Epidemiol.* 1992;45(6):621–626.

15 Zane RD. Are Cardiac Risk Factors of Value in ED Diagnosis of ACS? *Ann Emerg Med.* 2007; 49(2):145–152.

16 Thygesen K, Alpert JS, White HD. Joint ESC/ACCF/AHA/WHF Task Force for the Redefinition of Myocardial Infarction. Universal definition of myocardial infarction. *Eur Heart J.* 2007;28(20):2525–2538.

17 Lilly LS, ed. *Pathophysiology of Heart Disease.* 3rd ed. Baltimore: Lippincott, Williams, & Wilkins, 2003.

18 Diercks DB, Peacock WF, Hiestand BC, et al. Frequency and consequences of recording an electrocardiogram >10 minutes after arrival in an emergency room in non-ST-segment elevation acute coronary syndromes (from the CRUSADE Initiative). *Am J Cardiol.* 2006;97(4):437–442.

19 Behar S, Schor S, Kariv I, et al. Evaluation of electrocardiogram in emergency room as a decision-making tool. *Chest.* 1977;71:486–491.

20 Rude RE, Poole WK, Muller JE, et al. Electrocardiographic and clinical criteria for recognition of acute myocardial infarction based on analysis of 3,697 patients. *Am J Cardiol.* 1983;52(8):936–942.

21 Hamm CW, Goldmann BU, Heeschen C, et al. Emergency room triage of patients with acute chest pain by means of rapid testing for cardiac troponin T or troponin I. *N Engl J Med.* 1997;337(23):1648–1653.

22 Kudenchuk PJ, Maynard C, Cobb LA, et al. Utility of the prehospital electrocardiogram in diagnosing acute coronary syndromes: the Myocardial Infarction Triage and Intervention (MITI) Project. *J Am Coll Cardiol.* 1998;32:17–27.

23 Brush JE Jr, Brand DA, Acampora D, et al. Use of the initial electrocardiogram to predict in-hospital complications of acute myocardial infarction. *N Engl J Med.* 1985;312:1137–1141.

24 Cohen M, Hawkins L, Greenberg S, et al. Usefulness of ST-segment changes in greater than or equal to 2 leads on the emergency room electrocardiogram in either unstable angina pectoris or non-Q-wave myocardial infarction in predicting outcome. *Am J Cardiol.* 1991;67:1368–1373.

25 Slater DK, Hlatky MA, Mark DB, et al. Outcome in suspected acute myocardial infarction with normal or minimally abnormal admission electrocardiographic findings. *Am J Cardiol.* 1987;60(10):766–770.

26 Rouan GW, Lee TH, Cook EF, et al. Clinical characteristics and outcome of acute myocardial infarction in patients with initially normal or nonspecific electrocardiograms (a report from the Multicenter Chest Pain Study). *Am J Cardiol.* 1989;64(18):1087–1092.

27 Fesmire FM, Percy RF, Wears RL, MacMath TL. Risk stratification according to the initial electrocardiogram in patients with suspected acute myocardial infarction. *Arch Int Med.* 1989;149(6):1294–1297.

28 Zarling EJ, Sexton, H, Milnor P Jr. Failure to diagnose acute myocardial infarction. The clinicopathologic experience at a large community hospital. *JAMA.* 1983;250(9):1177–1181.

29 Fesmire FM, Percy RF, Bardoner JB, et al. Usefulness of automated serial 12-lead ECG monitoring during the initial emergency department evaluation of patients with chest pain. *Ann Emerg Med.* 1998; 31(1):3–11.

30 Savonitto S, Ardissino D, Granger CB, et al. Prognostic value of the admission electrocardiogram in acute coronary syndromes. *JAMA.* 1999;281(8):707–713.

31 Bakshi TK, Choo MK, Edwards CC, et al. Causes of elevated troponin I with a normal coronary angiogram. *Intern Med J.* 2002;32(11):520–525.

32 Roongsritong C, Warraich I, Bradley C. Common causes of troponin elevations in the absence of acute myocardial infarction: incidence and clinical significance. *Chest.* 2004;125(5):1877–1884.

33 Morrow DA, Antman EM, Tanasijevic M, et al. Cardiac troponin I for stratification of early outcomes and the efficacy of enoxaparin in unstable angina: a TIMI-11B substudy. *J Am Coll Cardiol.* 2000;36:1812–1817.

34 Antman EM, Tanasijevic MJ, Thompson B, et al. Cardiac-specific troponin I levels to predict the risk of mortality in patients with acute coronary syndromes. *N Engl J Med.* 1996;335(18):1342–1349.

35 Licka M, Zimmermann R, Zehelein J, et al. Troponin T concentrations 72 hours after myocardial infarction as a serological estimate of infarct size. *Heart.* 2002;87(6):520–524.

36 Bär FW, Verheugt FW, Col J, et al. Thrombolysis in patients with unstable angina improves the angiographic but not the clinical outcome. Results of UNASEM, a multicenter, randomized, placebo-controlled, clinical trial with anistreplase. *Circulation.* 1992;86(1):131–137.

37 Waters D, Lam JY. Is thrombolytic therapy striking out in unstable angina? *Circulation.* 1992;86:1642–1644.

38 Effects of tissue plasminogen activator and a comparison of early invasive and conservative strategies in unstable angina and non-Q-wave myocardial infarction. Results of the TIMI IIIB Trial. *Circulation.* 1994;89:1545–1556.

39 Kaplan K, Davison R, Parker M, et al. Intravenous nitroglycerin for the treatment of angina at rest

unresponsive to standard nitrate therapy. *Am J Cardiol.* 1983;51(5):694–698.

40 Karlberg KE, Saldeen T, Wallin R, et al. Intravenous nitroglycerin reduces ischaemia in unstable angina pectoris: a double-blind placebo-controlled study. *J Intern Med.* 1998;243(1):25–31.

41 Yusuf S, Collins R, MacMahon S, et al. Effect of intravenous nitrates on mortality in acute myocardial infarction: an overview of the randomized trials. *Lancet.* 1988;1(8594):1088–1092.

42 GISSI-3: effects of lisinopril and transdermal glyceryl trinitrate singly and together on 6-week mortality and ventricular function after acute myocardial infarction. Gruppo Italiano per lo Studio della Sopravvivenza nell'infarto Miocardico. *Lancet.* 1994;343(8906):1115–1122.

43 ISIS-4: a randomised factorial trial assessing early oral captopril, oral mononitrate, and intravenous magnesium sulphate in 58,050 patients with suspected acute myocardial infarction. ISIS-4 (Fourth International Study of Infarct Survival) Collaborative Group. *Lancet.* 1995;345:669–685.

44 Yusuf S, Peto R, Lewis J, Collins R, Sleight P. Beta blockade during and after myocardial infarction: an overview of the randomized trials. *Prog Cardiovasc Dis.* 1985;27(5):335–371.

45 Rydén L, Ariniego R, Arnman K, et al. A double-blind trial of metoprolol in acute myocardial infarction. Effects on ventricular tachyarrhythmias. *N Engl J Med.* 1983;308(11):614–618.

46 Mechanisms for the early mortality reduction produced by beta-blockade started early in acute myocardial infarction: ISIS-1. ISIS-1 (First International Study of Infarct Survival) Collaborative Group. *Lancet.* 1988;1(8591):921–923.

47 Everts B, Karlson BW, Herlitz J, et al. Effects and pharmacokinetics of high dose metoprolol on chest pain in patients with suspected or definite acute myocardial infarction. *Eur J Clin Pharmacol.* 1997;53:23–31.

48 Chen ZM, Pan HC, Chen YP, et al. COMMIT (ClOpidogrel and Metoprolol in Myocardial Infarction Trial) collaborative group. Early intravenous then oral metoprolol in 45,852 patients with acute myocardial infarction: randomized placebo-controlled trial. *Lancet.* 2005;366(9497):1622–1632.

49 Miller CD, Roe MT, Mulgund J, et al. Impact of acute beta-blocker therapy for patients with non-ST-segment elevation myocardial infarction. *Am J Med.* 2007;120(8):685–692.

50 Silvet H, Spencer F, Yarzebski J, et al. Communitywide trends in the use and outcomes associated with beta-blockers in patients with acute myocardial infarction: the Worcester Heart Attack Study. *Arch Intern Med.* 2003;163(18):2175–2183.

51 Randomised trial of intravenous atenolol among 16, 027 cases of suspected acute myocardial infarction: ISIS-1. First International Study of Infarct Survival Collaborative Group. *Lancet.* 1986;2(8498):57–66.

52 Metoprolol in acute myocardial infarction (MIAMI). A randomized placebo-controlled international trial. The MIAMI Trial Research Group. *Eur Heart J.* 1985;6(3):199–226.

53 Hjalmarson A, Elmfeldt D, Herlitz J, et al. Effect on mortality of metoprolol in acute myocardial infarction. A double-blind randomized trial. *Lancet.* 1981;823–827.

54 Timolol-induced reduction in mortality and reinfarction in patients surviving acute myocardial infarction. *N Engl J Med.* 1981;304(14):801–807.

55 A randomized trial of propranolol in patients with acute myocardial infarction: Mortality results. *JAMA.* 1982;247:1707–1714.

56 Hjalmarson A, Herlitz J, Holmberg S, et al. The Göteborg metoprolol trial. Effects on mortality and morbidity in acute myocardial infarction. *Circulation.* 1983;67(6 Pt 2):I26–I32.

57 Salpeter SR, Ormiston TM, Salpeter EE. Cardioselective beta-blockers in patients with reactive airway disease: a meta-analysis. *Ann Intern Med.* 2002;137(9):715–725.

58 Salpeter S, Ormiston T, Salpeter E. Cardioselective beta-blockers for chronic obstructive pulmonary disease. *Cochrane Database Syst Rev.* 2005;(4):CD003566.

59 Schulman SP. Antiplatelet therapy in non-ST-segment elevation acute coronary syndromes. *JAMA.* 2004;292:1875–1882.

60 Lewis HD Jr, Davis JW, Archibald DG, et al. Protective effects of aspirin against acute myocardial infarction and death in men with unstable angina. Results of a Veterans Administration Cooperative Study. *N Engl J Med.* 1983;309(7):396–403.

61 Cairns JA, Gent M, Singer J, et al. Aspirin, sulfinpyrazone, or both in unstable angina. Results of a Canadian multicenter trial. *N Engl J Med.* 1985;313: 1369–1375.

62 Théroux P, Ouimet H, McCans J, et al. Aspirin, heparin, or both to treat acute unstable angina. *N Engl J Med.* 1988;319(17):1105–1011.

63 Randomised trial of intravenous streptokinase, oral aspirin, both, or neither among 17,187 cases of suspected acute myocardial infarction: ISIS-2. ISIS-2 (Second International Study of Infarct Survival) Collaborative Group. *Lancet.* 1988;8607:349–360.

64 Risk of myocardial infarction and death during treatment with low dose aspirin and intravenous heparin in men with unstable coronary artery disease. The RISC Group. *Lancet.* 1990;336(8719):827–830.

65 Borzak S, Cannon CP, Kraft PL, et al. Effects of prior aspirin and anti-ischemic therapy on outcome of patients with unstable angina. TIMI 7 Investigators. Thrombin Inhibition in Myocardial Ischemia. *Am J Cardiol.* 1998;81(6):678–681.

66 Antithrombotic Trialists' Collaboration. Collaborative meta-analysis of randomized trials of anti-platelet therapy for prevention of death, myocardial infarction, and stroke in high risk patients. *BMJ.* 2002;324(7329):71–86.

67 Bertrand ME, Rupprecht HJ, Urban P, Gershlick AH, CLASSICS Investigators. Double blind study of the safety of clopidogrel with and without a loading dose in combination with aspirin compared with ticlopidine in combination with aspirin after coronary stenting: the clopidogrel aspirin stent international cooperative study (CLASSICS). *Circulation.* 2000;102(6):624–629.

68 Yusuf S, Mehta SR, Zhao F, et al. Clopidogrel in Unstable Angina to Prevent Recurrent Events Trial Investigators. Early and late effects of clopidogrel in patients with acute coronary syndromes. *Circulation.* 2003;107(7):966–972.

69 Yusuf S, Zhao F, Mehta SR, et al. Clopidogrel in Unstable Angina to Prevent Recurrent Events Trial Investigators. Effects of clopidogrel in addition to aspirin in patients with acute coronary syndromes without ST-segment elevation. *N Engl J Med.* 2001;345(7):494–502.

70 Mehta SR, Yusuf S, Peters RJ, et al. Clopidogrel in Unstable Angina to Prevent Recurrent Events Trial (CURE) Investigators. Effects of pretreatment with clopidogrel and aspirin followed by long-term therapy in patients undergoing percutaneous coronary intervention: the PCI-CURE study. *Lancet.* 2001;358(9281): 527–533.

71 Bhatt DL, Flather MD, Hacke W, et al. CHARISMA Investigators. Patients with prior myocardial infarction, stroke, or symptomatic peripheral arterial disease in the CHARISMA trial. *J Am Coll Cardiol.* 2007; 49:1982–1988.

72 Steinhubl SR, Berger PB, Mann JT 3rd, et al. CREDO Investigators. Clopidogrel for the Reduction of Events During Observation. Early and sustained dual oral antiplatelet therapy following percutaneous coronary intervention: a randomized controlled trial. *JAMA.* 2002;288(19):2411–2420.

73 Gluckman TJ, Sachdev M, Schulman SP, Blumenthal RS. A simplified approach to the management of non-ST-segment elevation acute coronary syndromes. *JAMA.* 2005;293(3):349–357.

74 Kandzari DE, Berger PB, Kastrati A, et al. Influence of treatment duration with a 600-mg dose of clopidogrel before percutaneous coronary revascularization. *J Am Coll Cardiol.* 2004;44(11):2133–2136.

75 Steinhubl SR, Berger PB, Brennan DM, et al. CREDO Investigators. Optimal timing for the initiation of pre-treatment with 300 mg clopidogrel before percutaneous coronary intervention. *J Am Coll Cardiol.* 2006;47(5):939–943.

76 Mehta RH, Roe MT, Mulgund J, et al. Acute clopidogrel use and outcomes in patients with non-ST-segment elevation acute coronary syndromes undergoing coronary artery bypass surgery. *J Am Coll Cardiol.* 2006;48(2):281–286.

77 Use of a monoclonal antibody directed against the platelet glycoprotein IIb/IIIa receptor in high-risk coronary angioplasty. The EPIC Investigation. *N Engl J Med.* 1994;330:956–961.

78 Lincoff AM, Califf RM, Anderson KM, et al. Evidence for prevention of death and myocardial infarction with platelet membrane glycoprotein IIb/IIIa receptor blockade by abciximab (c7E3 Fab) among patients with unstable angina undergoing percutaneous coronary revascularization. EPIC Investigators. Evaluation of 7E3 in Preventing Ischemic Complications. *J Am Coll Cardiol.* 1997;30(1):149–156.

79 Platelet glycoprotein IIb/IIIa receptor blockade and low-dose heparin during percutaneous coronary revascularization. The EPILOG Investigators. *N Engl J Med.* 1997;336:1689–1696.

80 Randomised placebo-controlled trial of effect of eptifibatide on complications of percutaneous coronary intervention: IMPACT-II. Integrilin to Minimise Platelet Aggregation and Coronary Thrombosis-II. *Lancet.* 1997;349:1422–1428.

81 Randomised placebo-controlled trial of abciximab before and during coronary intervention in refractory unstable angina: the CAPTURE Study. *Lancet.* 1997;349(9063):1429–1435.

82 EPISTENT Investigators. Randomised placebo-controlled and balloon-angioplasty-controlled trial to assess safety of coronary stenting with use of platelet glycoprotein-IIb/IIIa blockade. *Lancet.* 1998;352:87–92.

83 Cho L, Topol EJ, Balog C, et al. Clinical benefit of glycoprotein IIb/IIIa blockade with Abciximab is independent of gender: pooled analysis from EPIC, EPILOG and EPISTENT trials. Evaluation of 7E3 for the Prevention of Ischemic Complications. Evaluation in Percutaneous Transluminal Coronary Angioplasty to Improve Long-Term Outcome with Abciximab GP IIb/IIIa blockade. Evaluation of Platelet IIb/IIIa Inhibitor for Stent. *J Am Coll Cardiol.* 2000;36(2):381–386.

84 ESPRIT Investigators. Enhanced Suppression of the Platelet IIb/IIIa Receptor with Integrilin Therapy. Novel dosing regimen of eptifibatide in planned coronary stent implantation (ESPRIT): a randomized, placebo-controlled trial. *Lancet.* 2000;356:2037–2044.

85 Brener SJ, Barr LA, Burchenal JE, et al. Randomized, placebo-controlled trial of platelet glycoprotein IIb/IIIa blockade with primary angioplasty for acute myocardial infarction. ReoPro and Primary PTCA Organization and Randomized Trial (RAPPORT) Investigators. *Circulation*. 1998;98:734–741.

86 Anderson KM, Califf RM, Stone GW, et al. Long-term mortality benefit with abciximab in patients undergoing percutaneous coronary intervention. *J Am Coll Cardiol*. 2001;37:2059–2065.

87 Simoons ML. GUSTO IV-ACS Investigators. Effect of glycoprotein IIb/IIIa receptor blocker abciximab on outcome in patients with acute coronary syndromes without early coronary revascularisation: the GUSTO IV-ACS randomized trial. *Lancet*. 2001;357(9272):1915–1924.

88 Effects of platelet glycoprotein IIb/IIIa blockade with tirofiban on adverse cardiac events in patients with unstable angina or acute myocardial infarction undergoing coronary angioplasty. The RESTORE Investigators. Randomized Efficacy Study of Tirofiban for Outcomes and REstenosis. *Circulation*. 1997;96(5):1445–1453.

89 A comparison of aspirin plus tirofiban with aspirin plus heparin for unstable angina. Platelet Receptor Inhibition in Ischemic Syndrome Management (PRISM) Study Investigators. *N Engl J Med*. 1998;338:1498–1505.

90 Inhibition of platelet glycoprotein IIb/IIIa with eptifibatide in patients with acute coronary syndromes. The PURSUIT Trial Investigators. Platelet Glycoprotein IIb/IIIa in Unstable Angina: Receptor Suppression Using Integrilin Therapy. *N Engl J Med*. 1998;339(7):436–443.

91 Inhibition of the platelet glycoprotein IIb/IIIa receptor with tirofiban in unstable angina and non-Q-wave myocardial infarction. Platelet Receptor Inhibition in Ischemic Syndrome Management in Patients Limited by Unstable Signs and Symptoms (PRISM-PLUS) Study Investigators. *N Engl J Med*. 1998;338(21):1488–1497.

92 Valgimigli M, Percoco G, Barbieri D, et al. The additive value of tirofiban administered with the high-dose bolus in the prevention of ischemic complications during high-risk coronary angioplasty: the ADVANCE Trial. *J Am Coll Cardiol*. 2004;44:14–19.

93 International, randomized, controlled trial of lamifiban (a platelet glycoprotein IIb/IIIa inhibitor), heparin, or both in unstable angina. The PARAGON Investigators. Platelet IIb/IIIa Antagonism for the Reduction of Acute coronary syndrome events in a Global Organization Network. *Circulation*. 1998;97(24):2386–2395.

94 Mukherjee D, Mahaffey KW, Moliterno DJ, et al. Promise of combined low-molecular-weight heparin and platelet glycoprotein IIb/IIIa inhibition: results from Platelet IIb/IIIa Antagonist for the Reduction of Acute coronary syndrome events in a Global

Organization Network B (PARAGON B). *Am Heart J*. 2002;144(6):995–1002.

95 Boersma E, Harrington RA, Moliterno DJ, et al. Platelet glycoprotein IIb/IIIa inhibitors in acute coronary syndromes: a meta-analysis of all major randomized clinical trials. *Lancet*. 2002;359:189–198.

96 Heeschen C, Hamm CW, Goldmann B, et al. Troponin concentrations for stratification of patients with acute coronary syndromes in relation to therapeutic efficacy of tirofiban. PRISM Study Investigators. Platelet Receptor Inhibition in Ischemic Syndrome Management. *Lancet*. 1999;354:1757–1762.

97 Roffi M, Chew DP, Mukherjee D, et al. Platelet glycoprotein IIb/IIIa inhibitors reduce mortality in diabetic patients with non-ST-segment-elevation acute coronary syndromes. *Circulation*. 200;104(23):2767–2771.

98 Morrow DA, Antman EM, Snapinn SM, et al. An integrated clinical approach to predicting the benefit of tirofiban in non-ST elevation acute coronary syndromes. Application of the TIMI Risk Score for UA/NSTEMI in PRISM-PLUS. *Eur Heart J*. 2002;23:223–229.

99 Boden WE. "Routine invasive" versus "selective invasive" approaches to non-ST-segment elevation acute coronary syndromes management in the post-stent/platelet inhibition era. *J Am Coll Cardiol*. 2003;41(4):113S–122S.

100 Boersma E, Akkerhuis KM, Théroux P, et al. Platelet glycoprotein IIb/IIIa receptor inhibition in non-ST-elevation acute coronary syndromes: early benefit during medical treatment only, with additional protection during percutaneous coronary intervention. *Circulation*. 1999;100:2045–2048.

101 Bolognese L, Falsini G, Liistro F, et al. Randomized comparison of upstream tirofiban versus downstream high bolus dose tirofiban or abciximab on tissue-level perfusion and troponin release in high-risk acute coronary syndromes treated with percutaneous coronary interventions: the EVEREST trial. *J Am Coll Cardiol*. 2006;47(3):522–528.

102 Stone GW, Bertrand ME, Moses JW, et al. ACUITY Investigators. Routine upstream initiation vs. deferred selective use of glycoprotein IIb/IIIa inhibitors in acute coronary syndromes: the ACUITY Timing trial. *JAMA*. 2007;297:591–602.

103 Peterson ED, Pollack CV Jr, Roe MT, et al. National Registry of Myocardial Infarction (NRMI) 4 Investigators. Early use of glycoprotein IIb/IIIa inhibitors in non-ST-elevation acute myocardial infarction: observations from the National Registry of Myocardial Infarction 4. *J Am Coll Cardiol*. 2003;42:45–53.

104 Kaul S, Shah PK. Low molecular weight heparin in acute coronary syndrome: evidence for superior or equivalent efficacy compared with unfractionated heparin? *J Am Coll Cardiol*. 2000;35(7):1699–1712.

105 Telford AM, Wilson C. Trial of heparin versus atenolol in prevention of myocardial infarction in intermediate coronary syndrome. *Lancet*. 1981;1(8232):1225–1228.

106 Théroux P, Waters D, Qiu S, et al. Aspirin versus heparin to prevent myocardial infarction during the acute phase of unstable angina. *Circulation*. 1993;88:2045–2048.

107 Eikelboom JW, Anand SS, Malmberg K, et al. Unfractionated heparin and low-molecular-weight heparin in acute coronary syndrome without ST elevation: a meta-analysis. *Lancet*. 2000;355(9219):1936–1942.

108 Cohen M, Adams PC, Parry G, et al. Combination antithrombotic therapy in unstable rest angina and non-Q-wave infarction in nonprior aspirin users. Primary end points analysis from the ATACS trial. Antithrombotic Therapy in Acute Coronary Syndromes Research Group. *Circulation*. 1994;89:81–88.

109 Oler A, Whooley MA, Oler J, Grady D. Adding heparin to aspirin reduces the incidence of myocardial infarction and death in patients with unstable angina. A meta-analysis. *JAMA*. 1996;276(10):811–815.

110 Théroux P, Waters D, Lam J, Juneau M, McCans J. Reactivation of unstable angina after the discontinuation of heparin. *N Engl J Med*. 1992;327(3):141–145.

111 Antman EM, Cohen M, Radley D, et al. Assessment of the treatment effect of enoxaparin for unstable angina/non-Q-wave myocardial infarction. TIMI 11B-ESSENCE meta-analysis. *Circulation*. 1999;100(15):1602–1608.

112 Cohen M, Demers C, Gurfinkel EP, et al. A comparison of low-molecular-weight heparin with unfractionated heparin for unstable coronary artery disease. Efficacy and Safety of Subcutaneous Enoxaparin in Non-Q-Wave Coronary Events Study Group. *N Engl J Med*. 1997;337(7):447–452.

113 Antman EM, McCabe CH, Gurfinkel EP, et al. Enoxaparin prevents death and cardiac ischemic events in unstable angina/non-Q-wave myocardial infarction. Results of the thrombolysis in myocardial infarction (TIMI) 11B trial. *Circulation*. 1999;100(15):1593–1601.

114 Petersen JL, Mahaffey KW, Hasselblad V, et al. Efficacy and bleeding complications among patients randomized to enoxaparin or unfractionated heparin for antithrombin therapy in non-ST-segment elevation acute coronary syndromes: a systematic overview. *JAMA*. 2004;292(1):89–96.

115 Murphy SA, Gibson CM, Morrow DA, et al. Efficacy and safety of the low-molecular weight heparin enoxaparin compared with unfractionated heparin across the acute coronary syndrome spectrum: a meta-analysis. *Eur Heart J*. 2007;28(17):2077–2086.

116 Low-molecular-weight heparin during instability in coronary artery disease, Fragmin during Instability in Coronary Artery Disease (FRISC) study group. *Lancet*. 1996;347:561–568.

117 Klein W, Buchwald A, Hillis SE, et al. Comparison of low-molecular-weight heparin with unfractionated heparin acutely and with placebo for 6 weeks in the management of unstable coronary artery disease. Fragmin in unstable coronary artery disease study (FRIC). *Circulation*. 1997;96(1):61–68.

118 Gurfinkel EP, Manos EJ, Mejaíl RI, et al. Low molecular weight heparin versus regular heparin or aspirin in the treatment of unstable angina and silent ischemia. *J Am Coll Cardiol*. 1995;26:313–318.

119 Comparison of two treatment durations (6 days and 14 days) of a low molecular weight heparin with a 6-day treatment of unfractionated heparin in the initial management of unstable angina or non-Q wave myocardial infarction: FRAX.I.S. (FRAxiparine in Ischaemic Syndrome). *Eur Heart J*. 1999;20:1553–1562.

120 Goodman SG, Cohen M, Bigonzi F, et al. Randomized trial of low molecular weight heparin (enoxaparin) versus unfractionated heparin for unstable coronary artery disease: one-year results of the ESSENCE Study. Efficacy and Safety of Subcutaneous Enoxaparin in Non-Q Wave Coronary Events. *J Am Coll Cardiol*. 2000;36(3):693–698.

121 Ferguson JJ, Califf RM, Antman EM, et al. SYNERGY Trial Investigators. Enoxaparin vs unfractionated heparin in high-risk patients with non-ST-segment elevation acute coronary syndromes managed with an intended early invasive strategy: primary results of the SYNERGY randomized trial. *JAMA*. 2004;292(1):45–54.

122 Cohen M, Théroux P, Borzak S, et al. Randomized double-blind safety study of enoxaparin versus unfractionated heparin in patients with non-ST-segment elevation acute coronary syndromes treated with tirofiban and aspirin: the ACUTE II study. The Antithrombotic Combination Using Tirofiban and Enoxaparin. *Am Heart J*. 2002;144(3):470–477.

123 Goodman SG, Fitchett D, Armstrong PW, et al. Integrilin and Enoxaparin Randomized Assessment of Acute Coronary Syndrome Treatment (INTERACT) Trial Investigators. Randomized evaluation of the safety and efficacy of enoxaparin versus unfractionated heparin in high-risk patients with non-ST-segment elevation acute coronary syndromes receiving the glycoprotein IIb/IIIa inhibitor eptifibatide. *Circulation*. 2003;107(2):238–244.

124 Blazing MA, de Lemos JA, White HD, et al. A to Z Investigators. Safety and efficacy of enoxaparin vs unfractionated heparin in patients with non-ST-segment elevation acute coronary syndromes who receive tirofiban and aspirin: a randomized controlled trial. *JAMA*. 2004;292(1):55–64.

125 Mahaffey KW, Cohen M, Garg J, et al. SYNERGY Trial Investigators. High-risk patients with acute coronary syndromes treated with low-molecular-weight or unfractionated heparin: outcomes at 6 months and 1 year in the SYNERGY trial. *JAMA.* 2005;294:2594–2600.

126 de Lemos JA, Blazing MA, Wiviott SD, et al. A to Z Investigators. Enoxaparin versus unfractionated heparin in patients treated with tirofiban, aspirin and an early conservative initial management strategy: results from the A phase of the A-to-Z trial. *Eur Heart J.* 2004;25:1688–1694.

127 Berkowitz SD, Stinnett S, Cohen M, et al. ESSENCE Investigators. Prospective comparison of hemorrhagic complications after treatment with enoxaparin versus unfractionated heparin for unstable angina pectoris or non-ST-segment elevation acute myocardial infarction. *Am J Cardiol.* 2001;88(11):1230–1234.

128 Antman EM, McCabe CH, Braunwald E. Bivalirudin as a replacement for unfractionated heparin in unstable angina/non-ST-elevation myocardial infarction: observations from the TIMI 8 trial. The Thrombolysis in Myocardia Infarction. *Am Heart J.* 2002;143:229–234.

129 Randomized trial of intravenous heparin versus recombinant hirudin for acute coronary syndromes. The Global Use of Strategies to Open Occluded Coronary Arteries (GUSTO) IIa Investigators. *Circulation.* 1994;90:1631–1637.

130 Fuchs J, Cannon CP. Hirulog in the treatment of unstable angina. Results of the Thrombin Inhibition in Myocardial Ischemia (TIMI) 7 trial. *Circulation.* 1995;92:727–733.

131 Serruys PW, Herrman JP, Simon R, et al. A comparison of hirudin with heparin in the prevention of restenosis after coronary angioplasty. Helvetica Investigators. *N Engl J Med.* 1995;333:757–763.

132 Bittl JA, Strony J, Brinker JA, et al. Treatment with bivalirudin (Hirulog) as compared with heparin during coronary angioplasty for unstable or postinfarction angina. Hirulog Angioplasty Study Investigators. *N Engl J Med.* 1995;333:764–769.

133 A comparison of recombinant hirudin with heparin for the treatment of acute coronary syndromes. The Global Use of Strategies to Open Occluded Coronary Arteries (GUSTO) IIb investigators. *N Engl J Med.* 1996;335(11):775–782.

134 Comparison of the effects of two doses of recombinant hirudin compared with heparin in patients with acute myocardial ischemia without ST elevation: a pilot study. Organization to Assess Strategies for Ischemic Syndromes (OASIS) Investigators. *Circulation.* 1997;96(3):769–777.

135 Effects of recombinant hirudin (lepirudin) compared with heparin on death, myocardial infarction, refractory angina, and revascularisation procedures in patients with acute myocardial ischaemia without ST elevation: a randomized trial. Organisation to Assess Strategies for Ischemic Syndromes (OASIS-2) Investigators. *Lancet.* 1999;353:429–438.

136 Roe MT, Granger CB, Puma JA, et al. Comparison of benefits and complications of hirudin versus heparin for patients with acute coronary syndromes undergoing early percutaneous coronary intervention. *Am J Cardiol.* 2001;88:1403–1406.

137 Mehta SR, Eikelboom JW, Rupprecht HJ, et al. Efficacy of hirudin in reducing cardiovascular events in patients with acute coronary syndrome undergoing early percutaneous coronary intervention. *Eur Heart J.* 2002;23:117–123.

138 Direct Thrombin Inhibitor Trialists' Collaborative Group. Direct thrombin inhibitors in acute coronary syndromes: principal results of a meta-analysis based on individual patients' data. *Lancet.* 2002;359(9303):294–302.

139 Lincoff AM, Bittl JA, Harrington RA, et al. REPLACE-2 Investigators. Bivalirudin and provisional glycoprotein IIb/IIIa blockade compared with heparin and planned glycoprotein IIb/IIIa blockade during percutaneous coronary intervention: REPLACE-2 randomized trial. *JAMA.* 2003;289(7):853–863.

140 Lincoff AM, Bittl JA, Kleiman NS, et al. REPLACE-1 Investigators. Comparison of bivalirudin versus heparin during percutaneous coronary intervention (the Randomized Evaluation of PCI Linking Angiomax to Reduced Clinical Events [REPLACE]-1 trial). *Am J Cardiol.* 2004;93:1092–1096.

141 Sinnaeve PR, Simes J, Yusuf S, et al. Direct thrombin inhibitors in acute coronary syndromes: effect in patients undergoing early percutaneous coronary intervention. *Eur Heart J.* 2005;26(22):2396–2403.

142 Stone GW, McLaurin BT, Cox DA, et al. ACUITY Investigators. Bivalirudin for patients with acute coronary syndromes. *N Engl J Med.* 2006;355:2203–2216.

143 Gibson CM, Morrow DA, Murphy SA, et al. TIMI Study Group. A randomized trial to evaluate the relative protection against post-percutaneous coronary intervention microvascular dysfunction, ischemia, and inflammation among antiplatelet and antithrombotic agents: the PROTECT-TIMI-30 trial. *J Am Coll Cardiol.* 2006;47:2364–2373.

144 Stone GW, White HD, Ohman EM, et al. Acute Catheterization and Urgent Intervention Triage strategy (ACUITY) trial investigators. Bivalirudin in patients with acute coronary syndromes undergoing percutaneous coronary intervention: a subgroup analysis from the Acute Catheterization and Urgent Intervention Triage strategy (ACUITY) trial. *Lancet.* 2007;369:907–919.

145 Yusuf S, Mehta SR, et al. Fifth Organization to Assess Strategies in Acute Ischemic Syndromes Investigators, Comparison of fondaparinux and enoxaparin in acute coronary syndromes. *N Engl J Med.* 2006;354(14):1464–1476.

146 Mehta SR, Granger CB, Eikelboom JW, et al. Efficacy and safety of fondaparinux versus enoxaparin in patients with acute coronary syndromes undergoing percutaneous coronary intervention: results from the OASIS-5 trial. *J Am Coll Cardiol.* 2007;50(18): 1742–1751.

147 Alexander KP, Chen AY, Roe MT, et al. CRUSADE Investigators. Excess dosing of antiplatelet and antithrombin agents in the treatment of non-ST-segment elevation acute coronary syndromes. *JAMA.* 2005;294(24):3108–3116.

ST-segment elevation myocardial infarction

David F. M. Brown

Vice Chair, Department of Emergency Medicine, Massachusetts General Hospital,
Associate Professor, Harvard Medical School, Boston, Massachusetts, USA

Section I: Case presentation

A 45-year-old man developed chest tightness and nausea while watching TV. He also complained of jaw and left arm pain, but no back pain. EMS was called after the symptoms did not resolve over 30 minutes. Field vital signs were: heart rate 75 beats/min, blood pressure 100/66 mmHg, respirations 16 breaths/min, oxygen saturation 95%. The skin was diaphoretic with clear lungs, along with regular heart sounds without a murmur, a benign abdomen, and equal pulses. A field electrocardiogram (EKG) revealed evidence of acute inferolateral ST-segment elevation myocardial infarction (STEMI). The patient was then brought to the emergency department (ED). He arrived with ongoing chest pain, and continued diaphoresis.

The past medical history was notable for hypertension, for which he took lisinopril. He had no prior history of chest pain. He did not smoke nor use recreational drugs. His father had a coronary bypass surgery at age 50.

The ED vital signs were: heart rate 78 beats/min, blood pressure 110/60 mmHg, respirations 12 breaths/min, and oxygen saturation 99% on 2 liters of oxygen by nasal canula. The skin was moist and there was no jugular vein distention. The breath sounds were clear. The heart sounds were regular with a crisp S1 and S2. There were no murmurs. The extremities were without edema. The pulses were brisk. The neurological

examination was normal. An EKG was unchanged from the field tracing.

Section II: Case discussion

Dr Richard Harrigan: We stress the EMS presentation with acute myocardial infarctions (MIs) or patients with chest pain. With prolonged ED waiting times because of the backup in the waiting room or problems with triage, EDs need a protocol to obtain an emergent EKG for anyone who presents with chest pain, including those patients who arrive on their own (i.e., not via an ambulance). Without this, there is potential for critical delays in treatment.

Dr Peter Rosen: We had a patient present with chest pain. An EKG was taken and read by an ED attending. The EKG was not immediately diagnostic, and the patient was evaluated for a noncardiac cause. Subsequently, the patient developed more chest pain. A different attending was now responsible for that patient and said, "Let me see the patient's EKG." He had not seen the original one, and he wanted to see if there were changes on it. At that moment, a tech brought an EKG to be read and the attending thought he was reading the second EKG on the patient with chest pain, but was actually reading the first EKG on an entirely different patient. The error that was made was that the attending, who was very busy, didn't check the name of the patient against the name on the EKG. I could see how that would happen when you are busy, and you ask for a tracing and someone hands you one. You immediately assume it's the one you asked for rather than a separate one.

Dr William Brady: Thus, as with all diagnostic investigations, the confirmation of the patient's identity is a vital portion of the study interpretation.

Dr David Brown: Our policy is that an immediate EKG is done based on triage symptoms and handed to an attending, and that attending has to sign the tracing, stating "no STEMI." While that might avoid an error in recognition that this wasn't the patient's initial tracing, it would not identify an initial tracing for a separate patient. While it is understandable how such errors occur during busy times, there is no substitute for compulsive attention to the name on the tracing as part of interpretation.

PR: Hopefully this was a one-time error, but it seems to me that it is the kind of error that is easy to repeat. Perhaps, if we can computerize our patient care a bit better, then maybe the EKG will automatically appear rather than having to go hunt for the paper. On another note, not every state has a selective destination policy for potential acute MI patients, and not every EMS system has the ability to obtain 12-lead EKGs in the field.

Dr Shamai Grossman: Boston pioneered a selective destination policy for potential MI patients several years ago, and has successfully cut critical minutes away in treating STEMI patients by bringing them only to EDs with 24-hour catheterization laboratories.

WB: Prehospital diagnosis and prehospital notification prior to arrival using the 12-lead EKG can potentially shave as much as 20 to 30 minutes off the patient's total door-to-reperfusion therapy time just by having the hospital involved and ready to move quickly.

RH: In Philadelphia, there are five university hospitals all very close to each other, all percutaneous coronary intervention (PCI) capable, and many have arrangements with the smaller hospitals where they will, upon receiving a patient, fax an EKG to the University Hospital and activate the system there. The interventionalist will come into the catheterization laboratory in parallel with the patient arriving from the outside hospital. In the city of Philadelphia,

we do have prehospital EKG, but not prehospital lysis in place. EMS often show-up with a prehospital EKG, but we rarely get a call ahead of time to discuss.

DB: There are a number of papers that show prehospital EKGs, either interpreted by trained paramedics or sent to the receiving ED, are as accurate as those performed in EDs and interpreted by physicians, or at least close to as accurate. When we first went to paramedic performance of the EKG about a decade ago, the initial interpretations were somewhat spotty. However, with training and experience, the accuracy level has become very acceptable with rare false positives.

PR: My concern is that patients can be complex and at times not evolving MIs, but looking like they are, and this makes the problem somewhat harder when you can't get an answer until the patient is in the catheterization laboratory. To me, this emphasizes the need for early and easy access to the catheterization laboratory.

Let me ask you another question. We know that inferior wall MIs have better outcomes then anterior wall MIs. Do you think that we are unnecessarily reperfusing inferior wall MIs? Do you think they would do just as well if they were left alone?

SG: Ultimately, the anterior wall MI patients are far more likely to end up as cardiac cripples (with ejection fractions [EF] in the 15–20% range) if they are left without some form of reperfusion. For this reason, the fibrinolysis or primary intervention window is often extended beyond 6 hours for this group of patients. Inferior wall MI patients without concomitant right ventricle or posterior wall involvement will not only be more likely to survive their MI, but survive with minimal damage to their myocardium (EF of 40–45%). Nevertheless, there is some mortality benefit in reperfusing inferior wall MIs if they arrive within the 6-hour window. For this reason, one must weigh very carefully reperfusion in this population versus the adage of "do no harm."

PR: When would you do right-sided leads looking for a right ventricular infarction, and when would you add posterior leads looking for a posterior MI in the face of an EKG that was suggestive of inferior wall MI?

WB: The EKG in our case shows an extensive STEMI involving the lateral and inferior walls, with the

ST-segment elevation so extensive that it provides us with a diagnosis. If you are working in a system that primarily uses fibrinolysis, I would go ahead and start that process. If you work in a system that uses an invasive laboratory either at your institution or a neighboring institution, I would activate your team and move towards treatment. At this point, the patient's blood pressure is adequate, although at the low end of normal, at 100/66 mmHg.

With respect to a right-sided EKG, remember that between one-quarter and one-third of inferior wall STEMIs involve the right ventricle (RV) and exhibit RV infarction. Do you need to specifically diagnose it in an EKG? Not necessarily. I think you need to be aware of this possibility, and be cautious with vaso-dilatating medication like nitrates and morphine in inferior myocardial infarction patients, and perhaps be a little more aggressive with IV fluid. Placing a single lead on the right chest RV4 would be very appropriate. However, I would not delay time to lysis or to the cathetererization laboratory to perform these additional leads.

Posterior leads would be interesting, but again we already do have a diagnosis of an extensive MI here involving the lateral and inferior walls. This EKG already does show ST-segment depression in V1 and V2, so there could be a posterior wall as well. Unless I had some time on my hands waiting for the drugs to be mixed or for the patient to go to the catheter laboratory, I would not do posterior leads as how would it alter treatment? It may help you define a more ill patient with a greater degree of risk, yet this is already a high-risk EKG. Of the 12 leads, it looks like all but one have some form of ST-segment deviation. In a patient with a nondiagnostic 12-lead EKG, meaning that the ST-segments are not significantly abnormal other than V1 and V2, I would definitely perform a posterior lead analysis to look for the rare isolated posterior wall STEMI, which I think would alter your approach to treatment. That last scenario is where the real "added value" of the posterior lead analysis is found, in the detection of the "isolated" posterior wall infarction.

PR: If you knew that the patient had inferior and posterior involvement, would you be more inclined to transfer the patient to a facility with a catheterization laboratory instead of starting fibrinolysis in your own ED?

DB: This patient doesn't need any additional leads to push toward a treatment algorithm, and most U.S. hospitals have a treatment algorithm in place in advance of these patients' arrival. If you're at a place where either fibrinolysis onsite or transfer for PCI are options, then the extent of the MI might push you to think about transferring the patient. Nevertheless, there are also features here that favor fibrinolytic therapy; namely, the short duration of symptoms. That's the one situation where fibrinolysis might be considered the preferred therapy.

PR: We are all giving aspirin in the field, but do you feel that there is a need to start beta-blockers or nitrates in the field, or do you think this a case where faster transport to the definitive care site is really the optimal strategy?

RH: I favor "do less and get them there faster." This is colored by the environment I work in, which is an inner city where the transport times are much shorter then in a rural environment. Growing evidence about the risks of IV beta-blocker therapy lead me toward not asking prehospital personnel to make a decision about this therapy. IV beta-blockers must be given with extreme caution, even in patients who are hypertensive and don't have heart block or signs of cardiogenic shock. Prehospital aspirin is very appropriate. Nitrates have been given in the prehospital setting for a long time, and usually without ill effect; the caveat with nitrates being to be alert for a right ventricular infarction, where nitrates could cause hypotension. If the prehospital people are taking an appropriate history, checking blood pressures for hypotension, and know their patient is not taking medications such as sildenafil, then nitrates remain appropriate in the prehospital setting. Nevertheless, in contrast to aspirin, administering nitrates early has not been shown to alter mortality.

PR: The patient is now in your ED, and you have access to a catheterization laboratory. What medications would you start in the ED before you send the patient to the laboratory? Should you anticoagulate this patient with heparin or with platelet inhibitors?

WB: Aspirin is the key medication; if it hasn't been administered in the prehospital setting, I would make sure the patient receives aspirin.

SG: I favor four baby aspirin in lieu of enteric-coated aspirin, since baby aspirin has the most rapid absorption.

Most of the large studies used either 160 mg or 325 mg. Since there are few complications with the higher dose, that is what I would use.

WB: I would probably administer nitroglycerin whether it be sublingual or topical. At this point, I would probably hold off on any IV nitro, not because I have any concern about it, but because it will not lower mortality. Beta-blockers can wait until a later time during the first hospital day. Unless the patient had melenic stool by history or a positive hemaoccult test, I would use heparin, preferably unfractionated, with a bolus and drip, although I would have no problem in using low molecular weight heparin. This is one of the patient groups that benefits from a glycoprotein inhibitor. Nevertheless, I would not delay time to take the patient to the catheter laboratory to administer this medication. Lastly, I don't believe clopidogrel has a lot to offer this patient acutely in the ED, although I'm sure the patient will probably end up on this agent.

PR: Is morphine appropriate for the treatment of MI pain?

WB: If you look at several large databases, retrospective analysis has demonstrated that patients who receive morphine in a nonhospital setting actually don't fare so well compared to patients who receive the drug while in the hospital. In the ED, we need to be cautious with the administration of morphine, realizing that it is a very potent vasodilator, and can alter perfusion. In this patient, who has a reasonable chance of having a right ventricular wall infarction, we need to be even more cautious. Morphine is not only a pain medication, but also an anxiolytic. Therefore, in patients who are experiencing an acute coronary syndrome (ACS) event, a small dose of intravenous morphine, mainly as an anxiolytic, may still have a role. I continue to use morphine in selected individuals with potential ACS—but I do so cautiously.

PR: Besides a preference for fibrinolysis in a patient who has a short time period of symptoms, are there other indications that would make one want to fibrinolyse this patient rather than send him to the catheterization laboratory?

DB: The guidelines were written to encourage fibrinolytic therapy in those patients with early presentation. Having said that, the pendulum has swung in favor of primary PCI even for patients who present

to facilities that don't have interventional catheterization capability at their facility. I'm not sure that's a good thing, since we know that only a small percentage of patients with STEMI who are transferred from one institution to another have a door-to-balloon time of less than 90 minutes. Many of these community hospital patients are being transferred despite the fact that fibrinolytic therapy might be the preferred treatment.

SG: When would you transfer this patient from a community ED to a hospital with catheterization laboratory?

DB: A delayed presentation, an extensive MI, and the relative availability of PCI would all come into play in my decision. I think its incumbent on the community emergency physician to have some sense of door-to-balloon times of the receiving hospital if we select that therapy as our mainstay of treatment.

PR: Has the argument finally been resolved as to whether one worsens outcome if you both thrombolyse and subsequently PCI?

RH: The trials that looked at giving a dose of fibrinolytic agent in addition to follow up with PCI have not shown an improved outcome with both. There is a role for rescue PCI, but that's not the same thing as coming at the patient with a plan to both lyse and follow up with a PCI.

SG: Early data suggested that salvage angioplasty had a worsened outcome when compared to primary PCI. However, more recent data suggest that if a patient does not reperfuse with fibrinolytics (i.e., the patient has ongoing symptoms, EKG changes or hemodynamic instability), then that patient's outcome with salvage angioplasty is as good as one in whom primary PCI was instituted.

PR: Is there a standard fibrinolytic agent used universally now? There was a vicious debate between the use of streptokinase and tPA based on the cost of the relative drugs; people argued that tPA worked better than streptokinase.

WB: Today, most EDs use either t-PA, TNK, or, less often, rPA. I believe that although t-PA is more expensive than streptokinase, it has an incremental mortality benefit, particularly in early presenters who are both young and have anterior wall infarction. For all comers with STEMI, the data is less compelling. Many institutions have moved away from streptokinase because of the data and in part because of other issues, and have moved towards either rPA or tNK. tNK administered as a single dose, or rPA, which has two boluses without an infusion, have the benefit of having much simpler administration regimens—thus minimizing the potential for error and improving the efficiency of administration.

SG: Despite these small advantages, streptokinase remains the thromblytic agent of choice in Europe because of a very significant cost differential.

PR: Must the use of streptokinase be limited to one time only?

SG: Streptokinase is a protein produced by beta-hemolytic streptococcus. Because streptokinase is a bacterial product, one can develop immunity to it. Therefore, streptokinase should not be re-dosed after four days from the first administration, as it may not be as effective, and it can also cause an allergic reaction. In addition, streptokinase is contraindicated in patients who have had a strep throat in the prior 6 months.

PR: If this patient had signs of pump failure, given the extensiveness of the infarction as it appears on this EKG, would you consider primary surgical intervention for this patient instead of PCI or thrombolysis?

DB: That would depend on what we learned at angiography. In all likelihood, if this patient were taken to the catheterization laboratory, he would have a single vessel infarction that would be amenable to catheter-directed therapy and stent placement. He might need to be supported through the MI with intra-aortic balloon placement. The indications for emergency coronary artery bypass graft surgery (CABG) are limited to left main disease, left main thrombosis (which is not likely given this EKG), unexpected significant three-vessel disease, or complications of the procedure to place a stent (such as a coronary artery dissection or a coronary artery rupture). An unexpected rare aortic dissection complicated by retrograde flap propagation and occlusion of the right coronary artery would also require emergency surgery.

PR: This patient was treated with PCI, and received a metal stent. I believe that most cardiologists have moved toward drug-eluting stents. Are there differences in what we can expect to see in the ED in terms of

recurrent disease, or complications of the two different kinds of stents, and what should we be looking for?

RH: The argument can be made that, in a given patient at any given time, it doesn't matter. We should assume that a patient who has had a recent procedure with any kind of stent could have stent occlusion, or potentially dislodgment or propagation.

DB: The trend in our institution has moved toward bare-metal stents for PCI with acute MI, with the thinking that they are less likely to thrombose.

SG: Although the data are inconclusive, the GRACE registry finds that although acute MI survival appears similar in the first 6 months following discharge, thereafter mortality is greater in patients treated with drug-eluting stents due to an increased risk of late reinfarction. This suggests that in this patient population, late stent thrombosis is more likely with drug-eluting stents.

PR: I would stress that from an ED perspective, whatever the procedure, if the patient is having new symptoms and EKG changes, it is prudent to assume you are dealing with a new thrombosis and treat the patient accordingly. It seems as though we are seeing fewer STEMIs and more non-ST-segment myocardial infarctions. I don't know if that's because of better pre-infarction care, or if we are just getting people to the hospital earlier with their unstable angina?

WB: We are seeing fewer STEMIs in our region. This is likely related to much more aggressive control of risk factors, such as blood sugar, high blood pressure, serum lipids, cessation of smoking, etc.

PR: Years ago, the time from the onset of symptoms to coming to the ED averaged over three hours.

SG: Sadly, despite major public education initiatives, the lag time from symptom onset to arrival in the ED has not changed significantly in acute MI patients. Denial remains very powerful despite a growing public awareness of the disease.

Case resolution

The patient was recognized in the field to have an acute inferoposterior MI. This information was communicated to the emergency physician who, with a single page, activated the entire catheterization team.

In the ED, the patient received IV normal saline 1000 cc bolus, and the blood pressure increased to 120/80 mmHg. He was given IV unfractionated heparin 5000 unit bolus, and was started on an infusion of 1000 units/hr. He was given clopidogrel 600 mg p.o., and transferred to the cardiac catheterization laboratory. Coronary angiography revealed a proximal RCA thrombotic occlusion that was easily opened, and a bare-metal stent was placed without complications, resulting in TIMI grade 3 flow down the vessel. The patient was transferred to the critical care unit, and had an uncomplicated hospital course. The peak troponin level was 6.2. A cardiac ECHO on hospital day three showed an inferior hypokinesis with an EF of 52%. He was discharged on aspirin, clopidogrel, simvastatin, and metoprolol on hospital day four, and was doing well at 30-day follow up.

Section III: Concepts

Epidemiology and pathophysiology

ST-segment elevation myocardial infarction (STEMI) is at one end of the spectrum of ACS, which occurs as a result of coronary artery disease. Coronary artery disease continues to be the leading cause of death in the United States, despite marked advances in its prevention, diagnosis, and treatment over the past 60 years. The advances in the treatment of ACS and particularly of STEMI began with the use of cardiac monitoring and the development of external cardiac defibrillators in the 1950s, and progressed to widespread utilization of external cardiac massage and admission of ACS patients within cardiac care units in the 1960s. Pharmacologic developments in the management of STEMI began with the use of aspirin and beta-blockers, and have advanced to include more sophisticated antiplatelet and anticoagulant agents. In the 1980s, the widespread use of fibrinolytic therapy ushered in the reperfusion era of STEMI therapy. Also in the 1980s, coronary angiography was first performed in the setting of acute STEMI, demonstrating occlusion of the infarct-related epicardial coronary artery; subsequently, a variety of mechanical interventions to open the artery were developed. These advances have contributed to an overall decline in the age-adjusted mortality of ischemic heart disease by reducing the case fatality rate of STEMI. Nonetheless, there are approximately 500,000 STEMIs annually in the US

and of those who reach the hospital, at least 5–6% will still die within the following 30 days.[1]

A STEMI is strictly defined as a rise above the upper limit of normal and subsequent fall of cardiac biomarkers specific for myocardial necrosis (troponin or CK-MB) in a patient who also has new or presumed new ST-segment elevation in two or more contiguous leads. In practice for the emergency physician, who will not have the trending of cardiac biomarkers available in real time, the definition is generally considered to be a history consistent with ACS, and the electrocardiographic criteria as above. The definition of ST-segment elevation is >0.1 mV.[1] Contiguous leads are defined as V1-6 in the chest leads, while in the frontal plane, contiguity is defined as the lead sequence aVL, I, inverted aVR, II, aVF, and III. Patients who meet the clinical criteria for a STEMI and have either a left bundle branch block not known to be old, or electrocardiographic evidence of an isolated true posterior MI, are also considered, for treatment algorithm purposes, to have a STEMI.

The pathophysiology of a STEMI begins when an atherosclerotic plaque within a coronary artery becomes unstable due to plaque rupture or hemorrhage into the plaque; the degree of stenosis caused by atherosclerotic plaque need not be critical prior to the plaque becoming unstable. Plaque rupture or hemorrhage results in an inflammatory cascade that causes platelet adherence and subsequence activation. Activated platelets express glycoprotein (GP) 2b-3a receptors on their surface and are then cross-linked by fibrinogen, which is a bivalent molecule with binding sites on each end that are specific for the GP 2b-3a receptor. The resultant platelet-fibrinogen web is further stabilized by thrombin, which cross-links and modifies fibrinogen to fibrin. As the platelet-fibrin aggregation grows, it traps circulating red and white blood cells, and a thrombus forms. At the same time, the inflammatory process leads to the release of vasoactive mediators, which may cause local vasospasm, further compromising coronary blood flow. If this process results in complete occlusion of the epicardial coronary artery at the site of plaque rupture, a STEMI occurs.

Clinical presentation

Patients with a STEMI classically present with ongoing discomfort in the substernal (precordial) region of the *chest*. This discomfort may be described as pain, pressure, or tightness and may have started at rest or during exertion. It may also be located in the left or right anterior chest and may radiate to the shoulder, neck, jaw, arm, or back. There may be associated symptoms of dyspnea, nausea, vomiting, diaphoresis, weakness, dizziness, or fatigue. Note that patients may present atypically, with chest discomfort that is sharp, stabbing, pleuritic, or palpable. Occasionally there may be no discomfort at all, and the patient may present only with one or several of the associated symptoms. Other atypical presentations may include isolated discomfort in the back, neck, jaw, or arm; upper abdominal pain or burning; indigestion; and generalized weakness. Elderly patients, women, non-Caucasians, and diabetics are particularly likely to have atypical presenting symptoms.

The physical examination is frequently unrevealing in patients with a STEMI. The heart rate may be rapid, slow, or normal. A 4th heart sound (S4) may occasionally be present, and the skin may be diaphoretic. Most other findings relate to complications of a STEMI. Vital signs may show evidence of dysrhythmia, respiratory

compromise, or shock. Jugular venous distention, rales, and a third heart sound (S3) suggest congestive heart failure. If altered mental status and hypotension are additionally present, cardiogenic shock is likely.

Emergency department diagnosis

The differential diagnosis of chest discomfort and the associated symptoms described above are broad but, in the case of a STEMI, the diagnosis hinges on the findings on a 12-lead electrocardiogram (EKG). An EKG should be obtained immediately in the evaluation of any patient with chest discomfort or a suspected STEMI as the treatment (see below) is extremely time-sensitive. The initial EKG finding in patients with a STEMI is peaked hyperacute T waves in the distribution supplied by the infarct-related artery (IRA). These are uncommonly seen in isolation by the clinician because, while T waves will become tall and sharply peaked within minutes of IRA occlusion, within minutes thereafter ST-segment elevation will become evident as well (Figure 3-1). In order to be diagnostic, the

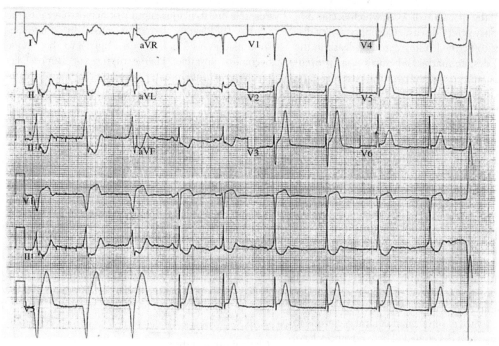

Figure 3.1 12-lead EKG shows hyperacute T waves in leads V2-V5 and ST elevations in leads I, avL, and V1-V5 consistent with acute anterolateral STEMI. Note also there is sinus node dysfunction with a ventricular escape rhythm for the first three beats, then normal sinus rhythm for the next two beats, and then a junctional escape rhythm for the rest of the tracing. Reproduced with the permission of David F. M. Brown, M.D.

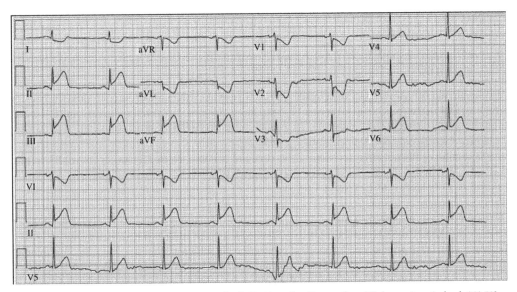

Figure 3.2 12-lead EKG shows ST elevation in leads II, III, and avF, as well as ST depressions in leads V1-V3 consistent with acute inferoposterior STEMI. Note also the reciprocal ST depressions in leads I and avL. Reproduced with the permission of David F. M. Brown, M.D.

ST-segment elevation must be at least one millimeter above the baseline, which generally is measured at the T-P segment. Most typically, the ST elevation in patients with a STEMI will be convex or domed; less commonly it may be straight or even rarely concave in appearance. Concave ST-segment elevations are more characteristic of conditions other than a STEMI, including pericarditis, benign early repolarization, left bundle branch block, left ventricular hypertrophy or aneurysm, paced ventricular rhythms, Prinzmetal's (variant) angina, hyperkalemia, hypothermia with Osborne waves, intracranial hemorrhage, Brugada's syndrome, and a normal variant.

In addition to the clinical history, another important feature that helps distinguish a STEMI from other conditions is the dynamic nature of the ST-segment abnormalities seen with a STEMI. The importance, therefore, of serial EKGs in patients with a suspected STEMI cannot be underscored enough. The EKG leads involved with the ST elevations generally correspond to anatomic location of the myocardial infarction, and the associated vessel. Anterior myocardial infarctions generally exhibit an ST elevation in leads V1-V4, while an ST elevation in leads V1-V2 is more specifically indicative of involvement of the septum. These infarctions are caused by acute occlusion of the left anterior descending (LAD) coronary artery.

If there are also ST elevations in leads V5, V6, I, and aVL, the location of the LAD occlusion is likely to be proximal to the first diagonal branch, resulting in an anterolateral MI (see Figure 3-1). Inferior infarctions (Figure 3-2) are characterized by ST elevations in leads II, III, and aVF, and are most commonly due to occlusion of the right coronary artery (RCA). With inferior MI, reciprocal ST depressions may also be present in leads I and aVL. Inferior MIs may be complicated by concomitant right ventricular (RV) infarction, which can be evident on right-sided EKG leads, particularly in RV4 and RV5. Inferior MIs may also be associated with posterior wall involvement, which is seen on an EKG as ST depressions in leads V1-V3, and often, early R wave progression with tall R waves in V1-V3 (Figure 3-2). Posterior MIs in isolation are the rarest of transmural MIs, and the most easily misdiagnosed. This is because the EKG will generally show ST depressions in V1, V2, V3 and sometimes V4 and V5, often with tall R waves in V1-V3, but without evidence of ST elevations. Such findings may be mistakenly attributed to non-transmural anterior wall ischemia. Clues to the diagnosis of isolated posterior wall infarction are the horizontal (rather than sloping) nature of the ST depressions, prominent R waves, and tall upright T waves in leads V1-V3.

Occasionally, isolated posterior wall MI will present with a nondiagnostic 12-lead EKG, and the diagnosis can only be confirmed when extended EKG leads, placed inferior to the tip of the left scapula (V8) and in the left paraspinal line at the same level (V9), reveal small pathognomonic ST elevations. Posterior wall MIs are the result of occlusion of the posterior descending coronary artery or the posterior left ventricular branch, either of which may be a branch from the RCA (more commonly) or the left circumflex coronary artery. Lateral wall MIs are characterized by an ST elevation in some or all of leads I, aVL, V5 and V6 (Figure 3-3). They may occur in isolation, or they may be associated with anterior MIs as described earlier or with inferior or posterior MIs. This is because the lateral wall of the heart is variably supplied with blood by the LAD, the left circumflex, and the RCA. Isolated lateral wall MIs are most frequently found with left circumflex occlusion, and the EKG often shows reciprocal ST depressions in leads II, III, and aVF.

Laboratory studies are generally unhelpful in the diagnosis of a STEMI. Although there are numerous cardiac biomarkers that will rise during myocardial infarction, none currently available are sufficiently sensitive or specific in a time frame that is useful for the emergency physician. The most sensitive and specific of these at the current time are troponins, which

are detectable 4–10 hours after the onset of myocardial cell death. In addition to troponins, creatine phosphokinase MB fraction and myoglobins are also frequently used.

Despite their limitations in the early stages of STEMI, cardiac biomarkers should nonetheless be sent along with a chemistry panel, complete blood count, and coagulation studies for ED laboratory analysis.

Imaging studies are also generally unhelpful in the diagnoses of a STEMI. Chest radiography is usually normal or unchanged from baseline. Nonetheless, it is indicated as it may help exclude other causes of chest pain, including pneumothorax, pneumonia, Boerhaave's syndrome, and, to a lesser degree, aortic dissection. In addition, the chest film can be valuable when a STEMI is complicated by congestive heart failure.

Treatment

After attending to the ABCs, the primary focus of treatment of a STEMI within 12-24 hours of symptom onset is urgent rapid revascularization of the IRA. This may be accomplished either with intravenous fibrinolytic therapy or with catheter-directed primary percutaneous coronary intervention (PCI). Although

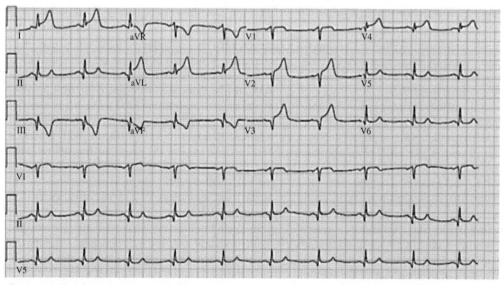

Figure 3.3 12-lead EKG shows ST elevation in leads I and avL consistent with acute lateral STEMI. Note also the reciprocal ST depressions in leads III and avF. Reproduced with the permission of David F. M. Brown, M.D.

fibrinolytic therapy remains the most common strategy worldwide, primary PCI is considered preferable in terms of safety and efficacy, and has become the more common choice in the US. When a primary PCI strategy is chosen, the IRA must be opened within 90 minutes of patient arrival to the hospital in order to achieve maximum efficacy.[2] This interval is referred to as the door-to-balloon (DTB) time. Note that the 90-minute DTB time includes time spent at the initial hospital if transfer to a PCI-capable facility is required. If a 90-minute DTB time cannot be routinely achieved, then revascularization with a fibrinolytic agent is preferable; this is particularly the case for those patients who present early (within 3 hours of symptom onset).[2] For patients in cardiogenic shock or in those with absolute contraindications to fibrinolytic therapy, primary PCI should be performed as soon as possible. In addition, those patients with a STEMI who fail to reperfuse with fibrinolytic therapy, as evidenced by ongoing anginal symptoms and persistent ST elevations an hour or more after treatment, should be referred for rescue PCI, which should be performed as soon as possible.

Patients with a STEMI who are treated with primary PCI should also receive aspirin, clopidogrel, and unfractionated heparin (UFH) as discussed below. While it is reasonable to also treat these patients with a GP 2b-3a inhibitor, which inhibits the final common pathway of platelet aggregation, there is no evidence that administering this in the ED is more efficacious than at the time of PCI in the catheterization laboratory.[3] None of these adjunctive therapies should delay transfer of the patient from the ED to the cardiac catheterization laboratory, which is the highest priority. A number of validated strategies should be utilized to decrease DTB time. Those that specifically involve the ED include (A) empowering the emergency physician to activate the entire cardiac catheterization laboratory team with a single page, (B) increasing the capacity to obtain prehospital EKG tracings on patients with chest pain, and allowing subsequent activation of the catheterization team for those patients with a field-identified STEMI while still en route to the hospital, and (C) providing prompt feedback to all clinical providers involved in the care of the patient.[4]

Despite the focus on primary PCI in recent years, fibrinolytic therapy remains a viable treatment option for patients with a STEMI; this is especially true for those who present to community hospitals that lack PCI capability. Rapid treatment is again important, with a target goal "door-to-needle" time of less than 30 minutes. Fibrinolytic therapy is indicated for patients who present with symptoms consistent with a STEMI within 12–24 hours of symptom onset, meet the EKG criteria (Table 3-1), and do not have an absolute contraindication (Table 3-2). The presence of relative contraindications (Table 3-3) must be weighed against the risk of treatment delay when primary PCI is not readily available.

Table 3-1. EKG criteria for fibrinolytic therapy.

1. ST segment elevation of >0.1 mV in two or more contiguous leads
2. Left bundle branch block not known to be old
3. ST-segment depressions and prominent R waves in leads V1-V4

Table 3-2. Absolute contraindications to fibrinolytic therapy.

1. Prior history of intracranial hemorrhage
2. Known cerebrovascular lesion (e.g., arteriovenous malformation)
3. Known malignant intracranial neoplasm
4. Suspected aortic dissection
5. Active bleeding (excluding menses) or known bleeding diasthesis
6. Significant closed head or facial trauma within 3 months
7. Ischemic stroke within 3 months (except if within 3 hours)

Table 3-3. Relative contraindications to fibrinolytic therapy.

1. Uncontrolled hypertension on presentation (SBP greater than 180 mm\Hg or DBP greater than 110 mmHg)
2. History of chronic severe poorly controlled hypertension
3. Prior ischemic stroke greater than 3 months
4. Traumatic or prolonged (> 10 minutes) CPR
5. Recent major surgery (less than 3 weeks)
6. Recent (within 2 to 4 weeks) internal bleeding
7. Noncompressible vascular punctures
8. Pregnancy
9. Active peptic ulcer
10. Current use of anticoagulants

There are several fibrinolytic agents available. Streptokinase, which is not fibrin specific and is administered as an intravenous infusion of 1.5 million units over an hour, is used mostly outside the United States, and has the advantage of being rather inexpensive. In the United States, fibrin-specific agents are used almost exclusively; the first of these to be developed was tissue plasminogen activator (t-PA), which is delivered as a bolus followed by two separate weight-adjusted infusions. This regimen is cumbersome, and it is easier and safer to administer one of the bolus fibrin-specific agents, retavase (r-PA) or tenecteplase (TNK), which have equivalent clinical efficacy and similar costs to t-PA. Dosing of r-PA is a non-weight adjusted double bolus of 10 units intravenously at time zero and again at 30 minutes. TNK is administered in a weight-tiered fashion as a single bolus of 30–50 mg. An additional advantage of the bolus agents is that they are easy to administer in the prehospital setting if that is a consideration. All STEMI patients who are treated with fibrinolytic therapy should also receive aspirin, clopidogrel, and beta-blockers in the absence of contraindications (see above). If a fibrin-specific agent is administered, UFH should also be given in a dose of 60 units/kg (maximum of 5000 units) and an infusion of 12 units/kg/hr (maximum 1000 units/hr). Enoxaparin can be safely and effectively substituted for UFH in patients with normal renal function who are less than 75 years of age.[5] Heparin preparations should not be given to patients treated with streptokinase.

There has been considerable interest in combination pharmacological therapy for a STEMI during the past decade. The most promising combination has been half-dose fibrinolytic therapy paired with full dose GP 2b-3a inhibitor. This combination provides better angiographic outcomes in the IRA at 90 minutes; however, no mortality benefit has been shown in large clinical trials.[6] Combination therapy does appear to confer a small reduction in the risk of recurrent MI, and in the need for rescue angioplasty.[6] However, it is more expensive than standard fibrinolytic therapy, and more cumbersome to administer. Hence, despite being an FDA-approved regimen for a STEMI, it should be utilized only in remote locations where transfer for rescue PCI is very difficult.

In addition to prompt revascularization treatment, a number of adjunctive agents are indicated in the treatment of a STEMI. Oxygen should be administered to all patients, even if the initial oxygen saturation is normal. This will reduce any areas of the lung that are poorly oxygenated, which in turn will reduce the possibility of shunting and subsequent hypoxia.

Platelet inhibitors are indicated as well, with aspirin remaining the most important of these agents. Aspirin is inexpensive, well tolerated, and independently reduces mortality by approximately 23%.[7] It should be administered orally (chewed and swallowed) or rectally in a standard dose of 162–325 mg. Enteric-coated preparations should be avoided. The only contraindication is a prior history of severe allergic reaction, in which case clopidogrel should be administered in its stead.

Clopidogrel is also indicated in the treatment of a STEMI. Clopidogrel is a thienopyridine, a class of drugs that inhibits ADP-mediated platelet aggregation. As an adjunct to fibrinolytic therapy, clopidogrel has been shown to improve clinical outcomes when a 300-mg oral loading dose is given with aspirin, as compared to aspirin alone.[8] For those STEMI patients undergoing a primary PCI, it is reasonable to administer clopidogrel with or without a loading dose, though this may instead be deferred until the time of catheterization.

Beta-blockers are an important therapy for patients with STEMI, although their role has been diminished in the most recent ACC/AHA guidelines.[9] Beta-blockers reduce the effects of catecholamines on the heart, slowing the heart rate, and reducing myocardial contractility, thereby reducing myocardial demand for oxygen. They are also effective antidysrhythmic agents, reducing the risk of ventricular fibrillation associated with a STEMI. However, beta-blockers also increase the risk of development of cardiogenic shock in patients with a STEMI, particularly in those patients over age 70, those with heart rate <60 beats/min, or blood pressure <120 mmHg.[10] In these latter subsets of patients, beta-blockers should not be given intravenously, though they may still be given orally. Absent these conditions, beta-blockers may still be given intravenously, though it may be more prudent to administer them only orally in patients with a STEMI. Several different agents are available, including metoprolol, atenolol, propranolol, and the ultra-short-acting esmolol. Beta-blockers in any form are contraindicated in patients with AV nodal block, bradycardia, hypotension, asthma, and acute severe congestive heart failure.

Anticoagulant therapy is indicated for patients with a STEMI who are being treated with fibrin-specific fibrinolytic agents, or with a primary PCI. At present, available agents include unfractionated heparin (UFH), low molecular weight heparin (LMWH), and direct thrombin inhibitors. The principal LMWH utilized in patients with ACS is enoxaparin. The heparins (UFH and enoxaparin) activate antithrombin-3, which in turn inhibits thrombin and factor Xa. Enoxaparin also directly inhibits factor Xa. Direct thrombin inhibitors, which include argatroban and bivalirudin, act directly on thrombin. The end result of therapy with any of these anticoagulant drugs, is the prevention of the conversion of fibrinogen to fibrin, thereby limiting thrombus propagation. These drugs are contraindicated in patients with active bleeding. In addition, the heparins are contraindicated in patients with a history of heparin-induced thrombocytopenia (HIT). For patients with a STEMI who are being treated with a primary PCI, UFH is administered as an intravenous bolus of 60 units/kg (maximum 5000 units) followed by an infusion of 12–15 units/kg/hr (maximum 1000 units/hr). If fibrin-specific fibrinolytic therapy is being utilized as the revascularization strategy, the maximum bolus dose of UFH should be reduced to 4000 units, and the infusion rate limited to 12 units/kg/hr (maximum 1000 units/hr).[1] Enoxaparin (1 mg/kg[2] b.i.d. with a 30 mg IV loading dose for those older than 75 years of age without increased bleeding risks) may be substituted for UFH as an adjunct to fibrin-specific fibrinolytic therapy.[5] Note that if streptokinase is utilized as the fibrinolytic agent, no adjunctive use of an anticoagulant is necessary. Use of direct thrombin inhibitors, which are very expensive and have not been shown to be superior to the heparins, should be limited to those patients with a known history of HIT.

Nitrates, which are available in a number of forms, may be used in patients with a STEMI. Most commonly, sublingual tablets are administered first, followed by an intravenous infusion of nitroglycerin as tolerated and needed. While nitrates may reduce symptoms of chest pain, there is no evidence that they reduce mortality. As such, since they may cause hypotension, they should be used judiciously, and withheld from patients with hypotension, RV infarction, and recent (within 24–48 hours) phosphodiesterase inhibitor use.

Morphine sulfate is an intravenous opioid analgesic agent that has a very limited role in the treatment of patients with a STEMI. It may be administered in small doses (2–5 mg increments) to patients with refractory ischemic pain or anxiety, but morphine may cause hypotension or sedation. The latter may compromise respiratory drive, and increase the risk of aspiration.

Prognosis

All patients with a STEMI should be admitted to a cardiac intensive care unit under the care of a cardiologist. The short-term prognosis for those patients with a STEMI who are treated with prompt revascularization and state of the art adjunctive therapies is quite good. Thirty-day mortality is between 5–6% in most studies, and is generally related to complications of a STEMI, which may be mechanical or electrical.

Complications of a STEMI

Bradyarrhythmias frequently complicate a STEMI, occurring in 25–30% of cases. The most common finding is sinus bradycardia, which is generally due to a predominance of vagal tone seen in a significant subset of STEMI patients. Sinus node dysfunction (sinus arrest or sinus exit block) may also complicate a STEMI (Figure 3-1), again generally related to increased vagal tone (rather than sinus node ischemia or infarction, which is rare). Sinus node-related bradyarrhythmias rarely need acute therapy, with pacing reserved for those with evidence of impaired cardiac output related to the slow heart rate. Generally, when the acute phase of the MI is over, balance between the sympathetic and parasympathetic nervous systems is restored, and the sinus node function recovers. Atrioventricular (AV) nodal block is a more ominous finding when it complicates a STEMI, particularly when associated with an acute anterior MI. While an AV block may be due to increased vagal tone in a subset of patients with acute inferior MI, it indicates extensive myocardial necrosis when complicating an acute anterior MI. High grade AV block (Mobitz type II second degree or third degree block) in the latter setting responds poorly to therapy, and carries a markedly increased mortality. First line therapy in the ED is directed at transcutaneous pacing. Atropine should be avoided, as it is not likely to be effective, and will increase the risk of a ventricular tachydysrhythmia by creating unopposed sympathetic stimulation of ischemic myocardium. Figures 3-4 and 3-5 are examples of 2:1 AV block and third degree AV block complicating an acute STEMI.

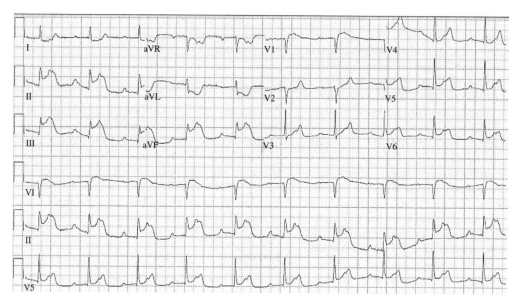

Figure 3.4 12-lead EKG shows ST elevation in leads II, III, and aVF consistent with inferior STEMI complicated by 2:1 AV block. Reproduced with the permission of David F. M. Brown, M.D.

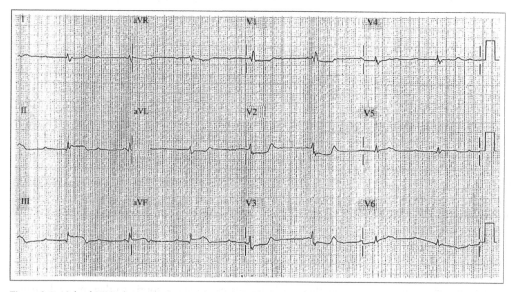

Figure 3.5 12-lead EKG shows ST elevation in leads II, III, and aVF with ST depressions in leads V1-V3 consistent with acute inferoposterior STEMI complicated by third-degree AV block. Reproduced with the permission of David F. M. Brown, M.D.

Tachydysrhythmias are frequent complications of a STEMI. Most are supraventricular in origin, with sinus tachycardia and atrial fibrillation the most common entities. Treatment for a sinus tachycardia may be pharmacological, with intravenous beta-blockers the drug class of choice, or directed at treating the underlying causative condition (e.g., congestive heart failure). Rapid atrial fibrillation of presumed new onset, complicating a STEMI is best treated with sedation and cardioversion. Ventricular tachydysrhythmias (ventricular tachycardia and ventricular fibrillation) occur less frequently as complications of an acute myocardial infarction (AMI). Primary ventricular fibrillation (VF) is seen in approximately 4% of patients, and more than half of these episodes occur in the first four hours after the onset of symptoms. Treatment is immediate defibrillation for VF and pulseless ventricular tachycardia (VT). For patients with a VT who are awake and maintaining a normal blood pressure, time may be taken for intravenous sedation followed immediately by synchronized cardioversion.

Pump failure or acute left ventricular dysfunction is a common complication of a STEMI. It can present across the spectrum of severity from mild congestive heart failure to cardiogenic shock. Cardiogenic shock is present if there is severe impairment of cardiac output that is unresponsive to efforts to increase preload, and causes impaired end-organ perfusion, as indicated by such findings as hypotension, pulmonary edema, altered mental status, and reduced urinary output. Generally, cardiogenic shock is associated with extensive myocardial necrosis of over half of the left ventricle, and carries a very poor prognosis. It must be distinguished from other conditions that may cause shock in the setting of a STEMI, including pericardial tamponade, acute valvular incompetence, and acute ventricular septal defect. Cardiogenic shock should be treated by mechanical intervention as rapidly as possible, which generally involves placement of an intra-aortic balloon pump and emergent revascularization via either PCI or coronary artery bypass grafting. Temporizing measures in the ED include intubation and mechanical ventilation with 100% oxygen, intravenous crystalloid to increase preload, inotropic agents (e.g., dobutamine) to improve cardiac contractility, and afterload reduction with an agent such as nitroprusside, if tolerated. Fibrinolytic therapy may be utilized as a last resort when mechanical intervention is not available, but there is little evidence that this improves mortality.

A RV infarction can complicate an acute inferior MI, or, much more rarely, may occur in isolation. Right-sided electrocardiographic chest leads, if obtained, may show pathognomonic ST elevations in lead R-V4 or R-V5, but the absence of this does not exclude the diagnosis. A RV infarction presents clinically with hypotension or a marked hypotensive response to agents that reduce preload, such as nitrates. A RV infarction is generally well treated with aggressive efforts to restore preload, which may require several liters of intravenous crystalloid, and should not require the use of inotropic agents. The presence of a RV infarction complicating an acute inferior MI increases the mortality rate to that of anterior MI.

Myocardial rupture may be a complication of an AMI. While the majority of cases occur several days after a STEMI, approximately one-third of cases will develop in the first 24 hours. Depending on the site of rupture, the patient may present with sudden death or with acute mitral valve regurgitation (due to papillary muscle rupture), acute ventricular septal defect (VSD) (due to septal infarction and rupture) or acute cardiac tamponade (due to free wall rupture). Acute mitral regurgitation (MR) and acute VSD will present similarly with severe and abrupt hemodynamic instability, coupled with acute pulmonary edema and a new very loud systolic murmur. Clinically, inferior and posterolateral MIs are associated with papillary muscle rupture, while anteroseptal MIs are associated with an acute VSD. Distinguishing between the murmurs of MR (a blowing systolic murmur loudest at the apex) and a VSD (a harsh systolic murmur heard best at the left sternal border) is difficult because of the marked pulmonary rales that are invariably present. Diagnosis is confirmed by echocardiography with doppler imaging, or by cardiac catheterization with left ventriculography. Both conditions are acute cardiac surgical emergencies, and require immediate surgical intervention. Temporizing measures in the ED include intubation and mechanical ventilation with 100% oxygen, and afterload reduction with an agent such as nitroprusside, if tolerated. Fibrinolytic therapy is not indicated. Acute mitral valve regurgitation may also complicate an ACS due to ischemia and dysfunction of a papillary muscle rather than infarction and rupture. In this situation, efforts should focus on the treatment of the myocardial ischemia as well as managing the acute pulmonary edema.

Free wall myocardial rupture may present as sudden death, or with findings of acute or subacute cardiac tamponade. The absence of classic EKG findings of a pericardial effusion (electrical alternans or low QRS voltage) does not exclude this diagnosis. Presenting symptoms include agitation, recurrent chest pain, and altered mental status. Signs include a precipitous fall in blood pressure, tachycardia, and jugular venous distention with signs of pulmonary edema. Mortality in this situation is high, and immediate cardiac surgical intervention is indicated. Aggressive intravenous crystalloid should be administered, and pericardiocentesis is indicated as a temporizing measure in the ED for patients in extremis. Be aware that intubation and positive pressure ventilation in the setting of tamponade (an extremely pre-load dependent state) can cause critical hemodynamic collapse because of the deleterious effect of positive pressure ventilation on preload.

Pericarditis can complicate AMI, either in the first week (infarct pericarditis) or in a more delayed fashion (a Dressler's syndrome). Infarct pericarditis presents with new chest pain that is often pleuritic or positional in nature. Pathologically, the pericardial inflammation is limited to the area adjacent to the transmural myocardial infarction. A Dressler's syndrome presents weeks to months after an AMI, and is characterized by fever and malaise as well as pleuritic or positional chest pain. In either case, there may be a pericardial friction rub, and the EKG may show the new characteristic ST changes and PR depressions seen in pericarditis. Non-steroidal anti-inflammatory drugs are first line therapy. Echocardiography can be performed to assess for the presence of pericardial effusion if there is a clinical concern for impending tamponade, and while not often necessary to determine in the ED, may enable the patient to be safely discharged home if there is no sign of an effusion.

An acute cerebrovascular accident (CVA) can complicate an AMI, with ischemic thromboembolic stroke being the most common kind of stroke seen. Sources of thromboembolism in AMI include the left ventricle, which may have mural thrombus in areas of hypokinesis; the left atrium, particularly if atrial fibrillation is present; and the carotid artery if there is concomitant carotid artery disease. A hemorrhagic CVA is a particular risk in patients with a STEMI who are treated with fibrinolytic therapy, occurring in approximately 0.9% of such cases, with the incidence sharply higher in the elderly. This accounts for the lower overall risk of stroke in patients with a STEMI treated with primary PCI (0.7%) compared with those treated with fibrinolytic therapy (1.6%).

The long-term prognosis after a STEMI is related to the size of the infarct, and the severity of the underlying coronary artery disease. Patients who develop congestive heart failure or ventricular dysrhythmias have higher mortality rates. Improved survival may be seen after aggressive risk factor modification.

Section IV: Decision making

- An immediate EKG should be performed in all patients with chest pain or other anginal equivalent symptoms.
- A revascularization strategy should be in place in all EDs that allows a DTB of less than 90 minutes or a door-to-needle time of less than 30 minutes in the vast majority of cases.
- Aspirin should be given to all patients with a STEMI except those with a true allergy.
- Clopidogrel, unfractionated heparin, and judicious use of beta-blockers are also indicated in appropriate patients with a STEMI.
- For patients treated with a primary PCI, no adjunctive treatment should be allowed to delay transfer to the catheterization laboratory.
- Anticipate and treat electrical and mechanical complications of a STEMI as they arise.
- All patients with a STEMI require admission to a coronary care unit.

References

1 Antman EM, Anbe, DT, Armstrong PW, et al. ACC/AHA guidelines for the management of patients with ST-elevation myocardial infarction—executive summary. *J Amer Col Cardiol.* 2004;44:671–719.

2 Alpert JS. Thygesen K. Antman E. Bassand JP. Myocardial infarction redefined—a consensus document of the joint European Society of Cardiology/American College of Cardiology Committee for the redefinition of myocardial infarction. *J Am Coll Cardiol.* 2000;36:959–969.

3 Ellis SG, Tendera M, de Belder MA, et al. Facilitated PCI in patients with ST-elevation myocardial infarction. *New Engl J Med.* 2008;358:2205–2217.

4 Bradley E, Herrin H, Wang Y,et al. Strategies to reduce the door-to-balloon time in acute myocardial infarction. *New Engl J Med.* 2006;355(22):2308–2320.

5 Antman EM, Morrow DA, McCabe CH, et al. Enoxaparin versus unfractionated heparin with fibrinolysis for ST-elevation myocardial infarction. *New Engl J Med.* 2006;354:1477–1488.

6 The GUSTO V Investigators. Reperfusion therapy for acute myocardial infarction with fibrinolytic therapy or combination reduced fibrinolytic therapy and platelet glycoprotein IIb/IIIa inhibition: the GUSTO V randomised trial. *Lancet.* 2001;57:1905–1914.

7 ISIS-2 (Second International Study of Infarct Survival) Collaborative Group. Randomised trial of intravenous

streptokinase, oral aspirin, both or neither among 17,187 cases of suspected acute myocardial infarction: ISIS-2. *Lancet*. 1988;2:349–360.

8 Sabatine MS. Cannon CP. Gibson CM. et al. Addition of clopidogrel to aspirin and fibrinolytic therapy for myocardial infarction with ST-segment elevation. *New Engl J Med*. 2005; 352(12):1179–1189.

9 Antman EA, Hand M, Armstrong PW, et al. 2007 focused update of the ACC/AHA 2004 Guidelines for the Management of Patients with ST-Elevation Myocardial Infarction. *J Am Coll Cardiol*. 2008;51: 210–247.

10 Chen ZM, Pan HC, Chen YP, et al. Early intravenous then oral metoprolol in 45,852 patients with acute myocardial infarction: randomised placebo-controlled trial. *Lancet*. 2005;366:1622–1632.

4

Unusual causes of myocardial ischemia

Robin Naples[1] & Richard Harrigan[2]

[1] *Assistant Professor of Emergency Medicine, Temple University School of Medicine, Philadelphia, Pennsylvania, USA*
[2] *Professor of Emergency Medicine, Temple University School of Medicine, Philadelphia, PA, USA*

Section I: Case presentation

A 31-year-old woman with a history of hypertension and a possible transient ischemic event presented with complaints of "not feeling well for four days." Specifically, she complained of intermittent mid-sternal to left precordial chest pain that was nonpleuritic, which had lasted for minutes before resolving spontaneously. Associated symptoms included dyspnea, diaphoresis, lightheadedness, and a near syncopal episode occurring shortly prior to presentation. She also complained of an increasing global weakness over that period of time. Enroute to the emergency department (ED), the blood pressure was noted to be 70/40 mmHg by the paramedic team.

The past medical history was significant for a cholecystectomy, hypertension, and a transient ischemic attack (TIA). An echocardiogram 2 months prior showed an ejection fraction of 60%, and trivial mitral regurgitation. Current medications included aspirin, clopidogrel, and irbesartan/hydrochlorothiazide. The social and family histories were noted for prior tobacco use, no illicit drug use, and no known coronary artery disease or coagulation disorders.

On physical examination, the vital signs were: temperature 36.8°C (98.2° F), pulse 84 beats/min, respirations 22 breaths/min, blood pressure 88/52 mmHg and O_2 saturation 100%. The skin was nondiaphoretic, the eyes had no conjunctival pallor, and the neck was without jugular venous distention. The lungs were clear. The cardiovascular examination showed a regular rate and rhythm without murmurs, gallops, or rubs. The abdomen was soft, nontender, and without masses or bruits. The extremities showed equal pulses and no peripheral edema. The neurologic examination showed a questionable ptosis, mild symmetric motor weakness, and normal deep tendon reflexes.

Laboratory studies were notable for a potassium of 2.5 mmol/L. A complete blood count, urinanalysis, BNP, troponin, and CPK were within normal limits. A chest X-ray study was normal, and CT angiography showed no pulmonary embolism. The electrocardiogram (EKG) is noted in Figure 4-1.

Section II: Case discussion

Dr David Brown: What would be your initial approach to a patient like this who presents with these complaints and the EKG findings as outlined?

Dr Shamai Grossman: This EKG is worrisome for cardiac ischemia and injury, and the story could be consistent with cardiac ischemia. Even 31-year-old women do have cardiac ischemia, although they don't represent the most common population for this disease. Particularly concerning in this case is that this patient is hypotensive with a blood pressure of 70 mmHg while with the paramedics, and still fairly hypotensive

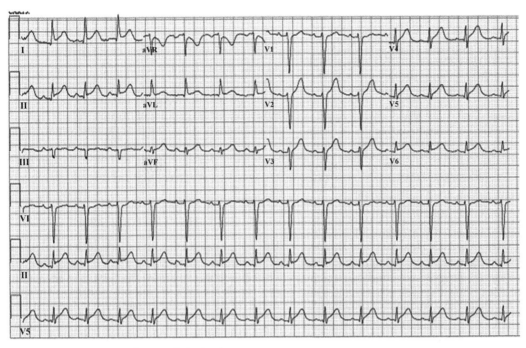

Figure 4.1 Unusual cause of myocardial infarction.

when she comes to the ED with a blood pressure of 88 mmHg. I don't know what her baseline is, but given that she has a history of hypertension, 88 mmHg is concerning. Therefore, I must assume that not only is this patient likely having cardiac ischemia based on her EKG, she is also in cardiogenic shock. Given all these things, my reflex would be to treat her as acute myocardial infarction and cardiogenic shock, and we'll see what happens.

DB: Going against the description of cardiogenic shock is that the lungs are clear on examination, and she doesn't appear to be in respiratory distress. Should this change your approach?

Dr Richard Harrigan: Given that our examinations are not always perfect, especially when trying to manage a complicated or potentially sick patient, an appropriate early approach to this woman would be covering your bases in terms of cardiac diseases, which means obtaining the relevant laboratory studies, starting aspirin, holding nitrates and beta-blockers with that blood pressure, and perhaps mixing some heparin while the situation gets clarified. Given the diffuse EKG changes, even with the absence of PR

depression and low voltage, it would be helpful to put the ED ultrasound probe on the chest, to look for a pericardial effusion, as the management would then be different, in terms of the use of heparin and how the blood pressure should be restored. It would be interesting to add a fluid bolus to the usual aspirin and heparin, in a patient who comes in like this, and see how she handles that. A 31-year-old woman would also be unusual to present with aortic dissection, but this still is a possible explanation for someone who presents with chest pain, hypotension, and with EKG changes that may or may not be ischemic. Pulmonary embolism, often a hard diagnosis to make, can also present similarly.

DB: Clearly, not all ST elevations are an ST elevation MI (STEMI). Even though we are in a current climate that pushes rapid diagnosis and treatment, at the same time, I think considering the differential diagnosis of ST elevations is important. You mentioned several: first, pericarditis or myopericarditis, which is associated with a pericardial effusion that would distinctly change the management, particularly with anticoagulation. You also mentioned pulmonary embolism that could also present like this, and would also change the management. Aortic dissection complicated by occlusion of one of the vessels could also present like this. So it's wise for our colleagues to consider the broader differential of ST elevations on an EKG, even though, in patients like these, most of the time we will all be moving faster towards early revascularization.

Dr Peter Rosen: One entity that I always forget is ventricular aneurysm. It seems unlikely in a young woman, but she did have a TIA sometime in the past, and it is possible that was caused by a myocardial infarction. An early chest X-ray study or cardiac echocardiogram might confirm that diagnosis.

DB: In most hospitals, access to formal echocardiography is somewhat limited to emergency physicians, as there are more emergency physicians who are comfortable performing a FAST examination, and have growing ability to interpret a trans-thoracic echo study. Even when formal cardiac echocardiography is present, the ability to accurately measure cardiac output or even left ventricle (LV) function would be limited to just a few physicians in each facility, so ED ultrasound may not be an option. Would you recommend a formal echocardiogram as part of the triage workup here?

SG: Part of my triage process here would entail involving cardiology early, since there are a number of things that cardiology can do besides activating the catheterization laboratory. Having cardiology involved for a formal detailed echocardiogram may help ensure that the patient doesn't end up with a procedure they don't need, such as a catheterization.

DB: If this person does, in fact, have a STEMI, are you concerned that if you obtain an emergent echocardiogram, you are going to be criticized for increasing door-to-balloon time beyond the expected treatment window of 90 minutes?

Dr Edward Ullman: The differential diagnosis for this patient is large, and I think this concern depends on how you focus in on it. If you say, "I'm worried that this is a STEMI," then I think you are going to be criticized if it goes over 90 minutes. You potentially can pursue multiple pathways by opening the laboratory, while at the same time telling cardiology "I'm not 100% sure, but my thinking is that a stat echocardiogram will slow you down, and you are going to have to give up the 90 minute window." Therefore,

you will need to be very careful about how you document your decision making, and how you verbalize your thought process with the cardiologists.

RH: In the end, unless cardiology is sitting in the ED with the echo machine, I would bypass that step. Using the bedside emergency ultrasound to see if you have a significant pericardial effusion without looking at wall motion will at least limit the differential causes of cardiogenic shock. Early cardiac catheterization is probably a very appropriate path here. I might take the time to run serial EKGs because, if you do see progressive ST-segments climbing or improving with nitrate therapy or heparin, that's important information that will sharpen your management.

DB: Ten years ago this case would be handled quite differently; she would get an echocardiogram because there are enough equivocal pieces to this case: young age, female gender, EKG findings perhaps in multiple regions of the heart, and enough atypical historical features to warrant getting an echocardiogram to look for a regional wall motion abnormality. I think the environment that we live in today makes that impossible. We are now judged for our sensitivity for STEMI, not our specificity,

SG: Yet, ultimately, our job as physicians, despite constant criticism from others with different agendas, is to do what is right for the patient. You have to think hard and fast as to whether you really believe that this patient needs to go to the catheterization laboratory emergently without an echocardiogram. What you don't want to do is put this patient through a potentially life-threatening procedure that she doesn't need. Although I agree that taking her to the catheterization laboratory might be the right decision here, you need to think it through very thoroughly before you activate the process for an emergent catheterization setup.

DB: Looking at the laboratory evaluations, the metabolic panel was normal, the complete blood count was normal, the pregnancy test was negative, a urinalysis was normal, the BNP was normal, the CK was 160, and the troponin I was 0.10, in the normal range for this laboratory. A chest X-ray study was normal, and she had been sent for a CT angiography (CTA) of the chest. Given our concerns for door-to-balloon time, I doubt we would have chosen a CTA as the advanced test here. Would you be satisfied with an

Elisa D-dimer that was negative, and forgoing the CTA in this patient?

EU: The clinical course evolved with hypotension, intermittent chest pain, EKG changes, and neurologic findings, including weakness in the upper extremities. This makes me wonder whether the CT angiography was chosen for pulmonary embolism (PE) or for dissection.

RH: As it turns out, these were not new focal neurological findings. Given concerns about her shortness of breath, her age group, and her chest pain, she went for a CTA utilizing a rule out PE protocol.

EU: Going after PE, in this case, strikes me as a little odd. I would not have gone there first, given an EKG with infero-lateral ST-segment elevation, a normal troponin, and hypotension. If someone was hypotensive from a PE, there should be some troponin or BNP elevation, indicating some kind of strain on the heart. I don't think I would have ordered a D-dimer either, as I might not believe the result and waiting for this result would also have consumed precious time needed to send the patient to the catheterization laboratory.

DB: This is a very challenging presentation, as there are some features that are atypical for just about all of the diagnoses we have considered so far. My concern with going to CTA for PE as the first test is that you use an opportunity to give IV contrast; when that CTA is negative, you are still left with "is this a STEMI or not," and you are going to end up taking this patient to the catheterization laboratory and subjecting her to a second round of contrast. I would prefer instead to proceed rapidly to cardiac catheterization, clear her coronary anatomy with angiography, do an LV-gram to understand what's going on with her LV function, and if all of that is normal, than we can move on to a right heart catheterization looking at right-sided pressures and an echocardiogram.

RH: If you are content that it's not an aortic dissection, you could say, "I'm going to cover my bases with heparin," because if this is a PE or coronary ischemia, heparin will be useful.

SG: Given that this is a patient who is hypotense, if she is having a PE, she may be an appropriate candidate for thrombolysis. We know that the sooner you lyse this patient, the more likely you are to have some benefit. If I am not going to send this patient for CTA, perhaps I should do an echocardiogram. Not only

looking for wall motion, but also looking at right ventricle (RV) function to give us prognostic information as to whether this is a massive pulmonary embolus causing the patient to be in shock, and to help guide the need for thrombolytic therapy.

RH: Echocardiography is a poor man's indicator of massive or sub-massive PE. Yet this type of PE is best identified by BNP or troponin elevation, and you don't have those, nor do you have a low O_2 saturation, unusual in the hypothetical setting of a PE causing hypotension. It seems like every time I pick an avenue to go on in this case, I am stymied by something leading me in another direction.

DB: We've talked a lot about the differential diagnosis and the initial diagnostic testing. What about response to therapy? This woman is treated initially with fluids. Would you be reassured if the patient became normotensive after 500 cc of normal saline? Would that reassure you that you weren't dealing with a massive PE or tamponade from some cause?

EU: With a PE, if she responded to 500 cc, my suspicion for a massive PE would drop, particularly given an O_2 sat of 100% and this person looking relatively well. I would still worry about tamponade, as I don't know what will happen 10 minutes after the fluid bolus. Did she become hypotensive again? If the pressure does drop again, then I'd be fairly concerned about tamponade. The EKG doesn't have low voltage or sinus tachycardia, and this further lowers my concerns for tamponade or PE.

DB: We still haven't completely excluded pericarditis with pericardial tamponade that resulted from hemorrhagic conversion of a pericardial effusion related to the aspirin and clopidigrel used, or less likely, although still possible, aortic dissection with rupture into the pericardium. Therefore, I would withhold giving this patient unfractionated heparin until I was more certain of what was going on, given that it adds very little to the treatment of STEMI in the absence of revascularization as well. It could be added at the time of revascularization in the catheter laboratory, if that turns out to be what we are dealing with. If this really is a massive PE, I don't think that unfractionated heparin would make that much of a difference and the patient becomes a candidate for thrombolytic therapy. My next step after the EKG in initial evaluation would be cardiac catheterization.

DB: The hypotension evident on admission improved with intravenous normal saline. During the admission process, the patient intermittently experienced chest pain. Repeat cardiac enzymes were elevated with a peak troponin I of 3.1, and the EKG remained abnormal. Unfractionated heparin was started in light of the EKG changes and presumed acute coronary syndrome (ACS), and plans for emergent cardiac catheterization were made. Since a second set of cardiac markers were obtained, was it wise to hold off on cardiac catheterization?

RH: Given that she looked better and the EKG was static, and despite a worrisome EKG here, the ST-segments were not classically territorial injury changes. Although all of us may have pushed for earlier catheterization, I understand somewhat how this unfolded.

PR: When you are facing a complex problem that has many contradictory and all life-threatening explanations, you have to expect that you can't get all of them eliminated in a timely fashion. Our best strategy is to select the course that will give us maximum information, while stabilizing the patient. That choice will also have to be dependent upon the local facility; in a tertiary care center, it may be easy to mobilize the catheter laboratory 24 hours a day, but in another institution the catheterization team may have to come in from home, and it might be more prudent to select a different imaging study such as a CTA, as was done here. Since there is no clear-cut correct answer, one must be guided by your institution, and your consultants, to do something. The clear wrong answer is to do nothing.

DB: An echocardiogram was obtained that showed moderate to marked LV dilatation, a decreased ejection fraction of 20% in each chamber, and akinesis of the apical walls and hypokinesis of the mid-apical, infraseptal, and antero-lateral walls of the LV. There was mild to moderate mitral regurgitation. Coronary angiography revealed no evidence of coronary artery disease, and confirmed the wall motion abnormality seen on echocardiogram. Ejection fraction was calculated to be 47%. Without being able to see the echo or the LV gram, what is being described here is akinesis of the apex and severe hypokinesis of the distal anterior wall and septal wall and lateral wall. What is the differential diagnosis at this point in this patient without coronary artery disease?

SG: The most likely etiologies at this point are either coronary vasospasm or a Takotsubo cardiomyopathy. There are other forms of cardiomyopathy that may cause depressed left ventricular function, but these myopathies are more likely to cause a global hypokinesis without regional wall variation.

DB: What would be the next step in management of this patient, as the patient leaves the catheterization laboratory?

RH: These patients are initially managed as acute coronary syndromes. With stable vital signs, now that you know there is no the coronary artery disease, you can withdraw the therapy that is given for ACS such as clopidigrel and heparin. Occasionally, a LV thrombus is described with apical ballooning syndrome, and in that instance, heparin might still be useful, but this is not the norm. If there is evidence by echocardiogram of outflow obstruction, then beta-blockade would be helpful for relaxation of the hyperkinetic segment. Beta-blockade would have been reasonable in coronary artery syndrome as well, and may have already been started. If there is overt cardiac failure with this diminished left ventricular function, then further beta-blockade acutely would probably not be helpful; instead, after load reduction, if the blood pressure tolerates it, would be more advantageous.

DB: This is a diagnosis that we are not likely to be able to make accurately in the ED. The pathognomonic features do not allow us or our colleagues to make this diagnosis definitively up front. Most of these cases will go to the catheterization laboratory for coronary angiography, and the diagnosis will be made when the coronaries appear normal and not obstructed, and the apical ballooning is found on left ventriculogram. In retrospect, since many of these cases are believed to be preceded by a period of intense stress or catecholamine excess, was there anything in the history that in retrospect could have been a clue?

RH: When we went back and talked to her some more, she did report more serious life stressors immediately preceding the development of symptoms. Unfortunately, this history was not elicited on presentation. Although this syndrome has been classically associated with a single antecedent event, these cardiac catheterization findings have also been described in people where a single precipitating event cannot be identified.

SG: Had the case been just slightly different where the EKG were a little less suggestive of an acute STEMI, and there were perhaps diffuse ST depressions or some less specific finding, this patient might have been an excellent candidate for a coronary CT scan. When there is no pressure for emergent catheterization, coronary CT scan may be very useful in helping to rule out cardiac ischemia completely. Perhaps this may be the ED test that we need to utilize more routinely in this patient population, particularly when you have a concomitant history of a major stressor that may have precipitated the event.

DB: I like the idea of doing a CT scan of the chest in this patient, because you may get information about the aorta and the pulmonary arteries as well as the coronary arteries. The one contraindication is that coronary CT is done with the co-administration of nitroglycerin, and her blood pressure may not tolerate this, unless it had responded to the IV fluid bolus. Most of these patients with documented Takotsubo cardiomyopathy tend to improve markedly. It appears that most of the LV dysfunction is myocardial stunning rather than myocardial infarction.

This is a very interesting case, and serves to highlight some of the challenges we face in those patients who present with ST elevations on EKG, but with symptoms that are conflicting in terms of the diagnosis. It is easy, in retrospect, to select the proper test in the proper order, but when your boots are on the ground in the ED, it is a lot more challenging. Do we have any longer follow-up on this patient to get a sense of whether she proved over time that her ejection fraction came back to normal?

Case resolution

The hypotension evident on admission improved with intravenous normal saline. During the admission process, the patient intermittently experienced chest pain; repeat cardiac enzymes were elevated with a peak troponin I of 3.1, and the EKG remained abnormal. Unfractionated heparin was started in light of the EKG changes and presumed acute coronary syndrome. An echocardiogram showed moderate to marked LV dilatation, a decreased ejection fraction (20%), akinesis of the apical walls, and severe hypokinesis of the mid-apical anteroseptal, inferolateral and anterolateral walls of the LV. There was mild-to-moderate

mitral regurgitation. Coronary angiography revealed no angiographic evidence of coronary artery disease and confirmed the wall motion abnormalities seen on echocardiogram, although the ejection fraction was calculated to be 47%.

A working diagnosis of Takotsubo cardiomyopathy was established. In retrospect, the patient reported significant life stressors coincident with her presenting event. Irbesartan/hydrochlorothiazide and clopidogrel were discontinued, and she was discharged on metoprolol, atorvastatin, aspirin, and lisinopril. Repeat echocardiogram at 11 days post-presentation showed normalization of the ejection fraction (50%) without any regional wall motion abnormalities. The motor weakness improved with potassium repletion, and neurology consultation and work-up revealed no alternative cause for the neurologic symptoms.

Section III: Concepts

Although there are numerous unusual causes of cardiac ischemia, this chapter focuses on eight salient causes: coronary embolism, coronary artery dissection, aortic dissection with coronary occlusion, congenital coronary artery anomalies, carbon monoxide poisoning, coronary vasospasm, thyrotoxicosis, and Takotsubo cardiomyopathy.

Coronary embolism

Coronary embolism has long been known as a non-atherosclerotic cause of cardiac ischemia, first being described by Virchow in 1856. Embolism may arise from many sources, including mural thrombi, valvular vegetations, atherosclerotic plaques, atrial myxomas, or paradoxically from the systemic veins.[1,2] Depending on the size of the embolus, symptoms of a coronary embolism can range from silent and undetected to a massive myocardial infarction (MI) leading to sudden death. Emboli are three to four times more likely to enter the left coronary artery than the right coronary artery because of its larger diameter.[3,4]

Emboli occur acutely in patients, unlike those with atherosclerotic changes where there is a gradual narrowing. The acute coronary occlusion causes transmural infarction with more extensive areas of damage. Even small emboli that lodge distally in the coronary arteries can cause infarction, although the vessel may undergo recanalization, which may lead to angiographically normal coronary arteries.[3] As a result of the complete occlusion, the EKG most often shows ST-segment elevation in cases of coronary embolism. Because the left coronary system is more commonly affected, ST-segment changes are seen in the anterior leads most frequently.

History and physical examination findings can provide clues that the cardiac event was caused by a coronary embolism instead of atherosclerotic disease. Patients with coronary embolism historically do not have preceding angina symptoms. These patients do not have risk factors for atherosclerotic disease, but may have a history of atrial fibrillation, left ventricle aneurysm, a prosthetic heart valve, or infective endocarditis.[4] If embolic infarction is suspected, it is important to ascertain symptoms that might suggest emboli to the cerebral and mesenteric vascular beds. The physical examination may suggest a source of the embolus; for instance, there may be findings consistent with infective endocarditis, atrial fibrillation, or deep venous thrombosis.

Treatment for cardiac infarction caused by coronary embolism is similar to that of infarction caused by atherosclerotic coronary artery disease (ASCAD). Morphine, aspirin, nitrates, oxygen, and anticoagulation are first line therapies for embolic occlusion. If the embolus is thought to have originated from the cardiac valves (either infective endocarditis or from a prosthetic valve thrombus), fibrinolytic therapy should be avoided because of the risk of cerebral embolism.[4,5] Coronary angiography may identify the embolus and allow for removal or lysis to restore coronary flow. A small embolus may undergo spontaneous lysis, resulting in normal coronary arteries at the time of angiography.

Coronary artery dissection

Coronary artery dissection can occur after blunt chest trauma, as a complication of coronary angiography, as an extension of an aortic dissection, or spontaneously. Similar to coronary embolism, coronary artery dissections may be small and clinically silent, or may involve the length of the vessel and cause complete occlusion and massive myocardial infarction and death.

Myocardial infarction from coronary vessel injury after blunt trauma is a rare occurrence, with traumatic coronary artery dissections consisting of only a small subset of all myocardial infarctions.[6] Motor vehicle collisions are the most common mechanism of injury.[6,7] The left anterior descending artery (LAD) is the most commonly injured artery (71%), followed by the right coronary artery (RCA) (19%), the left main artery (7%), and the left circumflex artery (3%).[6] Coronary artery dissection as a result of aortic dissection will be discussed separately.

Spontaneous coronary artery dissection is rare. It affects young women (mean age 38) in 80% of cases, one-third of whom are in their third trimester of pregnancy or postpartum period, and most of whom have no cardiac risk factors.[8-11] Men who experience spontaneous coronary artery dissection tend to be older, and have one or more risk factors for ASCAD. The LAD is the most commonly-affected artery with spontaneous coronary artery dissection; however, there does seem to be a predilection based on gender. Women tend to have left-sided dissections, while men have a higher involvement of the right coronary system, with up to two-thirds of men reported to have RCA dissections.[8,10,11] Men tend to have better survival rates after spontaneous dissection than women, although up to 70% of cases are diagnosed at autopsy after sudden death.[8,9,12]

Clinical presentation of coronary artery dissection can range from asymptomatic to unstable angina, cardiogenic shock, acute myocardial infarction, or sudden death depending on the location, extent, and rate of dissection.[10] The EKG changes will be consistent with the myocardial territory of the vessel involved, with anterolateral involvement correlating to the LAD being the most common. Traumatic coronary artery dissection should be considered in patients who complain of ischemic chest pain symptoms in conjunction with significant blunt trauma to the chest and presence of large chest wall contusions, sternal or thoracic vertebral fractures, or mediastinal hematomas. An EKG should be obtained after the patient is stabilized from a trauma perspective. Spontaneous coronary artery dissection should be strongly considered in a late pregnancy or postpartum woman with no ASCAD risk factors who presents with myocardial ischemia or infarction.

Myocardial injury from coronary artery dissection is treated similarly to injury with ASCAD with morphine, nitrates, aspirin, oxygen, and anticoagulation. Fibrinolytic therapy should be avoided in this patient population, as it may cause propagation of the dissection by restoring blood flow in the false lumen.[10] Distinguishing coronary artery dissection from atherosclerotic occlusion can only be done by coronary angiography. Placement of coronary stents during angiography is becoming more favored, especially with single-vessel dissections, while coronary artery bypass grafting (CABG) is being reserved for multi-vessel dissections or those complicated by atherosclerosis.[10] Medical therapy alone has also been shown to be successful.[8]

Aortic dissection with coronary occlusion

Aortic dissection is a disease that often occurs in patients who suffer from hypertension and atherosclerosis. Atherosclerotic plaques cause weakness in the vessel's intima and media, and false lumens form as a result of the increased pressure. There is also an association of aortic dissection in patients with connective tissue disorders such as Marfan's or Ehlers-Danlos syndromes. Weakness in the elastin and microfibrils cause the aorta to be susceptible to the constant pressure and turbulent flow of blood through the ascending aorta.[13]

Stanford type A aortic dissection, those involving the ascending aorta, can potentially propagate in a retrograde fashion to involve the coronary arteries, although this is uncommon.[14] When it does occur, occlusion of the coronary artery leading to ischemia or infarction may result from direct mural extension of the dissection, extravasation of blood into the pericardial and perivascular tissues, or via direct compression from the expanding hematoma.[15-17] When an aortic dissection does involve the coronary arteries, it is more likely to involve the right coronary artery.[15]

Classically, aortic dissection has a more acute onset of sharp, severe tearing chest pain than with the more dull, insidious pain associated with ASCAD. Additionally, young patients who have known connective tissue disorders should be suspected of having aortic dissection with coronary involvement when presenting with coronary ischemia or infarction. Physical examination findings consistent with ascending aortic dissection, such as unequal pulses and blood pressure measurements, neurologic deficits, a new aortic insufficiency murmur, or signs of pericardial tamponade, as well as with Marfan's-like physical features, should be sought.[4,14,18]

Diagnosis and treatment of aortic dissection with coronary artery occlusion is vastly different from ASCAD. One must obtain timely advanced imaging with computed tomography or transesophageal echocardiography.[14] Pain control and blood pressure management with morphine and beta-blockers should be initiated to prevent extension of the dissection, and to decrease myocardial demand. Anticoagulation and fibrinolysis are contraindicated, and can significantly worsen the patient's condition. Surgery is the definitive treatment strategy for patients with Stanford class A dissections with coronary involvement, often requiring CABG to restore myocardial blood flow.[14,15]

Congenital coronary artery anomalies

Congenital coronary artery anomalies are an elusive cause of myocardial ischemia and infarction. While coronary anomalies are known to occur in about 1% of the general population, it is not fully known what role they play in causing relevant clinical consequences.[19] Coronary anomalies often become symptomatic in young, otherwise healthy people who are involved in vigorous activity. They have been thought to be the cause of sudden death, myocardial infarction, chest pain, syncope, and rarely reproducible exercise-induced angina.[19,20]

In patients who present to the ED, symptoms are likely to have resolved with the cessation of vigorous activity. Look for myocardial ischemia from coronary anomalies in young athletes who present with exertional chest pain or syncope. Ischemia from coronary anomalies is thought to be caused by coronary spasm and lack of collateral flow.[19] There are data to suggest that thrombus formation is not an integral component of vascular occlusion.[21] Therefore, treatment for these patients begins with pain control and oxygen therapy, with coronary angioplasty for definitive diagnosis.

Carbon monoxide poisoning

Carbon monoxide (CO) has long been known to cause myocardial injury, and was first described in 1865.[22] Cardiotoxicity occurs after carbon monoxide exposure in patients with and without underlying atherosclerotic disease. At carboxyhemoglobin (CoHb) levels greater than 25%, myocardial ischemia is likely, although in patients with ASCAD, ischemia can occur at much lower levels.[23,24]

Carbon monoxide exerts its damage to the myocardium through multiple mechanisms. It has been shown to cause diffuse and punctuate hemorrhages involving the pericardium and endocardium, as well as myocardial fiber degeneration and necrosis.[22,23] While CO can act directly on the coronary arteries to reduce vascular resistance, it appears as though the subendocardial blood flow only marginally increases, resulting in tissue that remains hypoperfused.[25] Myocardial contractility is also decreased after CO exposure. This is due to a combination of tissue hypoxia from reduced oxygen delivery, as well as from direct myocardial depression and mitochondrial dysfunction.[22,23,26]

There are various EKG changes that can be seen with CO poisoning, ranging from sinus tachycardia to nonspecific ST-segment changes to ST-segment elevation. Cardiac biomarkers and an EKG should be obtained in all patients with significant CO exposure. A study by Satran, et al. finds that 30% of patients presenting with CO toxicity have ischemic EKG changes.[26] Of these patients, 64% have positive biomarkers. Overall, 35% of patients in this study had positive biomarkers, with 53% of them revealing ischemic EKG changes.[26]

Obtaining historical clues for CO poisoning will help differentiate patients with CO-induced myocardial ischemia. CO poisoning should be considered in patients who additionally complain of dyspnea, headache, nausea, or altered sensorium, or who present in clusters from the same environment. Patients without a history of cardiac disease who have cardiac ischemia from CO toxicity tend to be younger and have more profound CO poisoning (Glasgow Coma Scale [GCS] <14) and global left ventricular involvement. Those patients with known ASCAD tend to be older, and have a normal GCS with regional wall motion abnormalities.[26] There may be a history of worsening anginal symptoms in patients with previously stable angina.

Treatment of cardiac ischemia from CO poisoning requires early recognition. Aspirin and aggressive oxygen therapy should be initiated, followed by hyperbaric oxygen treatments. Hyperbaric oxygen is indicated for patients with ischemic chest pain, elevated biomarkers, ischemic EKG changes, or significant dysrhythmias. For those patients with known ASCAD who suffer ischemia after CO poisoning, there may be benefit in coronary angiography and revascularization after hyperbaric therapy.

Coronary vasospasm

Coronary vasospasm, also called Prinzmetal's angina was first described by Prinzmetal in 1959 as a "variant" cause of ST-segment elevation and chest pain. Vasospasm usually occurs at a single site in the blood vessel, and can occur in patients with and without underlying ASCAD.[27] While the etiology of Prinzmetal's angina is not entirely known, it is hypothesized that it occurs because of endothelial dysfunction and activation of the autonomic nervous system, specifically the alpha-adrenergic receptors.[27] Prinzmetal's angina has been associated with other vasospastic disorders such as Raynaud's disease and migraines; the vasospasm may be provoked by cocaine, alcohol, or nicotine abuse; hyperventilation; beta-blocker overdoses; and rapid eye movement sleep.[27-29]

Often, the ST-segment elevation seen on the EKG can be resolved with nitroglycerin, thus aborting the coronary vasospasm and preventing cardiac necrosis. However, myocardial infarction can result if the vasospasm occurs at the site of an atherosclerotic plaque, leading to complete occlusion; more commonly, myocardial infarction occurs if the spasm leads to endothelial injury, platelet aggregation, and thrombus formation.[30] In addition to ischemia and infarction, Prinzmetal's angina is also associated with sudden death and various dysrhythmias during periods of ST-segment elevation, including ventricular tachycardia, third-degree heart block, and asystole.[27]

Coronary vasospasm typically occurs in young females whose only cardiac risk factor is tobacco smoking.[27,31] The pain often occurs at rest in a circadian pattern, developing in the early morning hours. The pain is not affected by myocardial demand, and thus cannot be provoked with exercise stress testing. Historical clues of the timing of symptoms, other vasospastic symptoms such as headache patterns and cold intolerance with skin changes, or recent cocaine use, may aid in differentiation from typical ASCAD.

Medical therapy is the mainstay of treatment for Prinzmetal's angina. Nitroglycerin and calcium channel blockers are both highly effective at resolving the patient's chest pain and EKG changes associated with coronary vasospasm.[27,29] Aspirin and morphine are reasonable adjuncts. Beta-blockers should be avoided in patients with suspected coronary vasospasm because the unopposed alpha-adrenergic activity can worsen the spasm.[28] Anticoagulation and fibrinolysis may be of benefit if the patient's symptoms and ST-segment elevations do not resolve with nitroglycerin because of the potential for thrombus formation after prolonged vasospasm. Definitive diagnosis should be made with coronary angiography. Not only can provocative testing be done of suspect vasospastic arteries with ergonovine, but also it is important that underlying ASCAD be identified and treated.[27,29]

Thyrotoxicosis

Thyrotoxicosis is a complex disease with multiple pathologic effects that increase one's risk for cardiac disease, including congestive heart failure, dysrhythmias, and myocardial ischemia. Similar to the other unusual causes of myocardial ischemia, thyrotoxicosis can affect those patients with and without underlying atherosclerosis. Exercise intolerance and anginal complaints are common in this patient population.[32,33] Even those with only mild hyperthyroidism have a higher cardiovascular mortality than those who are euthyroid.[34]

In the thyrotoxic state, there is an increase in cardiac output and myocardial contractility, leading to higher myocardial oxygen demand. Increases in circulating blood volume cause increased wall stress on the heart and decreased contractile reserve, which may significantly affect the left ventricular workload, especially during exercise.[35] These factors can cause an otherwise insignificant atherosclerotic plaque to become symptomatic. Coronary spasm is well known to occur during thyrotoxicosis, although the mechanism is not clear. Vasospasm can affect both normal and diseased vessels. It is thought that there is increased sensitivity of the coronary arteries to catecholamines and higher concentrations of beta-adrenergic receptors, with a down regulation of alpha-adrenergic receptors limiting vasodilation and promoting vasoconstriction.[33] Additionally, elevated levels of fibrinogen have been found during hyperthyroid states, which may contribute to increased risk of thrombosis and coronary events.[36]

Historically, patients with angina secondary to thyrotoxicosis have a more rapid progression of their angina symptoms, and have more episodes occurring at rest than those patients with typical ASCAD.[32]

Similarly, they may be differentiated from those patients with Prinzmetal's angina in the timing of their symptoms; those with thyrotoxicosis-induced vasospasm have no association with the time of day, while those with Prinzmetal's angina have symptoms that most often occur in the early morning hours.[32] Additional symptoms of thyrotoxicosis may be elicited such as unintentional weight loss, hair loss, palpitations, insomnia, or tremor. Examination findings of exophthalmos and thyroid tenderness, enlargement, or bruit will support thyrotoxicosis as the cause of coronary ischemia.

Initial treatment of patients with myocardial ischemia from thyrotoxicosis should include the standard treatment for ASCAD-associated ischemia (aspirin, morphine, oxygen, and anticoagulation). If thyrotoxicosis as the cause of myocardial ischemia is not thought of and sought, and left untreated, the patient is at increased risk of thyroid storm.[33] Initial beta-blocker treatment will decrease myocardial oxygen demand, and may improve underlying vasospasm. Coronary angiography is useful in patients with suspected thyrotoxicosis-induced ischemia because of the potentially increased risk of thrombosis in those with underlying ASCAD as well as those with potential vasospasm. In most cases, treatment of the thyrotoxic state with antithyroid treatment (such as propylthiouracil and Lugol's solution) will reverse the cardiac effects.

Takotsubo cardiomyopathy

Recognized relatively recently, another clinical entity that presents virtually indistinguishably from acute coronary syndrome is Takotsubo cardiomyopathy (TC), also known as apical ballooning syndrome, stress cardiomyopathy, "broken heart" syndrome, and ampulla cardiomyopathy.[37,38] Originally described in 1990 in the Japanese literature, it has now been reported across the globe and has been recognized by the American Heart Association since 1996 as a primary acquired cardiomyopathy.[38] The name "tako-tsubo" derives from the Japanese fishing term for a round-bottomed, narrow-necked pot used to trap octopi (tako, "octopus" and tsubo, "jar"). This jar bears a striking resemblance to the systolic images of the left ventricle during cardiac catheterization in patients with TC, where the cardiac apex "balloons" out despite contraction of the hyperkinetic cardiac base.[38,39]

Although the true incidence is still unknown, it is estimated that, among individuals with an initial diagnosis of acute coronary syndrome or myocardial infarction, 1–2% are actually due to TC. Roughly 90% of cases occur in women, most of whom are postmenopausal, with an estimated 3% of cases occurring in women under 50 years of age.[38,40] Correspondingly, a hormonal-protective effect has been advanced to explain this age and gender bias.[38] Pathophysiology of the disease is still incompletely understood; various considerations include catecholamine-mediated myocardial stunning, epicardial microvascular spasm, and myocarditis, although the latter is considered unlikely.[37-40] A critical feature of the disease is the absence of significant obstructive coronary disease at cardiac catheterization, despite clinical evidence of acute coronary syndrome, manifested by patient symptoms, electrocardiographic changes, and serum cardiac enzyme elevations. A recent case registry demonstrates an increase in occurrence during the summer months (contrary to that seen in traditional acute MI), although cases do present throughout the year.[41]

On clinical presentation, TC presents like an acute coronary syndrome; bedside differentiation is not reliably possible. Anginal symptoms (chest pain, dyspnea) predominate, with or without clinical evidence of congestive heart failure. Syncope and prehospital cardiac arrest are unusual. Hypotension may be evident, but frank hemodynamic compromise is not the norm. The hypotension may be due to systolic reduction in stroke volume or dynamic obstruction of the left ventricular outflow tract. A prior history of hypertension and an antecedent stressful event (e.g., argument or altercation, significant medical illness—thus the term "stress cardiomyopathy") are more commonly associated, but not universal.[38,40-42] The classic presentation would be a postmenopausal woman presenting with chest pain or dyspnea after a stressful exchange, with electrocardiographic changes.

The Mayo Clinic criteria for TC are widely referenced for syndrome definition; they include the following[38]:

1 Transient hypokinesis, akinesis, or dyskinesis of the left ventricular mid-segments with or without apical involvement; the regional wall motion abnormalities extend beyond a single epicardial vascular distribution; a stressful trigger is often, but not always present;

2 Absence of obstructive coronary disease or angiographic evidence of acute plaque rupture;
3 New electrocardiographic abnormalities (either ST-segment elevation or T wave inversion) or modest elevation in cardiac troponin level;
4 Absence of pheochromocytoma and myocarditis.

The EKG in TC (Figure 4-1) traditionally demonstrates findings consistent with STEMI.[38-41] More recently, a spectrum of EKG changes have been elucidated. One series of 59 patients finds anterior ST-segment elevation to be the most common finding (56%), with T wave inversion being next most common (17%)[43]; another series of 105 patients finds ST-segment elevation/new left bundle branch block, T wave inversion (>3 mm in three contiguous leads), and nonspecific ST-T abnormalities. A normal EKG is present about one-third of the time.[44] The possibility that these variants are actually different electrocardiographic evolutionary stages is supported by Mitsuma and colleagues, who find four distinct electrocardiographic phases when following daily serial tracings in nine patients: (1) ST-segment elevation, (2) T wave inversion (days 1–3), (3) transient improvement in T wave inversion (days 2–6), (4) deeper T wave inversion (up until about 2 months), followed by recovery.[45] ST-segment elevation appears typically in the precordial leads, but may occur in the inferior or lateral leads.[38] Q waves and reciprocal changes are not the rule but may appear; QT prolongation occurs, but also tends to resolve over time.[38] Electrocardiographic presentation does not seem to predict outcomes.[44] Cardiac troponins are invariably elevated, although the degree of elevation is generally less than that seen with STEMI.[38,43]

The diagnosis is made at cardiac catheterization. Takotsubo cardiomyopathy typically features nonobstructive coronary artery disease or normal vessels; obstructive disease is rare. Hypokinesis or akinesis of the mid and apical segments of the left ventricle are seen on ventriculogram, while systolic function at the cardiac base is either spared or hyperkinetic. Wall motion abnormalities extend beyond the territory of a single coronary vessel. Right ventricular involvement is seen in roughly 30% of patients, and portends a more severe clinical course. Other imaging modalities may capture the characteristic ventricular findings, including echocardiography, computed tomography, and magnetic resonance imaging; echocardiography is useful to detect clinically significant left ventricular outflow tract obstruction.[38,46]

Variants of the disease present similarly to TC, including nonapical ballooning syndrome, where hypokinesis or akinesis is seen at the mid-ventricular segments on ventriculogram, but the apex and base are spared (compared to basal sparing with classic TC).[38,42] Patients with this variant have been reported to be younger and less likely to have cardiogenic shock or pulmonary edema than their TC counterparts.[42] An inverted Tako-tsubo syndrome also exists, where hypokinesis occurs at the cardiac base with apical sparing.[38] T wave inversion is less common in both these variants than it is in TC.[42]

Ideal initial management of TC has yet to be determined. Reasonable initial management includes aspirin, nitrates (blood pressure allowing), and heparin, managing as one would a patient with acute coronary syndrome. Beta-adrenergic blockade is helpful when a hyperkinetic base leads to outflow tract obstruction, but this is not apparent to the emergency physician at the bedside. The most common complication is congestive heart failure (20–30%), where ejection fraction is reduced and diuretics are usually helpful. Inotropic support and even intra-aortic balloon counterpulsation can be employed for cardiogenic shock if it occurs.[38,46] Complications include heart failure, left ventricular free wall rupture, left ventricular thrombus, outflow obstruction, mitral valve dysfunction, and rarely, dysrhythmia or death.[38,46] Complete recovery is the rule, with infrequent recurrence. Ejection fraction improves in days to weeks, and complete resolution of cardiac dysfunction is expected at 4–8 weeks. The role of pharmacologic management to prevent recurrence is unclear at this time.[37–39,46]

Section IV: Decision making

- Electrocardiographic manifestations (e.g., ST-segment elevation), as well as serum marker evidence (e.g., elevated cardiac troponins), of acute myocardial infarction are not absolute evidence of acute coronary occlusion; other disease processes may be the culprit but are diagnosed by exclusion of obstructive coronary disease.
- Traumatic and spontaneous coronary artery dissections are most likely to affect the left anterior descending artery; aortic dissection, if it involves a coronary artery ostium, most likely affects the right coronary artery.

- Takotsubo cardiomyopathy, also known as apical ballooning syndrome, classically presents in postmenopausal women complaining of chest pain or dyspnea after a stressful exchange, with electrocardiographic changes suggestive of acute myocardial infarction with ST-segment elevation.
- Consider coronary artery dissection and pulmonary embolism in pregnant women or women in the early postpartum period with chest pain and dyspnea.

References

1 Hamman L. Coronary embolism. *Am Heart J*. 1941;21:401–411.
2 Wegner NK, Bauer S. Coronary embolism: Review of literature and presentation of fifteen cases. *Am J Med*. 1958;25:549–557.
3 Prizel KR, Hutchins GM, Bulkley BH. Coronary artery embolism and myocardial infarction: A clinicopathologic study of 55 patients. *Ann Intern Med*. 1978;88:155–161.
4 Mirza A. Myocardial infarction resulting from nonatherosclerotic coronary artery disease. *Am J Emerg Med*. 2003;21:578–584.
5 Roudaut R, Labbe T, Lorient-Roudaut MF, et al. Mechanical cardiac valve thrombosis. Is fibrinolysis justified? *Circulation*. 1992;86(Suppl 5):II8–II15.
6 Christensen MD, Nielsen PE, Sleight P. Prior blunt chest trauma may be a cause of single vessel coronary disease; hypothesis and review. *Int J Cardiol*. 2006;108:1–5.
7 Oghlakian G, Maldjian P, Kaluski E, Saric M. Acute myocardial infarction due to left anterior descending coronary artery dissection after blunt chest trauma. *Emerg Radiol*. 2010;17:149–151.
8 DeMaio SJ, Kinsella SH, Silverman ME. Clinical course and long-term prognosis of spontaneous coronary artery dissection. *Am J Cardiol*. 1989;64:471–474.
9 Kay IP, Wilkins GT, William JA. Spontaneous coronary artery dissection presenting as unstable angina. *J Invasive Cardiol*. 1998;10:274–276.
10 Dhawan R, Singh G, Fesniak H. Spontaneous coronary artery dissection: the clinical spectrum. *Angiology*. 2002;53:89–93.
11 Vale PR, Baron DW. Coronary artery stenting for spontaneous coronary artery dissection: A case report and review of the literature. *Cathet Cardiovasc Diagn*. 1998;45:280–286.
12 Basso C, Morgagni GL, Thiene G. Spontaneous coronary artery dissection: a neglected cause of myocardial ischemia and sudden death. *Heart*. 1996;75:451–454.

13 Chen H. Marfan Syndrome. eMedicine. Available at: http://emedicine.medscape.com/article/946315-overview. Accessed April 21, 2009.

14 Hagan PG, Nienaber CA, Isselbacher EM, et al. The international registry of acute aortic dissection (IRAD). New insights into an old disease. *JAMA.* 2000;283: 897–903.

15 Zegers ES, Gehlmann JR, Verheugt FWA. Acute myocardial infarction due to an acute type A aortic dissection involving the left main coronary artery. *Neth Heart J.* 2007;15:263–264.

16 Coselli JS. Treatment of acute aortic dissection involving the right coronary artery and aortic valve. *J Cardiovasc Surg.* 1990;31:305–309.

17 Horszczaruk GJ, Roik MF, Kochman J, et al. Aortic dissection involving the ostium of right coronary artery as the reason for myocardial infarction. *Eur Heart J.* 2006;27:518.

18 Dorman SH, Barry J. Acute aortic dissection mimicking an acute coronary syndrome through occlusion of the right coronary artery. *Emerg Med J.* 2008;25:462–463.

19 Angelini PA, Velasco JA, Flamm S. Coronary anomalies. Incidence, pathophysiology, and clinical relevance. *Circulation.* 2002;105:2449–2454.

20 Angelini PA, Villason S, Chan AV, et al. Normal and anomalous coronary arteries in humans. In: Angelini PA, ed. *Coronary Artery Anomalies: A Comprehensive Approach.* Philadelphia: Lippincott Williams & Wilkins; 1999:27–150.

21 Basso C, Maron BJ, Corrado D, et al. Clinical profile of congenital coronary anomalies with origin from the wrong aortic sinus leading to sudden death in young competitive athletes. *J Am Coll Cardiol.* 2000;35:1493–1501.

22 Gandini C, Castoldi AF, Candura SM, et al. Carbon monoxide cardiotoxicity. *Clin Toxicol.* 2001;39:35–44.

23 Marius-Nunez AL. Myocardial infarction with normal coronary arteries after acute exposure to carbon monoxide. *Chest.* 1990;97:491–494.

24 Allred EN, Bleecker ER, Chaitman BR, et al. Short-term effects of carbon monoxide exposure on the exercise performance of subject with coronary artery disease. *N Engl J Med.* 1989;321:1426–432.

25 Einzig S, Nicoloff DM, Russel LV. Myocardial perfusion abnormalities in carbon monoxide poisoned dogs. *Can J Physiol Pharmacol.* 1979;58:396–405.

26 Satran D, Henry CR, Adkinson C, et al. Cardiovascular manifestations of moderate to severe carbon monoxide poisoning. *J Am Coll Cardiol.* 2005;45:1513–1516.

27 Keller KB, Lemberg L. Prinzmetal's angina. *Am J Crit Care.* 2004;13:350–354.

28 Petrov D, Sardowski S, Gesheva M. 'Silent' Prinzmetal's ST elevation related to atenolol overdose. *J Emerg Med.* 2007;33:123–126.

29 Opie LH. Calcium channel antagonist in the management of anginal syndromes: changing concepts in relation to the role of coronary vasospasm. *Prog Cardiovasc Dis.* 1996;38:291–314.

30 Vincent GM, Anderson JL, Marshall HW. Coronary spasm producing coronary thrombosis and myocardial infarction. *N Engl J Med.* 1983;309:220–223.

31 Sugiishi M, Takatsu K, Cigarette smoking is a major risk factor for coronary spasm. *Circulation.* 1993;87: 76–80.

32 Somerville W, Levine SA. Angina Pectoris and thyrotoxicosis. *Br Heart J.* 1950;12:245–257.

33 Lee SM, Jung TS, Hahm JR, et al. Thyrotoxicosis with coronary spasm that required coronary artery bypass surgery. *Intern Med.* 2007;46:1915–1918.

34 Parle JV, Maisonneuve P, Sheppard MC, et al. Prediction of all-cause and cardiovascular mortality in elderly people for one low serum thyrotropin result: a 10-year cohort study. *Lancet.* 2001;358:861–865.

35 Peter A, Ehler M, Blank B, et al. Excess triiodothyronine as a risk factor of coronary event. *Arch Intern Med.* 2000;160:1993–1999.

36 Dorr M, Robinson DM, Wallaschofski H, et al. Low serum thyrotropin is associated with high plasma fibrinogen. *J Clin Endocrinol Metab.* 2006;91:530–534.

37 Ramaraj R, Sorrell VL, Marcus F, Alpert JS. Recently defined cardiomyopathies: A clinician's update. *Am J Med.* 2008;121:674–681.

38 Prasad A, Lerman A, Rihal CS. Apical ballooning syndrome (Tako-Tsubo or stress cardiomyopathy): A mimic of acute myocardial infarction. *Am Heart J.* 2008; 155:408–417.

39 Kolkebeck TE, Cotant CL, Krasuski RA. Takotsubo cardiomyopathy: an unusual syndrome mimicking an ST-elevation myocardial infarction. *Am J Emerg Med.* 2007;25:92–95.

40 Gianni M, Dentali F, Grandi AM, et al. Apical ballooning syndrome or Takotsubo cardiomyopathy: a systemic review. *Eur Heart J.* 2006;27:1523–1529.

41 Regnante RA, Zuzek RW, Weinsier SB, et al. Clinical characteristics and four-year outcomes of patients in the Rhode Island takotsubo cardiomyopathy registry. *Am J Cardiol.* 2009;103:1015–1019.

42 Hahn JY, Gwon HC, Park SW, et al. The clinical features of transient left ventricular nonapical ballooning syndrome: Comparison with apical ballooning syndrome. *Am Heart J.* 2007;154:1163–1173.

43 Sharkey SW, Lesser JR, Menon M, et al. Spectrum and significance of electrocardiographic patterns, troponin levels, and thrombolysis in myocardial infarction frame count in patients with stress (tako-tsubo) cardiomyopathy and comparison to those in patients with ST-elevation

anterior wall myocardial infarction. *Am J Cardiol.* 2008; 101:1723–1728.

44 Dib C, Asirvatham S, Elesber A, et al. Clinical correlates and prognostic significance of electrocardiographic abnormalities in apical ballooning syndrome (takotsubo/stress-induced cardiomyopathy). *Am Heart J.* 2009;157; 933–938.

45 Mitsuma W, Kodama M, Ito M, et al. Serial electrocardiographic findings in women with takotsubo cardiomyopathy. *Am J Cardiol.* 2007;100:106–109.

46 Dorfman TA, Iskandrian AE. Takotsubo cardiomyopathy: state-of-the-art review. *J Nucl Cardiol.* 2009;16: 122–134.

SECTION TWO
Cardiac Dysrhythmias

5 Bradyarrhythmias

Colleen Birmingham[1] & Edward Ullman[2]

[1] *Fellow in Medical Toxicology, New York University Medical Center/ New York City Poison Center, New York, New York, USA*
[2] *Assistant Professor of Medicine, Harvard Medical School, Director of Medical Student Education, Division of Emergency Medicine, Beth Israel Deaconess Medical Center, Boston, Massachusetts, USA*

Section I: Case presentation

A 75-year-old man presented to the emergency department (ED) with a chief complaint of weakness. The patient reported feeling unwell for several days. He complained of some shortness of breath on ambulation and felt very lightheaded after walking, but there had been no loss of consciousness. He denied any cough, fever, chills, or chest pain. Prior to this episode, he could perform all of his activities of daily living without issue. The paramedics reported that the patient was found in a seated position in no apparent distress. His symptoms somewhat improved with oxygen.

The past medical history included a myocardial infarction 5 years prior with a preserved ejection fraction, hypertension, and hyperlipdemia. Medications included: aspirin, Lipitor, metoprolol, and Lasix.

Initial vital signs were: blood pressure 80/48 mmHg, heart rate 45 beats/min, respiratory rate 16 breaths/min, and temperature 36.7°C (98°F). The patient was in no apparent distress. The pulmonary examination was clear to auscultation. The cardiac examination showed a bradycardic rhythm with a 1/6 systolic murmur heard loudest at the apex. The extremities showed a trace pedal edema. The rectal examination was hemocult negative. The rest of the physical examination was unremarkable.

An EKG was performed (Figure 5-1).

Dr Peter Rosen: We often worry about tachycardias, but this case illustrates bradycardia, which is another potentially worrisome dysrhythmia. What is the formal definition of bradycardia? Does it include rate as well as symptoms, or is it rate alone?

Dr Richard Harrigan: I would split bradycardia into symptomatic and asymptomatic, with the generally accepted cutoff being 60 beats per minute as the threshold below which we define as bradycardia.

PR: What if you have a well-conditioned runner or bicyclist whose resting pulse is about 40 beats? Is that ever a concern, or can you just assume that it is the conditioning?

RH: This demonstrates the need for taking a more detailed history, such as asking "Have you ever been told that you run a slow pulse?" The conditioning history needs to be included when obtaining a medical history of a bradycardic patient. Further, we must remember that we are talking about a normal distribution, and although 59 beats per minute is termed bradycardia and 61 beats per minute is not, in truth it is relative and heart rate is a spectrum of findings. Also, bradycardia is relative to the person's conditioning. I've even seen people whose resting heart rate is in the high thirties, and they tolerate this well. Rather than treating a number, we have to look at the whole picture.

PR: One of the things that makes us a little anxious about asymptomatic bradycardia is that some

Cardiovascular Problems in Emergency Medicine: A discussion-based review, First Edition.
Edited by Shamai A. Grossman and Peter Rosen.
© 2011 John Wiley & Sons, Ltd. Published 2011 by John Wiley & Sons, Ltd.

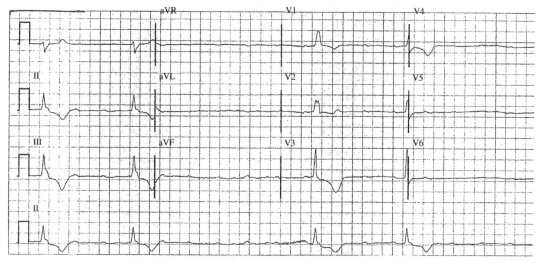

Figure 5.1 Case presentation EKG.

well-conditioned athletes have cardiomegaly. This probably represents the enlargement of exercise rather than the enlargement of disease. I'm not sure that there's an easy way to distinguish between the two beyond the onset of symptoms.

PR: We know that well-conditioned athletes can have a normal bradycardia at rest. Do they also sustain that bradycardia through mild exercise, or do they just accelerate as they need to? Will you see someone well-conditioned who fails to develop a tachycardia with exercise?

Dr Shamai Grossman: It will take more exertion for a well-conditioned athlete to reach a maximum heart rate. An unconditioned athlete may run 10 minutes, and reach a maximum heart rate, and a well-conditioned athlete may take 10 hours to reach that same maximum heart rate. The better the conditioning, the more reserve your heart has.

PR: Are there elderly patients who have bradycardia that is not symptomatic, or not representative of heart disease?

RH: Although there are elderly patients who have asymptomatic or benign bradycardia, medications may also be contributing to this. In this case the bradycardia may be inappropriate, yet the patient is still not symptomatic. They also may not be symptomatic because they lead a sedentary lifestyle, and are not

stressed. For this reason, it's important to ask an older person with a bradycardia not only about how he or she presently feels, but also how he or she feels when climbing stairs, running for a bus, or even doing daily activities around the house.

SG: This bradycardia may reflect simple senile degeneration of the conduction system. So, in truth, the bradycardia does represent heart disease, but very often disease that is well-tolerated and sustainable over many years.

PR: I remember first learning about drop attacks as a medical student, but I can't say I have ever seen a patient present with a history of "I'm feeling well but every once in a while I just fall over unconscious." I think that the more common symptoms of bradycardia are what our patient today experienced: lightheadedness, mild dyspnea on exertion, and weakness. It's interesting that this man had this condition develop rather rapidly. Does that suggest to you that this probably relates less to an acute heart attack that involves his conduction system and more to a medication?

SG: I would offer a third possibility: this can be related simply to the slow senile deterioration of his conduction system, and not related to any acute process. All three of these are possibilities. Generally, in something that is more abrupt, you would think that it would be related to either an acute myocardial infarction or a perhaps medication overdosage. It is, however, also conceivable that a patient reaches a certain threshold and this is when the symptoms commence.

PR: The abruptness may also reflect a change in physical activity. If it is the fall season, and the patient went out to rake leaves, which he hasn't done since a year ago, this might not really represent an acute change in exercise tolerance. With tachycardia, we are quick to slow it down, while with bradycardia, we are also quick to think of ways to speed it up. In the past, it seemed like everybody reached for atropine the minute they got a pulse count less than 60. Is that still an itch we scratch, or have we become a little more disciplined about who we try to pharmacologically speed up?

RH: I hope we have become more disciplined. What we should do when we have a heart rate like this, with 45 beats per minute reported to us by the nursing staff, is ask the time honored question of "How does the patient look?" followed by "What is the blood pressure?" If the blood pressure is adequate, and the patient looks well, I would not drop everything and run into the room to administer a medication. In cases where the patient has been symptomatic but is in no apparent distress, yet the blood pressure is low with a slow heart rate, I think you still should take some time to re-evaluate the situation, in order to repeat the vital signs before you cause more problems with your treatment than had you left the bradycardia alone.

PR: I wouldn't fault anyone urgently placing an intravenous line in this patient, but I would be very cautious in immediately attempting to speed up his rate.

PR: We have an electrocardiogram (EKG) in which there appears to be some nonconducting P waves; lead 2 looks like the second beat is different from the first beat, there is a P wave, and then there is another one subsequently, so it almost looks like there is a two-to-one block. I also see some extra beats. So it wouldn't be stretching too far to read this as some degree of high grade heart block with ventricular escape beats.

PR: Historically, whenever we found anything that looked like a premature ventricular contraction (PVC), we would try to eradicate it with lidocaine. Why isn't it a good idea to try to eradicate an escape ventricular beat?

RH: In this case, that may be what's maintaining your patient's blood pressure and cerebral perfusion. Escape beats are a compensatory measure of your heart for not being able to do what it's supposed to do from the sinus node. It's not a ventricular dysrhythmia. We don't want to make escape beats go away. It's very important not to eradicate them before you can fix what is making the heart beat so slowly.

PR: We have a patient who is bradycardic, with a blood pressure that undoubtedly represents an abnormally low pressure for him given his age and his history of hypertension. Since one of his medications is a beta-blocker, would you simply withdraw the beta-blocker and watch him, or would you administer some glucagon while you withdraw the beta-blocker?

SG: I don't think it's a good idea to leave this elderly patient with a history of coronary disease in a relatively hypotensive state. Presumably the hypotension is secondary to the bradycardia; therefore, I would like to increase the heart rate. The simplest thing to do with probably the fewest side effects is to try to reverse the beta-blockade with glucagon and calcium, and see if that helps.

PR: I am constantly surprised at how often people get into trouble with medications that they have been taking for a long period of time. Beta-blockers are a frequent culprit. I have seen numerous patients who claim they haven't altered the dose in years, yet suddenly they are symptomatic. Is there something associated with beta-blockade that suddenly precipitates symptoms, just as hypokalemia precipitates dig-toxicity? Is there anything that makes beta-blockade suddenly likely to have an overdose effect?

RH: Concomitant medications that also slow the atrioventricular (AV) node could be a culprit. In addition to taking extra beta-blocker, other medications like a calcium channel blocker, digoxin, or clonidine may have been co-administered to this patient. You can also have bradycardia and various degrees of heart block in hyperkalemia. In this case we are not seeing other signs of hyperkalemia, making this diagnosis unlikely.

PR: He has been treated with furosemide, which would make him more likely to be hypokalemic.

SG: I would not hastily rule out a metabolic abnormality. Hypokalemia and, less frequently, hypocalcemia and hypomagnesemia, can cause a variety of dysrhythmias including premature atrial contractions

(PACs) and PVCs, sinus bradycardia, and AV block, as well as ventricular tachycardia and ventricular fibrillation.

PR: It would be worthwhile to look at a basic metabolic panel while you straighten everything out. Regardless, this is a patient who is declaring himself as unsafe to send home. Historically, we used to try to treat these patients pharmacologically with bradycardia before reaching for a pacing wire. If atropine in sufficient doses didn't speed up the heart (and it almost never did), then we would try isoproterenol.

RH: The main concern with atropine in the face of ongoing cardiac ischemia is that it may increase myocardial oxygen demand with the resultant tachycardia, yet we still use it if we must. I can't think of the last time I used isoproterenol. I believe this is the case because of the lack of good data that it's helpful more than harmful, particularly with concerns again about increased myocardial oxygen demand, potentially worsening cardiac ischemia.

PR: If the patient hasn't responded to either calcium or glucagon, at what point would you consider reaching for a pacer?

SG: I would place external pacing pads on this patient the minute I realized he was bradycardic. Although right now he is bradycardic and is maintaining some blood pressure, I don't know what will happen in the very near future. Should the blood pressure drop further, or should he develop further bradycardia, for example, if the heart rate drops from 35 to 25 beats per minute, I would either administer atropine and see if there is a response, or pace him. At the same time, I would have someone on the phone with the cardiologist or, depending on the institution, I would have my nurses set up for me to float a transvenous wire. Most patients don't tolerate external pacing for prolonged periods of time. To review, I would first set up external pacing pads, have atropine at the bedside, and then watch the patient. I might then try glucagon or calcium to see if I can reverse the beta-blockade. Should he deteriorate, I would probably try atropine, and if that doesn't succeed, try external pacing with the plan to place a transvenous pacer either by cardiology, or if need be, by myself in the ED.

PR: I haven't floated a pacer wire in probably 20 years, likely because we have better support from our cardiology service than we used to have, but also I can remember that it was very hard to get capture in the ED without concomitant echo or fluoroscopy to help you guide the wire. Do you think that we just don't do it frequently enough to get good at it, and that's why we have so much trouble?

SG: The truth is that I've floated transvenous wires a number of times with success and good capture, but that happens less and less frequently because I work at institutions where cardiology is readily available. They strongly prefer to place wires under fluoroscopy control, which makes it a far easier and safer procedure. I think in an ideal world you would always float a wire under fluoroscopy, but in the real world, where sometimes we have to do things in less-than-ideal conditions (especially in the ED), it can still be accomplished. Unfortunately for emergency physicians, I don't think we get much opportunity, and therefore I don't think we have a lot of expertise. This may be why there isn't as much success as we would like to see.

PR: If you were at an institution where you didn't have a cardiologist readily available, but you did have access to an emergency ultrasound, would you use that to help you float the wire? Would you use external pacing while you were trying to place the internal wire?

RH: If the patient has a reasonable blood pressure and mental status, I would avoid external pacing as it may make it technically more difficult to place an internal wire. Ultrasound would be useful for two reasons. One, it makes placing an IJ line less risky because you can place it under ultrasound visualization; although this is not a procedure that we fear, it has complications, and in a sick, elderly patient, we don't need more complications. With ultrasound you feel better about placing that line, and placing it early. Two, ultrasound would also be useful to look for the appearance of the wire in the right ventricle. Given this patient's body habitus, you probably have a good chance of visualization. However, it's going to be hard to man the ultrasound probe and the pacing wire at the same time, so you are going to need another person with you. Rather than rely on looking up at the cardiac monitor to see when we have capture, this may be a useful adjunct.

PR: It's going to be the rural emergency physician who's stuck with this patient without much support.

SG: Traditionally, we would place alligator clips on the pacer wire and on an EKG V lead, then look for a current of injury (ST elevation) on EKG. As soon as we saw this, we would pull back ever so slightly away from what must have been the right ventricular wall, and know that the wire was in place. This can be done from any ED bedside.

PR: I still suspect beta-blockade to be the cause of his symptoms. It's not clear to me why this suddenly became too much for the man. I would still hope that after admitting him to the hospital he would turn around with relief from the beta-blockade, and not require permanent pacemaker placement. Clearly, what was done in this case was precisely that: to not rush to pace him, but to admit him, and to see what happens over a little time. When he continued to be bradycardic, a pacemaker was inserted. Of course, part of our problem is that we don't always have beds to admit such a patient to, and then one becomes a little bit more concerned about what to do in the ED. Do you believe that a patient like this would progress all right in an observation bed in the ED?

SG: Were telemetry to be the same in the ED as it is in the coronary care unit (CCU), then I would say yes. Unfortunately, most EDs, that I know, don't have someone watching the monitor 24 hours a day, 7 days a week. Even with all of the bells and whistles that we have in the modern ED, it's hard to closely monitor a dangerous dysrhythmia, even when only admitted to the ED for the short term. I would not keep this patient in an observation unit. I think the patient would benefit from being in a unit that has very close telemetry monitoring. Should the patient's rhythm deteriorate over the course of the observation process before the decision is made whether to place a permanent pacemaker, it could be appropriately recognized and dealt with quickly. Unfortunately, the reality of emergency medicine is that we don't have that kind of monitoring.

RH: When we make the decision of who to put in the observation unit in the ED, we have to decide whether there is a high, medium, or low likelihood to develop a problem. We are better off putting people with a low likelihood to have a problem, like those with low-risk chest pain, in the observation units. Here we have a 75-year-old man with low blood pressure, low heart rate, and third-degree heart block; even if it does

improve temporarily, there is a high probability for the patient to need further intervention, as well as for him to deteriorate while he is awaiting that intervention.

PR: I think that observation units within the ED are variable in their staffing and in their capabilities. Some don't have a nurse whose sole obligation is the patients in the observation unit; I wouldn't put any patient with a risk of deterioration in such a unit. But there are some heart units and observation units that do have good equipment and good nurses assigned, and in that case I don't know that there is much less observation than in the CCU. In the ED, you also have to worry about what kind of manpower you have to respond to the observation unit. Many EDs have a single physician responsible for both the patients in the main department and the patients in the observation unit, and that can stretch medical response time to an unacceptable length.

PR: Are there other conditions here that could be contributing to this problem and would need further workup or management? Are we looking at subtle sepsis, for example? What additional workup would you include in the management of this patient?

SG: You may want to tease out his initial complaints; he is lightheaded with exertion, short of breath, and weak. All of these are nonspecific complaints, but all of them are complaints that someone could develop with a concomitant infectious process. The complaint that we are not told about is whether the patient has been febrile; we are also not told if the patient has been coughing, having chest discomfort, or other symptoms that would be concerning for infection such as dysuria, changes in frequency of urination, rashes, etc. I think you have to take the pieces of history that you do know and say, what is the likelihood that this is going to be something else?

Given these known symptoms, how much do I have to pursue further workup? I would say, if the patient doesn't have a fever, and doesn't have any signs of infection on physical examination, then it's unlikely that the patient's going to have an infection. It's reasonable to do some very basic testing, such as a chest X-ray study and a urinalysis to make sure that we are not missing a very common but, in this case occult, infection, but I probably would stop there so long as the patient is afebrile, and doesn't have a profound leukocytosis or leukopenia.

The next thing I might consider is: does this patient actually have concomitant cardiac ischemia? Given his presentation, that is a reasonable thought. The EKG doesn't suggest cardiac ischemia. The EKG is the best test that we have, but unfortunately is not particularly sensitive for acute myocardial infarction; at best, it's in the 50% range. Serial cardiac enzymes in this patient would be reasonable to make sure this event is not a manifestation of a concomitant infarction. Then you get to more and more remote diagnoses, such as thyroid disease and so forth. The more remote the possibility, the less likely the diagnosis, especially when you have more likely diagnoses such as conduction diseases or beta-blocker toxicity.

PR: Are there medications that you would especially want to avoid should the patient deteriorate further? If his blood pressure drops and you want to intubate him, are there any respiratory management drugs that would make the bradycardia and heart block worse?

RH: Most of us are using succinylcholine preceded by etomidate, and I think we should be okay with these medications here.

SG: Intubation increases your vagal tone, and if you do need to intubate the patient, this patient may need pre-intubation atropine.

RH: That is written in every book, but do you really find that in practice your patients increase vagal tone and drop their heart rates when you intubate them?

PR: Only when they are hypoxic.

RH: Just because I am expected to see a drop in heart rate when the patient is instrumented, I don't know that I would reach for atropine now if I haven't already given atropine for the persistently low blood pressure and heart rate.

PR: Would you use isoproterenol to support the blood pressure while you were doing other things in this patient, as perhaps this might solve some of the concerns about atropine?

SG: Isoproterenol has fallen off the ACLS guidelines.

PR: Why did it fall out of favor?

SG: I suspect that it fell out of favor because there are better therapies. External pacing, as uncomfortable though it may be, is a better choice because it is more effective. Atropine is short lived so that if you

do get some ischemia, it is not likely to be sustained. Although isoproterenol can be shut off, it may take a little longer to clear from the system.

PR: If you got a call about this patient from the field from an ambulance that was coming a fairly long distance, which is typical for our more rural EDs, would you be inclined to start pharmacological therapy in the ambulance?

SG: This is one of those cases where you say "primo non nocere" or "first do no harm." You take a patient, who is relatively stable in an ambulance, and you start administering drugs; if they become far sicker and far more ill, they are still in an ambulance. For this reason I would say, "Wait until he gets here unless the blood pressure or heart rate deteriorates further, and then we can better assess him in an institution where we have more options available."

PR: This case fortunately has a good outcome. I wish all heart blocks looked this good when they arrive in the ED. Frequently they do not.

SG: I would suspect that this is likely related to a slow deterioration of his conduction system. He likely tolerated a relatively low heart rate for a while and that is why he had a good outcome.

Case resolution

The patient was admitted to the CCU with concern for third-degree block. Metoprolol was held for several days to identify whether this medication was the cause of the patient's bradycardia. However, bradycardic episodes persisted, and on hospital day three, a pacemaker was placed without complications. The patient was discharged the next day and on one month follow-up he had no complaints.

Section III: Concepts

Background/epidemiology

Bradycardia, defined as a heart rate of less than 60 beats per minute, is a relatively common finding during routine evaluation of patients in the ED. With a vast array of etiologies and related electrocardiographic manifestations, the clinical implications of bradycardias range from negligible incidental findings to life-threatening bradyarrhythmias. The first task is to determine whether the patient exhibits any signs or symptoms related to the bradycardia, and to treat accordingly.

Identifying the association between a slow heart rate and a patient's presentation proves challenging at times. The cardiac output is the product of left ventricular stroke volume and the heart rate. For example, in cases of an asymptomatic sinus bradycardia, often seen in seasoned athletes, increased stroke volume compensates for a slower heart rate; the result is a normal cardiac output and sufficient cerebral perfusion to leave the patient entirely asymptomatic. One study finds an incidence of sinus bradycardia in conditioned athletes to be as high as 50–80%, with a prevalence of 23% in the general population.[1]

In other cases, a bradyarrhythmias seems to be clearly temporally related to an episode of cerebral hypoperfusion, such as syncope, or obvious documented systemic hypotension. In one retrospective cohort study of 247 patients with bradycardia, 21% of patients with a hemodynamically significant bradycardia died within 30 days of presentation, with 41% of the deaths attributable to cardiovascular causes.[2] Thus, further diagnostic studies and interventions are clearly indicated in the case of hemodynamically significant bradycardia.

In the third category, a person presents with vague persistent complaints such as dizziness or weakness, and is found to have a bradycardia. In this case, the emergency physician must better describe the bradycardia in terms of the electrocardiographic rhythm and likely etiology; this information would be used to determine whether this slow heart rate could be the cause of the patient's symptoms, and therefore requires intervention. The first important responsibility, then, is to determine whether the bradycardia is the cause of the symptoms. Secondly, it must be determined whether or not a patient is symptomatic from a bradycardia. A rhythm strip should be obtained in order to further delineate the conduction abnormality causing the slow heart rate. Some bradycardias have the potential to deteriorate into an unstable rhythm even in the setting of a well-appearing patient, and these must be identified by EKG. Third, once the need to intervene is identified, a clinician must consider the risks and benefits of the available emergency therapies, including pharmacologic intervention, transcutaneous pacing, or transvenous pacing.

Initial workup history and physical

Similar to any emergency patient, the initial evaluation entails a rapid assessment of the patient's airway, breathing, and circulation. Also, for all critical patients, it involves promptly gaining intravenous access, providing supplemental oxygen, and cardiac monitoring. Unique to bradycardic patients, pacer pads should be applied to all patients until definitive management has been provided. Early preparation is necessary so that transcutaneous pacing can be initiated rapidly when necessary, as studies show decreased effectiveness of pacing after loss of spontaneous circulation.[3]

After immediate stabilizing interventions, a focused history and physical examination can be performed. Current symptoms that may indicate cerebral hypoperfusion in the setting of bradycardia, such as dizziness, presyncope, or syncope, must be elicited. Additionally, the clinician should identify symptoms of cardiac ischemia, including chest pain, shortness of breath, or nausea. Recent infectious illnesses should be noted as well as any travel history, as certain illnesses endemic to Central and South America may cause bradycardia. Given the wide range of etiologies in bradycardia, a thorough review of a patient's past medical history should be undertaken, with special attention paid to any history of structural heart disease, neoplastic disease, connective tissue disorders, or rheumatologic disorders. The patient's medication list should be reviewed, and any nodal blocking agents or cholinergic agents should be noted. The physical examination should focus on the overall appearance of the patient, as well as any abnormalities on cardiovascular examination, including those related to rhythm, murmurs, rubs, or an abnormal pulse rate.

Etiologies/differential diagnosis

The function of the cardiac conduction system is an integral step in creating the differential diagnosis. The sino-atrial (SA) node, located at the junction of the superior vena cava and the right atrium, consists of a group of specialized cells that spontaneously depolarize. Impulse is then conducted via the internodal pathway to the AV node, which is located in the lower septum of the right atrium. Electrical activation continues through the AV node, with a slight delay to ensure complete atrial contraction prior to ventricular contraction. Conduction continues via the Bundle of

His into the interventricular septum, where it travels for one to two centimeters before dividing into the right and left bundles. These bundles divide into branches as they run along the interventricular septum before terminating in Purkinje fibers that form interweaving networks on the endocardial surface of both the right and left ventricles. Rapid conduction of impulses across this network allows for nearly simultaneous contraction of both ventricles.[4]

In terms of perfusion, the sinus node is supplied by the right coronary artery in 65% of patients, the circumflex artery in 25% of patients, and both in 10% of patients. The AV node receives its blood supply from the posterior descending artery, which arises from the right coronary artery in 80% of patients, the circumflex artery in 10%, and both in 10%.[5] The conduction system is densely innervated by both the sympathetic and parasympathetic nervous systems. While increased adrenergic input increases SA automaticity during exercise and emotion, parasympathetic input predominates at rest in most healthy individuals, leading to an increased AV-nodal conduction time and refractoriness.[4]

Disorders of impulse formation or conduction through the cardiac conduction system can be caused by intrinsic or extrinsic factors. Intrinsic factors, those that involve some structural or functional abnormality of the SA node or conducting tissue itself, account for only 15% of bradyarrhythmias encountered in the ED.[6] The sick sinus syndrome encompasses the majority of these intrinsic abnormalities. Its characteristics include severe chronic and inappropriate bradycardia, sinus pauses, sinus arrest and exit blocks (with and without appropriate escape rhythms), alternating bradycardia and atrial tachydysrhythmias, and concurrent AV conduction disturbances in over 50% of patients.[7,8] This broadly-defined syndrome has a number of documented etiologies including vascular disease of the SA nodal artery, congenital and acquired cardiac disease, and genetic mutations, but its most common cause is the replacement of the sinus node with fibrous tissue, with or without degeneration and fibrosis of other conduction pathways (including the AV node).[9]

Extrinsic causes of bradycardia account for the majority of cases seen in the ED, and have a wide variety of etiologies. While any distribution of ischemia may be associated with bradycardia, inferior wall acute myocardial infarctions are most commonly associated with bradyarrhythmias. The resulting bradycardias in these cases are often due to ischemia at the AV node or increased parasympathetic tone in the setting of a right coronary artery- related infarction. They are often responsive to atropine or other pharmacologic intervention. The AV blocks that develop in the setting of an anterior myocardial infarction, on the other hand, often result from occlusion of the left anterior descending artery and lead to septal infarction and dysfunction of the Bundle of His and bundle branches, while often sparing the AV node. In these cases, complete heart block involves a wider QRS complex on electrocardiography, and confers a poorer prognosis with a more limited response to pharmacologic interventions.[6]

Other extrinsic causes of bradycardia include non-ischemic cardiac diseases such as cardiac amyloidosis, neoplasm, cardiomyopathy, collagen vascular disease, and pericarditis.[4] In particular, infiltrative sarcoidosis should be considered as a potential etiology of bradycardia, as up to 25% of patients with this disease demonstrate cardiac involvement on pathology. A highly unstable complete heart block is the most common presenting cardiac manifestation of infiltrative sarcoidosis.[6,10] Rheumatologic diseases that have been shown to cause AV conduction disturbances include Sjogren's syndrome, Wegener's granulomatosis and Behçet's syndrome.[6]

Infectious diseases can cause bradyarrhythmias whether in acute or chronic forms. Viral illnesses known to cause bradycardia or heart block include mononucleosis, hepatitis, varicella, respiratory syncytial virus, mumps, rubella, rubeola, and varicella, although influenza rarely involves the heart.[6] Bacterial endocarditis can also cause various degrees of heart block when the infection invades the conduction system.[6,11] Chagas disease, caused by protozoan infection of *Trypanosoma cruzi*, should be considered in the evaluation of any bradycardic patient who lives in Central or South America. While the disease has prominent gastrointestinal and cardiac manifestations, sudden cardiac death accounts for the death of 55–65% of people with this disease.[12] The cardiac arrest is usually precipitated by exercise, and results from ventricular tachycardia, ventricular fibrillation, asystole, or complete heart block.[13] Lyme disease, caused by the spirochete *Borrelia burgdorferi*, has cardiac manifestations during the early-disseminated phase of the disease, which usually occurs within weeks to months after infection. The primary manifestations of Lyme

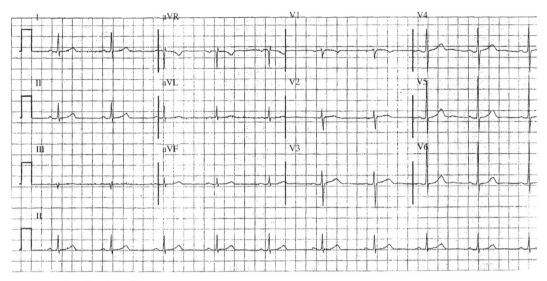

Figure 5.2 Sinus bradycardia.

disease carditis include conduction system dysfunction and decreased cardiac output due to myopericarditis. The conduction abnormalities range from first-degree AV block to complete heart block. One review of 52 patients with Lyme disease carditis finds that 87% of new Lyme disease patients have some degree of AV block, with the majority being symptomatic from this block.[14]

Another important extrinsic cause of bradycardia is medication, regardless of therapeutic or toxic doses. Nodal blocking agents such as beta-blockers, calcium channel blockers, or digitalis are extremely common causes. Alpha-2-agonists such as clonidine, as well as cholinergic agents and other antidysrhythmia agents, can also produce bradycardia.[5] In terms of toxicologic ingestions, botanicals such as foxglove, oleander, and lily of the valley contain cardiac-glycosides that can create a digitalis like toxicity.[6] Additionally, multiple medications, when taken in overdose (such as tricyclic antidepressants, carbamazepine, quinine, amantadine, cyclobenzaprine, thiordiazine, and chloroquine) act like class Ia antidysrhythmics and can produce serious heart block in addition to their more well-known sinus tachycardia.[6,15]

Other potential extrinsic causes of bradycardia include electrolyte abnormalities such as hyperkalemia, hypercalcemia, and hypermagnesemia. It is rarely associated with hypoglycemia. Iatrogenic causes exist, including post-heart transplantation or radiation therapy for malignancy. Neurologic causes include increased intracranial pressure and Cushing's syndrome, as well as an ictal-bradycardia syndrome.[6] Lastly, vagal events, such as vomiting or urination, may cause transient bradycardia, and are often implicated in cases of neurocardiogenic or "vaso-vagal" syncope.

Testing

The cornerstone for emergency testing in bradycardia is electrocardiography. The EKG will often identify the disorder of impulse formation or conduction. In sinus bradycardia, a disorder of impulse formation, the ventricular rate is less than 60 beats per minute. Importantly, each P wave is followed by a narrow QRS complex, the P-wave morphology does not change, and the PR interval remains consistent (Figure 5-2).

In an AV junctional rhythm, the rhythm is initiated by the AV node either due to lack of stimulation from the SA node or from an abnormally rapid AV node automaticity. Generally, the AV node has an intrinsic rate of 45–60, so it should not fire until sinus automaticity falls below this rate.[16] The QRS complex morphology should appear the same as in sinus rhythm, with the P waves falling before, during, or after the QRS complex (Figure 5-3).

A ventricular escape rhythm, also known as an idioventricular rhythm, occurs at a rate of less than

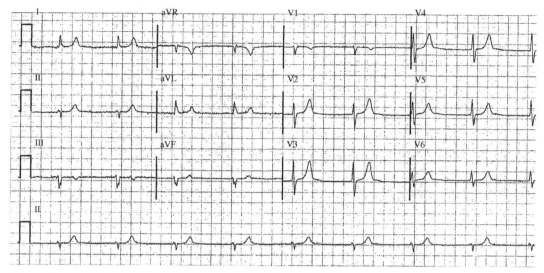

Figure 5.3 Atrioventricular junctional rhythm.

50 beats per minute. It acts as a safety net, demonstrating ventricular automaticity in the absence of proper conduction from above (i.e, sinus arrest, AV block). It produces a wide QRS, and should not be treated with lidocaine given the potential for cardiac standstill[16] (Figure 5-4).

First-degree AV block is a disorder of atrioventricular conduction, and is defined by a PR interval of more than 0.20 seconds. Importantly, all P waves are conducted with consistent PP and RR intervals. This is usually caused by a delay in the AV node, thus demonstrating a narrow QRS (Figure 5-5).

Mobitz type I (Wenckebach) second-degree AV block is a disorder of atrioventricular conduction characterized by progressive prolongation of the PR interval until a P wave is not conducted, resulting in a "dropped

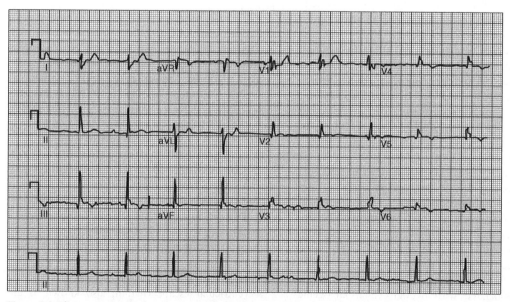

Figure 5.4 Idioventricular rhythm.

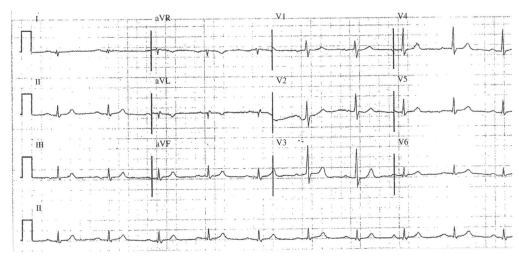

Figure 5.5 First-degree atrioventricular block.

beat." After the dropped beat, the cycle repeats itself, starting again with a normal PR interval. The rhythm strip often shows the appearance of "grouped beating" as the RR interval shortens progressively after a dropped beat. The RR interval decreases the same amount that the PR interval lengthens. This disorder is usually caused by slowed conduction at or above the AV node, resulting in a narrow QRS (Figure 5-6).

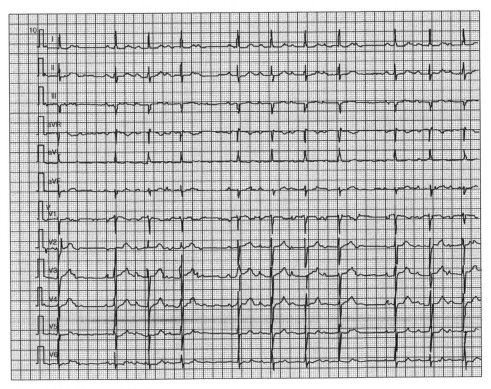

Figure 5.6 Mobitz type 1 block.

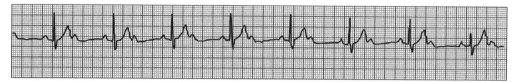

Figure 5.7 Mobitz type 2 block.

While this rhythm is often seen during acute myocardial infarction, it is usually a stable rhythm providing adequate perfusion, and is usually responsive to atropine.

Mobitz type II second-degree AV block is a disorder of atrioventricular conduction characterized by consistent PR intervals throughout (which may be normal or prolonged) and with intermittent nonconducted P waves. Thus, this rhythm does not have progressive PR prolongation demonstrated in Wenckebach. Since the conduction block usually occurs in the His Purkinje system, a wide QRS is usually seen (Figure 5-7). This rhythm has the potential to deteriorate into a third-degree block, and usually requires permanent cardiac pacing. Emergent pharmacologic interventions are often ineffective, and emergent pacing may be required. The magnitude of the AV block is described by the ratio of P waves to QRS complexes (i.e; 2:1 v. 3:2 conduction.) All ratios except for a 2:1 block are easy to distinguish from a Mobitz type I block by lack of prolonging PR segments (Figure 5-8). A 2:1 block may be either form of Mobitz block, and the patient should be monitored to see whether a higher degree of heart block develops.

Third-degree AV block is a disorder of atrioventricular conduction in which no atrial impulses reach the ventricles, and an escape pacemaker must emerge. There is no relationship between the P waves and the QRS complexes. The PP intervals and RR intervals are regular throughout. The block in this case may occur anywhere from the AV node to the Purkinje system, with the more severe symptoms occurring in lower blocks (Figure 5-9).

In addition to obtaining an EKG with a rhythm strip, serum electrolytes and chest radiography are useful tests to obtain in the ED for all patients with clinically significant bradycardia (Figure 5-10).

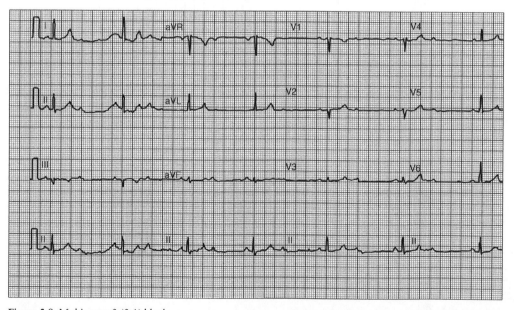

Figure 5.8 Mobiz type 2 (2:1) block.

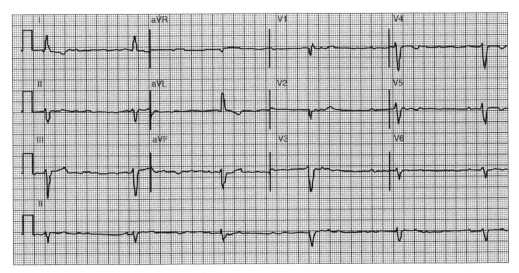

Figure 5.9 Third-Degree atrioventricular block.

Disposition

In cases of symptomatic bradycardia due to an extrinsic cause, patients require admission for treatment of that specific cause. In one study, a retrospective analysis of a bradycardia registry, it is reported that 51% of patients with compromising bradycardia have an inciting cause that requires specific treatment. These causes include: adverse drug effect (21%),

Bradycardia Algorithm

Heart Rate <60 bpm

Signs of poor perfusion (hypotension, altered mental status, chest pain)?

Yes	No
• Prepare for transcutaneous pacing • Give atropine while awaiting pacing • Attempt transcutaneous pacing ASAP for unstable rhythm OR if atropine fails • Consider giving epinephrine or dopamine	• Continue close monitoring

Heart rate improves?

Yes	No
• Continue close monitoring • Treat the primary problem	• Attempt transvenous pacing • Treat the primary problem

Figure 5.10 Management of bradycardia.

acute MI (14%), pacer dysfunction (6%), intoxication (6%), and electrolyte disorder (4%).[17]

In cases of idiopathic bradycardia, those who experience compromising symptoms from the bradycardia, and those whose rhythm on electrocardiography has the known predisposition to deteriorate into a more unstable rhythm (i.e; Mobitz type II) require admission to the hospital for further evaluation and treatment.

Regardless of the cause, hemodynamically unstable bradycardia should be treated medically with atropine, which is considered the first line treatment.[18] If unsuccessful, epinephrine or dopamine are second line agents that may be used as temporizing measures until pacing can be implemented or if pacing fails.[18] Glucagon may also be considered in the setting of a known or presumed beta-blocker or calcium channel blocker ingestion, and has been shown to improve heart rate and symptoms in such patients when atropine is ineffective.[18,19]

In the setting of an unstable patient and failure of medical management, transcutaneous pacing should be started with stimulation of the left ventricle (LV) through electrodes placed on the chest wall. Pain with impulse, skeletal muscle contraction, and difficulty with LV capture remain limitations to this intervention, but it can serve as a lifesaving bridge to transvenous or permanent pacing.[20]

Transvenous pacing requires catheter placement by central line (usually right internal jugular or left subclavian vein) into the heart with direct stimulation of the right ventricle. Complications of this procedure include myocardial perforation, pneumothorax, infection, ectopy, nonsustained ventricular tachycardia, or thromboembolism leading to a pulmonary embolism.[20]

While patients with isolated asymptomatic sinus bradycardia or asymptomatic stable AV blocks (first-degree AV block or Mobitz Type I second-degree AV block) require only electrocardiographic monitoring while in the ED; patients with higher grade block or new symptomatology require admission to the hospital. One study shows that 50% of patients presenting to the ED with compromising bradycardia ultimately require permanent pacing.[17]

Section IV: Decision making

- To establish the diagnosis of a benign bradycardia, an EKG should be obtained and the patient can be discharged home with routine follow up.

Table 5-1. Pharmacologic doses in symptomatic bradycardia.[18]

Drug	Dose
Atropine	0.5–1 mg IV q3-5 min (max 3 mg)
Epinephrine	2–10 μg/min
Dopamine	2–10 μg/kg/min
Glucagon	3 mg IV (followed by infusion at 3 mg/h if necessary)

- Asymptomatic unstable bradycardia (Mobitz type II second-degree AV block or third-degree AV block) should be admitted on telemetry monitoring for an EP evaluation.
- In symptomatic or compromising bradycardia, pacer pads should be placed on the patient while an EKG is obtained. See Table 5-1 for complete management.
- If reversible causes of bradycardia are identified, interventions such as potassium for hypokalemia, activation of the catheter laboratory in STEMI, antibiotics and aggressive fluid management in sepsis, active rewarming in hypothermia, glucagon in beta-blocker ingestion, or digi-bind in digitalis toxicity should be initiated emergently.

References

1 Bryan G, Ward A, Rippe JM. Athletic heart syndrome. *Clin Sports Med.* 1992:11:259.

2 Schwartz B, Vermeulen MJ, Idestrup C, Datta P. Clinical variables associated with mortality in out-of-hospital patients with hemodynamically significant bradycardia. *Acad Emerg Med.* 2004:11(6):656–661.

3 Barthell E, Troiano P, Olson D, Stueven HA, Hendley G. Prehospital external cardiac pacing: A prospective, controlled clinical trial. *Ann Emerg Med.* 1988:17: 1221–1226.

4 Vijayaraman P, Ellenbogen K. Bradyarrhythmias and pacemakers. In Fuster V, ed. *Hurst's The Heart Online.* 12th ed. New York: McGraw Hill; 2008. Available at: http://www.accessmedicine.com/content.aspx?aID=3051157&searchStr=atrioventricular+block. Accessed February 17, 2009.

5 Mangrum, JM, DiMarco JP. The evaluation and management of bradycardia. *N Engl J Med.* 2000: 342:703–709.

6 Brady, WJ, Harrigan PA. Evaluation and management of bradyarrhythmias in the emergency department. *Emerg Clin N Am.* 1998:16-2:361–388.

7 Ferrer, MI. The sick sinus syndrome in atrial disease. *JAMA.* 1968:206:645.

8 Narula, OS. Atrioventricular conduction defects in patients with sinus bradycardia. Analysis by His bundle recordings. *Circulation.* 1971:44:1096.

9 Thery C, Gosselin B, Lekieffre J, Warembourg H. Pathology of the sinoatrial node. Correlations with electrocardiographic findings in 111 patients. *Amer Heart J.* 1977:93:735.

10 Sharma OP, Maheshwari A, Thaker K. Myocardial sarcoidosis. *Chest.* 1993:103:253–258.

11 Huff JS, Syverud SA, Tucci MA. Case conference: Complete heart block in a young man. *Acad Emerg Med.* 1995:2:751–756.

12 Rassi A Jr, Rassi SG, Rassi A. Sudden death in Chagas' disease. *Arq Bras Cardiol.* 2001:76:75.

13 Mendoza I, Camardo J, Moleiro F, et al. Sustained ventricular tachycardia in chronic chagasic myocarditis: Electrophysiologic and pharmacologic characteristics. *Amer J Cardiol.* 1986:57:423.

14 McAlister HF, Klementowicz PT, Andrews C, et al. Lyme carditis: An important cause of reversible heart block. *Ann of Intern Med.* 1989:110:339.

15 Hessler R. Cardiovascular principles. In: Goldfrank LR, ed. *Goldfrank's Toxicologic Emergencies.* 5th ed. Norwalk, CT: Appleton & Lange: 1994:181–204.

16 Hartman D, Overton DT. Bradydysrhymias. In: Wolfson AB, ed. *Clinical Practice of Emergency Medicine.* 4th ed. Philadelphia: Lippincott Williams, and Wilkins; 2005: 260–265.

17 Sodeck GH, Domanovits H, Meron G, et al. Compromising bradycardia: Management in the emergency department. *Resuscitation.* 2007:73:96–102.

18 2005 American Heart Association Guidelines for Cardiopulmonary Resuscitation and Emergency Cardiovascular Care. *Circulation.* 2005:113:67–77.

19 Love JN, Sachdeva DK, Bessman ES, Curtis LA, Howell JM. A potential role for glucagon in the treatment of drug-induced symptomatic bradycardia. *Chest.* 1998:114:323–326.

20 Kaushik V, Leon AR, Forrester JS Jr, Trohman RG. Bradyarrhythmias, temporary and permanent pacing. *Crit Care Med.* 2000:28-10:N121–N128.

6 Atrial fibrillation

Kristin Cochran[1] & Shamai Grossman[2]

[1] Instructor in Medicine, Harvard Medical School, Beth Israel Deaconess Medical Center, Boston, Massachusetts, USA

[2] Director, Cardiac Emergency Center and Clinical Decision Unit, Beth Israel Deaconess Medical Center, Assistant Professor of Medicine, Harvard Medical School, Boston, Massachusetts, USA

Section I: Case presentation

A 78-year-old woman is brought in by her son after he visited her at home, and found her to be lethargic and complaining of "not feeling well." Her son stated that she looked like she was having trouble breathing, so he convinced her to let him take her to the emergency department (ED), but she refused to let him call an ambulance. The son cannot recall her medications, but states that she had a history of high blood pressure, high cholesterol, depression, "some kind of heart problem," and that he thought she was taking a "water pill." The patient on ED arrival was lethargic but arousable. She was oriented to place being the hospital, but didn't know the correct year. She needed to be constantly re-aroused to answer questions. She denied chest pain, but did complain of shortness of breath and cough. She did not recall fevers at home.

Upon examination, she appeared somewhat lethargic and tachypneic. The initial vital signs were: temperature 38.6°C (101.4°F), heart rate 146 beats/min with an irregular pulse, blood pressure 92/48 mmHg, respiratory rate 26 breaths/min, O_2 saturation 91% on room air. There was no jugular venous distention. The mucus membranes appeared somewhat dry. The chest examination revealed rhonchi at the right base. The heart sounds were irregularly irregular without a murmur. The abdomen was soft and nontender, and the rectal examination revealed hemoccult negative stool. The skin was warm and dry and the patient appeared to be perfusing well. There was 1+ pitting edema in the lower extremities. The patient was given 100% O_2 via a non-rebreather mask, and the oxygen saturation improved to 97%. An electrocardiogram (EKG) was performed, revealing atrial fibrillation at a rate of 142 beats/min without any clear ST changes. The blood pressure was then observed to be 83/40 mmHg with a heart rate of 148 beats/min and persistent atrial fibrillation.

Section II: Case discussion

Dr Peter Rosen: We have a patient who presents, as do many of our elderly patients, looking ill in a nonspecific way, and with nonspecific complaints. We have a fairly common ED scenario in that the patient appears somewhat confused, and the history-giver, her son, doesn't really know very much about her, so that we're basically performing geriatric veterinary medicine. Other than the history of hypertension, and that she may be on a diuretic, what in this particular clinical presentation would move you to consider a cardiac emergency?

Dr Amal Mattu: My first impression when I see her is that this is not necessarily a cardiac emergency. She has a fever of 38.6°C (101.4°F), she's short of breath, a bit tachypneic, and hypoxic, so the first thing I think of is that she probably has pneumonia. Next, I might consider a pulmonary embolus, which can also cause

Cardiovascular Problems in Emergency Medicine: A discussion-based review, First Edition.
Edited by Shamai A. Grossman and Peter Rosen.
© 2011 John Wiley & Sons, Ltd. Published 2011 by John Wiley & Sons, Ltd.

low-grade fevers. However, she's very tachycardic at 146 beats/min and the blood pressure is borderline at 92/48 mmHg, making septic shock more likely. Instead of dwelling on the diagnosis here, I would obtain IV access, begin fluid resuscitation, place her on a monitor, obtain an EKG and a quick chest X-ray study, though not because I thought this was a cardiac emergency. Even when I see the EKG, it seems like her primary problem is not a cardiac problem, but an infectious one, with a secondary cardiac problem.

Dr Shamai Grossman: I find that sometimes we become obsessed with one element of the patient's presentation, such as physical findings, history, or EKG, and we miss looking at the patient as a whole. This is a great example of a patient who looks like sepsis, but who also has a cardiac emergency and the cardiac emergency is the lesser evil. The priority here is to address the greatest life threat first. Here, this means treating what is likely an acute infectious process or sepsis inflammatory syndrome, and to succeed one needs to jump on the bandwagon early and begin therapy aggressively.

PR: One of the few physical findings that help you in making a cardiac diagnosis is the irregular irregularity of the pulse. Clearly, patients who have underlying atrial fibrillation can suffer from diseases that are not directly related to the heart, such as pulmonary embolism (PE), stroke, and even pump failure, all of which should be considered in this patient. This presentation must also make you consider metabolic disease, even though sepsis is higher on our list; a patient who is having complications of diabetes or adrenal insufficiency can also look like this. The initial approach to all of these problems is fluid resuscitation, antibiotics, and an attempt to find the source of the sepsis, looking at the urine as well as the chest, even though it sounds more like pneumonia. We find many patients in whom we end up concentrating on the dysrhythmia, when what we should be concentrating on is the tachycardia itself as a form of volume depletion. Do you see any utility in placing a central line in this patient?

AM: I would only use a central line if we need to administer vasopressors. As long as you can get good peripheral access with large bore IVs, you can rehydrate this patient and effectively administer antibiotics.

SG: There is growing evidence that goal-oriented treatment for sepsis significantly reduces mortality in sepsis. As part of this treatment regimen, there is value in placing a central line and measuring the central venous pressure (CVP) in a patient who does not respond to fluid, and who remains hypotensive. A CVP line would be very useful in this patient if she doesn't respond to two liters of fluid, and that's what should be the next step.

PR: How do you distinguish acute from chronic atrial fibrillation, when history is unavailable?

AM: Besides history and maybe a prior medication list, little else would definitely tell me if somebody has acute or chronic atrial fibrillation. In reading the EKG, a subtle clue is to look at the baseline atrial rhythm. Patients with new-onset atrial fibrillation often have a more coarse atrial rhythm; at times, it can look as if there is concurrent flutter co-existing with atrial fibrillation. If a person has atrial fibrillation of longer duration, the size of the atrial waves become smaller and smaller, and it becomes more of a fine atrial fibrillation rather than a coarse atrial fibrillation, but that's not always reliable.

PR: Is there any utility in looking for atrial enlargement on EKG to help determine chronicity or acuity of atrial fibrillation?

SG: If you find atrial enlargement, it would make chronic atrial fibrillation more conceivable, but finding it on the EKG is not enough to say this patient has chronic atrial fibrillation as many people have atrial enlargement without atrial fibrillation. Although I might look for atrial enlargement on the EKG, it is more useful to put an ultrasound probe on the patient to look for enlargement of the atrium; however, left atrial enlargement, even by ultrasound, remains a nonspecific marker for atrial fibrillation.

PR: Let's say you had a better history and knew that this was new-onset atrial fibrillation (AF); would you be inclined to immediately convert this person to a sinus rhythm?

AM: If the reminder of the presentation was unchanged, I would not attempt immediate cardioversion. When someone has new-onset AF, there are two questions that you ask yourself. Question number one: Did the new-onset AF cause the symptoms that the patient is having? Question number two: Is there some underlying condition that has caused the atrial fibrillation? In this case, I think the latter is correct. The patient has underlying sepsis and pneumonia, and that condition caused atrial fibrillation. When AF is caused by something else, initially you have to focus more on treating the underlying condition. The patient's infection needs to be treated aggressively; the patient needs fluid resuscitation, and if you under-resuscitate and just give medications to treat the AF, then you might allow the blood pressure to bottom out even more, and thus make a sick patient even sicker.

SG: I might add that if you try to treat the AF without trying to treat the underlying disease, most likely the atrial fibrillation will recur. Unless you change the circumstances that enabled the AF to start in the first place, you are not likely to successfully convert the patient to a sinus rhythm.

PR: We used to treat chronic AF patients with digoxin, which in turn would prompt a series of questions: is the patient adequately digitalized, or over-digitalized, is digoxin the cause of the tachycardia, or is digoxin playing its proper role? In order to see if the patient's tachycardia was capable of changing with medication management, we would give a dose of atropine, and if the heart rate speeded up, then the patient needed more digoxin; but, if the heart rate didn't speed up, then the patient was maximally digitized. In later years, we could do digoxin levels to help ensure that the patient was adequately dosed. If you found that one of our patient's medications was digitalis, what would make you concerned about toxicity?

AM: Usually with digoxin toxicity, you can have underlying atrial fibrillation or paroxysmal atrial tachycardia, with varying degrees of atrioventricular (AV) block. However, when a patient is digoxin toxic, the ventricular response is usually much slower than 100, let alone 146, so in this case I would not suspect digoxin toxicity.

SG: Beyond that, if the patient is maintaining this rhythm even if they are digoxin toxic, and even if you run a digoxin level and it's high, running a tachycardia in this case is not necessarily a bad thing. As an aside, this is why digoxin levels are often not useful. Many patients can be clinically therapeutic at seemingly toxic levels, while others can be clinically digitalized at very low levels.

PR: Is there utility in obtaining an early echocardiogram on this patient, potentially looking for a PE? Even though she has infiltrates, couldn't she have had a PE as the precipitating cause?

SG: Echocardiography should be limited to a patient whose CVP measurements do not respond to your initial volume-repletion or antibiotic therapy, and remain hypotensive and tachycardic.

PR: Here we have a patient who clearly looks and acts ill, has a source of fever, and even though she initially responds somewhat to therapy, she continues to look ill. Would you agree that it's well worth taking away the work of ventilation from this patient by intubating her?

AM: I think intubation in sick septic patients is useful not only by decreasing the work of breathing, but, as in our patient, to also help maximize the oxygenation. However, we must remember that when we intubate patients, we increase intrathoracic pressure, and if this patient is already hypotensive and hypovolemic, increasing intrathoracic pressure is going to decrease preload and decrease cardiac output and blood pressure even more. So when this type of patient gets intubated, we need to do everything possible to get fluids in as quickly as possible, otherwise that patient is going to drop the blood pressure further right after intubation.

PR: Although I wouldn't worry about the patient's atrial fibrillation until we felt that we had strongly and effectively managed the sepsis, atrial fibrillation always worries me with its potential for cerebral embolization. Is this a patient who you feel ought to be anticoagulated?

AM: I would anticoagulate a patient if there was uncertainty regarding how long the atrial fibrillation had been going on. Given the uncertainty in this patient's history, and I don't think that you are going to get more useful information here, I would start heparin.

SG: There is no rush to anticoagulate here since the AF may terminate itself over the course of the next few hours, while treatment for sepsis gets underway in earnest.

PR: It looks like the patient was thought to have sepsis. Aggressive management of the sepsis was undertaken, and the atrial fibrillation was thought to be less important in the management of this patient. Should this patient have any other cardiac evaluations, or are you content to just leave your money on sepsis?

AM: I would check the rest of the electrolytes and renal function, but the only additional test that I would do is to check thyroid function studies.

PR: I think that's a very good idea, as we forget that atrial fibrillation may be the presentation of hyperthyroidism in the elderly, and that cardiac manifestations often outweigh the peripheral manifestations that we see in younger patients with thyrotoxicosis. Nevertheless, this is not somebody who needs immediate management of a thyroid condition, unless this were thyroid storm.

AM: If we truly were considering thyroid storm, then I would start steroids, and maybe give earlier consideration to the use of a beta-blocker, but the rest of her treatment with propylthiouracil (PTU) and iodine, I would coordinate with the admitting team. I would still focus on fluid resuscitation.

SG: I'm very reluctant to give beta-blockers to patients in shock, and would be very judicious in their use in this population.

PR: In summary, we have a patient whose care could easily be blinded by the dysrhythmia, but the correct approach is the one that was taken here; go after the sepsis and worry less about the dysrhythmia until after your sepsis has been addressed, and by then hopefully your patient will have responded.

Case resolution

By the following morning, the patient had spontaneously converted to sinus rhythm, was off all pressors and oxygen support, and was able to transfer out of intensive care. She was discharged from the hospital 2 days later, and was doing well in sinus rhythm on her 6-month follow up.

Section III: Concepts

Background

The mechanism of atrial fibrillation is that of multiple disorganized re-entrant circuits within the atria. The atrial rate is often so fast (350–600) that P waves are not seen on an EKG, and since the atrial discharge rate may be in the 300s, many of these impulses will encounter refractory myocardium at the AV node. Only a portion of atrial impulses will reach the ventricles, causing an irregular and sometimes rapid ventricular rate (Figure 6-1). This affects hemodynamics predominantly in two ways: (1) rapid ventricular rates decrease the time of diastolic filling, and (2) the loss of an organized atrial impulse eliminates

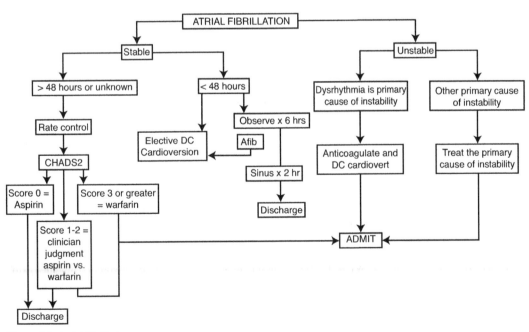

Figure 6.1 Atrial fibrilation.

the contribution of the atria to ventricular filling. Also, because of the loss of the organized atrial contraction, there is a stasis of blood in the atria that leads to a significant risk of thrombus formation and subsequent embolization of that thrombus. In part due to this mechanism, atrial fibrillation is a significant cause of morbidity and mortality in the US. The cardiovascular event risk for patients older than 60 with lone atrial fibrillation has been quoted as high as 5% per year.[1] Atrial fibrillation increases the risk of stroke fivefold and, even when adjusted for other cardiovascular conditions, atrial fibrillation is associated with as high as a 1.5 to 1.9-fold increase in mortality.[2,3] Furthermore, atrial fibrillation is estimated to be present in approximately 2.3 million Americans, and has been projected to affect 5.6 million by the year 2050.[4]

Initial atrial fibrillation workup

The first consideration when encountering a patient with atrial fibrillation, much like any other patient in the ED, is the question: Is the patient stable or unstable? Does the patient appear to be in distress? What are the vital signs? Is the patient tachycardic, hypotensive or hypoxic? Is the patient showing signs of hypoperfusion such as altered mental status, chest pain, or mottling? Does the patient show signs of pulmonary edema? Does the patient have other signs of heart failure such as jugular venous distention or pedal edema? As these assessments are being made, the patient should be placed on oxygen and monitoring. Laboratory tests should be drawn, and access should be obtained, preferably with the placement of two large bore IVs if the patient is unstable. An EKG should be obtained and interpreted fully, particularly for rhythm, rate, and signs of ischemia. Other clues from the EKG that may aid in management include signs of electrolyte abnormalities, atrial enlargement, left ventricular hypertrophy, and right heart strain. Look for delta waves or wide complex rhythms that may be due to an underlying Wolfe-Parkinson-White syndrome (WPW); this would change management decisions regarding pharmacologic rate control, as AV nodal blocking agents are contra-indicated in wide complex WPW tachycardias. The UK National Institute for Health and Clinical Excellence and the joint American-European Atrial Fibrillation guidelines, as well as the European Resuscitation Council guidelines, define instability as ventricular rates >150, persistent chest pain, systolic blood pressure <90 mmHg, heart failure, or reduced consciousness.[5,6,7]

If the patient is found to be unstable, then time is of the essence. Obtaining a few other key clues from history and physical examination will help direct you to the safest course of action, as not all unstable patients with atrial fibrillation are unstable because of the atrial fibrillation. Advanced cardiac life support guidelines recommend immediate DC cardioversion for all unstable patients with rapid atrial fibrillation; however, considering that the tachycardia may have been triggered by the body's effort to compensate for hypotension caused by another primary source (such as hypovolemia or sepsis), attempts to slow the rate in these cases have potential to worsen the patient's condition. In these specific situations, the safest course of action may be to direct therapy to the primary source of instability rather than at the atrial fibrillation (for instance, by providing volume or pressor support that may, in itself, reduce the ventricular response rate). A focused physical examination at this juncture should look for other sources of instability such as infection, other sepsis, gastrointestinal hemorrhage, hypovolemia, or signs of chronic heart disease like diffuse volume overload. Similarly, a focused history at this time, if obtainable, in addition to assessing for symptoms of instability like chest pain, should investigate symptoms suspicious for infection, gastrointestinal bleeding, hypovolemia, coronary artery disease, thyroid disease, alcohol use, and drug use, as well as the duration of the current symptoms. A history of symptoms for fewer than 48 hours may contribute to management decisions, given that anticoagulation has typically been recommended prior to cardioversion of patients with symptoms for longer than 48 hours. However, the risk of thromboembolic events in patients with atrial fibrillation for less than 48 hours has been shown to be less than 1%, and thus, in this instance, anticoagulation is generally not needed.[8] It is also important to know if this is the first episode of atrial fibrillation, or a recurrence of paroxysmal atrial fibrillation. If it is not new-onset atrial fibrillation, then it is also valuable to know the patient's history related to atrial fibrillation including home medications (including any anticoagulants), any history of cardioversion, and subsequent recurrence. Lastly, if the patient is unstable, and you anticipate having to initiate treatment rapidly, anticoagulation may be indicated, and it is important to know if the patient has any contra-indications to anticoagulation.

Etiologies of atrial fibrillation

The etiologies of atrial fibrillation are varied and numerous, including everything from infectious to ischemic, endocrine, toxicologic, postsurgical, and obstructive causes. In fact, anything that can precipitate sinus tachycardia can also precipitate atrial fibrillation; examples include infection, congestive heart failure, hypovolemia, anemia, pulmonary embolism, alcohol intake, hyperthyroidism, electrolyte abnormalities, valvular disease, and even electrocution. The Framingham study demonstrates diabetes, hypertension, congestive heart failure, valvular disease, and myocardial infarction to be significant risk factors in the development of atrial fibrillation.[3] In addition to all of the previously mentioned etiologies, atrial fibrillation can also be idiopathic.

Binge alcoholics frequently present with atrial dysrhythmias, the most common of which is an atrial fibrillation that usually converts to normal sinus rhythm within 24 hours. This syndrome, called a " holiday heart," should be considered in all ED patients presenting with new-onset atrial fibrillation without structural heart disease. Possible mechanisms include increased secretion of epinephrine and norepinephrine, increased sympathetic output, and a rise in the level of plasma-free fatty acids and acetaldehyde metabolites of alcohol. Calcium channel blockade is very effective if rate control is needed. If the patient is failing, has chest pain, or doesn't convert within 24 hours, then this may not be "holiday heart," and general protocols for atrial fibrillation management should be followed.[9,10,11]

Atrial fibrillation may be a consequence of inflammatory states that cause atrial structural remodeling. Correlation has been found between elevated C-reactive protein (CRP) levels and the atrial fibrillation burden, meaning that those patients with atrial fibrillation have higher levels of CRP than controls, and that those patients with persistent atrial fibrillation have higher CRP levels than those with paroxysmal episodes.[12,13] Patients with atrial fibrillation and underlying idiopathic dilated cardiomyopathy have higher serum levels of CRP than those without.[14] In addition, myocardial tissue samples from patients with atrial fibrillation demonstrate increased levels of oxidative damage as compared to controls without atrial fibrillation, supporting the theory that

inflammatory change underlies the development of atrial fibrillation.[15] This theory also explains why low-level chronic inflammatory states like diabetes and coronary artery disease are risk factors for the development of atrial fibrillation, as well as why acute inflammatory states (like postoperative recovery, ischemia or infection) can precipitate or exacerbate atrial fibrillation.

A particularly complicating fact is that in the case of congestive heart failure or hypotension, atrial fibrillation can be either the cause or the effect, and the correct sequence as to which came first can be hard to distinguish, especially in the acute care setting.

Testing

The testing indicated varies greatly with the clinical situation. The diagnosis of atrial fibrillation itself can be made simply by reviewing an EKG; however, diagnosing the etiology of the atrial fibrillation, or the acute episode of rapid ventricular response, is more of a challenge given the myriad of etiologies listed previously. In the patient presenting with a new-onset asymptomatic atrial fibrillation without obvious cause, an acceptable workup in the ED would include complete blood count, electrolytes, TSH, and chest X-ray study. Patients who are being maintained on anticoagulants should have a coagulation panel checked. For the remainder of patients, the workup is directed by a pertinent history and other complaints. For instance, in the diabetic patient with abdominal pain, mesenteric ischemia should be ruled out. For the cancer patient with sudden onset pleuritic chest pain, pulmonary embolism should be investigated. The patient who has significant chest pain and ST-segment changes on EKG should be ruled out for myocardial infarction (MI).

The patient with chest pain and ST changes on EKG can be a challenge, because depending on the rate of the atrial fibrillation, there may be chest symptoms and EKG changes that are simply related to rate. Zimetbaum, et al.[16] examined the incidence and predictors of myocardial infarction among 255 patients with atrial fibrillation in the ED. They find the incidence of acute MI in new-onset atrial fibrillation patients to be approximately 11%, agreeing with a prior study that cites the incidence at 11% for new onset AF.[17] The incidence of MI in all comers to the

ED with AF is 2.3% in the Zimetbaum study; however, this does not exclude patients who had preexisting atrial fibrillation. The sensitivity and specificity of chest pain for acute MI in atrial fibrillation are 100% and 65%, respectively, with a positive predictive value of 14%. The most sensitive and specific predictor of MI is the presence of major ST-segment deviation—defined as >2 mm of ST-segment depression or any ST-segment elevation—on the presenting EKG. This factor has a positive predictive value of 86% and a negative predictive value of 100%. This study does not note the average heart rate on the presenting EKG for these patients.

There is controversy about whether to measure levels of cardiac enzymes in patients with atrial fibrillation, and specifically with rapid atrial fibrillation. Troponins may be elevated as the result of demand ischemia, the mechanism for which is twofold. Tachycardia causes an increase in the myocardial oxygen demand, while also decreasing the time for diastolic subendocardial perfusion. The clinical significance of this subendocardial demand ischemia is largely dependent on the degree of ischemia. This can also be further modified by the patient's underlying coronary artery disease, diastolic dysfunction, and length of time in tachycardia. As such, the next challenging decision for the emergency physician is what to do about the elevated troponin when it results. In some scenarios, it may be hard to differentiate ischemia as the cause or the effect of the rapid ventricular response. Some would argue that if cardiac ischemia is unlikely to be the cause of the atrial fibrillation, and if clinically significant demand ischemia is unlikely, measuring cardiac enzymes may provide more questions than useful answers. Appropriate rate or rhythm control should be undertaken as needed, and measurement of cardiac enzymes may be undertaken depending on the clinical scenario. Decisions regarding how to treat elevated enzymes may necessitate cardiology consultation, and hospital admission for further observation or testing.

Acute management

Atrial fibrillation with rapid ventricular response is a common occurrence in the ED, and can be appropriately treated with rate control, rhythm control, directed therapy for the underlying cause, or anticoagulation,

depending on the clinical situation. Critical decision points are whether the patient is stable or not, and whether the patient has been in atrial fibrillation for longer than 48 hours.

Determination of instability has been outlined above. Current clinical guidelines dictate direct current cardioversion for patients determined to be unstable.[6] Given these guidelines, it is unethical to randomize acutely unstable patients to other treatments, and, as such, there are no prospective clinical trials investigating other therapies (e.g., fluids or pressors) directed toward treating underlying causes of unstable atrial fibrillation, such as sepsis or hypovolemia. DC cardioversion is recommended over chemical cardioversion in this setting because of the delayed effect of chemical cardioversion. Furthermore, even for the stable patient who has been in atrial fibrillation for under 48 hours, DC cardioversion is often preferred to chemical cardioversion, not only because of the immediate effect of electrical cardioversion, but also because of the higher success rate and lower incidence of prodysrhythmic complications with DC cardioversion.[18] Current ACC/AHA guidelines also recommend administration of heparin prior to emergent cardioversion; however, this should not significantly delay cardioversion.[19]

Once the patient in AF has been determined to be stable, the choice becomes rate control or rhythm control. If the patient has been in atrial fibrillation for less than 48 hours, the risk of atrial thrombus is less than 1%; therefore, attempts may be made at elective cardioversion to sinus rhythm in the ED without necessitating anticoagulation for three weeks prior to cardioversion.[8] However, atrial thrombi are reported to be present on transesophageal echocardiography (TEE) in 15% of patients whose symptoms were reported to be less than 48 hours in duration.[20] In addition, atrial fibrillation very frequently has "silent" or asymptomatic episodes, so a patient's description of duration of symptoms may inaccurately predict actual duration of the dysrythmia.[21] Therefore, current ACC/AHA guidelines do recommend starting anticoagulation with heparin or lovenox at presentation even for patients with atrial fibrillation of less than 48 hours duration, as there may still be thrombus formation even after sinus rhythm is restored.[6,22–24] Current guidelines suggest that anticoagulation be used postcardioversion for all patients who have other stroke risk factors (based

Table 6-1. The CHADS2 score.

A decision tool guiding long-term anticoagulation in patients with atrial fibrillation based on stroke risk.

C	Congestive heart failure	1
H	Hypertension	1
A	Age >75	1
D	Diabetes	1
S	Prior stroke	2

Score 0: aspirin therapy only
Score 1–2: physician judgment
Score 3 or greater: coumadin

on CHADS2, see Table 6-1) or if the patient has had more than one episode of paroxysmal atrial fibrillation.[6] The AFFIRM trial in 2002 demonstrates that rate control is at least equivalent to rhythm control in the management of atrial fibrillation.[25] Considering this, and the frequency with which the length of the dysrythmia is unknown, many ED patients, including all who have stable symptoms of greater than 48 hours duration, are treated with rate control and some form of anticoagulation. Patients may electively be cardioverted as outpatients after an adequate period of anticoagulation. For patients who have a significant contra-indication to anticoagulation, TEE should be performed to assess the presence of thrombus before any attempt at elective cardioversion is made.

There are several options for rate control of atrial fibrillation in the ED, including calcium channel blockers (e.g., diltiazem, verapamil), beta-blockers (e.g., esmolol, metoprolol), magnesium, and amiodarone (Table 6-2). The use of digoxin acutely in the ED is limited due to its delayed effect on rate control. The use of IV amiodarone for acute rate control has a high incidence of side effects including hypotension.[26] Magnesium has been shown to be safe and effective for rate control, and has been demonstrated to be as effective as amiodarone and diltiazem for this purpose regardless of underlying magnesium depletion.[27] The two most popular options are calcium channel blockade and beta-blockade. Diltiazem has been shown to be superior to both digoxin and amiodarone for acute rate control in atrial fibrillation.[28] In addition, another study demonstrates that diltiazem and metopolol are both safe and effective for ventricular rate control; however, the effect with diltiazem is greater and is seen earlier than that of metoprolol.[29] Depending on the clinical situation, one class may be more beneficial

Table 6-2. Rate control medications for atrial fibrillation with rapid ventricular response.

Drug	Patient Population	Loading Dose	Maintenance Dose	Onset	Approximate Half-life	Side Effects
Diltiazem	Stable patients	0.25mg/kg IV over 2 min	5–15 mg/hr	2–7 min	Moderate (hours)	Hypotension, decreased AV nodal conduction
Metoprolol	Ischemia, thyrotoxicosis	2.5–5mg IV bolus over 2 min. Up to 3 doses	n/a	5 min	Moderate (hours)	Hypotension, decreased AV nodal conduction, bronchospasm
Esmolol	Ischemia, thyrotoxicosis	0.5mg/kg over 1 min	0.05–0.2 mg/kg/min	5 min	Short (minutes)	Hypotension, decreased AV nodal conduction, bronchospasm
Magnesium	Mg-depleted (alcoholics)	1g over 20 min	Variable	5 min	Short (minutes)	Hypotension
Amiodarone	Wide complex tachycardia	150mg IV bolus over 10 min	1mg/min for 6 hr, then 0.5mg/min for 18hr	20 min	Long (days)	Hypotension
Digoxin	Refractory to first line therapy	0.25mg IV Q2hrs up to 1.5mg	n/a	2 hours	Long (days)	Digoxin toxicity, heart block

than the other. For instance, in the case of myocardial ischemia or postcardiac surgery patients, beta-blockade may have additional benefit. In the case of the patient with systolic dysfunction, calcium channel blockade may be more likely to precipitate hypotension. There are some studies, however, that report that pretreatment with IV calcium may blunt the hypotensive effect of calcium channel blockers while preserving the rate controlling effects.[30] In the patient with underlying reactive airway disease, calcium channel blockade may be chosen over beta-blockade to prevent the precipitation of bronchospasm.

In addition to controlling rate or rhythm, attention needs to be paid to decreasing the incidence of secondary embolic events with anticoagulation. The CHADS2 scoring system (Table 6-1) has been validated as a tool to determine which patients in atrial fibrillation need chronic anticoagulation.[31,32] Patients get one point each for congestive heart failure, hypertension, age greater than 75 years, and diabetes, and two points for having a prior stroke. By this scoring system, patients with a score of 0 may be managed with aspirin therapy only. Scores of 1–2 are left up to the physician's clinical judgment (though current guidelines favor warfarin therapy), and a score of 3 or greater indicates chronic warfarin therapy.[6]

Disposition

Emergency department patients with new-onset atrial fibrillation who have other significant comorbidities (particularly cardiac disease), instability, or concurrent ischemia should be admitted to the hospital for further management. Furthermore, patients for whom anticoagulation is indicated benefit from inpatient admission for initiation of anticoagulation and rate controlling therapy. Patients who have significant contraindications to anticoagulation may need to be admitted to the hospital for TEE to assess for thrombus formation, and to weigh the risks and benefits of cardioversion versus chronic rate control.

Patients who have been in stable atrial fibrillation for less than 48 hours and who convert back to a sinus rhythm in the ED may be observed for a short period and discharged with close follow up. Another choice in managing patients with stable atrial fibrillation for less than 48 hours is to simply observe the patient for a period, as approximately 50% of patients who

have been in atrial fibrillation for less than 48 hours will spontaneously revert back to a sinus rhythm.[33] Current guidelines recommend administering heparin or lovenox upon presentation for these patients.[6] One study evaluated a protocol for observation of these patients in the ED, with electrical cardioversion at 6 hours if not already spontaneously converted. Eighty-five percent of patients are able to be discharged from the observation unit after converting to a sinus rhythm, and remaining in a sinus rhythm for 2 hours. Thirty-two percent convert spontaneously with only rate controlling medications.[34] The utility of ED observation protocols for this clinical scenario greatly depends on the volume and resources of each individual ED.

Section IV: Decision making

- Decide if the patient is stable or unstable.
- Treat the underlying cause of instability first.
    If the rapid ventricular rate is the cause, emergently cardiovert and anticoagulate.
    If there is a more likely physiologic cause of instability, initial treatment should be directed here.
- In the stable ED patient with atrial fibrillation, attempt rate control or DC cardioversion if within 48 hours of onset.
- Admission may not be necessary unless there are underlying signs of ischemia or concurrent acute medical issues.
- Most patients should have anticoagulation postcardioversion.

References

1 Kopecky SL, Gersh BJ, McGoon MD, et al. Lone atrial fibrillation in elderly persons: a marker for cardiovascular risk. *Arch Intern Med.* 1999;159:1118–1122.

2 Wolf PA, Abbott RD, Kannel WB. Atrial fibrillation as an independent risk factor for stroke: the Framingham Study. *Stroke.* 1991;8:983–988.

3 Benjamin EJ, Wolf PA, D'Agostino RB, et al. Impact of atrial fibrillation on the risk of death: the Framingham Heart Study. *Circulation.* 1998;98:946–952.

4 Go AS, Hylek EM, Phillips KA, et al. Prevalence of diagnosed atrial fibrillation in adults: national implications for rhythm management and stroke prevention: the

Anticoagulation and Risk Factors in Atrial Fibrillation (ATRIA) Study. *JAMA*. 2001;285:2370–2375.

5 National Collaborating Centre for Chronic Conditions. *Atrial fibrillation: national clinical guideline for management in primary and secondary care.* London, UK: Royal College of Physicians; 2006.

6 Fuster V, Ryden LE, Cannom DS, et al. ACC/AHA/ESC 2006 guidelines for the management of patients with atrial fibrillation: full text: a report of the American College of Cardiology/American Heart Association Task Force on practice guidelines and the European Society of Cardiology Committee for Practice Guidelines (Writing Committee to Revise the 2001 guidelines for the management of patients with atrial fibrillation) developed in collaboration with the European Heart Rhythm Association and the Heart Rhythm Society. *EuroPACE*. 2006;8:651–745.

7 Nolan JP, Deakin CD, Soar J, et al. European Resuscitation Council Guidelines for Resuscitation 2005. Section 4. Adult advanced life support. *Resuscitation*. 2005;67(S1): S39–S86.

8 Weigner MJ, Caulfield TA, Danias PG, Silverman DI, Manning WJ. Risk for clinical thromboembolism associated with conversion to sinus rhythm in patients with atrial fibrillation lasting less than 48 hours. *Ann Intern Med*. 1997;126:615–620.

9 Thornton JR. Atrial fibrillation in healthy non-alcoholic people after an alcoholic binge. *Lancet*. 1984;2: 1013–1015.

10 Engel TR, Luck JC. Effect of whiskey on atrial vulnerability and "holiday heart." *J Am Coll Cardiol*. 1983;1:816–818.

11 Menz V, Grimm W, Hoffmann J, Maisch B. Alcohol and rhythm disturbance: the holiday heart syndrome. *Herz*. 1996;21:227–231.

12 Chung MK, Martin DO, Sprecher D, et al. C-reactive protein elevation in patients with atrial arrhythmias: inflammatory mechanisms and persistence of atrial fibrillation. *Circulation*. 2001;104:2886–2891.

13 Psychari SN, Apostolou TS, Sinos L, et al. Relation of elevated C-reactive protein and interleukin-6 levels to left atrial size and duration of episodes in patients with atrial fibrillation. *Am J Cardiol*. 2005;95:764–767.

14 Dai S, Zhang S, Guo YH, et al. C-reactive protein and atrial fibrillation in idiopathic dilated cardiomyopathy. *Clin Cardiol*. 2009;32(9):E45–50.

15 Mihm MJ, Yu F, Carnes CA, et al. Impaired myofibrillar energetics and oxidative injury during human atrial fibrillation. *Circulation*. 2001;104:174–180.

16 Zimetbaum PJ, Josephson ME, McDonald MJ, et al. Incidence and predictors of myocardial infarction among patients with atrial fibrillation. *J Am Coll Cardiol*. 2000;36:1223–1227.

17 Friedman H, Weber-Bornstein N, Deboe S, Mancini JGB. Cardiac care unit admission criteria for suspected acute myocardial infarction in new-onset atrial fibrillation. *Am J Cardiol*. 1987;59:866–869.

18 Flaker GC, Blackshear JL, McBride R, et al. The Stroke Prevention in Atrial Fibrillation Investigators. Antiarrhythmic drug therapy and cardiac mortality in atrial fibrillation. *J Am Coll Cardiol*. 1992;20:527–532.

19 Michael JA, Stiell IG, Agarwal S, et al. Cardioversion of paroxysmal atrial fibrillation in the emergency department. *Ann Emerg Med*. 1999;33:379–387.

20 Stoddard MF, Dawkins PR, Prince CR, Ammash NM. Left atrial appendage thrombus is not uncommon in patients with acute atrial fibrillation and a recent ambolic event: a transesophageal echocardiographic study. *J Am Coll Cardiol*. 1995;25:452–459.

21 Page RL, Tilsch TW, Connolly SJ, et al. Azimilide Supraventricular Arrhythmia Program (ASAP) Investigators. Asymptomatic or "silent" atrial fibrillation: frequency in untreated patients and patients receiving azimilide. *Circulation*. 2003;107:1141–1145.

22 Manning WJ, Silvermann DI, Katz SE, et al. Impaired left atrial function after cardioversion: relation to the duration of atrial fibrillation. *J Am Coll Cardiol*. 1994;23:1535–1540.

23 Falcone RA, Morady F. Armstrong WF. Transesophageal echocardiographic evaluation of left atrial appendage function and spontaneous contrast formation after chemical or electrical cardioversion of atrial fibrillation. *Am J Cardiol*. 1996;78:435–439.

24 Kinch JW. Davidoff R. Prevention of embolic events after cardioversion of atrial fibrillation: current and evolving strategies. *Arch Intern Med*. 1995;155:1353–1360.

25 Wyse DG, Waldo AL, DiMarco JP, et al. The Atrial Fibrillation Follow-up Investigation of Rhythm Management (AFFIRM) Investigators. A comparison of rate control and rhythm control in patients with atrial fibrillation. *N Engl J Med*. 2002;347:1825–1833.

26 Kosinski EJ, Albin JB, Young E, Lewis SM, LeLand OS Jr. Hemodynamic effects of intravenous amiodarone. *J Am Coll Cardiol*. 1984;4:565–570.

27 Onalan O, Crystal E, Daoulah A, et al. Meta-analysis of magnesium therapy for the acute management of rapid atrial fibrillation. *Am J Cardiol*. 2007;99:1726–1732.

28 Siu CW, Lau CP, Lee WL, Lam KF, Tse HF. Intravenous diltiazem is superior to intravenous amiodarone or digoxin for achieving ventricular rate control in patients with acute uncomplicated atrial fibrillation. *Crit Care Med*. 2009;37:2174–2179.

29 Demircan C, Cikriklar HI, Engindeniz Z, et al. Comparison of the effectiveness of intravenous diltiazem and metoprolol in the management of rapid

ventricular rate in atrial fibrillation. *Emerg Med J.* 2005; 22:411–414.

30 Haft JI, Habbab MA. Treatment of atrial arrhythmias. Effectiveness of verapamil when preceded by calcium infusion. *Arch Intern Med.* 1986;146:1085–1089.

31 Go AS, Hylek EM, Chang Y, et al. Anticoagulation therapy for stroke prevention in atrial fibrillation: how well do randomized trials translate into clinical practice? *JAMA.* 2003;290:2685–2692.

32 Gage BF, Waterman AD, Shannon W, et al. Validation of clinical classification schemes for predicting stroke:

results from the National Registry of Atrial Fibrillation. *JAMA.* 2001;285:2864–2870.

33 Dell'Orfano JT, Patel H, Wolbrette DL, Luck JC, Naccarelli GV. Acute treatment of atrial fibrillation: spontaneous conversion rates and cost of care. *Am J Cardiol.* 1999;83:788–790, A10.

34 Decker WW, Goyal DG, Boie ET, et al. A prospective, randomized trial of an emergency department observation unit for acute onset atrial fibrillation. *Acad Emerg Med.* 2003;10:543–544.

7

Superventricular tachycardia

Theodore Chan

Medical Director, Department of Emergency Medicine, University of California,
San Diego Medical Center, Professor of Clinical Medicine, University of California,
San Diego, San Diego, California, USA

Section I: Case presentation

A 28-year-old woman with a history of asthma presented to the Emergency Department (ED) complaining of shortness of breath and increased wheezing over the prior several days. Her symptoms worsened progressively during this time, despite repeated use of the patient's albuterol inhaler. On the day of presentation, she also noted intermittent chest tightness, lightheadedness, and palpitations particularly when exerting herself.

In addition to her inhaler, the patient's only medication was an oral contraceptive. She denied any recent travel or preceding illnesses. She did not smoke, and denied any illegal drug use. The family history was notable for a cardiac condition in her father, the specifics of which were unknown to the patient.

The triage vital signs included: blood pressure 125/62 mmHg, respiratory rate 22 breaths/min, temperature 37.2°C (98.9°F). The triage nurse noted that the "pulse rate was too fast to count." The oxygen saturation was 93% on room air. On initial evaluation, the patient was a young woman in mild respiratory distress, who was able to speak only in short sentences. On chest auscultation, there were diffuse wheezes bilaterally with a prolonged expiratory phase. The cardiac examination was notable for a rapid regular tachycardia with no murmurs, gallops, or rubs. The remainder of the examination was otherwise unremarkable.

The patient was given oxygen by nasal canula, and placed on a cardiac monitor. A 12-lead EKG was obtained demonstrating a rapid, regular narrow QRS complex tachycardia at a rate of 212 beats/min with ST depressions in the infero-lateral leads (Figure 7-1). There were no prior EKGs available for comparison.

Section II: Case discussion

Dr Peter Rosen: This is an interesting tachydysrhythmia case because there is a confounding disease that might force us to alter our approach. If this were simply a patient who developed a tachycardia, and came in with an EKG like this, I suspect most of us would reach immediately for pharmacologic therapy. However, this patient's symptomatology suggests that either she's not tolerating this tachycardia very well, or her problem is her bronchial airway disease. How does this change your approach to this patient?

Dr Amal Mattu: The first thing I would do to treat this patient is to attempt vagal stimulation such as a Valsalva maneuver, avoiding potential interactions between medications and her underlying condition. If this didn't work, then I would go directly to a calcium channel blocker if the patient's blood pressure remains as stable as it is right now. I would avoid adenosine as this may produce worsening bronchospasm in a patient who is already bronchospastic.

Cardiovascular Problems in Emergency Medicine: A discussion-based review, First Edition.
Edited by Shamai A. Grossman and Peter Rosen.
© 2011 John Wiley & Sons, Ltd. Published 2011 by John Wiley & Sons, Ltd.

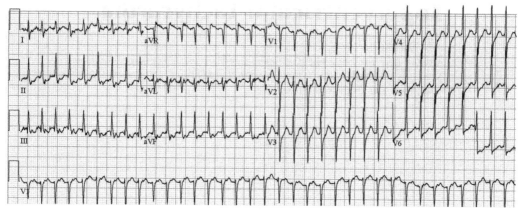

Figure 7.1 Initial 12-lead EKG demonstrating regular, narrow QRS complex tachycardia.

Dr Shamai Grossman: Adenosine also counteracts the effects of theophylline. Formerly, when theophylline was used more regularly in asthma therapy, if patients were given adenosine, it sometimes blocked the effects of the theophylline, and that alone could exacerbate the patient's asthma symptoms. Today, we think about this when patients manifest ischemia during pharmacologic stress tests with adenosine, as here, and we would employ theophylline as the antidote.

PR: I grew up practicing medicine when theophylline was virtually the only treatment we had for asthma, and there are still some practitioners who use it. One of the side effects of theophylline is that it produces tachycardia that persists long after the reactive airway disease is still active. The patients on chronic theophylline therapy often walked around with a pulse rate of 150–180 beats/min. Although this patient denies taking other medications, I would keep in mind that patients frequently do not accurately remember which medications they take.

Dr David Brown: I recall the most characteristic tachycardia associated with theophylline toxicity as MAT, multifocal atrial tachycardia.

SG: You might be thinking of the chronic obstructive pulmonary disease (COPD) patient who takes theophylline, but in general, theophylline is more likely to cause sinus tachycardia or supraventricular tachycardia (SVT).

PR: Along these lines, I wouldn't give this patient a beta-blocker for the supraventricular tachycardia because of the effect on bronchospasm.

PR: What forced you to conclude that this isn't a sinus tachycardia caused by hypoxia?

SG: The first thing that is striking is the rate. A ventricular rate of greater than 200 beats/min is not typical of a sinus tachycardia, which is what you would expect if the patient were having symptoms that were related to the asthma alone. Then you must think, what sort of narrow complex dysrhythmias cause a heart rate in the 200 beats/min range? There aren't too many, besides either an AV nodal reentry (AVRT) or AV reentry tachycardia (AVNRT).

DB: There are retrograde P waves that you can see in the inferior leads just after the QRS complex that further suggest that this is AVRT or AVNRT. Although there is some overlap between those two conditions in terms of where the retrograde P waves show up, the small positive deflections right after the QRS complex in II, III, and AVF suggest that this reentry tachycardia is most likely the less common AVRT.

PR: Is there an upper limit to sinus tachycardia? What rate would you use for a cut-off?

AM: The formula generally used to predict maximum heart rate in stress testing is 220 minus the age. Assuming the patient is neither abusing cocaine nor is hyperthyroid, I would think this formula could be used in this scenario as well.

PR: How effective are vagal maneuvers? All I seem to get when I use one is patients with cold faces and cold limbs, and with hearts still beating very rapidly.

AM: It's difficult to know for sure how effective these maneuvers are. The patients we see represent a very skewed population because, in most patients in whom vagal maneuvers work, they convert themselves at home and never come to the ED. As a result, the vagal maneuvers we do in the ED often don't work because they already failed at home. Nevertheless, although we have a skewed patient population, when a patient presents with an SVT, I think it's still reasonable to give vagal maneuvers a try.

DB: There was a study about 10 years ago that compared the Valsalva maneuver to carotid sinus massage for SVT. It did not show significant differences between the techniques. The study further found that a quarter of these patients converted with vagal maneuvers.[1]

PR: There are a large number of alternative vagal maneuvers that have been described, some of which I would have a hard time getting a patient to allow, such as a digital rectal examination, or putting a patient's face or even one of the limbs in ice water. One maneuver that I found particularly effective is to place a MAST suit on the patient. Many patients would convert because of the blood pressure rise obtained from inflating the MAST suit. However, it's hard to find a MAST suit anymore.

PR: For how long would you try vagal maneuvers before starting pharmacotherapy?

DB: I usually start doing vagal maneuvers while the nurse is drawing up the adenosine or diltiazem. In other words, I generally do not give vagal maneuvers more than a few minutes to work.

PR: I almost never do vagal maneuvers anymore; I just can't see risking a stroke from a carotid massage. I think adenosine is safer, and far more effective. Diltiazem is a good alternative, especially if the dysrhythmia turns out to be rapid atrial fibrillation rather than a supraventricular tachycardia. What would make you want to electrically cardiovert this patient?

Dr Theodore Chan: In this case, as she is hemodynamically stable, the blood pressure is adequate, the mental status is at baseline, and I think the respiratory symptoms are more likely related to her asthma, you have time. In many cases with these types of tachycardias you do have more time, and no need to jump to cardioversion. In this case, it's also useful to

remember she has recently used a beta-agonist, so to allow this medication to wear off, I would probably delay electrical cardioversion a bit longer.

PR: What if the paramedics call this case into you, and say she's beginning to complain of chest pain. It's a rainy night, and it is going to be 30 minutes before they can bring the patient in.

AM: If she's still hemodynamically stable, with a normal mental status and clear lungs, I would still give diltiazem. The alternative would be to sedate her and cardiovert her. In terms of safety, diltiazem has such a good safety profile, and is so effective that, in a person who is hemodynamically stable, it's just a matter of getting to the right dose. However, if she's starting to drop her blood pressure, develop heart failure, or a decreased level of consciousness, then electrical cardioversion would be my first choice.

PR: What dose would of diltiazem would you start with?

AM: I usually start with about 15 mg in an average size person, rather than the weight-based manufacture recommendation, which usually comes to about 20 mg. I prefer to start lower, as given its half-life, it will last for about 45 minutes. If it doesn't work, I would give a second dose 5–10 minutes later. Eventually you will achieve the dose that that will work.

PR: If you gave this patient diltiazem in the field, and she converted to the second EKG here, would you still bring her to the ED?

TC: I am unaware of any EMS agencies that would give a treatment like diltiazem, and not bring her to an ED. In part this is because the diltiazem will remain in her system for a while during which she should be monitored, and in part because the symptoms may recur. Given her ongoing asthma exacerbation, she will probably require hospital admission regardless.

PR: Now that you have converted her tachycardia, is there any interference with your approaches to treating her asthma flare-up? Are you afraid that as you treat her asthma flare, she might revert right back into this supraventricular tachycardia?

SG: I believe that if you treat her asthma flare-up you will make her less likely to revert back to the SVT. Although beta-agonists can cause tachycardia, in this case the asthma likely increased her heart rate in the first place, and if you treat the asthma, her baseline heart rate will actually decrease. I might emphasize here that I would discharge patients who have no other concomitant symptomatology with their SVT and who remain in a sinus rhythm for at least the amount of time it takes to check a set of electrolytes, and ensure that a repeat EKG is normal. Perhaps you might set the patient up with outpatient monitoring, but in a patient who doesn't have a concomitant disease process or signs of ischemia, hospitalization is not particularly useful

PR: Are you aware of any reason why steroids would be contraindicated, or would cause a dysrhythmia recurrence?

DB: I think that they are indicated here for the treatment of asthma, and I would have no hesitation for delivering them.

PR: I might hesitate if I thought the patient was in heart failure, as the steroids could make that a little worse, but I don't think that's the case here. Do you think this patient needs an electrophysiology work-up?

DB: The original tracing showed retrograde P waves that were no longer visible when the patient converted to a sinus rhythm. This confirms that these were retrograde P waves, and clinches the diagnosis of a reentry tachycardia. Given that she has a condition that can be treated definitively with radiofrequency ablation or some similar technique, I would refer her to an electrophysiologist. This way, she may avoid life-long suppressant therapy such as with beta-blockers, which cause depression, or antidysrhythmics that have a host of other side effects. I would also keep in mind that, at age 28, a recurrent SVT is far better tolerated then at 70.

PR: Assuming that she has converted successfully to a sinus rhythm, whether it be through vagal maneuvers or from pharmacology, are there any medications that you like to put the patient on to prevent immediate relapse in the next 48 hours, or are you comfortable with allowing nature to declare itself?

AM: If this is a first time episode, and the patient is not currently on medications, I would check the history for a trigger. Perhaps the patient has been taking a lot of caffeine lately. I've seen chocolate set this off. Perhaps the patient is taking over-the-counter cold

medicines or some other sympathomimetic agent. If it's a first episode, I would tell the patient to stay away from those medicines, and ensure follow up. As long as this is a first, isolated episode that converted easily, I wouldn't start outpatient medication. If this is a recurrent episode where I can't come up with a precipitant, and they are not already on medication for an SVT, then I would probably start a low-dose beta-blocker if there are no contraindications. I would not use a beta-blocker for this patient because of the asthma. Instead, I might start a low-dose calcium channel blocker, and arrange close follow up with a primary care physician, or, preferably, with a cardiologist. Some of my colleagues, however, prefer to initiate medications even with a first episode, if there are no obvious precipitants.

TC: Another option, particularly with recurrent episodes, is to prescribe a calcium channel blocker or beta-blocker that could be taken only when the patient senses that she's having a recurrence of the SVT. This so-called "pill-in-the-pocket" approach could obviate the need for long-term prophylactic therapy.

PR: Are we missing subtle cases of Wolff-Parkinson-White (WPW), or the other congenital accessory tract diseases if the second EKG looks normal? Is there some sort of special diagnostic workup that those patients need to be revealed as having this problem?

SG: If you don't pick up findings consistent with WPW on EKG, either on their posttreatment EKG or on their pretreatment EKG, it is hard to identify WPW in the ED without the patient telling you that they have a history of WPW. The only way you may ultimately know whether this patient has WPW may be with an event or Holter monitor, or if she ends up having an electrophysiology (EP) study.

DB: During the EP study, she could be injected with adenosine when not acutely bronchospastic. This will poison the AV node for a few seconds, and allow her to conduct through a bypass track if it actually exists and is functional. About 70% of reentry tachycardias are caused by AV nodal reentry tachycardia, where the electrical circuit is confined completely to the AV node. However, about 30% are related to AV reentry tachycardia, where the circuit involves a bypass track with orthodromic conduction around this bypass track. These patients have WPW with a functioning bypass track. If these patients go into atrial fibrillation

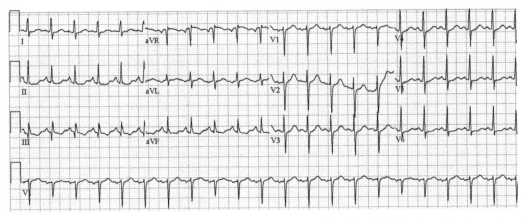

Figure 7.2 Repeat 12-lead EKG following pharmacologic conversion with adenosine. Note the patient is now in a sinus tachycardia with clear P wave activity in a 1:1 AV pattern.

at some point in the future, they could have hemodynamic compromise by rapidly conducting down their bypass tract. This, in my mind, reinforces the need to refer these patients for an EP study.

Case resolution

Despite the patient's asthma exacerbation, the patient underwent cautious treatment in the ED for a supraventricular tachycardia with intravenous adenosine administration, after which she converted to a sinus tachycardia at a rate of 128 beats/min (Figure 7-2). She was also treated for the acute asthma exacerbation with inhaled nebulized albuterol and systemic steroid administration. The asthma symptoms did not improve significantly, perhaps in part due to the administration of adenosine, and she was subsequently admitted to the hospital for further treatment and evaluation. After a two-day hospitalization, during which time the patient's asthma exacerbation resolved and she had no additional episodes of SVT, she was discharged to home in good condition.

Section III: Concepts

Background/epidemiology

Supraventricular tachycardia (SVT), by definition, includes all forms of tachycardia that involve the atria or atrioventricular (AV) node for initiation and continuance. Technically, SVT includes sinus tachycardia, atrial fibrillation, atrial flutter, and multifocal atrial tachycardia, but the term is generally used to refer to the three most commonly encountered forms of paroxysmal, or sudden-onset, SVT, which are atrial tachycardia, AVNRT and AVRT.[2]

Published data on the incidence of SVT in the general population varies widely and depends on what cardiac rhythm disturbances are included in the definition. When referring to paroxysmal tachydysrhythmias, the prevalence is approximately 2.25 per 1,000.[3] Age and gender may influence the prevalence of certain types of SVTs. AVRT often initially presents at a younger age (mid-20s) compared with AVNRT (mid 30s).[4] So-called "lone" paroxysmal SVT (not associated with any cardiac structural disease) is also more commonly present in younger patients. Paroxysmal SVT is more commonly diagnosed in women than men, whereas the opposite is true for atrial flutter.[4]

Paroxysmal SVT can be classified in a number of different ways. First, these tachydysrhythmias can be classified by their underlying etiology, as noted above, as atrial tachycardia, AVNRT, or AVRT. Atrial tachycardias comprise approximately 10% of cases, usually from an atrial focus origin either due to abnormal automaticity or triggered activity. A reentry mechanism is more common, with 60% of cases caused by a reentry circuit located within the AV node (AVNRT), and the other 30% involving an atrioventricular reentry circuit mediated by an accessory pathway (AVRT).[5]

SVTs can also be classified by whether the condition requires AV nodal conduction to maintain the tachydysrhythmia, referred to as AV node-dependent or AV node-independent. This information can be of clinical utility by indicating whether the SVT can be terminated by AV blocking measures. Finally, paroxysmal SVTs can be classified by EKG appearance, such as the duration of the RP interval (long RP tachycardia or short RP tachycardia).

Initial workup history and physical examination

The initial tasks in the ED for patients with SVT are to obtain vital signs, determine the patient's overall hemodynamic and cardiovascular status, and initiate any immediate stabilization measures as warranted. Patients commonly present with a variety of complaints and symptoms, including palpitations, lightheadedness, fatigue, syncope and presyncope, weakness, chest pain or discomfort, anxiety, shortness of breath, diaphoresis, and a pounding sensation in the neck or chest.[6] Increased urinary frequency and polyuria, resulting from the diuretic effect of increased atrial natriuretic factor release in response to elevated atrial pressures (from contraction against a closed AV valve), has been reported with SVT as well.[7] Syncope can be observed in up to 15% of patients with SVT; this is usually just after the initiation of the tachydysrhythmia, or as a result of a long pause following termination of the abnormal rhythm.[4] In addition, syncope may also occur not as a direct result of the SVT, but from a vasovagal response to the dysrhythmia.[8]

Classically, patients complain of sudden onset and occasionally abrupt termination of their symptoms associated with SVT. This paroxysmal quality can assist in differentiating SVT from other tachycardias, including sinus tachycardia, which often has a more gradual onset and termination. However, some patients may not perceive a sudden onset of their associated symptoms; similarly, an abrupt termination may not be obvious, particularly if the patient converts to a rapid sinus tachycardia as a result of anxiety-related increased adrenergic drive or hemodynamic compromise associated with the previous SVT rhythm.

On history, patients should be asked about the duration and frequency of symptomatic episodes and any possible triggers. In particular, patients should be asked about caffeine intake, alcohol consumption, and recreational drug use, which are known precipitants.[5] An SVT can occur in patients of all ages, and is not usually associated with underlying structural heart disease. However, accessory pathways that can play a role in certain types of AVRTs are associated with structural heart conditions, such as Ebstein's anomaly and hypertrophic cardiomyopathy. Similarly, atrial tachycardias may be associated with congenital or acquired heart disease involving the atria. In addition, while SVT is uncommonly associated with myocardial ischemia, this possibility should be considered in older patients who may have a history of underlying coronary atherosclerosis.[2] Finally, an SVT may be the result of an underlying metabolic disorder, such as hyperthyroidism, or electrolyte abnormalities, and additional history should focus on determining if these conditions may be present.

The physical examination should first focus on the patient's vital signs and underlying hemodynamic status. Tachycardia in adults, by definition, is a heart rate greater than or equal to 100 beats/min, and classic SVTs usually present with rates varying from 120–220 beats/min. Higher rates may occur, but these raise concern for other etiologies, including ventricular tachycardia or the conduction of an atrial tachycardia, such as atrial fibrillation, directly down an accessory pathway. Slower ventricular rates can also be seen in the presence of an atrial tachydysrhythmia where AV block or delay is present, such as from pharmacologic beta-blockade.

In many cases, the remainder of the physical examination is often normal, particularly if the patient has converted to a sinus rhythm by the time of the evaluation.[5] During an episode of SVT, examination of the neck veins may reveal intermittent prominent jugular venous A waves from right atrial contractions against a closed tricuspid valve, the so-called "Frog sign."[9] The examination should otherwise focus on evidence of acute cardiac compromise as a result of the dysrhythmia, underlying structural heart disease, or sequelae of possible etiologies (i.e., hyperthyroidism). Rarely, patients who have persistent or long-standing tachycardia (weeks to months) may present with evidence of cardiomyopathy and chronic cardiac failure on examination.[2]

Etiologies

As noted above, SVTs are frequently classified as AV node-independent or node-dependent, which can be helpful in not only determining potential etiologies, but also in providing guidance as to management.

AV Node-Independent: These forms of SVT are independent of AV nodal conduction and arise from a source above the AV node. Most commonly, these types of atrial tachydysrhythmias are caused by a small atrial focus with abnormal automaticity or triggered activity (such as can occur with digoxin toxicity). Although rare, a microreentry circuit within the atrial tissue (such as with Sinus Node Reentry Tachycardia) can occur.

AV node-independent dysrhythmias comprise approximately 10% of all SVTs. Technically, AV node-independent SVTs include sinus tachycardia, atrial flutter, atrial fibrillation, and multifocal atrial tachycardia; these are tachycardias that all arise above the AV node and are independent of AV conduction, but are generally not included in the general use of the term SVT.

Clinically, atrial tachydysrhthmias typically have a regular rhythm and rate, ranging from 100–250 beats/min. Because they are not dependent on the AV node, blockade or delay has little effect on the tachydysrhythmia. AV blockade can slow the ventricular response to the SVT, but does not terminate the atrial tachydysrhythmia.

AV Node-Dependent: The more common forms of SVTs are AV node-dependent. These tachydysrhythmias arise from a reentry circuit that involves the AV node. As a result, AV nodal conduction is necessary to maintain the tachydysrhythmia. Blockade of conduction at the AV node will, in fact, terminate these types of SVTs.

AVNRT occurs when there is a small microreentry circuit located within or near the AV node, and it comprises approximately 50–60% of SVTs. The reentry circuit loop itself is made up of slow and fast pathways with different refractory periods. The SVT is triggered when a premature atrial impulse conducts antegrade to the ventricles down one pathway, and subsequently conducts retrograde back to the atria up the other pathway, thus completing the reentry loop. Because the microreentry circuit is located within or very near the AV node, there is a near simultaneous, rapid activation of both the atria and ventricles.

The other primary form of AV node-dependent SVT is AVRT, which tends to present at an earlier age and more frequently in men than AVNRT.[10]

AVRT has also been associated with certain structural heart diseases, such as congenital Ebstein's anomaly.

AVRT occurs when there is a larger macroreentry circuit that involves the normal conduction pathway through AV node and an accessory bypass tract between the atria and ventricles. Impulses travel from the atria to the ventricles down one of these pathways, and then back to the atria up the other pathway, thus completing the circuit loop.

Orthodromic conduction in an AVRT occurs when antegrade conduction proceeds from the atria to the ventricles through the normal conduction system and AV node, and retrograde conduction takes place from the ventricles back to the atria through the accessory bypass tract. Because activation of the ventricles occurs through the normal conduction pathway (unless there is a preexisting aberrancy), the QRS complex is narrow in orthodromic AVRT. In this case, differentiation from AVNRT can be difficult. Antidromic conduction occurs when antegrade conduction from the atria to the ventricles occurs through the bypass tract, and retrograde conduction occurs from the atria to the ventricles through the normal AV node and conduction system. Because the ventricular activation occurs via the abnormal bypass tract, the QRS complex is abnormally wide and can have a bizarre morphology in antidromic AVRT (Figure 7-3). In this case, differentiation from ventricular tachycardia or other tachycardias with aberrant ventricular conduction can be difficult.

Other less common forms of SVT include focal junctional tachycardia, also known as junctional ectopic tachycardia, and nonparoxysmal junctional tachycardia. These rare AV tachydysrhythmias originate from abnormal automaticity or triggered activity in the AV node, and are often associated with congenital heart disease, presenting in early childhood. Abnormal junctional tachycardias have also been associated with digoxin toxicity, cardiac ischemia and infarction, or following cardiac surgery.

Testing

After the initial physical examination and vital signs, the EKG is the most important test to obtain in a patient with suspected SVT. Whenever possible, it is best to obtain a 12-lead EKG during the SVT, but doing so should not delay immediate therapy to

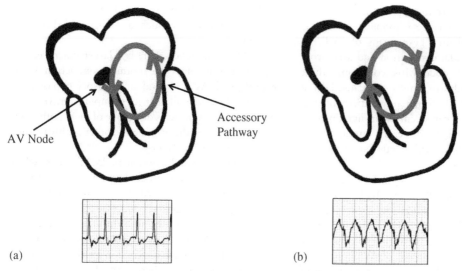

Figure 7.3
A. Reentry mechanism for orthodromic AVRT. Atrioventricular conduction occurs down the AV node and ventriculoatrial conduction up the accessory pathway, resulting in a narrow QRS complex tachycardia.
B. Reentry mechanism for antidromic AVRT. Atrioventricular conduction occurs down the accessory pathway and ventriculoatrial conduction up the AV node, resulting in a wide QRS complex tachycardia.

terminate the abnormal cardiac rhythm if there is hemodynamic instability.[4]

The approach to the 12-lead EKG demonstrating an abnormal tachycardic rate should focus on the regularity of the rhythm and the QRS complex morphology. An irregular tachycardia may be the result of atrial fibrillation, atrial flutter and other atrial tachycardias with variable block, and MAT. A regular tachycardia can occur with sinus tachycardia, atrial tachycardias or atrial flutter (without variable block), and SVTs, including both AVNRT and AVRT.

The QRS complex can be prolonged, regardless of the underlying rate, in the presence of aberrant ventricular conduction, bundle branch block, or preexcitation (in addition to rhythms arising from ectopic ventricular foci, such as VT). In fact, rate-related bundle branch block is relatively frequent in patients with SVT.[2] As noted above, antidromic AVRT results in a wide QRS complex regular tachycardia that is often difficult to distinguish from VT.

In addition to rate, regularity, and QRS complex morphology, the other EKG findings that may be of interest in the setting of SVT include the P-wave morphology, relative position of the P wave in the RR interval (RP and PR interval durations), onset and termination of the dysrhythmias if seen electrocardiographically, and presence or absence of preexcitation on the baseline 12-lead EKG.

Atrial tachycardias typically present as a regular narrow QRS complex tachycardia (except in the presence of aberrant conduction) and have a long RP interval.[11] Atrial tachycardias also most commonly terminate with a ventricular complex, and not an atrial complex or P wave as seen on a 12-lead EKG. Atrial tachycardias can be differentiated from sinus tachycardia by the change in P-wave morphology during sinus and tachycardic rates.

AVNRT classically presents with a regular narrow complex tachycardia, but rate-related aberrant or bundle branch block conduction is common and can result in a wide complex tachycardia. Usually, P waves are not discernable, particularly at rapid rates, but in some cases P waves can be seen superimposed within the QRS complex as pseudo-R, pseudo-Q, or pseudo-S waves. These waves, which are not seen during normal sinus rhythm, can be quite specific for AVNRT.[12] AVNRT is typically a short RP tachycardia, though this again can be difficult to determine with rapid tachycardias. In addition, AVNRT is usually initiated by a premature atrial beat, and terminates with a P wave, unlike atrial tachycardias.

The appearance of AVRT on the 12-lead EKG is dependent on whether conduction is orthodromic or antidromic. Orthodromic AVRT presents as a narrow complex tachycardia (unless aberrant or bundle branch block conduction is present) as ventricular activation occurs down the normal conduction system. Most patients have visible retrograde P waves best seen in V1 and the inferior leads.[13] AVRT is typically a short-RP tachycardia, but if retrograde conduction is significantly delayed, the RP interval can be prolonged. Other electrocardiographic findings more commonly seen with orthodromic AVRT include QRS alternans (alternating QRS complex amplitude) and ST-segment depression more than 2 mm in several leads.[14]

Antidromic AVRT, where ventricular activation occurs through the accessory pathway, results in a wide complex tachycardia. Retrograde P waves are frequently seen, often in a 1:1 ventriculoatrial relationship.[12] The P wave and PR interval are variable, depending on the retrograde conduction through the AV node for atrial depolarization.

With AVRT, evidence of the accessory pathway or ventricular preexcitation may be seen as a shortening of the PR interval and an initial slurring of the QRS complex upstroke on the baseline 12-lead EKG. These so-called delta waves have been reported to be present on EKGs in up to 0.15–0.25% of the general population.[4] Most accessory pathways are capable of bidirectional conduction (anterograde and retrograde). However, a small subset only allow retrograde conduction, and are referred to as "concealed."[5] These accessory pathways do not produce preexcitation or delta waves on the EKG and can only result in orthodromic AVRT. Wolff-Parkinson-White (WPW) syndrome refers to patients who have both preexcitation and tachydysrhythmias. AVRT is the most common dysrhythmia seen in these patients, accounting for 9% of reentry tachycardias in patients with accessory pathways.[4]

Detecting underlying atrial rhythms can be difficult on a standard 12-lead EKG in the setting of SVT because of the rapid ventricular activity. Recording continuous electrocardiographic activity during periods of enhanced AV blockade (thus decreasing the ventricular activity as with vagal maneuvers) can be important in determining the underlying atrial rhythm. In addition, diagnosis can be enhanced by doubling the EKG machine paper speed (from 25 mm/sec to 50 mm/sec), which artificially slows the recording of the cardiac cycle on the paper so that the underlying cardiac rhythm may be easier to detect.[16]

Beyond the standard 12-lead EKG and monitoring, additional testing may not be necessary, depending on the clinical presentation of the patient with SVT. For example, in otherwise healthy patients with prior episodes of AVNRT following a given trigger and no other history of cardiac disease, additional laboratory and radiology testing has a low yield.

Alternatively, if the patient's history and presentation suggest another underlying etiology for the SVT, such as thyroid disease or structural heart disease, further testing is warranted. Additional testing can include serum electrolytes (particularly potassium levels), thyroid function tests, digoxin level, chest radiograph, echocardiogram, and event monitor as indicated. Some of these tests, such as the echocardiogram and event monitor, can be obtained as an outpatient after treatment in the ED.

Treatment and disposition

The initial treatment should focus on acute resuscitative measures as needed if the patient is in a state of cardiovascular collapse. If the patient is otherwise stable, the approach to the patient is to terminate the SVT as safely and expeditiously as possible, using either vagal maneuvers, pharmacologic intervention, or electrical cardioversion. Vagal maneuvers and the pharmacologic interventions generally increase AV block, and in doing so, terminate AV node-dependent SVTs including AVRNT and AVRT. In some cases, AV node-independent atrial tachycardias may also respond to these measures as well, either by slowing of the ventricular response rate or actual termination of the dysrhythmia itself. Because of the potential for rapid deterioration into a life-threatening dysrhythmia, resuscitative equipment, including a defibrillator, should be close at hand.

Vagal maneuvers include carotid massage, Valsalva, and facial immersion in cold water. These measures increase vagal tone and prolong the AV nodal refractoriness, leading to AV block and termination of AV node-dependent SVTs. Carotid massage in the elderly should be undertaken with caution, and only after auscultation to determine the absence of a carotid bruit. Pressure is applied at the level of the cricoid cartilage for approximately five seconds in a firm circular movement, and repeated on the other side if needed.

If these measures are unsuccessful, pharmacologic intervention should be considered. Adenosine induces a transient, but intense, AV blockade that is highly effective in terminating the majority of SVTs. A 6 mg dose has been shown to terminate 62.3% of cases, and the larger 12 mg dose, 91.4% of AV node-dependent SVTs.[17] While the half-life of the medication is quite short, patients should be warned that the medication will cause intense, but transient, chest tightness, nausea, and flushing sensations. The medication should also be used cautiously in the setting of asthma or COPD, as it can cause acute bronchospasm. Adenosine blocks the action of theophylline, and can be potentiated by dipyridamole.

Other pharmacologic agents that may be useful in SVT include calcium channel blocking agents (verapamil, diltiazem) and beta-blocking agents (esmolol, metoprolol). These medications increase AV block, and can be useful in treating AVNRT and AVRT. However, these agents should be used cautiously in the setting of hypotension, history of heart block, or congestive heart failure because of their potential to exacerbate the patient's cardiovascular status.

In addition, these agents should not be used in the setting of WPW or an accessory pathway, where blockade of the AV node can actually increase transmission of impulses down the accessory pathway, leading to potentially lethal ventricular tachydysrhythmias or even ventricular fibrillation. Other antidysrhythmic agents that can be used for SVT, and in particular in the setting of WPW, include procainamide, propafenone, or flecainide.[5] If these measures fail, or if the patient deteriorates and becomes hemodynamically unstable, electrical cardioversion should be performed expeditiously.

If treatment is successful, most patients can be safely discharged home from the ED. Patients should be admitted for further evaluation if they are hemodynamically unstable; have evidence of cardiac injury, ischemia, or compromise such as acute heart failure; or have another underlying condition requiring inpatient care. If discharged, most patients can follow up with their regular provider for further evaluation and testing. Conditions warranting referral to an electrophysiologist include wide complex tachycardias or evidence of a preexcitation syndrome, significant presenting symptoms such as syncope, or recurrent episodes that are having a significant detrimental effect on the patient's life. Subsequent need for further testing (such as an event monitor), and the utility of further treatment including pharmacologic prophylaxis or catheter ablation, can be determined at that time.

Section IV: Decision making

- Accurate diagnosis is the major challenge, as other potentially life-threatening tachydysrhythmias and etiologies must be considered and evaluated.
- The EKG should be assessed for the regularity of the rhythm, QRS width and morphology, and P-wave activity (Table 7-1).
- Treatment options include vagal maneuvers, pharmacologic interventions, and electrical cardioversion.

Table 7-1. Differential diagnosis for tachydysrhythmia.

Regular Rate	Narrow QRS Complex	Sinus Tachycardia
		Sinus Node Reentry Tachycardia
		Atrial Tachycardia
		Atrial Flutter
		AVNRT
		AVRT—orthodromic
		Focal Junctional Tachycardia
		Nonparoxysmal Junctional Tachycardia
	Wide QRS Complex	Regular tachycardias with aberrancy or BBB or preexcitation
		Paced Tachycardia
		AVRT—antidromic
		Ventricular Flutter
		Ventricular Tachycardia
		Hyperkalemia
		Drug Toxicity (tricyclics, cocaine)
Irregular Rate	Narrow QRS Complex	Atrial Fibrillation
		Atrial Flutter with variable block
		Atrial Tachycardias with variable block
		Tachycardia with PACs, PVCs, PJCs
		Digitalis toxicity
		Multifocal Atrial Tachycardia
	Wide QRS Complex	Irregular tachycardias with aberrancy or BBB or preexcitation
		Polymorphic VT (torsades de pointes)

Table 7-2. Emergency department interventions for patients in svt.

Vagal Maneuvers	Valsalva
	Carotid Sinus Massage
	Facial Ice Water Immersion
Pharmacologic Interventions	Adenosine
	Calcium Channel Blocking Agents
	– Diltiazem
	– Verapamil
	Beta-Blocking Agents
	– Metoprolol
	– Propranolol
	– Esmolol
Pharmacologic Interventions in setting of:	Procainamide
	Flecainide
	Propafenone
– Refractory SVT	Ibutilide
– Atrial Fibrillation with Preexcitation	
Electrical Cardioversion	

- Avoid drugs like digoxin that increase conduction via the accessory pathway, given the risk of precipitating very rapid ventricular rates or ventricular fibrillation (Table 7-2).
- Most patients treated in the ED for SVT can be discharged to home safely, assuming hemodynamic stability and no co-morbid conditions.

References

1 Lim SH, Anantharaman V, Teo WS, Goh PP, Tan ATH. Comparison of treatment of supraventricular tachycardia by valsalva maneuver and carotid sinus massage. *Ann Emerg Med.* 1998;31:30–35.
2 Fox DJ, Tschenko A, Krahn D, et al. Supraventricular tachycardia: diagnosis and management. *Mayo Clin Proc.* 2008;83:1400–1411.
3 Orejarena LA, Vidaillet H Jr, DeStefano F, et al. Paroxysmal supraventricular tachycardia in the general population. *J Am Coll Cardiol.* 1998;31:150–157.
4 Blomstrom-Lundqvist C, Scheinman MM, Aliot EM, et al. ACC/AHA/ESC guidelines for the management of patients with supraventricular arrhythmias—executive summary. *J Amer Coll Cardiol.* 2003;42:1493–1531.
5 Delacretaz E. Supraventricular tachycardia. *New Engl J Med.* 2006;354:1039–1051.
6 Brembilla-Perrot B, Marcon F, Bosser G, et al. Paroxysmal tachycardia in children and teenagers with normal sinus rhythm and without heart disease. *Pacing Clin Electrophysiol.* 2001;24:41–45.
7 Tikkanen I, Metsarinne K, Fyhrquist F. Atrial natriuretic peptide in paroxysmal supraventricular tachycardia. *Lancet.* 1985;2:40–41.
8 Leitch J, Klein G, Tee R, Murdock C, Teo WS. Neurally mediated syncope and atrial fibrillation (letter). *N Engl J Med.* 1991;324:495–496.
9 Gursoy S, Steuer G, Brugada J, Andreis E, Brugada P. The hemodyamic mechanism of pounding in the neck in atrioventricular nodal reentrant tachycardia. *N Engl J Med.* 1992;327:772–774.
10 Kazzi AA, Wong H: Other supraventricular tachy-dysrhythmias. In: Chan TC, Brady WJ, Harrigan RA, Ornato JP, Rosen P, eds. *ECG in Emergency Medicine and Acute Care.* Philadelphia: Elsevier; 2005.
11 Kalbfleisch SJ, el-Atassi R, Calkins H, Langberg JJ, Morady F. Differentiation of paroxysmal narrow QRS complex tachycardias using the 12-lead electrocardiogram. *J Am Coll Cardiol.* 1993;21:85–89.
12 Kumar UN, Rao RK, Scheinman MM. The 12-lead electrocardiogram in supraventricular tachycardia. *Cardiol Clin.* 2006;24:427–437.
13 Chen SA, Tai CT, Chiang CE, et al. Electrophysiologic characteristics, electropharmacologic responses and radiofrequency ablation in patients with decremental accessory pathway. *J Am Coll Cardiol.* 1996;28:723–727.
14 Jaeggi ET, Gilljam T, Bauersfeld U, et al. Electrocardiographic differentiation of typical atrioventricular node reentrant tachycardia from atrioventricular reciprocating tachycardia mediated by concealed accessory pathway in children. *Am J Cardiol.* 2003;91:1084–1090.
15 Zhong YM, Guo JH, Hou AJ, et al. A modified electrocardiographic algorithm for differentiating typical and atrioventricular node re-entrant tachycardia from atrioventricular reciprocating tachycardia mediated by concealed accessory pathway. *Int J Clin Pract.* 2006;11:1371–1377.
16 Accardi AJ, Holmes JF. Enhanced diagnosis of narrow complex tachycardias with increased electrocardiograph speed. *J Emerg Med.* 2002;22:123–127.
17 DiMarco JP, Miles W, Akhtar M, et al. Adenosine for paroxysmal supraventricular tachycardia: dose ranging and comparison with verapamil: assessment in placebo-controlled, multicenter trials. *Ann Intern Med.* 1990;113:104–110.

The differential diagnosis of wide complex tachycardia—ED diagnostic and management considerations

Nathan Charlton[1] & William J. Brady[2]

[1] Assistant Professor of Emergency Medicine, Department of Emergency Medicine, Consultant in Toxicology, Division of Medical Toxicology, Department of Emergency Medicine, Medical Director, Blueridge Poison Center, University of Virginia Health System, Charlottesville, VA, USA

[2] Vice Chair, Department of Emergency Medicine, Professor of Emergency Medicine and Medicine, University of Virginia Health System, Charlottesville, VA, USA

Section I: Case presentation

A 54-year-old woman drove to the emergency department (ED) with complaints of palpitations and weakness. The patient noted the onset of these symptoms approximately 1 hour prior. She also complained of mild dyspnea. Her medical history was significant for a myocardial infarction with stent placement, congestive heart failure, diabetes mellitus, and hypertension. On examination, the emergency physician found an alert, mildly distressed woman appearing her stated age. The vitals signs were: blood pressure 115/70 mmHg, pulse 180 beats/min, respirations 24 breaths/min, and oxygen saturation of 95% on room air. The cardiac examination revealed a rapid regular rate without murmur or gallop; the lungs were clear to auscultation with appropriate aeration. The cardiac monitor demonstrated a wide complex tachycardia (WCT), rapid and regular (Figure 8-1); the 12-lead EKG showed similar findings (Figure 8-2).

Based upon the patient's age, medical history, and electrocardiographic findings with a WCT, the emergency physician felt that the rhythm was likely ventricular tachycardia (VT). The patient remained hemodynamically stable, but with persistence of the WCT. Intravenous amiodarone (150 mg) was given over approximately 15 minutes, and then repeated. No response was noted after the second dose of amiodarone. Intravenous procainamide was prepared, but,

unfortunately, the patient's respiratory status worsened and the blood pressure dropped to 80 mmHg systolic. Given continued tachycardia recalcitrant to medical therapy and a worsening hemodynamic status, the patient was electrically cardioverted with a return to a sinus rhythm.

Section II: Case discussion

Dr Peter Rosen: I think the most interesting question in the management of an acute tachycardia is, "What do you do first?" Is it necessary to get a 12-lead EKG? How do you decide whether you are going to treat the patient chemically versus giving a counter-shock? What sedation, if any, would you use if you thought the patient needed immediate counter-shock? How much time would you be willing to spend trying to sort out the kind of tachycardia your patient has prior to initiating therapy?

Dr Amal Mattu: I would begin by looking for signs of hemodynamic instability. If the patient is in an unstable tachycardia, then I would consider rapid electrical cardioversion. Hemodynamic instability in the presence of a tachycardia can by defined by four parameters: the presence of hypotension, the presence of a decreased level of consciousness, the presence of acute congestive heart failure, and the presence of ischemic chest pain. Any one of these four parameters would

Cardiovascular Problems in Emergency Medicine: A discussion-based review, First Edition.
Edited by Shamai A. Grossman and Peter Rosen.
© 2011 John Wiley & Sons, Ltd. Published 2011 by John Wiley & Sons, Ltd.

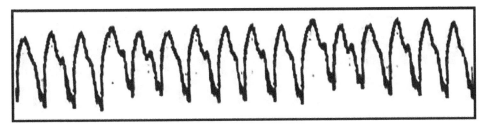

Figure 8.1 Wide complex tachycardia in lead II.

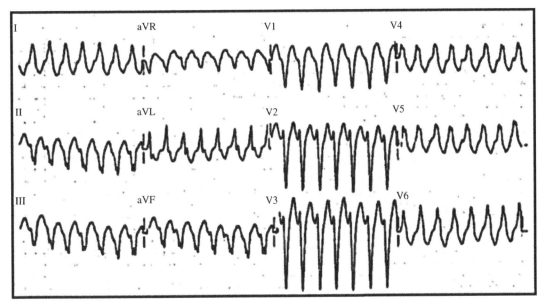

Figure 8.2 Wide complex tachycardia. The rate is approximately 170 bpm with a regular rhythm. Evidence of atrioventricular dissociation is seen in multiple leads.

potentially define an unstable tachycardia. If a patient has an unstable tachycardia, then that patient would likely need electrical cardioversion. A possible exception would be if the patient has minimal symptoms or instability, and the wide complex rhythm is most likely a supraventricular tachycardia; then, in that case, I might try adenosine first if it's readily available.

Regardless of whether I have a 12-lead EKG or not, I can make a decision to cardiovert simply by observing the monitor. The two primary exceptions that I would make are the two tachycardias that one does not cardiovert: sinus tachycardia (ST) and multifocal atrial tachycardia (MAT). Any other tachycardia, narrow or wide, in an unstable patient ought to be cardioverted without worrying about whether it is

ventricular or supraventricular. Of course, the treating physician is the most appropriate person to determine the initial therapeutic strategy.

Dr Shamai Grossman: I would do a 12-lead EKG simply to verify that this is a wide complex rhythm, and that you are not dealing with something artifactual, which is more common than we like to think. This would be particularly appropriate in the hemodynamically stable patient.

PR: What about sedation in this patient?

AM: If the patient can tolerate waiting several minutes for sedation, then ideally I would like to administer etomidate, propofol, or ketamine. If those agents are not readily available, then I would consider a small dose of midazolam. If the patient is markedly unstable, then I would not wait for the sedation, but rather would proceed directly to electrical cardioversion.

PR: Does the patient's age make any difference in this particular protocol? In other words, if you had a very young patient, for example, less than a year old, or an elderly patient, in his late eighties, would that make you move toward cardioversion more quickly?

Dr William Brady: One really must look at the entire patient. The patient's age is another piece of data that must be included along with the other clinical findings, including the patient's complaints, the focused examination, and the electrocardiogram. However, I would not look at age as the primary determinant to drive the decision to electrically cardiovert instead of utilizing medical therapy. Certainly, an older person may be less physiologically able to withstand a dysrhythmia for a long period of time. But, if the patient did present in a stable fashion, and was tolerating the dysrhythmia, I would likely proceed with chemical therapy. Nevertheless, I would be watching that elderly patient even more closely than our patient today, the 54 year old.

PR: Do you think that it's necessary to raise the patient's blood pressure before you attempt to convert chemically or electrically? We know that in paroxysmal atrial tachycardia (PAT), sometimes just a mild raise in blood pressure can cause a conversion. I have seen patients with PAT converted by placing cardioversion pads on them, and getting a 20 mmHg rise without any other therapy whatsoever. Does that play any role in the management of this type of tachycardia, where you have not bothered to distinguish whether it is a ventricular or a supraventricular tachycardia?

SG: No, I would generally not make any effort to raise the blood pressure if the patient is truly hemodynamically unstable. The dysrhythmia is more likely the cause of the hemodynamic instability. I think that the focus has to be on managing the dysrhythmia. Focusing on dysrhythmia management should then increase the blood pressure.

PR: If you had a history that this patient had prior episodes of tachycardia, and that she said she had a congenital condition but cannot remember what it was, would you be inclined to start with a drug other than amiodarone? For example, would you give her procainamide on the grounds that perhaps she had a Wolf-Parkinson-White (WPW) Syndrome?

AM: Assuming that the patient is hemodynamically stable with a wide complex tachycardia, I would look at the rhythm strip first and then a full 12-lead EKG. Of primary importance to me is whether the rhythm is regular or irregularly irregular. If it is a wide regular tachycardia, then I would feel comfortable using amiodarone or procainamide. If it is irregularly irregular, than there are really only two things in the differential: atrial fibrillation with a bundle branch block or atrial fibrillation with WPW. To tell the difference between these two, you must look at the morphology of the QRS complex. If the QRS morphology remains the same beat-to-beat, then the rhythm is likely atrial fibrillation with a bundle branch block, and you can use any agent you want. If the QRS complex has changing morphologies in a beat-to-beat, then that suggests atrial fibrillation with WPW. In caring for this patient, one should avoid using amiodarone. Instead, this patient should be treated chemically with procainamide or cardioverted electrically.

Procainamide is an excellent choice because it is appropriate for ventricular tachycardia, atrial fibrillation with a bundle branch block, and atrial fibrillation with WPW. Although procainamide seems to have fallen out of favor, it is an excellent medication to consider in the stable wide complex tachycardia patient. Regarding other treatments, such as magnesium, I do not think empiric magnesium is very helpful unless the patient has torsades de pointes, or has some type of underlying condition that makes one consider hypomagnesemia.

PR: It seems to me that every time I try to give procainamide, the blood pressure immediately falls. Is that because I run it too fast, or is that just one of the consequences of using that drug?

WB: Procainamide is a very effective medication. It has the ability to treat dysrhythmias that are supraventricular or ventricular in origin. The major drawback to procainamide is it cannot be used rapidly because patients will develop hypotension, and in certain cases can develop worsening intraventricular conduction, such as further widening of the QRS complex.

There are two different methods of procainamide administration that depend on the acuity of the patient and the acuity and volume of rest of your ED. Assuming the patient is stable, if you have the luxury of having a quiet ED and a fair amount of staff to help, you can infuse the drug at a load of 17 mg/kg over about 45 minutes while carefully monitoring the blood pressure and the clinical situation. If the patient is more ill or you must administer the medication more rapidly, one can follow a different protocol by giving the drug in 100–200 mg increments over approximately 2–3 minutes, and repeating that every 5–10 minutes up to a total loading dose. Utilizing this protocol, a full load can be infused much more rapidly. Nevertheless, with both administration strategies, you can develop hypotension. In this case, it may be difficult to determine if the hypotension is related to the tachycardia, or related to your intervention. I would err on the side of caution; if the patient develops hypotension, I would likely call that tachycardia unstable, and consider electrical therapy.

PR: If the patient gave you a history of being on digitalis but came in unstable, would that make you reluctant to use cardioversion?

SG: I think that if that patient is unstable, the therapy of choice, regardless of the patient's past medical or medication history, needs to be electrical cardioversion.

PR: Once the patient is stabilized from a rhythm standpoint, laboratory testing can be pursued. If the first troponin should be slightly elevated, or if the second troponin is slightly elevated, would you then deem it necessary to arrange for immediate angiography on this patient?

WB: The abnormal troponin value must be interpreted within the context of the clinical situation. Thus, if the patient's presentation suggests an acute coronary syndome (ACS) event, then I would pursue therapy as appropriate for ACS, considering the postconversion 12-lead EKG—such, of course, was the case with our presentation in this chapter. If the situation does not suggest ACS, however, then I would likely monitor the patient's situation closely with repeat troponin testing. It must be remembered that a dysrhythmia with or without stability can cause an elevation of the serum troponin.

PR: Two questions: first, going back to the original assessment of this patient, is there any help in the physical examination of the neck in terms of distinguishing the type of tachycardia? The second question is: given the reality that this women almost certainly has an ischemic coronary syndrome, would you place her on antiplatelet therapy?

SG: To answer your first question, I think that starting to look at the neck when you have a patient who is potentially unstable with a wide complex tachycardia would be moving in the wrong direction. Here, I think the focus needs to be on the wide complex tachycardia, and not to be led astray by the question: "Is this an SVT with aberrancy?" This rhythm needs to be considered a ventricular dysrhythmia alone. I think that especially in the extreme conditions of the ED, it is an error to spend prolonged periods of time looking at the physical examination or other adjuncts, with the hope of diagnosing the rhythm disturbance, when you have a potentially unstable patient in front of you.

As far as starting antiplatelet therapy, I think that this depends on the patient's history, and age. The case we are discussing today is someone with known coronary disease who comes in with symptoms that are suggestive of ischemia. This patient most likely has a ventricular tachycardia secondary to either myocardial excitability from an acute ischemic process, or from scarring from the previous infarction. So starting this patient on antiplatelet therapy, especially if she were not already on it, is clearly appropriate given the likelihood that she is actually having an acute ischemic event. If the patient is young with no history of coronary artery disease, or clearly has another etiology for the dysrhythmia, then, starting antiplatelet therapy without a more thorough investigation is not a good idea.

PR: If an EMS unit is en route to your ED with a wide complex tachycardia patient, when would you ask them to perform electrical cardioversion?

WB: I would use the same markers of stability in and out of the hospital. If the patient is unstable or the ETA to the ED is excessive, I would consider a sedative-assisted electrical cardioversion prior to ED arrival. It must be stressed, however, that each case is individual and the management decisions are best made by the treating clinicians.

PR: In summary, I like to remember that an important management decision in any acute tachycardia focuses on the stability of the patient. Further, the urge to over-interpret EKGs must be avoided—recall that the ultimate rhythm diagnosis may not be possible even with the performance and review of a 12-lead EKG. In most instances, it does not matter if the dysrhythmia is ventricular or supraventricular in origin if the patient is unstable: electrical cardioversion is required for both kinds of unstable tachycardia.

WB: I must reiterate the last point, do not focus entirely on the EKG, but interpret it within the context of the clinical presentation. Do not consider the situation a diagnostic failure if you are unable to confirm the rhythm diagnosis in the initial presentation.

To review, many people find themselves in the situation where they feel they must determine the cause of the tachycardia before they can treat it. In this case you have a patient who comes in who does have a wide complex tachycardia. She has several historical features, including her age and her cardiovascular history, which suggest that VT is the likely origin. Certain electrocardiographic features can suggest VT, yet they are uncommon; these are discussed within the chapter. Regardless of the specifics of the presentation, what one must initially determine is the need for emergent electrical cardioversion.

The clinician must also consider the other forms of wide complex tachycardia in this differential, including sinus tachycardia with a bundle branch block, sodium channel blocker poisoning as seen with a tricyclic antidepressant drug overdose, or the unusual case of a hyperkalemia with a very rapid, wide complex rhythm. These scenarios would be rhythm presentations that you would not want to treat electrically. The clinician should be able to sort out these rhythms based on historical clues, with the exception of the sinus tachycardia with a bundle branch block, and this occurrence is quite rare.

When you are left with an SVT with aberrant conduction versus VT, the key is to treat the patient. If the patient presents in an unstable fashion, electrical cardioversion is the therapy of choice. If the patient is stable, observe closely while therapy is initiated. If you are not worried about a Wolf-Parkinson-White-type rhythm disturbance, then amiodarone is a reasonable choice. If you have concern about WPW, then procainamide is a great choice. Realize that the patient can become unstable at any time, if your medications do not work, and that you may need to move rapidly and use electrical therapy to address the problem. I think

that in a situation like this, we always have to keep in mind the rest of what is going on in the ED. If you have a patient who is borderline stable, but have an ED that is very chaotic, then you have another very legitimate reason to move forward, give the patient a sedative agent, and perform electrical cardioversion.

Case resolution

The patient was admitted to the hospital without further WCT. Serial cardiac biomarkers were elevated with a typical rise-and-fall pattern characteristic of an acute myocardial infarction. Cardiac catheterization revealed occlusion of the right coronary artery; this occlusion was stented. The patient was discharged on hospital day three with non-ST-segment elevation myocardial infarction complicated by ventricular tachycardia.

Section III: Concepts

The patient with a wide complex tachycardia (WCT) can present both a diagnostic and a therapeutic challenge to the emergency physician (EP). WCT results from a number of etiologies and produces a variety of patient presentations. The term wide complex tachycardia describes the rhythm scenario characterized by a broad, or widened, QRS complex (greater than 0.12 seconds) and a ventricular rate over 120 beats per minute in the adult patient (Figures 8-1 and 8-2). In children, heart rates and QRS complex widths vary with age. Consequently, children may present with WCT, including ventricular tachycardia, with a QRS duration of less than 120 ms; age-related values of the QRS complex duration and ventricular rate define WCT in younger children (Figure 8-3).[1]

The electrocardiographic differential diagnosis of WCT classically includes VT and supraventricular tachycardia (SVT) with aberrant intraventricular conduction (Table 8-1 and Figures 8-4 and 8-5). Electrocardiographically, VT can be described as either monomorphic (one primary QRS complex type) or polymorphic (greater than one QRS complex type) ventricular tachycardia (Figure 8-4). Supraventricular tachycardia with aberrant conduction includes any supraventricular tachycardia (sinus tachycardia, atrial fibrillation, atrial flutter, or paroxysmal supraventricular tachycardia) occurring with abnormal conduction

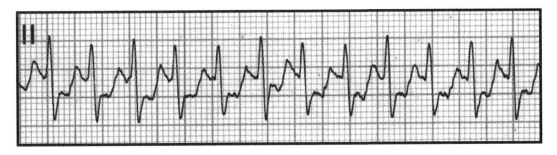

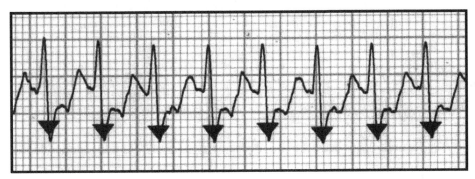

Figure 8.3 Ventricular tachycardia in the pediatric patient (four-month-old male). The QRS complex duration is 0.10 msec and the ventricular rate is 225 bpm.

within the ventricle (Figure 8-5). This abnormal intraventricular impulse transmission can occur via bundle branch block (fixed and rate-related), ventricular pre-excitation, and toxic-metabolic adverse effect on the conduction system.

Numerous strategies aimed at assisting the clinician with the proper diagnosis of WCT have been proposed, emphasizing various data including patient age, medical history, and the electrocardiogram.[2–9] Other factors, such as the physical examination or

Table 8-1. Electrocardiographic rhythm diagnoses in wide QRS complex tachycardia.

Ventricular Tachycardia	Supraventricular Tachycardia with Aberrant Intraventricular Conduction
Monomorphic ventricular tachycardia	Sinus tachycardia**
Polymorphic ventricular tachycardia	Atrial fibrillation**
Torsade de pointes*	Atrial flutter**
	Paroxysmal supraventricular tachycardia**
	Multifocal atrial tachycardia**
	Atrial tachycardias**
	WPW-related atrial fibrillation/atrial flutter
	WPW-related AV reentry (antidromic) tachycardia
	Hyperkalemia-related tachycardia
	Sodium-channel blockade toxicity-related tachycardia

* Note that torsade de pointes is a subtype of polymorphic ventricular tachycardia associated with abnormal ventricular repolarization (prolonged QT interval).

** Occurring with associated bundle branch block.

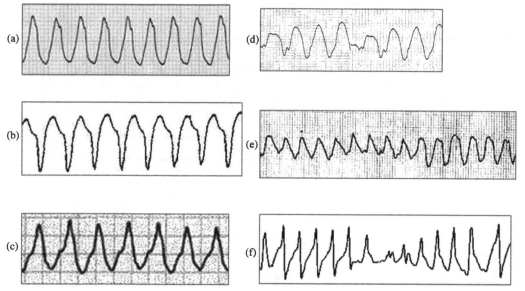

Figure 8.4 (a) Monomorphic ventricular tachycardia. (b) Monomorphic ventricular tachycardia. (c) Monomorphic ventricular tachycardia. (d) Polymorphic ventricular tachycardia. (e) Polymorphic ventricular tachycardia. (f) Polymorphic ventricular tachycardia (torsade de pointes).

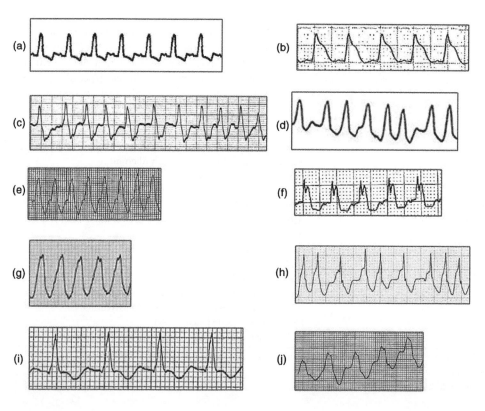

response to therapeutic maneuvers, are of little value in this diagnostic determination.

If one considers all patients encountered with WCT from the perspective of the cardiologist, approximately 80% will be diagnosed with VT; this preponderance of VT, however, probably reflects the bias of difficult cases referred to electrophysiology centers.[2,4,10,11] The emergency physician, however, likely encounters a much broader range of causes of the WCT presentation: VT as well as numerous other causes of the WCT. A review of WCT encountered in the ED demonstrates the exact opposite distribution of rhythm etiologies: 80% supraventricular tachycardia with aberrant conduction and 20% ventricular tachycardia; sinus tachycardia and atrial fibrillation, both with bundle branch block morphology, are the most frequent forms of WCT seen in the greater ED population.[12]

Many clinical decision rules have been suggested as guides to the determination of the cause of the wide complex tachycardia.[6,9,10,13] Certain aspects of these guides and decision tools can be valuable; however, some of the rules have used aberrantly conducted SVT as the default diagnosis. Such an approach is potentially problematic, as it defaults to the less severe diagnosis of SVT. Utilizing therapies aimed at SVT when VT is occurring can result in cardiovascular collapse and death.[13,14] Also, these decision rules are somewhat cumbersome to apply, and are associated with poor rates of interobserver reliability (demonstrated in that different physicians use the same decision tool in different fashion).

If VT is the likely diagnosis based upon an analysis of the presentation (history and electrocardiogram), then therapy can be tailored to this entity. In other cases, if the rhythm distinction is not possible, whether because of an unclear medical history or an unrevealing EKG, the approach in the ED should focus on the patient, not just the electrocardiogram. In many cases, discovering the specific etiology of the WCT may not be possible in the ED.

Clinical presentation

Historical features

Features of the past medical history that can help identify VT as the etiology of a WCT include older patient age (over age 35 years), history of myocardial infarction or congestive heart failure, and recent angina. Even though older age is associated with VT, geriatric patients can still frequently present with sinus tachycardia or atrial fibrillation with bundle branch block as the cause of WCT. Thus, increasing patient age, while associated with VT, cannot be relied upon as a primary diagnostic feature.

Medical history of abnormal left ventricular function, such as from a past myocardial infarction or congestive heart failure, is of significant value and can support a diagnosis of VT; as with age, however, these features do not "guarantee" VT and their absence does not support SVT with aberration.

Past dysrhythmia with prior EKG, if available, is a critical piece of history. Other potentially important history that can guide the diagnostic evaluation includes automatic internal defibrillator, renal insufficiency (hyperkalemia), the use of cardioactive medications, or overdose. A history of coronary revascularization (either coronary artery bypass grafting or interventional coronary procedure), is not helpful in the diagnosis of WCT unless there has been associated infarction or scarring of the myocardium that would make VT a more likely diagnosis. Gender and valvular or congenital heart disease are also not helpful in distinguishing SVT from VT.[3]

Physical examination

The physical examination does not provide useful information in the distinction of SVT from VT. The physical examination, however, is of considerable importance in the identification of hemodynamic stability, which will then guide therapy. The presence of systemic hypoperfusion, ischemic chest discomfort,

Figure 8.5 (a) Sinus tachycardia with bundle branch block. (b) Sinus tachycardia with a giant R wave of an early ST-segment elevation myocardial infarction. (c) Atrial fibrillation with a bundle branch block. (d) Atrial fibrillation with a bundle branch block. (e) Paroxysmal supraventricular tachycardia with a rate-related bundle branch block. (f) Paroxysmal supraventricular tachycardia with a preexisting bundle branch block. (g) Wolff-Parkinson-White syndrome-related wide QRS complex (antidromic) tachycardia. (h) Wolff-Parkinson-White syndrome-related atrial fibrillation. (i) Sodium channel toxicity with a wide QRS complex sinus tachycardia. (j) A wide complex tachycardia related to hyperkalemia.

pulmonary edema, or extremely rapid ventricular response are potential indicators of hemodynamic instability, and should be utilized in determining the most appropriate treatment course at the bedside.

Physicians often associate hemodynamic instability with VT and stability with SVT with aberrant conduction. However this association is incorrect. Patients can present with WCT, ultimately be diagnosed with VT, and tolerate the dysrhythmia clinically while conversely, SVT can cause marked hemodynamic instability, requiring emergent electrical cardioversion.[11] One study of patients presenting with VT finds that patients are hemodynamically stable 77% of the time.[15]

Electrocardiographic features
The EKG, whether as a single-lead rhythm analysis or a complete 12-lead electrocardiogram, plays a pivotal role in the evaluation of the patient with WCT; yet, it still may not reveal the specific rhythm diagnosis. In the patient in extremis, single-lead analysis is usually adequate, but if possible, a 12-lead EKG may further assist in this evaluation. In the stable patient, both rhythm monitoring and 12-lead electrocardiography is recommended. Prior EKG studies, if available in timely fashion, can be very helpful.

Inspection of the EKG should begin with evaluation of rate, regularity, evidence of AV dissociation, and QRS complex morphology.[16] However, the utility of ventricular rate in differentiating among the many causes of WCT is unclear. In one such study, heart rate in ventricular tachycardia is most often between 130–170 beats per minute, while patients with SVT are more likely to have heart rates between 170–200 beats per minute.[7] This study also finds, however, that both groups of patients have individuals with rates above 200 beats per minute.[7] Therefore, in clinical practice, both VT and SVT can result in a broad range of heart rates; this significant overlap of heart rates and variability of various dysrhythmias' rates markedly reduces the value of this finding.

Significant irregularity of the ventricular response can suggest several different rhythm diagnoses: atrial fibrillation with bundle branch block, WPW-related atrial fibrillation, and polymorphic ventricular tachycardia (Figures 8-4d–f, 8-5c, 8-5d, and 8-5h). Other dysrhythmias to be considered are regular in terms of the ventricular response. Determining the presence of irregularity at extremely rapid heart rates is difficult, as the "naked" eye often does not discern irregularity

at such rapid heart rates; the use of an electrocardiographic caliper or other measuring methods is useful in these situations.

Atrial fibrillation with a bundle branch block commonly presents in the ED with tachycardia and marked irregularity of the ventricular response.[12] In situations with normal atrioventricular conduction (i.e., no ventricular preexcitation), each QRS complex is similar in morphology to its neighbors. In WPW-related atrial fibrillation, the rate is extremely rapid with some degree of beat-to-beat variation in QRS complex morphology; furthermore, delta waves can be seen. With polymorphic ventricular tachycardia, there is both irregularity and differences in QRS complex morphology. In this situation, the degree of beat-to-beat variation is usually very prominent, more so than seen in WPW with atrial fibrillation.

Once the rate and regularity have been reviewed, certain features of the QRS complex may be of value. Combinations of the QRS complex width and axis are reportedly of significant import, but yet, when evaluated real-time in the ED, do not demonstrate significant utility; these features are cumbersome to apply and thus of lower diagnostic yield.[7,9,17] One feature of the QRS complex, however, which is both valuable and straightforward is QRS complex concordance. Concordance is defined as the conformity of the QRS complexes in an all-positive or an all-negative direction across the precordial leads (from leads V1-V6). Positive (Figure 8-6) and negative (Figure 8-7) concordance of the QRS complexes in the precordial leads has been shown to usually be VT.[18,19]

Three other features of the EKG, though rare, are of value as their presence supports a VT diagnosis: atrioventricular dissociation, fusion beats, and capture beats. Multiple studies have reported that the presence of AV dissociation approaches 100% specificity for VT.[9,17] AV dissociation is identified by the presence of P waves distinct from the QRS complex, but not in direct relationship to each QRS complex (Figure 8-8). AV dissociation is reportedly uncommon, occurring in only 10% of presentations; yet, it is likely present more frequently if the EKG (rhythm monitoring and 12-lead electrocardiogram) is scrutinized closely. Aktar et al. note that the presence of AV dissociation on EKG correctly diagnoses VT in all of their study patients in whom these features were present on EKG.[4] Vereckei et al. also note that the presence of AV dissociation correctly diagnoses VT in all

Figure 8.6 Ventricular tachycardia with positive QRS complex concordancy.

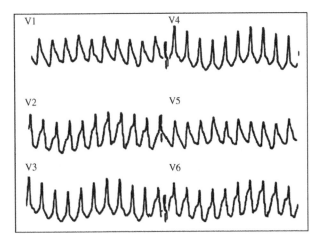

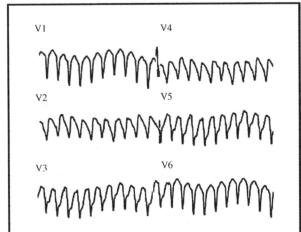

Figure 8.7 Ventricular tachycardia with negative QRS complex concordancy.

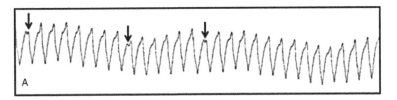

Figure 8.8 A. Ventricular tachycardia with atrioventricular dissociation (note obviously dissociated P waves [arrows]). B. Insert from the EKG rhythm in "A" with irregularities of the QRS complex (arrows) likely representing "less obvious" atrioventricular dissociation.

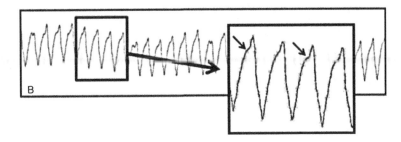

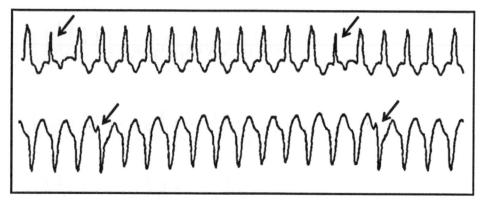

Figure 8.9 Ventricular tachycardia with fusion beats (arrows).

35 patients in whom the EKG findings were present.[17] Brugada et al. include the presence of AV dissociation in their criteria, although these same studies also confirm the rare occurrence of the findings on EKG even in the presence of a known VT.[9]

Fusion and capture beats, also rare in the WCT patient, strongly support a VT diagnosis. A fusion beat (Figure 8-9) results from simultaneous ventricular activation from a normally-conducted supraventricular beat through the AV node, along with beat of ventricular origin. The resulting QRS complex is a fusion of the ventricular and supraventricular beats; it is "more narrow" with a different morphology than the underlying WCT tachycardia.[18] Capture beats (Figure 8-10) result from a completely-conducted supraventricular depolarization that passes through the His-Purkinje system, electrically activating the ventricular myocardium.[16,18] A capture beat has the morphology of the native narrow sinus rhythm.

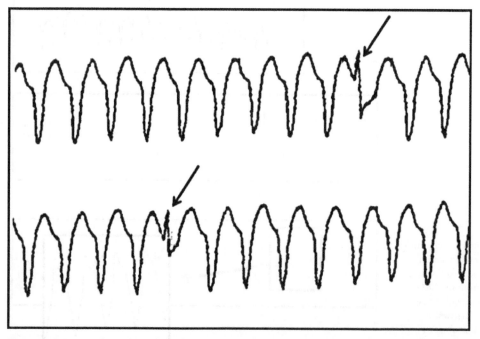

Figure 8.10 Ventricular tachycardia with capture beats (arrows).

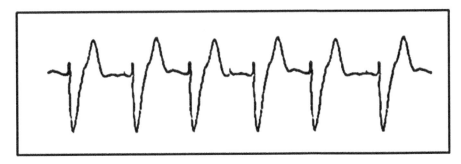

Figure 8.11 A widened QRS complex in a patient with hyperkalemia.

Beyond the traditional electrocardiographic findings noted above, a variety of diseases can lead to unique rhythm presentations. Patients in renal failure often develop hyperkalemia. Elevated serum potassium can cause several different electrocardiographic abnormalities, including prominent T waves, QRS complex widening, and a sinoventricular rhythm. Prominent T waves are considered the first significant electrocardiographic manifestation of hyperkalemia. At progressively higher serum levels, the QRS complex widens (Figure 8-11), at times resembling a bundle branch block; eventually, the QRS complex blends with the T wave, forming a "sine-wave," or sinusoidal, structure on the EKG.

At this point, the P wave further lessens in amplitude, ultimately disappearing with continued serum potassium elevation; the sine wave with loss of the P wave characterizes the "sinoventricular" rhythm of hyperkalemia.

Purposeful and accidental overdose of numerous medications can affect the EKG. Sodium channel blocking agents such as tricyclic antidepressants can cause sinus tachycardia, widening of the QRS complex, and an extreme right axis deviation of the terminal QRS complex with a deep S wave in lead I and prominent R` wave in lead aVr (Figure 8-12).

The Wolff-Parkinson-White (WPW) syndrome can cause several different wide complex tachycardias,

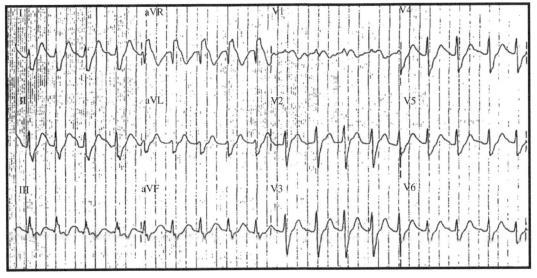

Figure 8.12 A 12-lead EKG in tricyclic antidepressant ingestion, demonstrating a sinus tachycardia, a widened QRS complex, and a rightward axis deviation of the terminal portion of the QRS complex (deep S wave in lead I and prominent R wave in lead aVr).

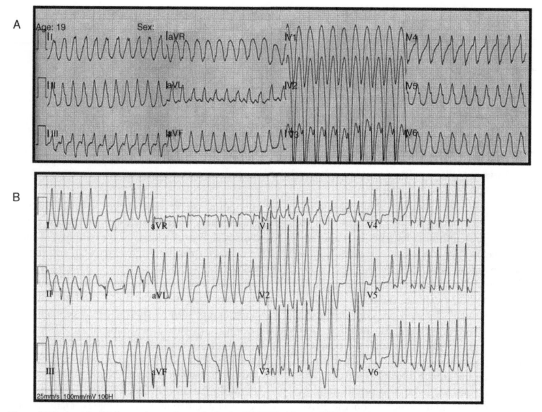

Figure 8.13 A wide QRS complex tachycardia in the Wolff-Parkinson-White syndrome. A. An atrioventricular reentry (antidromic) tachycardia. B. Atrial fibrillation.

including AV reentry (antidromic) tachycardia (Figure 8-13A) and preexcited atrial fibrillation (Figure 8-13B). In both cases, the rate will be extremely rapid with a markedly widened QRS complex and delta wave. In WPW with atrial fibrillation, the beat-to-beat variation in the QRS complex morphology is clear.

Management

Patients presenting with a WCT and significant hemodynamic compromise should be prepared for an immediate electrical cardioversion. This approach is appropriate for VT and most forms of SVT with aberrant conduction. Patients with sinus tachycardia complicated by bundle branch block, sodium channel blockade-related tachycardia, or hyperkalemia-associated tachycardia should not undergo electrical cardioversion, but instead should receive therapy targeted at these various conditions. In patients refractory to standard WCT therapy, a

metabolic or drug-induced cause of dysrhythmia should be considered.

Even in hemodynamically stable patients with undifferentiated WCT, the rhythm should be considered VT until proven otherwise, unless sinus tachycardia with bundle branch block pattern, sodium channel blockade-related tachycardia, or hyperkalemia-associated tachycardia is likely. Patients who are hemodynamically stable on presentation can be managed initially with medication. Should the clinical status deteriorate, electrical cardioversion can be utilized as secondary therapy.

In a stable patient with an undifferentiated WCT, procainamide is very effective in terminating the dysrhythmia. Using a dose of 10 mg/kg, one study finds that procainamide terminates approximately 80% of stable WCT (in this case, monophorphic ventricular tachycardia); in contrast, the same study finds that lidocaine dosed at 1.5 mg/kg terminates only 20%

of stable WCT.[20] Procainamde has the added benefit of being a relatively safe agent for use in preexcitation syndrome-related tachycardia (atrial fibrillation and AV reentry tachycardia). A common adverse effect and significant limitation of procainamide is hypotension, which is usually an infusion-related problem. For this reason, procainamide is not suggested for use in patients with significantly impaired left ventricular function or acute pulmonary edema. Standard procainamide dosing is as follows: a maximum of 17 mg/kg infused at a rate of 20 mg/min; alternatively, 100–200 mg increments of procainamide can be infused in slow intravenous "push" fashion over 2–5 minutes, thus allowing for a full loading dose in more rapid fashion. The method of administration is dependent upon both the patient's situation and the clinician's resources. Therapeutic endpoints for procainamide include full loading dose achieved, development of clinically significant hypotension, or dysrhythmia termination.

Amiodarone should be considered the second line agent for treatment of an undifferentiated WCT in which procainamide has failed to produce a cardioversion. It can be considered a first line agent in patients with pronounced left ventricular dysfunction. A recent study finds that 150 mg/kg of amiodarone terminates only 29% of stable ventricular tachycardias.[21] Few studies, however, have investigated the efficacy of amiodarone in stable WCT. In the hemodynamically stable patient, the initial dose of amiodarone is 150 mg intravenously over 10 minutes, which may be repeated every 10 minutes as necessary to a maximum daily dose of 2.2 grams. It should not be used for wide complex rhythms related to Wolff-Parkinson-White syndrome because of its AV-node blocking abilities.

Two common WCTs include sinus tachycardia and atrial fibrillation, both with bundle branch block configuration. Sinus tachycardia with a bundle branch block should be approached with an investigation of the underlying cause of the dysrhythmia. As this rhythm is likely a reactive dysrhythmia, issues such as hypovolemia, hypoxia, or fever should be considered as possible causes, and therapies should be aimed at the correction of the underlying disease process. Atrial fibrillation, either with or without a bundle branch block pattern, can be challenging to manage as hemodynamic instability in atrial fibrillation may or may not be related to the rapidity of the ventricular response. A patient with chronic atrial fibrillation may be dependent upon the rapid rate to maintain cardiac output in the face of pronounced hypovolemia or inadequate vascular tone; attempts at rate control in this setting, rather than management of the underlying process, can lead to patient deterioration.

The QRS complex widening from both sodium channel blockade and hyperkalemia must be approached in a different fashion from traditional WCTs. The QRS complex widening with tachycardia in the setting of poisoning with a sodium channel-blocking agent should be treated with intravenous sodium bicarbonate. An initial bolus of 1–2 mEq/kg should be followed by a repeat EKG to evaluate for narrowing of the QRS complex. Repeat sodium bicarbonate boluses, continuous infusion, or both can be used to improve conduction and increase contractility. The QRS complex duration can be monitored to determine the response to therapy.

The primary goals in treating a WCT due to hyperkalemia are to stabilize the myocardium and lower the serum potassium concentration. Intravenous calcium chloride or calcium gluconate will assist in stabilization of the myocyte. Several different agents can transiently lower the serum potassium. Beta-adrenergic agonists push potassium into cells through activation of a membrane potassium pump; albuterol is the most commonly used beta-agonist in this setting. Insulin works to activate the sodium potassium ATPase, thereby shifting potassium into cells; 10 units of regular insulin are administered intravenously initially along with 25 grams of dextrose to avoid hypoglycemia. Sodium bicarbonate both shifts potassium into cells and increases renal excretion of potassium; the initial recommended dose is 1 mEq/kg intravenously. Magnesium sulfate, given at a dose of 8 mEq intravenously, will also cause internal shifting of potassium. As these measures primarily serve to temporarily decrease serum potassium concentrations, definitive measures must be taken to decrease overall potassium body burden (i.e., hemodialysis or sodium polystyrene, Kayexalate). Furthermore, repeat therapy may be necessary if the time to definitive management is prolonged.

Section IV: Decision making

- For a WCT with hemodynamic compromise, electrical cardioversion is the first line treatment.

- In sinus tachycardia with a bundle branch block, sodium channel blockade-related tachycardia, or hyperkalemia-associated tachycardia, target the underlying condition.
- In a hemodynamically-stable WCT, the rhythm should be considered VT until proven otherwise, but can be managed initially with procainamide.
- Amiodarone should be used as a second line agent for an undifferentiated WCT, except in patients with significantly impaired left ventricular function or acute pulmonary edema.
- A QRS complex widening sodium channel blockade (TCA overdose) should be treated with sodium bicarbonate.
- Treatment for a WCT due to hyperkalemia requires stabilizing the myocardium and lowering the serum potassium, using calcium, beta-agonists, insulin, sodium bicarbonate, magnesium, and ultimately hemodialysis or sodium polystyrene, Kayexalate.

References

1 Meldon SW, Brady WJ, Berger S, Mannenbach M. Pediatric ventricular tachycardia: a review with three illustrative cases. *Pediatr Emerg Care*. 1994; 10:294–300.

2 Tchou P, Young P, Mahmud R, et al. Useful clinical criteria for the diagnosis of ventricular tachycardia. *Am J Med*. 1988;84:53–56.

3 Baerman JM, Morady F, DiCario LA, de Buitleir M. Differentiation of ventricular tachycardia from supraventricular tachycardia with aberration: Value of the clinical history. *Ann Emerg Med*. 1987;16:40–43.

4 Akhtar M, Shenasa M, Jazayeri M, Caceres J, Tchou PJ. Wide QRS complex tachycardia. Reappraisal of a common clinical problem. *Ann Int Med*. 1988;109: 905–912.

5 Levitt MA. Supraventricular tachycardia with aberrant conduction versus ventricular tachycardia: Differentiation and diagnosis. *Am J Emerg Med*. 1988;6:273–277.

6 Antunes E, Brugada J, Steurer G, et al. The differential diagnosis of a regular tachycardia with a wide QRS complex on the 12-lead ECG: Ventricular tachycardia, supraventricular tachycardia with aberrant intraventricular conduction, and supraventricular tachycardia with anterograde conduction over an accessory pathway. *PACE*. 1994;17:1515–1524.

7 Wellens HJ, Bar FW, Lie KI. The value of the electrocardiogram in the differential diagnosis of a tachycardia with a widened QRS complex. *Am J Med*. 1978;64:27–33.

8 Steurer G, Gursoy S, Frey B, et al. The differential diagnosis on the electrocardiogram between ventricular tachycardia and preexcited tachycardia. *Clin Cardiol*. 1994;17:306–308.

9 Brugada P, Brugada J, Mont L, Smeets J, Andries EW. A new approach to the differential diagnosis of a regular tachycardia with a wide QRS complex. *Circulation*. 1991;83:1649–1659.

10 Steinman RT, Herrera C, Schluger CD, et al. Wide QRS tachycardia in the conscious adult: Ventricular tachycardia is the most frequent cause. *JAMA*. 1989; 261:1013–1016.

11 Morady F, Baerman JM, DiCarlo LA, et al. A prevalent misconception regarding wide complex tachycardias. *JAMA*. 1985;254:2790–2792.

12 Brady W. Unpublished data. University of Virginia 2009, Charlottesville, VA.

13 Herbert ME, Votey SR, Mortan MT, et al. Failure to agree on the electrocardiographic diagnosis of ventricular tachycardia. *Ann Emerg Med*. 1996;27: 35–38.

14 Stewart RB, Bardy GH, Greene HL. Wide complex tachycardia: misdiagnosis and outcome after emergent therapy. *Ann Intern Med*. 1986; 104:766–771.

15 Domanovits H, Paulis M, Nikfardjam M, et al. Sustained ventricular tachycardia in the emergency department. *Resuscitation*. 1999;42:19–25.

16 Brady WJ, Skiles J. Wide QRS complex tachycardia: ECG differential diagnosis. *Am J Emerg Med*. 1999;17:376–381.

17 Vereckei A, Duray G, Szénási G, et al. New algorithm using only lead aVR for differential diagnosis of wide QRS complex tachycardia. *Heart Rhythm*. 2008;5: 89–98.

18 Goldberger ZD, Rho RW, Page RL. Approach to the diagnosis and initial management of the stable adult patient with a wide complex tachycardia. *Am J Cardiol*. 2008;101:1456–1466.

19 Gupta AK, Thakur RK. Wide QRS complex tachycardias. *Med Clin North Am*. 2001;85:245–266.

20 Gorgels AP, van den Dool A, Hofs A, et al. Comparison of procainamide and lidocaine in terminating sustained monomorphic ventricular tachycardia. *Am J Cardiol*. 1996;78:43–46.

21 Marill KA, deSouza IS, Nishijima DK, et al. Amiodarone is poorly effective for the acute termination of ventricular tachycardia. *Ann Emerg Med*. 2006;47:217–224.

Cardiac arrest

Benjamin J. Lawner[1] & Amal Mattu[2]

[1] *Clinical Assistant Professor, Department of Emergency Medicine, University of Maryland School of Medicine, Deputy EMS Medical Director, Baltimore City Fire Department Baltimore, Maryland, USA*
[2] *Professor and Residency Director, Department of Emergency Medicine, University of Maryland School of Medicine, Baltimore, Maryland, USA*

Section I: Case presentation

A 56-year-old woman was brought to the emergency department (ED) by EMS personnel for evaluation of a "possible cardiac arrest." The patient had been sitting with family members watching TV when she began to complain about substernal chest pressure and dyspnea. She became diaphoretic, and then collapsed to the floor. The family members, who were untrained in CPR, immediately began chest compressions without checking for a pulse. After approximately a minute, the patient began moving spontaneously, though she remained unconscious. Someone dialed 911.

The paramedics found the patient unconscious, but breathing; she was spontaneously moving and localizing pain, but not following commands. The vital signs were: blood pressure 80/60 mmHg, pulse 110 beats/min, respirations 22 breaths/min, pulse oximetry 97%. A finger stick glucose was 140 mg/dl. The EKG showed sinus tachycardia, 2 mm ST-segment elevation in leads II, III, and aVF, and 1 mm ST-segment depression in leads V1-V3. The paramedics placed the patient on a cardiac monitor, applied 100% oxygen via non-rebreather facemask, initiated a normal saline bolus, and transported the patient, a trip of ten minutes, to the ED.

The vital signs did not change during transport. The past medical history included a history of renal failure, with the patient receiving hemodialysis 3 times per week; the last time was 2 days prior to the current event. The patient also had insulin-dependent diabetes mellitus and hypertension. She had been doing well until the arrest.

Shortly after arrival in the ED, the patient became limp. The cardiac monitor showed a rhythm change to a wide complex regular tachycardia with a rate of 160 beats/min. She had no palpable pulse and agonal respirations.

Section II: Case discussion

Dr Peter Rosen: This case illustrates a number of my prejudices about cardiac arrest. It's a problem that probably drove the origin of emergency medicine, but I think it's the wrong end of the disease to be treating. I don't really think we've made great progress in the management of cardiac arrest since we first started doing emergency medicine about 30 years ago. There's been a lot of controversy about the value of citizen CPR, touted mostly by the Seattle system. Nevertheless, when you talk to the people in Seattle, they tell you some odd things, such as CPR doesn't work in asystole, and when they study the quality of citizen CPR, there isn't any difference between providers. It doesn't seem to matter what citizens do, so long as they do something; they haven't been able to define whether citizen CPR is having an effect on the patient directly, or whether the benefits involve an earlier call to the 911 system.

There does seem to be an advantage to defibrillators in public buildings and airports, and it would seem, over time, that our best success with cardiac arrest is when it probably isn't a cardiac arrest, in terms of asystole or a ventricular fibrillation (VF), but probably ventricular tachycardia (VT) or perhaps a seizure that's assumed to be a cardiac arrest, and the patient gets shocked. These patients do very well; they come back with great cerebral function. However, in terms of true cardiac arrest, I think the outcome is still dismal, and it would appear that all of our efforts to improve citizen CPR have failed because we are treating the wrong end of the disease. Currently or in 2009 (Since the guidelines have since been published), the best treatment for cardiac arrest is immediate defibrillation, and if that can't be achieved, these patients don't fare well.

Dr David Brown: I largely agree: survivors of out-of-hospital cardiac arrest are most likely to be those who can be successfully defibrillated in the field. There are a few subsets of patients who have a chance; this case is one example, an ischemic-related VF arrest, or, less likely, VT arrest. These kinds of arrest are more likely to be successfully defibrillated than some other kinds of out-of-hospital cardiac arrest, such as asystole or primary respiratory arrest leading to cardiac arrest.

Dr Amal Mattu: I would add that good compressions may help, but the best chance for recovery is when the patient has a rhythm that can respond to defibrillation. Otherwise, just focus on basic life support (BLS), and transport as quickly as possible. Today, there is a lot less emphasis on ventilation, instead focusing on good compressions en route and hoping that the patients may have a rhythm that can respond to defibrillation, but not much else can be done in the field.

PR: Do you think the dog experiments or other animal experiments on arrest, with the different positioning of the thumpers and the different rates of compression, have any clinical relevance in humans?

Dr Shamai Grossman: The American Heart Association (AHA) goes back and forth as to the appropriate rate of compressions; however, I think that rescuers aren't very good at compressions to start with, and aren't very compliant with the continuous compressions either. Currently, the AHA recommends 100 compressions

per minute, yet I think that to actually get someone to do 100 compressions per minute and have good compressions is really difficult. This limits the value of ongoing animal experiments.

The one advance in out-of-hospital care that is likely beneficial, which paramedics can do and routinely do now in Massachusetts, is to call ahead to the ED with a 12-lead EKG. If the patient is restored to a regular rhythm, and if the 12-lead EKG demonstrates an ST elevation myocardial infarction (STEMI), we can send them directly to the cardiac catheterization laboratory, bypassing other hospitals that do not have this availability. There are data that suggest that the best option for this patient is immediate revascularization.[1-3] If that's true, then when you call ahead and let the ED know you have an ST elevation MI in a patient who is in cardiac arrest, they can potentially have the cardiac catheterization laboratory available more quickly, and you may significantly improve this person's mortality.

PR: Since this case sounds to me like a dysrhythmic event with probable VT and loss of consciousness, as opposed to VF or asystole, what is the outcome of VT arrest? I have not been impressed that VT arrest fares much better than VF. I have seen a couple of patients with VT who developed the rhythm in the ED instead of in the field, but when they were returned to a sinus rhythm, they still never woke up nor regained meaningful cardiac function.

Dr Edward Ullman: I think your real best chance is to arrest in the ED. An article reports that in-hospital cardiac arrests have an equal to or worse door-to-defibrillation time compared to out-of-hospital cardiac arrests. Clearly this is going to significantly affect outcome.[4] One advance that may help is to initiate cooling of patients who suffer out-of-hospital cardiac arrest, even while in the prehospital arena and during transport.[5] In Boston, EMS is now starting to commence hypothermia treatment.

DB: There is a prognostic difference between an ischemic-related VT or VF versus a patient who is dying of sepsis who has a hypotensive cardiac arrest. But if we lump together every outcome of in-hospital cardiac arrest, it's hard to interpret that data. In particular, I would make the distinction that most of the cardiac arrests associated with acute MIs are VF and not VT, and usually respond to immediate defibrillation.

These are the patients who we really might be able to help. The likelihood of success in any cardiac arrest depends on what is the underlying disease.

PR: When I started in medicine, we were taught to respond to an arrest by opening the chest. Our results weren't as dismal as many of the results of patients who arrive in the ED with VF or asystole, yet once closed-chest defibrillation became widespread in use, open chest resuscitation was reserved for patients who already had their chest open. I've never understood what the difference was, although perhaps direct defibrillation works a little better than defibrillation through the chest wall. I've always been puzzled as to why those patients survived with open chest massage when they don't with closed.

SG: We are more leery of opening a chest today, typically because of the risk it entails to the provider, particularly if you are not used to opening the chest. Risks can include blood and body fluid exposure and exposure to sharps, and the risks that the patient will go through, such as infection and wound healing. In addition, I am not aware of results that show that it's a better therapy.

DB: If you were in a community hospital and you opened the chest and resuscitated the patient, what would you do if you didn't have a cardiothoracic surgeon there?

PR: I would not open the chest if you don't have the capacity to fix the obstructed vessel; all you could do is close the chest and hope that the patient survives, which is what we were formerly doing because we didn't have the capacity to fix the problem. The bypass graft surgical techniques were just being developed, so we just closed the chest and admitted the patient to the medical service, with a surgical consultation to manage the chest wound.

DB: I wonder if a lack of surgical resources is what moved us towards closed-chest compression?

PR: I think this was more because there were fewer people who knew how to open a chest, and it was much easier to learn how to defibrillate. Unfortunately, it was an excellent technologic improvement, but not an excellent outcome improvement. I continue to wonder what we could do to improve our results. We spend too much time trying to resuscitate a patient with cardiac arrest; if they don't defibrillate right away and you

haven't gotten control of their rhythm and blood pressure right away, I think they should be pronounced.

DB: That's the way clinical care has evolved. Our codes are much shorter than they were when I first was on staff or in training 20 years ago.

PR: I think that's reasonable. I believe this led us to the high dose epinephrine, which was supposed to have been the magic bullet breakthrough for cardiac arrest. Then we discovered all it did was keep the patients alive long enough to have a three-day stay in the coronary care unit, and markedly increase the cost of dying. Is there a drug that has enabled you to salvage a patient in arrest? I am underwhelmed by the use of the antidysrhythmic drugs. I don't think amiodarone or lidocaine have saved lives. Perhaps epinephrine has converted a couple of people from fine VF into a VF more amenable to defibrillation.

AM: The AHA guidelines from 2005 do admit that there are no antidysrhythmic drugs that improve survival to discharge, in contrast to 2000 when the recommendations favored amiodarone. The 2005 guidelines express a similar sentiment toward the utility of vasopressors.[6]

PR: This patient who we presented today with renal failure is part of a subset of cardiac arrest that strangely, often, has a good outcome. I have been surprised at how easily these patients resuscitate from what's most likely a hyperkalemic arrest, although I'm also surprised at how often they go into arrest, even when they are being regularly dialyzed.

EU: I think hyperkalemia is easier as an electrocardiographic abnormality to correct, but I think that when they arrest, these patients may perhaps be even more difficult to fully resuscitate because there is always extensive concomitant pathology present.

AM: Renal disease is associated with a very poor prognosis in many conditions. Patients with strokes and renal disease, patients with MIs and renal disease, and patients with heart failure and renal disease all have worse outcomes. It's not the renal disease itself that makes the cardiac arrest more intractable, but the underlying other medical illnesses that makes the cardiac arrest more intractable.

PR: Do you think that the standard antipotassium pharmacologic therapy is indicated for the renal failure patient who arrests? Would you start them all on insulin and bicarbonate and calcium?

DB: I think that, in this particular case, the likelihood is that the patient is having ischemic cardiac arrest. My experience with hyperkalemic arrest is that these patients don't have abrupt VT; instead, they tend to sequentially peak their T waves, broaden out their PR interval, lose their P waves, and then finally broaden out their QRS in a slow, sinusoidal, brady-systolic arrest. I find those patients easier to resuscitate because one generally has more time while they are getting worse. If you catch the very end, then resuscitation can be more difficult. Calcium chloride is very effective if you catch hyperkalemic dysrhythmias early. A patient who presents with abrupt VT like this patient, in the setting of a STEMI, is unlikely to also have acute hyperkalemia causing the arrest. In this patient I probably wouldn't reach for antihyperkalemic therapy. Instead, I would look to shock this patient, move to the catheterization laboratory as soon as possible for revascularization, and at the same time cool the patient as much as I could while I'm waiting.

AM: If the patient were refractory to therapy, then I would consider treating this patient for acute hyperkalemia with calcium and bicarbonate, and then all the other appropriate hyperkalemia therapies.

PR: One area that causes dysrhythmic arrest that we used to see more frequently is digitalis toxicity. I used to think that virtually all patients we saw who came in with dysrhythmias were digitoxic, but that seems to be a lot less common today. Do you think they do better if you have the opportunity to reach for Fab fragments therapy?

AM: I think we are seeing fewer cardiac arrest. Fewer and fewer patients are being treated with digoxin. I've given Fab fragments to patients who were taking digoxin and had life-threatening dysrhythmias, although they were still perfusing, and I have witnessed dramatic successes.

PR: Other severe electrolyte disturbances can also lead to dysrhythmia. It seems like our treatment of hypertension has helped us to see fewer arrest patients with hypokalemia, since we're not using thiazide diuretics as much to treat hypertension. Yet, none seem to turn around as magically as hyperkalemia.

PR: One of the things that always used to irritate me when I practiced in San Diego was our helicopter being called for a large number of cardiac arrests. It seemed to me that was a dreadful misuse of the helicopter. I never could understand why those patients couldn't be pronounced dead on site. I would wonder if it isn't time that we stop racing cardiac arrest patients through the streets in ambulances. I would consider pronouncing patients in the field, if they could not be defibrillated immediately.

AM: I think that we should probably be more willing to pronounce patients in the field. Transporting with lights and sirens is associated with traffic crashes and dangers to the public as well as to the responders, and the arrested patient is difficult to treat in a moving ambulance. There are studies that have looked at reasonable indications to pronounce a patient in the field. Several years ago, the OPALS study group proposed criteria for termination of prehospital resuscitation for victims of cardiac arrest.[7] There are five different criteria, including event not witnessed by EMS personnel, no shock in the prehospital setting, no return to spontaneous circulation in the prehospital system, event was not witnessed by a bystander, and the bystanders did not administer CPR. Common sense would dictate that, considering those five criteria together, there is no way a person is going to survive to discharge. Unfortunately, the prehospital medical directors often have tried to employ these rules, but their responders frequently will not follow them and transport the patient in any event.

I think that the prehospital care providers often times feel a lot of pressure pronouncing the patient in the field when the family is hovering over them, yelling at them, "Please do something!" It's a lot harder to convince the family in the field that the patient has no chance of survival. In addition, I think that a big problem we have in our society is that we have a tremendous societal expectation or misperception of resuscitation rates. Society really thinks that people who are in cardiac arrest who are getting CPR are probably going to survive. This may be related to the media, but I don't think the public has any concept that the chance that a patient will survive a prehospital arrest is, at best, 5%.

PR: We had a few rules for withholding resuscitation that we added in Denver, including decapitation, decomposition, and rigor mortis on a warm night.

The one exception is pediatric arrests, which I believe are better pronounced at the hospital, not because they do better, but because the social requirements of dealing with a pediatric death are such that it's best to start at the hospital.

PR: This particular patient was lucky in that she probably survived the dysrhythmia at home; maybe the efforts to do CPR were comparable to the cough technique or doing a chest thump. The cough technique has been shown to be efficacious as long as the patient is still conscious and can institute the cough. You can get people to do this as they're suddenly descending into a dysrhythmia, but it doesn't work once the patient has lost consciousness.

SG: Sometimes, the couple of joules of energy with a chest thump may be all you need to convert an early VT to sinus rhythm, and can save valuable time wasted trying to employ a defibrillator.

PR: Perhaps we as emergency physicians are going to feel even more futility in trying to resuscitate out-of-hospital cardiac arrests, because now a number of high-risk patients who have implanted defibrillators don't have cardiac arrests anymore; these were the patients who would present with VT and VF amenable to defibrillation, and most likely to survive an out-of-hospital cardiac arrest if they had access to defibrillation. With these patients no longer part of the denominator, the patients that we are seeing as emergency physicians with out-of-hospital arrest are even more likely to have heart rhythms that are not amenable to defibrillation, and so they will be more likely to die.

AM: In addition, the growing number of people with underlying heart disease placed on chronic beta-blocker therapy has decreased significantly the overall incidence of VF cardiac arrest. Instead, we are seeing an increase in asystolic and PEA cardiac arrest. Overall, we are probably seeing fewer cardiac arrests, and the ones that we see are presenting with rhythms that are not amenable to defibrillation.

PR: This case may ultimately be frustrating because you think that you've had a salvage, but this is a patient, given her comorbidities, who is probably not going to survive in the hospital, and if she gets out of the hospital, the chances are that her final outcome will be death. However, we must try to respond, keeping in mind is that if this is an ischemic arrest, the patient must go for an intervention very quickly once the rhythm is stabilized. Part of this problem involves how to get the patient from the field to a hospital that has the catheterization laboratory. Given our ever increasing hospital crowding, we simply are probably losing some of these patients because we don't have open access to an institution that has a 24-hour catheterization laboratory.

EU: In Boston, where it was initially studied, we are bypassing the EDs that do not have a 24-hour catheterization laboratory with patients with ST-elevation MIs.[8] When EMS calls ahead, and the paramedic has already done a 12-lead EKG, the ED itself can call the catheterization laboratory to open up. They will not go to a hospital that does not have a catheterization laboratory. I think that this model will likely generalize as we continue to show improved outcomes for these patients.

DB: In Massachusetts we also just abolished diversion for all hospitals statewide, so that diversion should no longer be an impediment to getting patients to the right hospital.

Case resolution

Upon arrival to the ED, the patient had a repeat cardiac arrest with a cardiac rhythm of pulseless ventricular tachycardia. She received an immediate defibrillation, and converted back to sinus tachycardia (rate 110/minute). The EKG continued to demonstrate the previously noted ST-segment changes. Empiric calcium was administered via IV in the event that she was hyperkalemic, though laboratory studies later revealed a normal serum potassium value.

The patient met criteria for induced hypothermia (unconscious with spontaneous circulation after resuscitation from cardiac arrest), so she was intubated, kept sedated, and paralyzed to prevent shivering. Cooling was initiated with cooling blankets and cool IV fluids. The cardiology service was consulted emergently because of the EKG evidence of STEMI, and 45 minutes after arrival she was transported to the cardiac catheterization lab. A 100% right coronary artery blockage was opened, and a stent was placed, after which she was admitted to the coronary care unit. Therapeutic hypothermia was discontinued after approximately 18 hours, and the patient made a steady improvement. She was discharged home 6 days later with minimal cognitive deficits, and was able to care for herself independently. Outpatient occupational therapy follow up was arranged. The family members who performed chest compressions prior to paramedic arrival can be credited with saving her life.

Section III: Concepts

Background

Cardiac arrest remains an expensive resource-intensive condition that requires input from providers across the disciplines of emergency medicine and critical care.[9] Survival from cardiac arrest remains poor despite prolonged and extensive resuscitation research initiatives. Despite revisions in prehospital treatment protocols and an increased awareness among the general public, this condition is still associated with an extremely high mortality. Paramedics routinely encounter cardiac arrest patients in the prehospital setting, and emergency physicians are charged with orchestrating initial resuscitative efforts.

Dismal rates of neurologic recovery from cardiac arrest have encouraged continued and thoughtful reexamination of resuscitation strategies. Protocols that minimize interruptions to chest compressions, and focus on the maintenance of cerebral blood have gained recent emphasis. The initial evaluation and stabilization of the patient in cardiac arrest now focuses less on pharmacology, and more on the mechanics of circulation. Time tested modalities like defibrillation and chest compression are reemerging as powerful tools in the emergency physician's resuscitative arsenal.[10,11]

Cardiac arrest poses unique challenges to the delivery of emergency health care. Cardiac arrest is never entirely predictable, but the survival clock starts ticking once circulation ceases. Access to trained and willing bystanders is not universal, and automated external defibrillators may not be immediately available. The inverse relationship between survival and time has remained constant; consequently, meaningful neurologic recovery is predicated upon the timely delivery of chest compressions, and access to definitive care.[12-14]

Epidemiology

In the United States, sudden cardiac death accounts for approximately 200,000–400,000 deaths per year. Precise statistics represent unique epidemiological challenges because of subtle differences in the classification of sudden death. Studies on sudden cardiac death detail different inclusion criteria; nevertheless, current research estimates that 50% of all deaths from cardiovascular disease are sudden and unexpected, occurring shortly (instantaneous to 1 hour) after the onset of symptoms. Predictably, data suggest two peak ages of incidence for sudden cardiac death: infants under 6 months comprise one peak, and the other involves adults from 45–75 years of age. Most sudden deaths occur outside of the hospital, and may therefore remain unwitnessed.[9,15]

The occurrence of sudden cardiac death heralds an inexorable march towards global cellular destruction. The neurologic disability among survivors is often devastating, and patients may require varying types of artificial life support to maintain vital functions. Out-of-hospital cardiac arrest is associated with low survival to hospital discharge (2–9%) and even lower rates of functional neurologic recovery. Though recent years have borne witness to an expansion of resuscitation research, the emphasis still remains on time-tested interventions such as: (1) bystander CPR, (2) defibrillation, and (3) adequate compressions. Current treatment recommendations will detail this renewed "back to basics" focus.[16]

Initial patient assessment

Brain death and irreversible neurologic dysfunction begin within minutes of circulatory collapse; the likelihood of survival with a functional neurologic outcome decreases with every minute that passes prior to the initiation of resuscitative efforts. The treatment of the patient in cardiac arrest should be focused on the restoration and maintenance of perfusion. Return of spontaneous circulation (ROSC) is most likely in those patients who receive prompt bystander CPR, technically adequate compressions, and rapid defibrillation of a ventricular dysrhythmia.[10,14]

Obtaining information about the events surrounding cardiovascular collapse is exceedingly difficult for the emergency physician. Bystanders may give details about resuscitative efforts, and emergency medical services personnel may have valuable information about the incident scene. The presence of pill bottles, for example, prompts a consideration of toxic overdoses in the initial differential diagnosis; alternatively, patients transported from a nephrologist's office may have an electrolyte derangement that precipitated a lethal dysrhythmia. With respect to pulseless electrical activity, the consideration of toxidromes is vital to articulating a comprehensive treatment plan. The initial history must necessarily encompass relevant scene details, if possible, and understanding of preceding events.

The absence of central pulses, respirations, and responsiveness defines cardiac arrest. Agonal or gasping respirations may persist after the cessation of cardiac activity, but effective breathing is absent during circulatory collapse. Patients presenting to the ED in cardiac arrest must be completely undressed. The physical examination proceeds in a detailed but rapid fashion. Priorities include airway maintenance, circulatory assessment, and an investigation for any potential underlying causes of cardiac arrest. The history and physical examination are performed concurrently with resuscitative interventions.

Current recommendations place less of an emphasis on advanced airway techniques.[11,17] For patients intubated prior to ED arrival, confirmation of tube placement is important, as movement of the patient's neck during transport or transfer has been implicated in tube migration, and efforts should be directed at verification of tracheal location. Capnography, direct laryngoscopy, and auscultation of lung sounds are confirmatory techniques that can be rapidly performed while minimizing any interruption in chest compressions. Some paramedic systems have implemented continuous carbon dioxide capnometry to warn providers of inadvertent dislodgement. A rapid respiratory assessment can also uncover potentially reversible etiologies of cardiac arrest such as tension pneumothorax. Chest X-ray studies contribute little information beyond what is discovered at the patient's bedside.

Heart tones are generally absent in cardiac arrest patients, but the clinical examination can yield important clues about contributing factors. The presence of chest wall trauma may signal an underlying tamponade. Patients with chronic renal failure and metastatic disease harbor more subtle signs of tamponade, and benefit from bedside emergency echocardiography. Utilizing the focused assessment for sonography in trauma, or FAST window, emergency practitioners can obtain a "quick look" at cardiac activity and establish the presence or absence of a large pericardial effusion (Figure 9-1). The parasternal long axis represents an alternative and easily accessible cardiac

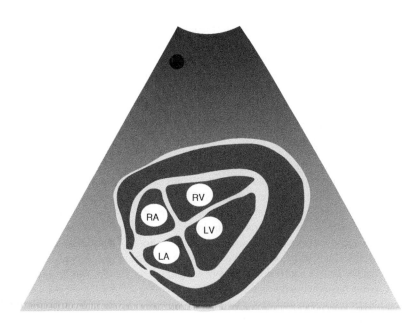

RA: Right Atrium   RV: Right Ventricule
LA: Left Atrium   LV: Left Ventricle

Figure 9.1 Schematic of FAST/ subxiphoid ultrasound window.

The bright, hyperechoic lining represents the pericardium. The dark and hypoechoic fluid contained within the pericardial sac indicates a large effusion.

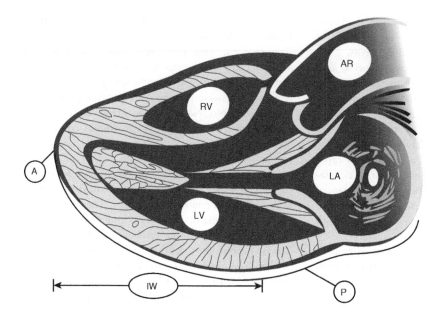

AR: Aortic root and arch
RV: Right ventricle
LV: Left ventricle

LA: Left atrium
IW: Inferior wall of left ventricle
A: Apex
P: Pericardium

Figure 9.2 Diagram of the parasternal long axis in bedside emergency echocardiography.

window (Figure 9-2). Furthermore, ultrasound images may complement performance of therapeutic pericardiocentesis. Similar to the respiratory assessment outlined above, bedside ultrasound complements ongoing resuscitative efforts.[9,18]

Basic life support (BLS) and out-of-hospital cardiac arrest (OOHCA)

When the American Heart Association (AHA) detailed its "chain of survival" metaphor, early CPR and early defibrillation were featured components. Though the chain also encompassed advanced care and interventions, it remains clear that intact neurologic survival is not possible without understanding basic life support as the foundation of effective treatment. Until recently, the goal of survival from out-of-hospital cardiac arrest has remained less than tangible. Intensive resuscitation research and newer technology have not been accompanied with complementary improvements in patient outcome.[11]

The document highlights the importance of minimally interrupted compressions, compression-to-ventilation ratios are changed to emphasize faster

compressions, and advanced life support providers are encouraged to delay certain interventions if they interfere with the delivery of chest compressions. This shift in focus to BLS has particular relevance to emergency medical services systems, as the majority of advanced life support treatment (ALS) protocols embrace the full scope of advanced cardiac life support. Previous resuscitation paradigms embraced a drug-shock, drug-shock approach to life support, and a large number of prehospital studies sought to attribute survival benefits to one drug over another. The widespread implementation of prehospital ALS did not correlate with increased survival from cardiac arrest. One of the largest prehospital studies, the Ontario Prehospital Life Support (OPALS) initiative, reports that paramedic-staffed EMS systems do not convey any survival benefit. In fact, better outcomes are associated with BLS crews who are trained in early defibrillation.[19] The renewed focus on BLS techniques, coupled with data from studies similar in spirit to OPALS, has produced a new approach to the treatment of the patient in cardiac arrest.

"Push hard and push fast" captures the thrust of newer resuscitation guidelines. The AHA advocates compression rates of at least 100 per minute that also allow for full and complete chest recoil. Uninterrupted compressions are thought to maintain a baseline level of perfusion that is consistent with survival, and EMS systems are now beginning to embrace this shift back to basics. In his editorial on improving survival from out-of-hospital cardiac arrest, Eisenberg, reflecting on the 40th anniversary of out-of-hospital cardiac care in 2006, notes the paucity of "dramatic breakthroughs," and affirms that "there is ample evidence that every minute saved in delivering CPR and defibrillation translates directly into a higher survival rate." Eisenberg encourages emergency practitioners to focus on system-specific initiatives that are designed to deliver CPR and defibrillator-capable providers as fast as possible to the patient in cardiac arrest.[16]

Several landmark prehospital studies confirm the survival benefit of a treatment algorithm that features rapid compressions, and touts BLS interventions as its corner stone. A large review by Ewy in 2008 examines the impact of newer treatment initiatives started in Tucson, Arizona and in rural Wisconsin communities.[20] Acknowledging the dismally low rate of neurologically intact OOHCA survivors, several medical directors collaborated to demonstrate the impact of a push hard and push fast strategy. Called "cardiocerebral resuscitation," this subset of protocols encompasses: (1) compression-only bystander CPR, (2) minimally interrupted compressions, and (3) modified ALS protocols. Specifically, bystanders are advised to initiate compressions at approximately 100 per minute. Paramedics delay intubation, applying only passive oxygenation, until three series of compression/defibrillation/chest compressions can be completed. A retrospective study by Kellum and Kennedy, et al.[14] details the results of such protocol modifications. Neurologically intact survival following OOHCA prior to the adoption of "cardiocerebral CPR" was 15% (14/92). In the 3 years that followed the implementation of newer guidelines, 39% of patients (35/89) were neurologically intact.

Several physiological and practical principles inspired these seemingly drastic alterations in the treatment of OOHCA. First, a study conducted by Valenzuela et al. notes that patients in cardiac arrest do not receive compressions for approximately 50% of the time they are being actively treated by paramedic personnel.[21] Second, a novel three-phase model of cardiac arrest reveals that, "the generation of adequate cerebral and coronary perfusion pressure" is the key to a good neurologic outcome. The researchers confirm that defibrillation is most successful in the "electrical phase" of cardiac arrest, which is thought to occur within the first 5 minutes following collapse. Not surprisingly, resuscitative efforts begun during the "metabolic," or third phase of arrest, are not likely to result in success or meaningful neurologic recovery.[22] Clearly, basic life support interventions have rightfully recaptured their place at the forefront of cardiac arrest management. Contemporary resuscitation paradigms must necessarily advocate for early, rapid, and uninterrupted cardiac compressions.

Advanced life support and emergency care for cardiac arrest

The 2005 AHA guidelines for the management of cardiac arrest begin with a reminder that drug therapy and other advanced interventions are of "secondary importance" to BLS. The guidelines instruct rescuers to "establish intravenous access, administer any drug therapy, and insert an advanced airway" after CPR and early defibrillation has been attempted.[11] A discussion of advanced life support in cardiac arrest must begin with an acknowledgment that typical advanced cardiac life support (ACLS) strategies have failed to show improvements in intact neurological survival.

Antidysrhythmics

Neurologically favorable outcomes do not correlate with newer drug therapies for cardiac arrest. Several antidysrhythmic drugs that had been recommended in the prior ACLS algorithms fail to confer a survival benefit. In 1999, an out-of-hospital trial of amiodarone was reported to demonstrate a possible improvement in survival to admission; nevertheless, the benefits of amiodarone do not extend to hospital discharge.[23] Rea et al. compared intravenous amiodarone to lidocaine for the treatment of adults with pulseless ventricular dysrhythmias.[24] The patients treated with amiodarone exhibit a decreased likelihood of survival, and no difference can be detected in the number of patients alive in the 24-hour period after cardiac arrest. Despite its placement in several AHA algorithms, research fails to corroborate the benefits attributed to amiodarone. A retrospective case series that concluded in 2005 indicates that amiodarone does not effectively terminate sustained monomorphic ventricular tachycardia.[25] Procainamide has some utility in the treatment of refractory ventricular fibrillation, and is favored in other clinical scenarios (i.e., atrial fibrillation and Wolff-Parkinson-White syndrome) because of its lack of atrioventricular nodal blockade. The AHA cautions rescuers to avoid multiple drug therapies, as the chances of dysrhythmia and side effects increase with each added medication. Overall, the preferred and most time-tested therapies for pulseless ventricular dysrhythmias remain defibrillation and effective cardiac compressions.[11]

Vasopressors

Intermediate, escalating, and high dosages of epinephrine (HDE) had been given a class IIb classification ("possibly useful and effective") in previous editions of the AHA guidelines, largely based on animal studies and small human trials.[26-33] These studies demonstrated an improved ROSC and survival to hospital admission when adult cardiac arrest patients are treated with HDE versus standard dosages of epinephrine (SDE). It was assumed that this improvement in ROSC and survival to hospital admission would translate into increased rates of survival to hospital discharge and neurologic recovery as well. However, this was not the case. Subsequent studies confirm that HDE is not associated with improved survival to hospital discharge, and there is some evidence that HDE is actually associated with a worse neurologic outcome in survivors.[34-40] No subgroups of cardiac arrest patients have been identified who benefit from HDE, and, as a result, HDE is no longer recommended.

In the 2000 AHA guidelines, the use of vasopressin was incorporated as an alternative to the use of epinephrine (EPI) in the protocols for cardiac arrest.[41] Vasopressin is a naturally occurring antidiuretic hormone that acts upon receptors in the renal collecting ducts, as well as upon receptors in vascular smooth muscle. In high dosages, the vascular smooth muscle effect produces potent peripheral vasoconstriction. This results in the beneficial effect of increased diastolic aortic blood pressure and coronary perfusion pressure, similar to the alpha-agonist effect of EPI.

However, vasopressin does not have the adverse beta-agonist effect of EPI, which is associated with increased myocardial oxygen consumption. In theory, therefore, vasopressin appeared to have the beneficial effects of EPI but without the drawbacks. Early studies utilizing a pig model for cardiac arrest appeared to support to this idea.[42-45] These studies demonstrate improved coronary perfusion pressure, improved vital organ blood flow, improved cerebral oxygen delivery, no increase in myocardial oxygen demand, and improved return of spontaneous circulation. However, other large studies failed to demonstrate a survival benefit or improvement in neurological outcome among survivors, and so vasopressin cannot be recommended as a preferred vasopressor.[46-48] The 2005 AHA guidelines also concede that, to date, no vasopressor has demonstrated a survival advantage to hospital discharge or improvement in neurological outcome.[6]

Specific clinical situations

Specific clinical situations mandate consideration of alternative medications. Chronic alcoholics and patients with congenital syndromes (Romano Ward, Lown-Ganong-Levine) may exhibit conduction abnormalities on the routine or pre-arrest EKG. A specific type of polymorphic ventricular tachycardia, torsades de pointes, results from prolongation of the QT interval. Patients presenting with torsades de pointes require empiric treatment with magnesium sulfate, though hemodynamic instability may demand electrical countershock first. Magnesium is commonly administered as an IV push medication at a dose of 2–4 g. Magnesium has minimal side effects for the patient in arrest, and has the potential to increase the chances of successful cardioversion or defibrillation. Patients who exhibit intermittent torsades de pointes who are unresponsive to magnesium require overdrive pacing with a pacemaker or isoproterenol.

Electrolyte abnormalities, such as hyperkalemia, are extremely important to consider in the differential diagnosis of pulseless arrest. Patients with renal insufficiency, diabetes, or hypertension may develop dysrhythmias from altered cardiac repolarization. Hyperkalemia may manifest in a wide variety of electrocardiographic abnormalities. The hyperkalemic patient in cardiac arrest may exhibit peaked T waves, failure to capture, and a peculiar rhythm that appears as a "sine wave" pattern. Though these features may not be readily apparent on a rhythm strip or pre-arrest EKG, the diagnosis is often suggested from the patient history. Patients transported from dialysis centers, for example, are at high risk for hyperkalemia. Empiric calcium gluconate or calcium chloride should be administered if the diagnosis of hyperkalemia is probable. Sodium bicarbonate may also be useful during the initial resuscitation, but it is widely accepted that calcium stabilizes irritable myocardial membranes, and therefore has the most rapid onset of therapeutic effect. Calcium precipitates in solution, so it should not be given concurrently in the same intravenous line as other resuscitation drugs.

Drug overdose is also known to cause cardiac arrest. A full discussion of toxin-induced cardiac arrest is beyond the scope of this chapter, but it is well-known that AHA guidelines fall short in their treatment protocols when they are applied to patients with drug overdose. Most of the usual antidysrhythmics have a limited role in the treatment of cardiac arrest due to toxic ingestion. Though not generally recommended early in most protocols, the early consideration of sodium bicarbonate, glucagon, and calcium should be included in the early management of patients with presumed drug overdose.

Sodium bicarbonate is the treatment of choice for toxicity from tricyclic antidepressant (TCA) drugs and other drugs that are sodium-channel blockers. Sodium-channel blockade results in prolongation of the QRS complex. If untreated, ventricular tachycardia and ventricular fibrillation can ensue. If overdose of these types of drugs is considered, it is important to avoid class IA and IC antidysrhythmics, such as amiodarone or procainamide.[49] Although sodium bicarbonate is not routinely recommended in the AHA guidelines for most cases of cardiac arrest, its use is critically important in the setting of sodium-channel toxicity. An overdose of either beta-blockers or calcium-channel blockers also has dire clinical consequences. Untreated overdose results in pulseless electrical activity or bradyasystolic cardiac arrest. Intravenous bolus dosing of glucagon is used in beta blocker toxicity to assist with the regeneration of metabolites necessary for effective cardiac contraction; intravenous dosing of large quantities of calcium is critical for reversal of calcium-channel blockade in the setting of calcium-channel blocker overdose.

Post-cardiac arrest ED care: therapeutic hypothermia and critical care interface

Arguably the most important recent intervention to emerge out of contemporary postarrest resuscitation research is that of therapeutic hypothermia (TH). The history of therapeutic hypothermia dates back to its use in cardiac surgery. Animal studies demonstrate a survival benefit, and the first human trials for postarrest hypothermia by Bernard and colleagues took place in 1997.[13] Conducted in Australia, the study enrolled out-of-hospital victims of ventricular fibrillation cardiac arrest. Of the 43 enrolled patients, 21 (49%) had a good outcome that was described as "discharge to home or to a rehabilitation facility."[13] A multicenter European study confirms clinical benefit, and the American Heart Association gives a class IIa recommendation to induced hypothermia for victims of ventricular fibrillation arrest.[11,13]

Protocols for postarrest hypothermia are by no means consistent. Some studies exclude rhythms other than ventricular fibrillation, and cooling methods vary according to hospital preference and resources. A 2006 study by Oddo et al. reports that the benefits of therapeutic hypothermia extrapolate to patients in hemorrhagic shock. This 2006 study enrolled patients with all-cause cardiac arrest and describes hypothermia that is initiated in the emergency department. Teams led by critical care physicians "apply ice bags on the neck, axillae, torso, and groin," targeted to achieve a temperature of 33°C. Other methods of inducing TH include the application of cooling blankets, and the insertion of specialized vascular catheters. Patients in the Oddo et al. study underwent pulmonary artery catheterization in order to continuously monitor core temperature and had external cooling continued in the critical care unit. The study demonstrates both survival and neurological benefits from cardiac arrest due to ventricular fibrillation and shock. The benefits of therapeutic hypothermia appear unrelated to the specific cooling method (i.e., ice packs versus vascular devices). Any postarrest hypothermia initiative must necessarily involve a coordinated and multidisciplinary approach. Patients cooled in the ED require definitive care in a critical care environment that can monitor and maintain desired core body temperature. Side effects from TH such as dysrhythmia and infection have been documented.[50,51] A sample protocol for the initiation of hypothermia following cardiac arrest is detailed in Table 9-1.

Table 9-1. Sample protocol for postarrest/therapeutic hypothermia (TH) induction.

- Out of hospital:
  - Begin external cooling for cardiac arrest survivors with return of spontaneous circulation.
  - Apply external cooling with ice packs to axillae and groin and infusion of cold IV fluids.
  - Transport expeditiously to appropriate receiving facility.
- Emergency department
  - Continue induction of TH for patients who remain comatose.
  - Monitor core temperature; cool to 32–34°C.
  - Continue usual postresuscitation care (inotropic, ventilator support as required).
- Critical Care Unit
  - Maintain core temperature at 32–34°C for 24 hours.
  - Consider invasive monitoring.

Discussion of cardiac arrest treatment cannot take place without considering resource allocation. Victims of cardiac arrest at all stages of their clinical course demand meticulous attention to detail, significant expertise, and intensive monitoring. Those who survive the initial insult may depend upon a whole host of support providers for their rehabilitation and recovery. The costs associated with cardiac arrest are staggering. Few patients survive neurologically intact; survivors with hypoxic brain injury or encephalopathy often require long-term, specialized nursing care.[13,14]

Future directions in cardiac arrest care

Cardiocerebral resuscitation
The success of cardiocerebral resuscitation protocols implemented in Arizona and Wisconsin prehospital systems will likely result in modifications to advanced cardiac life support treatment priorities.[12,14,17] Further research into the optimal interplay of airway support and circulatory support is ongoing, and if the results of that research continue to support the principles of cardiocerebral resuscitation, the traditional emergency medicine focus on early airway support will be further deemphasized for patients in cardiac arrest.

Urgent percutaneous intervention
Early coronary angiography and percutaneous coronary intervention (PCI) is accepted as a valuable treatment modality for patients who demonstrate EKG evidence of STEMI, either before the cardiac arrest or after resuscitation.[1–3] However, more recent data show that early PCI may also improve the outcomes for survivors of cardiac arrest without definite evidence of STEMI on their EKG.[52,53] If further studies confirm these findings, it would strongly argue for a significant change in prehospital systems of care to recommend that all survivors of cardiac arrest should be immediately transported to hospitals that have the capability to perform urgent PCI.

Out-of-hospital termination of resuscitation (TOR)
Finally, decades of research have established that survival rates for victims of cardiac arrest with nonshockable rhythms are extremely poor. Patients surviving asystolic arrest are not likely to exhibit functional neurologic recovery. Modern discussion of cardiac arrest, therefore, incorporates the idea of termination of efforts. Rules for out-of-hospital termination of resuscitation have shown reproducible results, and several EMS systems already utilize preestablished protocols for cessation of efforts.[54,55] Some of these so-called "TOR rules" have been prospectively studied, but are by no means without controversy. This strategy acknowledges the high mortality associated with asystolic arrest. Though the decision to stop resuscitation is exceedingly complex, it makes little sense to reflexively mandate emergent transport for every victim of prehospital cardiac arrest. There is general consensus about which patients are unlikely to survive, and the allocation of intensive care monitoring and personnel to a clearly unsalvageable patient is impractical, costly, and of questionable ethics. While each decision must be made in the context of the individual patient and family, it is part of the modern practice of Emergency Medicine to not undertake futile expensive treatments. This means increasing willingness to not extend futile resuscitations, neither in the field, nor in the ED. Table 9-2 provides a sample TOR protocol.[56,57]

Section IV: Decision making

- Patients who suffer a witnessed cardiac arrest and have immediate bystander/EMS chest compressions have the best chance at intact neurological survival.
- Prehospital care must deliver early defibrillation, and avoid interruptions in compressions.

Table 9-2. Sample out-of-hospital termination of cardiac arrest protocol.[56,57]

Consider withholding or discontinuing resuscitation in the following:
- Victims of blunt trauma found in the field without signs of life
- Victims of blunt trauma with obviously nonsurvivable injuries (decapitation, hemicorpectomy)
- Victims with dependent lividity, rigor mortis, and decomposition
- Patients who are asystolic or are in a wide complex pulseless bradycardic rhythm with a rate less than 60, are normothermic, and fail an adequate trial of resuscitation therapy

- Advanced life support should be deferred until several cycles of BLS are completed.
- Patients who require drug therapy are less likely to survive than those who achieve return of spontaneous circulation after early defibrillation.
- Survivors of witnessed arrest warrant treatment with therapeutic hypothermia.

References

1 Quintero-Moran B, Moreno R, Villarreal S, et al. Percutaneous coronary intervention for cardiac arrest secondary to ST-elevation acute myocardial infarction. Influence of immediate paramedical/medical assistance on clinical outcome. *J Invasive Cardiol.* 2006;18:269–272.

2 Gorjup V, Radsel P, Kocjancic ST, Erzen D, Noc M. Acute ST-elevation myocardial infarction after successful cardiopulmonary resuscitation. *Resuscitation.* 2007;72:379–385.

3 Garot P, Lefevre T, Eltchaninoff H, et al. Six-month outcome of emergency percutaneous coronary intervention in resuscitated patients after cardiac arrest complicating ST-elevation myocardial infarction. *Circulation.* 2007;115:1354–1362.

4 Chan PS, Krumholz HM, Nichol G, Nallamothu BK. Delayed time to defibrillation after in-hospital cardiac arrest. *N Engl J Med.* 2008;358:9–17.

5 Kim F, Olsufka M, Longstreth WT, et al. Pilot randomized clinical trial of prehospital induction of mild hypothermia in out-of-hospital cardiac arrest patients with a rapid infusion of 4 degrees C normal saline. *Circulation.* 2007;115:3064–3070.

6 Hazinski MF, Nadkarni VM, Hickey RW, et al. Major changes in the 2005 AHA guidelines for CPR and ECC: Reaching the tipping point for change. *Circulation.* 2005;112:IV206–IV211.

7 Morrison LJ, Verbeek PR, Vermeulen MJ, et al. Derivation and evaluation of a termination of resuscitation clinical prediction rule for advanced life support providers. *Resuscitation.* 2007;74(2):266–275.

8 Anderson PD, Mitchell PM, Rathlev NK, Fish SS, Feldman JA. Potential diversion rates associated with prehospital acute myocardial infarction triage strategies. *J Emerg Med.* 2004;27:345–353.

9 Neumar RW, Ward KR. Adult resuscitation. In: Marx JA, Hockberger RS, Walls RM, Adams J, Rosen P, eds. *Rosen's Emergency Medicine: Concepts and Clinical Practice.* 6th ed. Philadelphia: Mosby/Elsevier; 2006.

10 Ristagno G, Gullo A, Tang W, Weil MH. New cardiopulmonary resuscitation guidelines 2005: Importance of uninterrupted chest compressions. *Crit Care Clin.* 2006:22;531–538.

11 American Heart Association. 2005 American Heart Association Guidelines for Cardiopulmonary Resuscitation and Emergency Cardiovascular Care. *Circulation.* 2005:IV1–IV5.

12 Ewy G, Kern K, Sanders A, et al. Cardiocerebral resuscitation for cardiac arrest. *Am J Med.* 2006;119:6–9.

13 Geocadin RG, Koenig MA, Jia X, Stevens RD, Peberdy MA. Management of brain injury after resuscitation from cardiac arrest. *Neurol Clin.* 2008;26:487–506.

14 Kellum MJ, Kennedy KW, Barney R, et al. Cardiocerebral resuscitation improves neurologically intact survival of patients with out-of-hospital cardiac arrest. *Ann Emerg Med.* 2008;52(3):244–252.

15 Myerburg RJ, Castellanos A. Cardiac arrest and sudden cardiac death. In: Libby P, Bonow RO, Mann DL, Zipes DP, eds. *Libby: Braunwald's Heart Disease: A Textbook of Cardiovascular Medicine.* 8th Ed. Philadelphia: Saunders; 2007.

16 Eisenberg MS. Improving survival from out-of-hospital cardiac arrest: back to the basics. editorial. *Ann Emerg Med.* 2007;49(3):314–316.

17 Ewy GA, Kern KB. Recent advances in cardiopulmonary resuscitation: cardiocerebral resuscitation. *J Am Coll Cardiol.* 2009;53(2):158–160.

18 Breitkreutz R, Walcher F, Seeger F. Focused echocardiographic evaluation in resuscitation management: concept of an advanced life support-conformed algorithm. *Crit Care Med.* 2007;35(Suppl 5):150–161.

18a 2010 American Heart Association Guidelines for Cardiopulmonary Resuscitation and Emergency Cardiovascular Care Science. *Circulation.* 2010;122:S639, doi:10.1161/CIR.0b013e3181fdf7aa

19 Stiell IG. Advanced cardiac life support in out of hospital cardiac arrest *N Engl J Med.* 2004;351(7):647–656.

20 Ewy GA. Cardiocerebral resuscitation: a better approach to cardiac arrest. *Curr Opin Cardiol.* 2008;23(6): 579–584.

21 Valenzuela TD, Kern KB, Clark LL, et al. Interruptions of chest compressions during emergency medical systems resuscitation. *Circulation.* 2005;112(9): 1259–1265.

22 Weisfeldt ML. A three phase model for cardiopulmonary resuscitation following cardiac arrest. *Trans Am Climatol Assoc.* 2004;115:115–122.

23 Kudenchuk PJ, Cobb LA, Copass MK, et al. Amiodarone for resuscitation after out-of-hospital cardiac arrest due to ventricular fibrillation *N Engl J Med.* 1999;341:871–878.

24 Rea RS, Kane-Gill SL, Rudis MI, et al. Comparing intravenous amiodarone or lidocaine, or both, outcomes for inpatients with pulseless ventricular arrhythmias. *Crit Care Med.* 2006;34(6):1617–1622.

25 Marill KA, deSouza IS, Nishijima DK, et al. Amiodarone is poorly effective for the acute termination of ventricular tachycardia. *Ann Emerg Med.* 2006;47(3):217–224.

26 Cummins RO, ed. *Advanced Cardiac Life Support.* Dallas, TX: American Heart Association; 1994.

27 Cummins RO, ed. *Advanced Cardiac Life Support.* Dallas, TX: American Heart Association; 1997.

28 Koscove EM, Paradis NA. Successful resuscitation from cardiac arrest using high-dose epinephrine therapy. Report of two cases. *JAMA.* 1988;259:3031–3034.

29 Martin D, Werman HA, Brown CG. Four case studies: high-dose epinephrine in cardiac arrest. *Ann Emerg Med.* 1990;19:322–326.

30 Barton C, Callaham M. High-dose epinephrine improves the return of spontaneous circulation rates in human victims of cardiac arrest. *Ann Emerg Med.* 1991; 20:722–725.

31 Cipolotti G, Paccagnella A, Simini G. Successful cardiopulmonary resuscitation using high doses of epinephrine. *Int J Cardiol.* 1991;33:430–431.

32 Paradis NA, Martin GB, Rosenberg J. The effect of standard- and high-dose epinephrine on coronary perfusion pressure during prolonged cardiopulmonary resuscitation. *JAMA.* 1991;265:1139–1144.

33 Wortsman J, Paradis NA, Martin GB, et al. Functional responses to extremely high plasma epinephrine concentrations in cardiac arrest. *Crit Care Med.* 1993; 21:692–697.

34 Brown CG, Martin DR, Pepe PE, et al. A comparison of standard-dose and high-dose epinephrine in cardiac arrest outside the hospital. *N Engl J Med.* 1992;327:1051–1055.

35 Stiell IG, Hebert PC, Weitzman BN, et al. High-dose epinephrine in adult cardiac arrest. *N Engl J Med.* 1992;327:1045–1050.

36 Lipman J, Wilson W, Kobilski S, et al. High-dose adrenaline in adult in-hospital asystolic cardiopulmonary resuscitation: a double-blind randomised trial. *Anaesth Intensive Care.* 1993;21:192–196.

37 Rivers EP, Wortsman J, Rady MY, et al. The effect of the total cumulative epinephrine dose administered during human CPR on hemodynamic, oxygen transport, and utilization variables in the postresuscitation period. *Chest.* 1994;106:1499–1507.

38 Sherman BW, Munger MA, Foulke GE, Rutherford WF, Panacek EA. High-dose versus standard-dose epinephrine treatment of cardiac arrest after failure of standard therapy. *Pharmacotherapy.* 1997;17:242–247.

39 Behringer W, Kittler H, Sterz F, et al. Cumulative epinephrine dose during cardiopulmonary resuscitation and neurologic outcome. *Ann Intern Med.* 1998; 129:450–456.

40 Gueugniaud PY, Mols P, Goldstein P, et al. A comparison of repeated high doses and repeated standard doses of epinephrine for cardiac arrest outside the hospital. *N Engl J Med.* 1998;339:1595–1601.

41 Cummins RO et al, eds. *Guidelines 2000 for cardiopulmonary resuscitation and emergency cardiovascular care.* Dallas, TX: American Heart Association; 2000.

42 Lindner KH, Brinkmann A, Pfenninger EG, et al. Effect of vasopressin on hemodynamic variables, organ blood flow, and acid-base status in a pig model of cardiopulmonary resuscitation. *Anesth Analg.* 1993;77:427–435.

43 Lindner KH, Prengel AW, Pfenninger EG, et al. Vasopressin improves vital organ blood flow during closed-chest cardiopulmonary resuscitation in pigs. *Circulation.* 1995;91:215–221.

44 Prengel AW, Lindner KH, Keller A, Lurie KG. Cardiovascular function during the postresuscitation phase after cardiac arrest in pigs: a comparison of epinephrine versus vasopressin. *Crit Care Med.* 1996; 24:2014–2019.

45 Prengel AW, Lindner KH, Keller A. Cerebral oxygenation during cardiopulmonary resuscitation with epinephrine and vasopressin in pigs. *Stroke.* 1996;27:1241–1248.

46 Stiell IG, Hebert PC, Wells GA, et al. Vasopressin versus epinephrine for inhospital cardiac arrest: a randomized controlled trial. *Lancet.* 2001;358:105–109.

47 Wenzel V, Krismer AC, Arntz HR, et al. A comparison of vasopressin and epinephrine for out-of-hospital cardiopulmonary resuscitation. *N Engl J Med.* 2004;350:105–113.

48 Gueugniaud PY, David JS, Chanzy E, et al. Vasopressin and epinephrine vs. epinephrine alone in cardiopulmonary resuscitation. *N Engl J Med.* 2008;359:21–30.

49 Pentel P, Keyler D. Cyclic antidepressants. In: Ford M, Delaney KA, Ling L, Erickson T, eds. *Clinical Toxicology.* Philadelphia: Saunders; 2001.

50 Oddo M, Schaller M, Feihl F, Ribordy V, Liaudet L. From evidence to clinical practice: effective implementation of therapeutic hypothermia to improve patient outcome after cardiac arrest. *Crit Care Med.* 2006;34(7):1865–1873.

51 Arrich J, The European Resuscitation Council Hypothermia After Cardiac Arrest Registry Study Group. Clinical application of mild therapeutic hypothermia after cardiac arrest. *Crit Care Med.* 2007;35(4):1041–1047.

52 Sunde K, Pytte M, Jacobsen D, et al. Implementation of a standardized treatment protocol for post resuscitation care after out-of-hospital cardiac arrest. *Resuscitation.* 2007;73:29–39.

53 Reynolds JC, Callaway CW, El Khoudary SR, et al. Coronary angiography predicts improved outcome following cardiac arrest: propensity-adjusted analysis. *J Int Care Med.* 2009;24:179–186.

54 O'Brien E, Hendricks D, Cone DC. Field termination of resuscitation: analysis of a newly implemented protocol. *Prehosp Emerg Care.* 2008;12(1):57–61.

55 Richman PB. Independent evaluation of an out-of-hospital termination of resuscitation (TOR) clinical decision rule. *Acad Emerg Med.* 2008;15(6):517–521.

56 American College of Emergency Physicians. Discontinuing resuscitation in the out of hospital setting. Available at: http://www.acep.org/practres.aspx?id=29180. Accessed September 2009.

57 Hopson LR, Hirsh E, Delgado J, et al. Guidelines for withholding or termination of resuscitation in prehospital traumatic cardiopulmonary arrest: a joint position paper from the National Association of EMS Physicians Standards and Clinical Practice Committee and the American College of Surgeons Committee on Trauma. *Prehosp Emerg Care.* 2003;7(1):141–146.

Strategies in out-of-hospital cardiac arrest: automatic external defibrillator and cardiopulmonary resuscitation

Catherine Cleaveland[1] & William J. Brady[2]

[1] *Fellow, Division of EMS, Attending Physician, Department of Emergency Medicine, University of Virginia Health System, Charlottesville, VA, USA*
[2] *Vice Chair, Department of Emergency Medicine, Professor of Emergency Medicine and Medicine, University of Virginia Health System, Charlottesville, VA, USA*

Section I: Case presentation

A 46-year-old man complained of chest pain and collapsed while attending a university lecture. Bystanders (nonmedical personnel) found the patient pulseless and apneic. They initiated compression-only CPR, and located an automatic external defibrillator (AED) placed at the entrance of the building; 911 was called. The AED was applied approximately 90 seconds after collapse; a shock was advised and delivered. The patient began to make spontaneous movements, regaining consciousness 3 and a half minutes after the onset of the cardiac arrest. At this point, university police arrived with an AED.

The patient continued to experience chest pain, but remained alert and oriented. Six minutes after the cardiac arrest, an engine company arrived on scene with emergency medical technician basic staffing; they also carried an AED. One minute later, a paramedic-staffed EMS transport unit arrived and uneventfully transported him to the emergency department (ED) with prehospital notification of anterior wall ST-segment elevation myocardial infarction (STEMI), suggested by 12-lead electrocardiogram (EKG). Upon arrival at the ED, the patient was rapidly evaluated with a 12-lead EKG. The probability of a STEMI was confirmed, necessitating transfer to the catheterization laboratory where a proximal left anterior descending artery occlusion was successfully stented;

left ventricular function was impaired with anterior wall hypokinesis.

Section II: Case discussion

Dr Peter Rosen: There's has been some suggestion in the literature that bystander CPR improves survival from cardiac arrest, but also that bystander CPR, and even CPR by medical personnel, is not performed in the recommended fashion. It appears that the greatest advantage of CPR is early mobilization of the 911 system, as opposed to CPR itself. How do you interpret the discrepancy between these two findings?

Dr Edward Ullman: I think the advantage of bystander CPR is that it activates a 911 call and enables relatively early defibrillation, which I feel is the real beneficial step. That no one does CPR correctly is, at least in part, due to lack of reinforcement. You're often taught CPR once, and it's assumed that you know it from then on. Speed and compression depth are not adequately emphasized.

PR: The evidence for the benefit of CPR is poor. Most of it is based on efficacy in other animal species and often includes a form of therapy that cannot be applied to humans. I believe the only action that makes a difference in prehospital cardiac arrest is rapid defibrillation. It seems that AEDs have made

Cardiovascular Problems in Emergency Medicine: A discussion-based review, First Edition.
Edited by Shamai A. Grossman and Peter Rosen.
© 2011 John Wiley & Sons, Ltd. Published 2011 by John Wiley & Sons, Ltd.

an enormous difference in some instances, yet there's some literature that suggests they don't make much difference at all. Do you have any explanation for this discrepancy? It would appear in this case that an AED is a good way to get early defibrillation. Yet, when you study AEDs in various other locations, they don't seem to be helpful. Is this why AEDs haven't really caught on?

Dr William Brady: I think the widespread application of the AED is a very worthwhile endeavor, but just like in the ED and everywhere else in the hospital, we need to use therapies in patient populations that are likely to need it, and therefore benefit from it. For example, if you put an AED in an elementary school, which many systems do, the likelihood of a cardiac arrest is markedly lower because children don't frequently have cardiac arrests. If it is used, it is used on the teachers, administrative staff, or the parents who are visiting. You have to look at the demographics of the area where you are placing the AED. Conversely, if you put an AED in an office where you have a large number of workers who are 40, 50, or 60 years of age, you have a much greater likelihood of using the AED. Although I believe the public access defibrillation (PAD) approach is very worthwhile, the literature is only somewhat supportive. If you look at the 2002 public access defibrillation trial, it demonstrates a higher rate of cardiac arrest resuscitation, but its impact is limited for a couple of reasons.[1] This trial was criticized because the AEDs were used in workplace areas where some cardiac arrest does occur, but the most typical cardiac arrest occurs in the home setting. Only two defibrillations took place in home settings in this study. Nonetheless, the PAD model of AED application can and does provide safe, early defibrillation to patients with out-of-hospital cardiac arrest.

PR: I've never used an AED, but I have trouble figuring out how to use a fire extinguisher. If you have to use a fire extinguisher in a hurry, you often need a sledgehammer to get at it, since they're usually locked up so securely. Have you had any experience with personal use of an AED? Is one of the problems hindering their success that people aren't trained to use them, and trying to use them for the first time is very difficult?

WB: I've used an AED in a cardiac arrest in one of the public hallways of our hospital, and I found that the most recent versions of these machines are so simple and easy to use that if you can connect your DVD player to a television set, then you can certainly use an AED successfully. There are a number of applications where the AED has been shown to be very safely, and potentially very effectively, used, such as in Las Vegas gaming casinos or airports. AEDs are safe for the provider, and safe for the patient. It basically requires someone to be able to connect the pads, and push the button. The machines are so sophisticated that incorrectly delivered shocks essentially don't occur anymore. The machines will also guide you through the entire process of checking for signs of life, instruct you on how to perform CPR in a correct fashion, and remind you to call 911. Although they are not endorsed by the American Heart Association, lay providers not trained in CPR or AED use have used them successfully. I believe the most appropriate approach is to be trained; yet, I don't want to dissuade anyone from shocking someone in cardiac arrest with an AED. Regarding access, most PAD settings have AEDs placed in cabinets that are very visible and provided with easy access.

Dr Shamai Grossman: I remember a study from about 7 or 8 years ago that examined 2 years' worth of resuscitations from a Chicago airport, and reports that they were able to resuscitate 11 people, and 6 of the resuscitations were done by people who had no training whatsoever in the use of an AED. Clearly, you can resuscitate patients without ever having touched an AED before.[1]

WB: That same study also documents that time to first defibrillation is markedly shorter when used by the lay provider, compared to public safety response with local fire rescue, and that there is almost a 6–7 minute difference in the application of a shock. If someone is going to survive cardiac arrest, they're going to have to be defibrillated very early in the process.

PR: I think airports are the optimal places for these devices, especially the way they schedule flights so close together, causing people to be running in airports who haven't run in 20 years. Public buildings are another useful location; one of the problems we used to have in Denver was how to get to an office in time to resuscitate a patient when you have to find the right elevator and ride it for 30 floors. The real question today is, "Where do you place AEDs, how many do you need, and who pays for them?"

EU: The cost saving is significant in the right setting, but they have to be in places with relatively high visibility. That's why airports and casinos, with all of the cameras, deserve defibrillators.

SG: I would make an argument that the average cost of a defibrillator today is about $1500, and that's for a new defibrillator. You can probably get a used defibrillator for half that price. That said, I would say half of the United States could probably afford to have a defibrillator in their home. Would it make sense to actually start a public access defibrillation program that was based on home-owned defibrillators, and really try to train the overwhelming majority of the United States to use a defibrillator that they would have in their home like a fire extinguisher?

WB: Thus far there's no conclusive data to support routine home placement of AEDs for people with a cardiac history or an increased chance of cardiac arrest, but the trials are ongoing. It would make sense for somebody who has had some cardiac issue who is at high risk for ventricular dysrhythmias (for example, someone with reduced ventricular function who does not qualify for an AICD) to have an AED in the home. Remember, most cardiac arrests occur in or near the home. In the near future, home use will probably be the third or fourth deployment of AEDs to be considered, with public access defibrillation being the first model, followed by hospital use, followed by targeted first responder use.

SG: I believe the greatest challenge to home defibrillation may be an inability to self defibrillate. To effectively utilize home defibrillation, someone else needs to be at home to apply the device.

PR: I think defibrillation is the primary answer to cardiac arrest, but this is still treating the wrong end of the disease. If you can't defibrillate quickly, then it takes luck for the patient to survive. Defibrillators should be more available than they have been, especially in places where we're more likely to see cardiac arrest.

WB: I agree. Early defibrillation, regardless of the mode of defibrillation (i.e., either via a lay bystander with an AED or EMS with a standard multifunction device), is the key. But early and adequate CPR is also important. The new description of compression-only CPR is a new and important intervention that hopefully will increase the use of bystander interventions for out-of-hospital cardiac arrest.

Case resolution

The patient experienced an uneventful hospital course with confirmation of a STEMI via elevated cardiac biomarkers. An internal cardiac defibrillator was placed. The patient returned to employment as a university history professor at his prearrest level of function. He was well at 6-month follow up.

Section III: Concepts

The problem of sudden cardiac arrest

The preceding case scenario highlights many of the key factors surrounding sudden cardiac arrest (SCA), automatic external defibrillators (AED), current cardiopulmonary resuscitation (CPR) recommendations, and the public access defibrillation (PAD) initiative supported by the American Heart Association (AHA). Cardiac arrest causes nearly 500,000 deaths per year in the United States, with nearly half of these events occurring outside the hospital setting.[2] While individuals with known advanced cardiac disease have a greater than 50% incidence of cardiac death, they constitute only a fraction of sudden cardiac deaths that occur. With a majority of SCA events occurring in individuals without known cardiac disease, prevention measures are difficult to implement. Thus focusing on improvements in the treatment of sudden cardiac arrest could be a more cost-effective means to decrease the negative impact of sudden cardiac death.[3] However, despite advances in prehospital advanced life support, most American communities have out-of-hospital cardiac arrest survival rates of less than 5%.[4]

Therapies of value in sudden cardiac arrest

The AHA has promoted the "Chain of Survival" concept as a strategy to improve outcomes: early access, early CPR, early defibrillation, and early advanced life support.[5] Recent research suggests that among these "links," early defibrillation is a very effective, if not the most effective, intervention in improving outcomes in sudden cardiac arrest.[6,7] Given this observation, efforts have been made to decrease the interval from sudden cardiac arrest onset to defibrillation. Among these efforts is the promotion of the Public Access Defibrillation initiative.[8]

Multiple studies have shown that defibrillation improves outcomes in sudden cardiac arrest.[7,9–11] In fact, defibrillation immediately after witnessed ventricular fibrillation (VF) arrest results in survival rates greater than 90%.[12–15] However, this benefit declines precipitously with increasing time from VF onset to initial defibrillation.[7,10–12] Common medical opinion estimates that each minute of VF leads to a 10% reduction in survival; in cases of prolonged cardiac arrest greater than 10 minutes, outcomes are universally dismal.

Defibrillation, while extremely important in the early management of cardiac arrest, should not be employed in isolation of other lay interventions. CPR is one such other therapy. CPR, when begun immediately upon the recognition of sudden cardiac arrest, has been shown to improve outcome when defibrillation is not immediately available. CPR provides some degree of perfusion to the central nervous system and myocardium to maintain temporary viability, thus increasing the chance of maintaining a "shockable" rhythm (e.g., ventricular tachycardia [VT] or VF), until a defibrillator arrives.[6,16–18] CPR also increases the likelihood that defibrillation will be successful once it is delivered, and improves the chances of a positive neurological recovery if return of spontaneous circulation is achieved.[18,19] However, despite the benefit of early CPR, outcomes remain poor if the defibrillation delivery is delayed (i.e., greater than 8–12 minutes after collapse), and the combination of late CPR (greater than 4 minutes) and late defibrillation (greater than 12 minutes) is particularly poor.[20,21]

The improved survival seen with early CPR has been theorized to be due to increasing the likelihood of VF being present when a defibrillator arrives (i.e., the "shockable rhythm" concept).[17,18,20] In Seattle, a system frequently cited for its superior outcomes in cardiac arrest, investigators report that 80% of sudden cardiac arrest victims who receive early bystander CPR are in VF or VT, compared to 68% if CPR is delayed.[18] In Stockholm, the presence of VT or VF is 22% more likely in victims who receive bystander CPR, and, in Belgium, it is 13% more likely.[20,21]

Furthermore, victims with a shockable rhythm upon EMS arrival are more likely to convert to a perfusing rhythm, and enjoy a better outcome, if they receive early CPR. In Seattle, patients in VF have a 37% rate of long-term survival if they have bystander CPR prior to EMS arrival, but only 29% survival rate if not.[18] In Houston, patients with ventricular fibrillation or tachycardia have a 40% survival to hospital discharge rate if they receive bystander CPR compared to 19% without.[20] While studies show the benefit of bystander-initiated CPR in the setting of delayed defibrillation in unwitnessed arrest, immediate defibrillation in the setting of witnessed sudden cardiac arrest with available AED is still recommended and well supported.[22]

Interestingly, recent studies show that the fourth link—early access to advanced life support—in the "chain of survival" may be of less importance than previously believed.[19,23] In the final phase of the Ontario Prehospital Advanced Life Support, it is reported that, in a community where early CPR and early defibrillation are achieved, there is no survival benefit to the addition of prehospital advanced life support interventions. This finding should be of interest to communities with limited resources seeking to maximize gain from their investments in their EMS system.

The importance of early therapy

The importance of early therapy suggested by the studies mentioned earlier in this chapter is described numerically by Larsen et al.: Rate = 0.67 − 0.023 [min CPR] − 0.011 [min defibrillation] − 0.021 [min ACLS].[24] This time-sensitive difference in response to therapy has been explained in a physiologically-based model.[24] In this model, the timeline in ongoing cardiac arrest is separated into three phases: electrical, circulatory, and metabolic. This separation is based on the physiologic changes that occur during prolonged cardiac arrest, and how these changes impact outcome. In the electrical phase, within the first 4 minutes of cardiac arrest, immediate defibrillation alone is very effective, and multiple studies show success rates near 50%; after the initial 4 minutes, however, immediate defibrillation is not as successful, and is perhaps detrimental.[25]

In the circulatory phase, 4–10 minutes after onset of sudden cardiac arrest, the ischemic heart has been deprived of oxygen, and metabolic byproducts accumulate in the myocardium. Immediate defibrillation is indicated for patients with downtime less than 4 to 5 mnutes. In either unwitnessed arrest or prolonged downtimes (greater than 4 to 5 minutes), at the present time, there is disagreement with regards to the most appropriate time for defibrillation relative to the time of cardiac arrest onset. Certain researchers suggest that the initiation of CPR prior to defibrillation allows for the partial replenishment of necessary myocardial energy substrates, such as oxygen, and the removal of anoxic metabolites, improving the metabolic milieu prior to defibrillation attempts; this increases the likelihood of defibrillation success.[26] Others note that the data is inconclusive in this area of defibrillation and suggest that defibrillation occur as soon as possible while appropriate compressions and other therapies are applied. In fact, a recent meta-analysis of this topic demonstrates no benefit to providing CPR before defibrillation as compared to immediate defibrillation in those patients with prolonged down-times. They also noted that no harm to performance of CPR before defibrillation. Thus, the time to defibrillation is best determined by the patient's needs, arrest situation, and provider abilities.

After approximately 10 minutes, at the onset of the *metabolic phase*, resuscitation rates are universally poor regardless of the order of steps in attempted resuscitation. The proponents of the model suggest that the circulation of cytokines, accumulated during the electrical and circulatory phase, contribute to cell death in the metabolic phase. It is not known whether by this point that irreversible injury has occurred, or whether known therapeutic approaches simply fail to correct important reversible factors in this phase.

The challenge of EMS timely response

The preceding physiological discussion of cardiac arrest is important foundation information in the discussion of the "hard truths" of sudden cardiac arrest, as well as public assumption that the local EMS system is solely responsible for the response to and resuscitation of these patients. It has been propounded that EMS systems that achieve response times of 5 minutes or less after collapse have dramatically higher survival rates than those with longer response times.[27] They appear to have survival rates twice as high as systems with response times of 8 minutes long, which is the standard response interval goal for out-of-hospital cardiac arrest.

The lay public often considers their proximity to fire-rescue stations as a "fail safe" guaranteeing a timely response, yet they fail to understand the need to include several other steps that must occur between onset of sudden cardiac arrest and initiation of resuscitation attempts by EMS. This interval includes: (1) recognition of a medical emergency by bystanders; (2) the decision to make a call for emergency medical assistance; (3) locating a telephone; (4) calling the emergency number; (5) interrogation of the caller by an emergency dispatcher; (6) the decision to send an emergency vehicle; and (7) the time to transfer the call to a proper response station or vehicle. Multiple minutes may pass before one even reaches step (8) ambulance response time, the interval between response unit notification by dispatcher and unit arrival at the scene (6). Once this occurs, depending on the community size and type of location, it may still be several minutes longer before emergency personnel actually reach the patient. This analysis also assumes that all local EMS units are in service and available for the call.

Over the last two decades, the establishment of a common 3-digit emergency number used to gain access to the dispatch system has done much to shave minutes off this time consuming process, strengthening the early access link in the chain of survival. Nevertheless, depending on the geography of the local community and current economic state of the local system, there may not be funds available for cost-effective improvement to shorten the time to EMS arrival to below this crucial 5-minute threshold. Studies show that after a certain point, an increase in the number of ambulances fails to decrease response time intervals.[28]

Public access defibrillation

PAD is a strategy to decrease the interval between onset of sudden cardiac arrest and initial defibrillation, by placing the means of safe defibrillation into the hands of the public. With this strategy, AEDs are distributed to areas where sudden cardiac arrest occurs more frequently (i.e., areas where there are large numbers of people and where older people tend to gather, such as malls, casinos, and airports). Nonmedical personnel are trained in the use of AEDs in order to provide early defibrillation in the event of sudden cardiac arrest. The training involved is rather minimal; in most instances, a lay provider CPR course requiring no more than 4 hours of instruction and demonstration is sufficient. Not only are "minimally-trained" personnel capable of safely managing cardiac arrest seconds after occurrence, but also persons with no training are able to intervene effectively. While training is encouraged, numerous cases have been reported in which the untrained, lay provider has safely and effectively saved a life using an AED seconds after the onset of cardiac arrest.

Public access defibrillation is commonly divided into four levels, based on the medical training of the responder as well as the assumed "duty to respond" to such an emergency.[4]

Level 1: Traditional First Responder Defibrillation: This level includes defibrillation by law enforcement and fire department personnel. In many locations, police officers and firefighters are the first responders to cardiac emergencies, but until recently, were often prohibited by regulations and state codes from providing early defibrillation.

Level 2: Non-Traditional First Responder Defibrillation: This level includes defibrillation efforts by lifeguards, security personnel, and airline flight attendants.

Level 3: Citizen CPR Defibrillation: This level includes laypersons in the community who have received AED training. They are interested in providing emergency cardiac care, often in the setting of a home or workplace where a family member or colleague is a high risk for cardiac arrest.

Level 4: Minimally-Trained Witness Defibrillation: This level includes individuals who witness a potential cardiopulmonary emergency, have an AED available, yet have no formal training in AED application. As PAD is becoming more available, this level of application often occurs in public locations where AEDs are displayed prominently and are available to the public much like fire extinguishers.

Public access defibrillation programs

A cardiac arrest management strategy to decrease time to defibrillation intervals has been to place AEDs in the hands of other first responders (Level 1 PAD), such as police and fire department personnel. Several studies evaluating the effectiveness of this type of strategy, as implemented in various sized communities, report mixed results.[29–31] Miami-Dade County reports increased survival rates from 9.0% to 17.2% for victims with shockable rhythms with the addition of a police-equipped AED program.[32]

To the contrary, the urban community of Cincinnati and rural and suburban communities in Indiana report no improvement.[31,33] This failure may be due in part to a lack of police confidence in assuming these new roles. Officers participating in the PARADE study were questioned regarding possible reasons for the poorer than expected response by police in out-of-hospital cardiac arrest. The reasons proffered included police comfort level, lack of confidence in providing medical care, and officers' concerns about personal liability issues related to treating the cardiac arrest victim.[33] Low population density could also limit the success of such programs in rural communities where arrest-to-defibrillation intervals, while improved with Police-AED programs, continue to fall beyond the 10-minute threshold.

Several studies show success with implementation of Level 2 PAD programs in locations such as on airlines and in casinos.[32,33] In 1997, American Airlines began equipping its aircraft with automated external defibrillators, as well as training its flight attendants in their use, and in 2000 they published the results of their measures.[34] The AED identifies ventricular fibrillation and recommends defibrillation in 100% of patients with electrocardiographic evidence of ventricular fibrillation, but does not recommend shock in any other instance, making its use on aircraft 100% sensitive and specific. A similar program was instituted in casinos where AEDs were placed and security officers were trained in their use, as well as in CPR. During the study period, 105 of 148 cardiac arrest victims were found in ventricular fibrillation. Of these, 56 (53% of VF and 38% of all cardiac arrest victims) survived to hospital discharge after being successfully defibrillated.[35]

Level 3 PAD, defibrillation by previously trained private citizens, was implemented and reported successful in the public access defibrillation trial.[34] Locations were randomized to CPR only versus CPR with AED. Volunteers were recruited and trained in CPR at all locations. In the AED locations, they were also trained in the use of AEDs. Victims of cardiac arrest have a survival-to-hospital discharge rate of 38.4% in the CPR/AED group compared to 14% in the CPR only group. In Piacenza, Italy, a program of mobile lay volunteers equipped with AEDs and trained in the use of AEDs alone, without CPR, more than tripled the survival rate to hospital discharge in victims with shockable dysrhythmias.

Level 4 PAD is also safe and effective, as reported in the Chicago HeartSave Program.[35] In this program, AEDs were distributed to the Chicago area airports O'Hare, Midway and Meigs Field. They were housed in glass-faced cabinets, 90-second walking intervals apart, and were prominently marked by signs placed in highly visible positions. During the study period, the AEDs were used on 22 unresponsive patients, and 18 of whom were found to be in ventricular fibrillation. Of these, 11 were successfully defibrillated, regained spontaneous circulation, and ultimately regained consciousness; a survival rate of 50%, which is 10 times the estimated survival rate with traditional EMS response alone.[36] Over half of these arrest patients were resuscitated by individuals who had never before operated an AED nor been trained in its use. In no situation where an AED was used did it permit inappropriate defibrillation, showing that such programs can be safe and effective even in the hands of untrained volunteers.

Thanks to the manufacturers' responses to the American Heart Association's call to develop smaller, simpler, more lightweight, and lower cost designs, AEDs are now more accessible, as well as more affordable, to purchase and maintain. The simplification of their design has made them easy for untrained individuals to use. The self adhesive pads are printed with diagrams showing how to apply them, and are designed to transmit electrocardiac activity to the device for analysis as well as to deliver the defibrillating current when indicated. Once activated, they have voice prompts to guide the user through the few simple steps. A programmed algorithm interprets the rhythm automatically, and advises "shock" or "no shock." These simplifications in design and operation have made it possible for untrained laypersons to safely, quickly, and effectively provide life-saving defibrillation. In one study involving a group of untrained sixth graders, the average time to defibrillation is only 90 seconds.[37] Early AEDs used monophasic waveforms, in which current is delivered to the patient in a single direction. More recently, biphasic waveforms, where the direction of current is reversed during the delivery of the shock, have been found to achieve equivalent or superior defibrillation rates at lower energy levels. This feature has resulted in biphasic waveforms becoming the most common type used in AEDs.[7] The development of smaller, lighter, lithium-based batteries that can last up to 5 years without

requiring service, and devices that perform regular self-tests and alert users when service is required, have led to marked reduction in the cost to maintain AEDs, as well as an improvement in their portability.

Public Access Defibrillation programs are cost effective in comparison to other common treatments for life-threatening illnesses in industrialized countries.[38,39] It is estimated that PAD programs, when added to an established EMS system, cost $44,000 per additional quality-adjusted life-year saved, but the results from Chicago's HeartSave Program show far more efficient results, costing on average $3000 per individual treated, and $7000 per life saved. This program's cost efficiency is largely due to the uniquely diverse and densely populated environment found within the concourses of an international airport. Educational settings (e.g., schools, universities, etc.) have been proposed as promising locations for the establishment of PAD programs.[40] While such settings, like the one in the proceeding case scenario, account for only 2.6% of all public-location cardiac arrests, the survival rate to hospital discharge for cardiac arrest in school settings is significantly higher (39% compared to 27% in other public locations).[41] The arrests are more likely to be witnessed (79% vs. 62%), to receive bystander CPR (74% vs. 51%), and to present with an initial rhythm of ventricular fibrillation or pulseless ventricular tachycardia (78% vs. 56%). Also, the effect of establishing PAD and CPR training in school environments could positively affect the establishment of similar programs, and public health in general, as graduates go to other areas of a community with AED and CPR knowledge and ability.

Barriers to early therapy—bystander CPR and public access defibrillation

In the past, many members of the lay community have been hesitant to provide bystander CPR to unknown individuals out of concern for risk of infection, as well as fear of performing this potentially lifesaving therapy incorrectly and the possibility of incurring a liability. The new AHA guidelines for compression only CPR alleviates two of these three concerns. The new recommendations, which eliminate the need to remember compression to ventilation ratios, are easier to recall, allowing lay-responders to be more confident in their care. The elimination of "mouth-to-mouth" ventilation eliminates the contact that made many people afraid of and adverse to providing aid. Many organizations and individuals have voiced safety concerns as well as liability issues in purchasing and providing access to AEDs. Nevertheless, AEDs are safe and effective even in untrained hands. Over the past several years, as more and more evidence supporting the safety and efficacy of AED and PAD has been published, state legislatures have promoted PAD by writing legislation specifically to protect responders using AEDs. Some states and the federal government have gone further to even mandate AEDs be placed in special environments, such as aboard commercial aircraft, in health clubs, and in schools. There have even been cases in which a business corporation has been found negligent for not having AEDs available.[42]

Section IV: Decision making

The "local site" personnel should consider the following issues when deciding upon AED deployment:

- Will the individual location is occupied by a good-sized number of persons for a significant portion of the 24-hour day?
- Will the persons potentially present at the site are of the appropriate age and risk for sudden cardiac death (middle-aged and older adults)?
- Will EMS (and AED-equipped public safety officer) response times to the patient's side likely be greater than 4 minutes?

References

1 Caffrey SL, Willoughb PJ. Pepe PE. Becker LB. Public use of automated external defibrillators. *N Engl J Med.* 2002;347:1242–1247.
2 Zheng Z-J, Croft, JB, Giles WH, Mensah, GA. Sudden cardiac death in the United States, 1989 to 1998. *Circulation.* 2001;104;2158–2163.
3 Nicol G, Hallstrom AP, Kerber R, et al. American Heart Association Report on the Second Public Access Defibrillation Conference, April 17-19, 1997. *Circulation.* 1998;97:1309–1314.
4 Eisenberg MS, Horwood B I, Cummings RO, Reynolds-Haertle R, Hearne TR. Cardiac arrest resuscitation: a tale of 29 cities. *Ann Emerg Med.* 1990;19:179–186.
5 Cummins RO, Ornato JP, Thies WH, Pepe PE. Improving survival from sudden cardiac arrest: The chain of survival concept. *Circulation.* 1991;83:1832–1847.

6 Marenco JP, Wang PJ, Link MS, Homoud MK, Estes NAM. Improving survival from sudden cardiac arrest: The role of the automated external defibrillator. *JAMA.* 2001;285:1193–1200.
7 Nichol G, Stiell IG, Laupacis A, et al. A cumulative meta-analysis of the effectiveness of defibrillator-capable emergency medical services for victims of out-of-hospital cardiac arrest. *Ann Emerg Med.* 1999;34:517–525.
8 Weisfeldt ML, Kerber RE, McGoldrick RP, et al. Public access defibrillation: a statement for health care professionals from the American Heart Association Task Force on Automatic External Defibrillation. *Circulation.* 1995;92:2763.
9 Eisenbert MS, Bergner L, Hallstrom AP, Cummins RO. Sudden cardiac death. *Sci Am.* 1986;254:37–43.
10 Weaver WD, Cobb LA, Hallstrom AP. Factors influencing survival after out-of-hospital cardiac arrest. *J Am Coll Cardiol.* 1986;7:752–775.
11 Eisenberg MS, Hallstrom A, Bergner L. The ACLS score: predicting survival from out-of-hospital cardiac arrest. *JAMA.* 1981;246:50–52.
12 Kouwenhoven DR, Brady WJ. The development of the defibrillator. *Ann Intern Med.* 1969;71:449–458.
13 Haskell WL. Cardiovascular complications during exercise training of cardiac patients. *Circulation.* 1978;57:920–924.
14 Hossack KF, Hartwig R. Cardiac arrest associated with supervised cardiac rehabilitation. *J Card Rehabil.* 1982;2:402–08.
15 VanCamp SP, Peterson RA. Cardiovascular complications of outpatient cardiac rehabilitation programs. *JAMA.* 1986;256:1160–1163.
16 Weaver WD, Cobb LA, Dennis D, Ray R, Hallstrom AP. Amplitude of ventricular fibrillation waveform and outcome after cardiac arrest. *Ann Intern Med.* 1985;102:53–55.
17 Cummins RO, Eisenberg MS, Hallstrom AP, Litwin PE. Survival of out-of-hospital cardiac arrest with early initiation of cardiopulmonary resuscitation *Am J Emerg Med.* 1958;3:114–119.
18 Jakobsson J, Nyquist O, Rehnqvist N. Cardiac arrest in Stockholm with special reference to the ambulance organization. *Acta Med Scand.* 1987;222:117–122.
19 Larsen MP, Eisenberg MS Cummins RO, Hallstrom AP. Predicting survival from out-of-hospital cardiac arrest: a graphic model. *Ann Emerg Med.* 1993;22:1652–1658.
20 Eisenberg M, Bergner L, Hallstrom A. Paramedic programs and out-of-hospital cardiac arrest: I. Factors associated with successful resuscitation. *Am J Public Health.* 1979;69:30–38.
21 Bossaert L, VanHoeywghen R. Cerebral resuscitation study group: Bystander cardiopulmonary resuscitation

(CPR) in out-of-hospital cardiac arrest. *Resuscitation.* 1989;17(suppl):S55–S69.

22 Connolly SJ, Hallstrom AP, Cappato R, et al. Meta-analysis of the implantable cardioverter defibrillator secondary prevention trials. *Eur Heart J.* 2000;21:2071–2078.

23 Stiell IG, Wells, GA, Field, B, et al. Advanced cardiac life support in out of hospital cardiac arrest. *N Engl J Med.* 2004;351:647–656.

24 Weisfeldt ML, Becker LB. Resuscitation after cardiac arrest: A 3-phase time-sensitive model. *JAMA.* 288;23:3035–3038.

25 Niemann, JT, Carins CB, Sharma J, Lewis RJ. Treatment of prolonged ventricular fibrillation : Immediate countershock versus high-dose epinephrine and CPR preceding countershock. *Circulation.* 1992;85:281–287.

26 Simpson PM, Goodger MS, Bendall JC. Delayed versus immediate defibrillation for out-of-hospital cardiac arrest due to ventricular fibrillation: A systematic review and meta-analysis of randomized controlled trials. Resuscitation 2010;81:925–931.

27 DeMaio AJ, Stiell IG, Wells GA, Spaite DW. Optimal defibrillation response intervals for maximum out-of-hospital cardiac arrest survival rates. *Ann Emerg Med.* 2003;42:242–250.

28 Hallstrom AP. Improving the EMS system, in Eisenberg MS, Bergner L, Hallstrom AP (eds): *Sudden Cardiac Death in the Community.* Philadelphia: Praeger Pubs; 1984:126–139.

29 Sayre MR, Evans J, White LJ, Brennan TD. Providing automated external defibrillators to urban police officers in addition to a fire department rapid defibrillation program is not effective. *Resuscitation.* 2005;66:189–196.

30 Groh WJ, Newman MM, Beal PE, Fineberg NS, Zipes DP. Limited response to cardiac arrest by police equipped with automated external defibrillators: lack of survival benefit in suburban and rural Indiana. The olive as responder automated defibrillation evaluation (PARADE). *Acad Emerg Med.* 2001;8:324–333.

31 Myerburg RJ, Fenster J, Velez M, et al. Impact of community-wide police car deployment of automate external defibrillators on survival from out-of-hospital cardiac arrest. *Circulation.* 2002;106:1058–1064.

32 Valenzuela TD, Roe DJ, Nichol G, et al. Outcome of rapid defibrillation by security officers after cardiac arrest in casinos. *N Engl J Med.* 2000;343:1206–1209.

33 Page RL, Joglar JA, Kowal RC, et al. Use of automated external defibrillators by a U.S. airline. *N Engl J Med.* 2000;343:1210–1216.

34 Hallstrom AP, Ornato JP, Weisfeldt M, Travers A, Christenson J. Public-access defibrillation and survival after out-of-hospital cardiac arrest. *N Engl J Med.* 2004; 351:637–646.

35 Caffrey SL, Willoughby PJ, Pepe EP, Becker LB. Public use of automated external defibrillators. *N Engl J Med.* 2002;347:1242–1247.

36 Becker LB, Ostrander MP, Barrett J, Kondos GT. Outcome of CPR in a large metropolitan area—where are the survivors? *Ann Emerg Med.* 1991;20:355–361.

37 Gundry JW, Comess KA, De Rook FA, Jorgenson D, Bardy GH. Comparison of naïve sixth-grade children with trained professionals in the use of an automated external defibrillator. *Circulation.* 1999;100:1703–1707.

38 Jermyn BD. Cost-effectiveness analysis of a rural/urban first-responder defibrillation program. *Prehosp Emerg Care.* 2000;4:43–47.

39 Nicholg, Hallstrom AP, Ornato JP, et al. Potential cost-effectiveness of public access defibrillation on the United States. *Circulation.* 1998;97:1315–1320.

40 Estes NAM. Prediction and prevention of sudden cardiac arrest: Lessons learned in schools. *Circulation.* 2007; 116:1341–1343.

41 Lofti K, White L, Rea T, et al. Cardiac arrest in schools. *Circulation.* 2007;116:1374–1379.

42 England H, Weinberg PS, Estes NAM. The automated external defibrillator: clinical benefits and legal liability. *JAMA.* 2006;295:687–690.

11 Pacemakers and AICDS in emergency medicine

Theodore Chan

Medical Director, Department of Emergency Medicine, University of California, San Diego Medical Center, Professor of Clinical Medicine, University of California, San Diego, San Diego, California, USA

Section I: Case presentation

An 82-year-old woman with a history of Alzheimer's dementia was brought to the emergency department (ED) from her nursing home by paramedics. She was complaining of weakness and bilateral lower extremity swelling, but could not provide much history beyond that. A review of records sent from the nursing home indicates that she had these complaints for the prior 3 days. In addition, her appetite and intake had been poor during this time, but she had no vomiting, diarrhea, fevers, or other symptoms noted by the nursing home staff. The staff became concerned when they recorded a pulse rate of 48 beats/min, so they called 911.

The nursing home records indicate the patient was taking hydrochlorothiazide, diltiazem, potassium supplementation, and thyroid hormone replacement, with no recent changes to her medications. The past medical history from the nursing record was notable for hypertension, hypothyroidism, pacemaker placement, and a remote history of breast cancer.

The triage vital signs were: blood pressure 106/52 mmHg, pulse rate 50 beats/min, respiratory rate 16 breaths/min, and temperature 37.2°C (98.9°F). On initial evaluation, the patient was an elderly woman in mild distress, lying on a gurney. Physical examination findings were notable for a healed bilateral mastectomy scar, a palpable pacemaker device along the

left upper chest wall, and clear breath sounds on chest auscultation. Cardiac examination revealed a slow, occasionally irregular heart beat with a faint systolic murmur, best heard along the base. The abdomen was soft and benign, and the extremities were nontender with no edema.

The patient was placed on a cardiac monitor and a 12-lead EKG was obtained, which demonstrated pacer spikes with intermittent QRS wave forms with T wave inversions in the anterolateral leads (Figure 11-1). There was no prior EKG available for comparison. A complete blood count, serum electrolytes and TSH level were unremarkable, and the cardiac troponin-I level was < 0.02 ng/ml.

Section II: Case discussion

Dr Peter Rosen: Assuming that this is a patient capable of independent living, and we want to improve the quality of her life, do you believe many of her symptoms can be explained by the pacemaker?

Dr David Brown: The description of the EKG doesn't specifically tell me whether each QRS is preceded by a pacemaker spike, nor whether every pacemaker spike is followed by a QRS. It doesn't describe whether it is atrioventricular (AV) pacing or ventricular pacing. I think we need to know a little more about precisely what the EKG showed. Is there evidence of pacemaker

Cardiovascular Problems in Emergency Medicine: A discussion-based review, First Edition.
Edited by Shamai A. Grossman and Peter Rosen.
© 2011 John Wiley & Sons, Ltd. Published 2011 by John Wiley & Sons, Ltd.

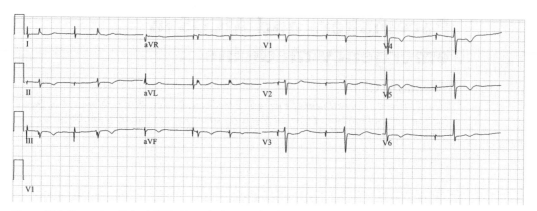

Figure 11.1 Presenting 12-lead EKG. Note the low amplitude pacing spikes not associated with the QRS complexes.

malfunction, or is she at a rate of 50 simply because that is what the pacemaker is set at as a default for when she goes into some other kind of bradycardia, native bradyarrhythmia, for some other reason.

DB: Looking at her EKG with pacer spikes at a regular rate of about 65, QRS waveforms at about 0.10 msec, but with T wave inversions laterally and pacer spikes that do not appear to be associated with the QRS waveforms, I would think her bradycardia is at least in part related to pacemaker malfunction. We have evidence of a pacemaker that was set at 65, not capturing the ventricles, and there's what may be a junctionally-derived escape rhythm at 50 beats/min that is maintaining cardiac output. It is likely the bradycardia that is causing her to be sick.

PR: In this situation would you recommend obtaining a chest X-ray study immediately to look for a pacemaker wire fracture, or do you just reach for a magnet to define whether or not there is pacemaker function?

Dr Amal Mattu: I would probably do both simultaneously. Getting a quick chest X-ray study certainly doesn't take long, and might give you information about whether there's a break in the lead insulation or dislodgement. In the meantime, I would be on the phone with an electrophysiologist or a technician from the pacemaker manufacturers who also might be able to assess the pacer. I would place a magnet as well.

PR: This patient doesn't sound like she's in a great deal of distress from the pacemaker dysfunction. Given she's functioning adequately in this case, despite the pacemaker dysfunction, we don't need to immediately reach for an external pacemaker. What would your indications be for external pacing?

Dr Theodore Chan: If the nursing records note a significant change in her mental status, or any suggestion that she's hemodynamically unstable, then external pacing might be useful. It would be important to look at the nursing records to see what her previous hemodynamic status was. If she had a history of hypertension, then a blood pressure of 106 may be significantly low for her, and indicate hemodynamic instability.

PR: My experience with external pacing has been dismal. I've had patients capture with it, but if they were at all alert, they hated the experience, and required heavy sedation. If the clinical circumstances were forcing your hand, would you ever consider floating another temporary transvenous pacemaker wire on someone who has a nonfunctioning pacemaker?

Dr Shamai Grossman: I would always start with an external pacemaker. The only real contraindication to an external pacemaker, aside from failure to capture, is patient discomfort. Patients often are very uncomfortable. The major problem with an external pacemaker is it requires more amperage to pace someone than a transvenous or an implanted pacemaker. We use far more electricity externally to pace someone, and clinically that causes discomfort. If the blood pressure can tolerate it, you can concomitantly give analgesia and that may help, but if you can't get capture with an external pacer or the patient is so uncomfortable he or she refuses to allow you to externally pace him or her, then you can try to float a temporary transvenous pacemaker wire in the ED.

PR: It's been a long time since I've floated a wire, since I've been lucky enough to work at places where many resources are readily available, but if you're in a more remote community hospital, do you have any suggestions for us in terms of floating a wire without fluoroscopic guidance?

DB: When one is forced to proceed because of lack of resources or instability of the patient, ideally, you want to place the introducer in the right internal jugular vein since it's a more direct route, straight down through the superior vena cava and into the right atrium and then into the right ventricle. Although some EDs may have a portable c-arm, fluoroscopy is often unavailable to emergency physicians; however, ultrasound is very useful. A portable ultrasound should be available in most EDs these days to watch the wire progress to the right ventricle.

PR: Do you think that this patient, on a thiazide diuretic, could have a metabolic abnormality, such as hypokalemia, that's interfering with the pacemaker function? Could the pacemaker perhaps be in place, but the heart can't respond?

AM: Metabolic abnormalities would definitely be in the differential when the pacemaker's not being sensed. Several electrolyte or metabolic abnormalities are notorious for causing problems with pacemakers, and are the most common cause of transcutaneous pacemaker dysfunction that I've seen. Any patient presenting with a pacemaker problem must have a set of electrolytes and metabolic panel performed looking for this relatively simple reversible cause.

PR: Could you take us through the use of a magnet? What kind of magnet, where do you put it, what do you expect to see, and how do you interpret the monitor strip when the magnet is in place?

TC: We usually keep a donut-shaped magnet in the ED. It should be placed directly on top of the pacemaker generator where, once in place, the magnet turns off sensing. This temporarily puts the pacemaker into the asynchronous mode, where pacing is initiated at a set rate. This may allow you to assess whether capture is occurring, and helps assess function when the native heart rhythm is faster than the rate the pacemaker is set at.

PR: So you'd see a series of spikes with or without a QRS following.

TC: Correct.

SG: Application of a magnet can also determine if the pacemaker's battery needs to be replaced. Each pacemaker type has a unique asynchronous rate for beginning-of-life of the unit (BOL), elective replacement indicator (ERI), and end-of-life of the unit (EOL).

PR: How can you tell if the pacemaker is single- or dual-chambered, or what kind of pacemaker your patient has?

TC: Dual-chamber pacemakers will often have both atrial and ventricular spikes on the EKG.

SG: On chest X-ray study, if you see a lead going into the atrium, and a lead going into the ventricle, then clearly it's a dual-chamber pacemaker. Often the specific type of pacemaker can be verified by identifying the generator on the chest X-ray study. In addition, most patients carry a card with them verifying essential pacemaker information, such as the model type and the magnet rates. Patients who have atrial fibrillation generally don't get DDD (atrial and ventricular lead) pacemakers, because in atrial fibrillation the pacemaker itself is not able to pace the atrium.

PR: Is it possible that the atrium can capture, but not the ventricle, or vice versa with a dual chamber? What would that look like?

TC: That depends on the underlying rhythm. If the atrium were capturing and the ventricle not capturing, and the native AV conduction intact, you would see the atrial spike and subsequent P wave, followed by the native QRS complex from conduction through the intact AV pathway. If the native AV conduction pathway is not intact or there is a block, you would again see the atrial spike with P wave, followed by a ventricular spike, but no corresponding paced QRS complex due to the lack of ventricular capture.

PR: Would anybody set a pacemaker at a rate of 50?

DB: Perhaps not in an 82-year-old, but patients with intermittent bradyarrhythmias who, for the most part, are in sinus rhythm, might have a pacemaker placed and set at a low rate to avoid competing with their native sinus rhythm. The pacemaker would provide a safety backup.

SG: A trained athlete might also have the pacemaker set at a slow rate.

PR: What would be your next step in evaluating this person after getting an EKG, a chest X-ray study, and a magnet strip?

DB: I think it's clear that the pacemaker is not functioning, and that's why this patient is in a junctional escape rhythm. Whether it's not functioning because the wire is broken, the battery has run out, or the wire has become dislodged, almost doesn't matter. She needs to be admitted to the hospital to a monitored bed, and to have this addressed by whoever takes care of pacemakers in this hospital, whether it's general cardiology, or cardiac electrophysiology. Particularly in this case, since her electrolytes and renal function are normal, and the cardiac troponin testing is negative, I don't think we have to suspect an underlying disease causing the heart muscle to respond inappropriately to the pacemaker.

SG: I might consider in this case whether the brady-dysrhythmia is related to an overdose of diltiazem.

DB: If she were living at home that would be a real concern, but in a nursing home, where she has no control over her medications, this would be less likely.

PR: Even in nursing homes, there are dosage errors, or even dosing changes that could be responsible; for example, she also could have been given another patient's medication. If something can go wrong, it certainly will. How would you test for this clinically? Would you give her some glucagon?

DB: I would not. She's maintaining a reasonable blood pressure. Her mental status appears close to her baseline, and giving her glucagon will often cause emesis and make her miserable. Instead, I would simply observe her on a monitor to assess whether the pacemaker works or not. The diltiazem should wear off over 12–24 hours, so she ought to be back in a paced rhythm by morning if the pacemaker looks like it is intact.

SG: I might add that if the patient should deteriorate, it should remain in the back of your mind, particularly if you're not finding success with external pacing or transvenous pacing. I would give her glucagon or perhaps some calcium. However, in a patient who appears hemodynamically stable with normal cerebral perfusion, trying medications that can have new side effects may further compromise the patient's current status and hinder more than help.

PR: Do you ever see pacemaker dysfunction that causes tachycardia rather than bradycardia?

AM: You can get a pacemaker-mediated tachycardia, even from a normally functioning pacemaker. Retrograde conduction of a ventricular beat may cause the atrium to trigger a second ventricular contraction that falls during the pacemaker's refractory period. Because this contraction is not sensed by the pacemaker, the pulse generator fires, initiating a reentry tachycardia.

SG: Treatment consists of lengthening the atrioventricular time by any of the following methods: (1) programming an increase in the atrial refractory time, (2) administering adenosine or verapamil, (3) increasing atrial sensory threshold, and (4) applying a magnet to stop atrial sensing by the pacemaker.

PR: There are patients who come to the ED to "have their pacers interrogated." I never know what they mean by that, and I'm not sure what to do to help them. Can you explain that for me?

TC: Interrogation is really a more in-depth assessment of their pacemaker functioning, and usually requires the technician or electrophysiologist to come in to assess the sensing and the pacing functions, and also review prior incidents. For example, in a pacemaker with an automatic implantable cardioverter defibrillator (AICD), they can look at the recent history of the device to see if there were any shocks delivered to the patient.

PR: One of the problems with longstanding pacemakers, like any other foreign body, is extrusion of the pacemaker and infection at the site of the pacemaker pocket. Obviously, you deal with the infection the way you would with any localized abscess, but is there any way to preserve the function while you're draining the abscess?

DB: If you have an infection generally, the pacemaker, like any foreign body causing infection, needs to be removed because it continues to be a nidus for infection. As with most infections or abscesses, the chances of it healing properly are diminished unless you remove the foreign body.

PR: While we're on the subject of internal defibrillators, what do you do about patients who come in

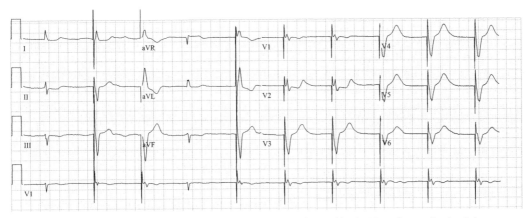

Figure 11.2 Follow-up 12-lead EKG after replacement of pacemaker and leads. Note the amplitude of the ventricular pacing spikes followed by the typical paced QRS complexes.

complaining that they're getting thumps all the time, and it really bothers them?

TC: In the patient with a complaint that the device is firing multiple times, and these are new events, the question is whether or not the device is firing appropriately. The device may be firing frequently, but appropriately, if the patient's underlying cardiac rhythm is abnormal or life threatening. Alternatively, the device may be malfunctioning and firing inappropriately when the patient has a normal or stable baseline cardiac rhythm. In this case, I would have the device interrogated to assess the patient's underlying rhythm when these shocks occurred, and to discern whether the device is firing appropriately. If it is firing appropriately, I would treat the underlying rhythm as appropriate; if not, I'd have the device settings adjusted or replace the device.

Case resolution

Additional records were obtained from an outlying hospital where the patient had formerly been admitted. The prior EKG demonstrated that the T wave inversions in the anterolateral distribution were old. It was determined that she had a VVI pacemaker; accordingly, the initial ED 12-lead EKG demonstrated a failure to capture for the patient's pacemaker. A chest radiograph was obtained on this patient that revealed a lead fracture in one of the pacemaker wires. The patient was admitted to a telemetry bed on the electrophysiology service, and underwent replacement of her pacemaker the following day. She was discharged

back to the nursing home with a normally functioning VVI pacemaker 2 days after admission. She was at her baseline condition (Figure 11-2).

Section III: Concepts

Background

Nearly three million pacemakers or implantable cardioverter-defibrillators (ICDs) have been implanted in the past decade (1990–2002) in the United States.[1] As a result, patients with pacemakers and ICDs are now very commonly seen in the ED. The indications for cardiac pacemakers have expanded broadly since these devices were first introduced in the 1950s to prevent Stokes-Adams attacks. Recently revised guidelines from the American College of Cardiology and American Heart Association now list a wide variety of cardiac conditions as indications for pacemakers, including sinus node and atrioventricular node dysfunction, atrioventricular block, chronic bifascicular block, neurocardiogenic syncope and hypersensitivity carotid sinus syndrome, hypertrophic cardiomyopathy, and atrial fibrillation, to name a few.[2,3] Similarly, the indications for ICDs have expanded to include ventricular tachycardia (VT) and ventricular fibrillation (VF), familial or inherited conditions with high risk for life-threatening ventricular tachydysrhythmias (i.e., long QT syndrome), and syncope in patients with advanced structural heart disease or Brugada syndrome (RBBB pattern with ST-segment elevation in lead V1).[4]

Pacemakers and ICDs have become increasingly complex, with memory requirements of less than 1 KB in the early 1990s up to more than 512 MB today.[5] These sophisticated medical devices have very low rates of malfunction, but when these failures occur, the clinical impact on the patient can lead to significant morbidity and even death.

The specific actions, functions, and capabilities of a given pacemaker are delineated by a letter code (NPG code) developed by the North American Society of Pacing and Electrophysiology (NASPE) and the British Pacing and Electrophysiology Group (BPEG), and revised in 2002.[6] The NASPE/BPEG pacemaker code is often shortened to the first three letter positions, such as DDD or VVI.

The first letter position indicates the chamber of the heart that is paced, such as the atrium (A), ventricle (V), both or dual (D), or none (O).

The second letter position indicates where the pacemaker senses native electrical activity of the heart (again: A, V, D, or O).

The third letter position indicates the pacemaker's response to sensing native electrical activity, such as triggering the pacemaker (T), inhibiting the pacemaker (I), both (D), or none (O).

Commonly encountered pacemakers in the ED include the VVI type (in which the pacemaker paces the ventricle, senses native ventricular electrical activity, and inhibits pacing when it does so), and the DDD type (in which the pacemaker paces both the atrium and ventricle, senses native and electrical activity in both chambers, and both inhibits and triggers pacing depending on the type of native activity sensed).

The fourth and fifth letter positions of the NPG code are less commonly noted, but do indicate potentially important functions.

The fourth letter position was used in the past to indicate programmability of the pacemaker in a hierarchical fashion, but now only indicates the presence or absence of rate modulation (automatic adjustment of the pacing rate), denoted as R or O respectively.

Similarly, the fifth letter position was used in the past to indicate any antitachydysrhythmic functions, but now only specifies the location or absence of multisite pacing (O, A, V, or D).[7]

ICDs have a similar identification code (NBD) where the first letter indicates the chamber shocked (O, A, V, or D); the second letter the chamber where antitachycardia pacing takes place (O, A, V, or D); the third letter the means of detection either by electrogram signal (E) or by other hemodynamic variables, such as blood pressure or transthoracic impedance, in addition to the electrogram signal (H); and the fourth letter the chamber where antibradycardia pacing takes place (O, A, V, or D). A short form of the NBD code has been developed to signify the ICD function as one of three types: shock capability only (ICD-S); shock and bradycardia pacing (ICD-B); and shock, bradycardia pacing, and tachycardia pacing (ICD-T).[8]

Initial workup: history and physical examination

Patients with pacemaker dysfunction can present to the ED with a myriad of complaints. If the pacemaker fails, the patient's hemodynamic status is dependent on the underlying native cardiac rhythm; as a result, patients may present with symptoms similar to those that precipitated the need for the pacemaker in the first place. Common presenting symptoms include palpitations or "fluttering" or "pounding" sensations, lightheadedness, dizziness, presyncope, actual syncope, weakness, fatigue, and shortness of breath.

As with any ED patient, the initial step is to obtain vital signs and determine the need for stabilization. Pacemaker malfunction and reversion to an abnormal underlying native cardiac rhythm has the potential to result in significant hemodynamic compromise and instability. As such, the emergency physician must determine if the clinical presentation and hemodynamic status of the patient with device failure require immediate intervention, such as with external pacing, electrical cardioversion/defibrillation, or pharmacologic pressor support.

Provided that the patient is stable, additional history should be obtained to determine if the patient's pacemaker and its malfunction are the cause of the individual's clinical presentation. Does the patient know the original indication for the pacemaker, the name of the manufacturer, or the make and type (NPG code) of the device? If they do not know this information, they may have a pacemaker identification card, which usually is provided when the pacemaker is implanted. This card includes information on the manufacturer, make, model, and type of pacemaker implanted (NPG code).

The patient should also be asked when the pacemaker was implanted, as many complications, such as a site infection, occur within a few weeks or months of implantation. In addition, if the patient has knowledge of any recent changes to the pacemaker settings or other device interventions or interrogations, this information may be useful in determining the potential for any complications or malfunction. Knowing the age of the battery and the date its function was last checked would be similarly useful.

Careful physical examination is important in the assessment of the device. The implantation site should be inspected for any signs of infection or migration, as well as evidence of a mechanical problem with the device generator. The chest wall should be examined for any extracardiac stimulation by the pacemaker, such as chest wall twitching or diaphragmatic irritation (manifesting as hiccups).

The examination should focus, in particular, on an assessment of cardiac status and functioning. Abnormally slow, fast, or irregular pulse rates may indicate a malfunction has occurred. Inspection of the neck veins may reveal distension and the presence of so-called "cannon" A-waves, indicating asynchrony of the atria and ventricles. Cardiac auscultation may reveal abnormal first and second heart sounds (i.e., paradoxical splitting), which could indicate abnormal pacing. In addition, a pericardial friction rub may be present if the pacemaker lead has perforated the myocardium. Evidence of heart failure, such as rales on chest examination or lower extremity edema that is new, may also indicate pacemaker failure.

The approach to the history and examination of patient with an ICD should be similar to that of a patient with a pacemaker, though the clinical presentation is more limited in scope. The most common complaint of patients with ICDs is an increase in shock frequency.[9] This presentation may represent a normally functioning ICD responding to increased episodes of triggering dysrhythmias (such as VT or VF), or an abnormally functioning ICD firing inappropriately. Alternatively, malfunction may occur when the ICD does not shock when it should. In this case, patients will present with clinical manifestations of the underlying abnormal cardiac rhythm (VT or VF), including syncope, pre-syncope, lightheadedness, weakness, shortness of breath, chest pain, and cardiac arrest.

Etiologies and differential diagnosis

Pacemaker malfunction can occur as a result of a failure to pace, failure to capture, and failure to sense.

In addition, patients may present to the ED with pacemaker-mediated dysrhythmias, and the so-called "pacemaker syndrome."

Failure to pace, also known as output failure, occurs when the pacemaker fails to deliver an electrical stimulus to the heart. This can occur for a variety of reasons, including battery or component failure, lead fracture, dislodgement or disconnection, and oversensing. Battery depletion is the most commonly reported cause of pacemaker malfunction, and component or generator failure has been reported with blunt trauma to the chest wall.[10,11] However, abrupt failure is rare with today's lithium-iodine batteries.[12] Typically, a gradual deterioration occurs over weeks to months as the battery is depleted, initially manifesting as a decrease in programmed pacing rate, and subsequent decrease in stimulus voltage. These changes may be noted on regularly scheduled checks of the pacemaker and, as a result, emergent replacement is uncommon.

Complete lead fracture or disconnection can cause failure to pace by preventing delivery of the pacing impulse to the myocardium. Lead fractures typically occur at the attachment to the generator, or at various lead stress points, particularly abrupt angulations. In addition, poor contact between the pulse generator and lead can also result in failure to pace.

Oversensing occurs when the pacemaker senses other electrical activity and misinterprets that activity as native cardiac depolarizations, causing the device to initiate its programmed activity—triggering or inhibiting pacing. For pacemakers that inhibit upon sensing native cardiac activity, oversensing can result in a failure to pace. Common non-cardiac activities that can result in pacing inhibition include chest wall and skeletal muscle myopotentials, particularly from the pectoralis and rectus abdominis musculature.[13] In fact, succinylcholine has been reported to cause pacemaker malfunction from oversensing of skeletal muscle fasciculations.[14] Intermittent contact from lead disconnections, also known as "make-break" signals, can also generate electrical activity resulting in pacing inhibition.[15] In addition, normal native cardiac signals may be misinterpreted by the pacemaker, resulting in pacing failure. For example, a VVI pacemaker may oversense T wave activity as a QRS complex and thus inhibit the ventricular pacing stimulus.

Environmental electrical activity can also result in oversensing and pacemaker malfunction. Wireless cellular phone signals and electrical cautery have been reported to cause abnormal pacemaker function from oversensing; in the case of cellular phones, malfunction is seen most commonly when the device is held to the ear on the same side of the pacemaker pocket.[16,17]

Failure to capture occurs when the pacemaker generates a pacing impulse, but the stimulus fails to trigger or "capture" the myocardium to cause cardiac depolarization. This failure can occur because the pacemaker is unable to generate a sufficient current to trigger depolarization, or the voltage threshold required for capture at the electrode-myocardial interface has changed. As noted above, a failing battery can manifest gradually with decreasing impulse voltage that can result in pacer activity, but is insufficient to capture the myocardium. Similarly, partial lead fractures, or breaks in the electrode insulation, can result in current leakage and inability to capture despite delivery of the pulsing stimulus.

Exit block occurs when a pacing stimulus at an appropriate voltage current fails to trigger depolarization, commonly from electrode-myocardium interface alterations changing the pacing threshold. An elevated threshold can be seen soon after initial implantation because of tissue changes and inflammation at the lead insertion sites, resulting in a failure to capture within weeks of implantation. However, advances in steroid-eluting leads and initial pacemaker programming voltage outputs set significantly higher than threshold levels have reduced this risk.[18]

Ischemia and infarction can also alter the electrode-myocardium interface, elevate pacing thresholds, and result in failure to capture. External defibrillation on patients with pacemakers has been well documented to increase the risk of failure to capture, presumably from tissue damage at the electrode-myocardial interface.[19] Similarly, metabolic and electrolyte derangements, including systemic hyperkalemia, hypoxemia, hypothyroidism, and acidemia, can result in a failure to capture.[20,21] Antidysrhythmic agents, such as flecainide and amiadarone, have been reported to elevated pacing thresholds and result in failure to capture.[22] Underlying prolonged myocardial refractoriness, such as in long QT syndrome, may also result in failure to capture if pacing impulses are delivered during the longer native refractory periods.

Failure to sense, or undersensing, occur when the pacemaker fails to sense underlying native cardiac activity. Undersensing can be complete or intermittent,

depending on changes in the amplitude, vector, and frequency of myocardial potentials. Thus, changes in the myocardium that cause an impact upon intracardiac electrical signals, such as from acute infarction (especially right ventricular infarction), bundle branch blocks, or other rhythm disturbances, can cause undersensing. In addition, changes in the electrode-myocardium interface, from inflammation or external defibrillation, can also result in failure to sense native activity. As with failure to pace or capture, lead fracture, dislodgement, insulation defects, or disconnections can result in a failure to sense. Finally, undersensing can be caused by simple programming errors where the pacemaker-sensing threshold is set well above normal baseline cardiac activity.

While initially designed to treat abnormal bradydyshrythmias, pacemakers themselves can actually cause heart rhythm disturbances. These pacemaker-mediated dysrhythmias include pacemaker-mediated tachycardias (PMTs), runaway pacemakers, sensor-induced tachycardias, and dyshrhythmias due to lead dislodgement. PMT can occur in dual-chamber pacemakers with atrial sensing where the pacemaker itself acts as part of a large reentry "endless loop" circuit. PMT is usually initiated by a premature ventricular contraction conducted retrograde through the AV node, causing atrial depolarization that is sensed by the pacemaker as native atrial activity, and results in a pacing stimulus to the ventricle, thus completing the circuit loop. In PMT, the rate does not exceed the pacemaker's programmed upper limit.[23] Similarly, atrial tachycardias, such as atrial flutter, can be sensed by these pacemakers, and result in a ventricular tachycardia that does not exceed the upper limit.

Pacemakers with rate modulation usually vary the pacing rate on specific sensors that detect vibration, temperature, or even minute ventilation as a measure of physiologic activity. Sensor-induced tachycardias occur when these sensors are stimulated by other stimuli, such as vibrations from external factors (i.e., loud noises, machinery, helicopters), febrile illness, or arm or chest movement.[24,25] Runaway pacemaker is an uncommon, but life-threatening, malfunction in which the pacemaker fires inappropriately rapid discharges, potentially inducing VT or VF. Fortunately, modern pacemakers are programmed to prevent such rapid discharges, and this complication is exceedingly rare today.[26] Another pacemaker malfunction that can cause abnormal cardiac rhythms occurs when a dislodged or disconnected lead has varying and inter-mittent contact with the ventricular myocardial wall, resulting in ectopy and ventricular dysrhythmias.

Pacemaker syndrome is a constellation of signs and symptoms similar to those of a true pacemaker malfunction. The syndrome is most commonly associated with VVI pacemakers, and the onset is usually soon after implantation. Pathophysiologically, the syndrome is thought to be the result of loss of AV synchrony or suboptimal synchronization of the atria and ventricle by the pacing device, resulting in an inadequate cardiac pump function.[27]

ICD malfunction can occur when there is an abrupt change in shock frequency or failure to shock or pace (antitachycardic or antibradycardic) when indicated. "Electrical storm" refers to a high frequency of shocks over a short period of time.[28] A sudden increase in shock frequency can be the result of normal appropriate ICD functioning in the face of frequent episodes of shockable native rhythms (i.e., VT or VF); however, increased shocks can also indicate a malfunction of the device itself, possible lead displacement or break, as well as oversensing of supraventricular tachydysrhythmias, T wave morphologies, or other non-cardiac signals misinterpreted by the device as malignant rhythms.[29] Alternatively, the device may fail to shock or pace appropriately when indicated in the setting of battery failure, lead problems (break, dislodgement, disconnection), or suboptimal programmed-threshold settings.

Testing

The 12-lead EKG is indispensable in the evaluation of pacemaker function, as single lead rhythm strips and telemetry monitoring may not display low level amplitude pacemaker impulses. The EKG should be evaluated for pacing spikes (atrial, ventricular, or both), as well as the usual cardiac waveforms, both native and paced, and their temporal relation to pacing stimuli (if any). Because the ventricular pacing lead is usually placed in the right ventricle, the normal paced ventricular beat demonstrates a wide QRS complex waveform similar to left bundle branch block with left axis deviation, but with a preceding ventricular pacing spike. ST-segments and T waves should typically be discordant with the QRS complex.[30]

When evaluating the 12-lead EKG, it is important to know the type of pacemaker the patient has, to determine what electrocardiographic findings to expect. For example, with a dual-chamber pacemaker, one might expect to see atrial spikes followed by a P wave and ventricular spikes followed by a QRS complex. However, if the atrial depolarization is transmitted to the ventricle normally, there may be a normal native QRS complex with no preceding ventricular spike. Similarly, if the native heart rate is above that of the threshold for pacing and AV conduction is not delayed, both the native P wave and QRS complex will appear with no preceding pacer activity, provided the pacemaker is sensing this native activity and is programmed to inhibit its impulses.

In order to evaluate pacemaker function in this setting, vagal maneuvers and even short-acting medications such as adenosine, which slow the patient's heart rate, have been employed to induce pacing activity for device evaluation. However, the most effective method for the emergency physician to assess the device when native cardiac activity inhibits pacing is the use of a magnet. A magnet placed over the pacemaker generator will typically stop the sensing function and put the device into an asynchronous, fixed pacing mode. In this mode, the 12-lead EKG can be assessed to determine if the pacemaker has malfunctioned as a result of failure to pace from device or battery failure (no pacing spikes seen despite the asynchronous mode), or from failure to capture (no atrial or ventricular depolarizations despite pacing spikes). However, if the asynchronous pacing stimulus occurs during the refractory period (atrial or ventricular), there will not be a corresponding paced complex (P wave or QRS complex respectively), and this finding would not necessarily indicate failure to capture. Removal of the magnet will cause the device to revert back to its normal programmed mode with sensing.

Sensing malfunctions are more difficult to assess on the 12-lead EKG. The physician must consider the type of device and the expected response to sensing to determine what would be expected on the surface EKG. For example, in dual-chamber pacing, lack of an intrinsic or paced QRS complex following a P wave at an appropriate AV interval may indicate atrial undersensing with the resulting failure to trigger a ventricular stimulus. Alternatively, if the pacemaker is programmed to inhibit impulses when native activity is sensed, undersensing could lead to more asynchronous pacing spikes with variable capture, depending on whether the stimulus falls during the refractory periods.

Similarly, the 12-lead electrocardiogram may provide clues to the presence of oversensing, depending on what signals are being detected and the programmed response of the pacemaker. For example, if cardiac signals such as the T wave are oversensed as native QRS complexes, there may be intermittent, irregular, or loss of normal pacing spikes. If skeletal myopotentials are sensed as native cardiac activity, isometric movement of the chest wall or arm musculature may trigger or inhibit pacing activity inappropriately.

The 12-lead EKG is also helpful in determining the presence of pacemaker-mediated dysrhythmias. For ICD devices, 12-lead EKG or continuous monitoring can be helpful to determine if the device is firing in error, such as from oversensing, or is shocking the patient appropriately in response to a life-threatening dysrhythmias. In addition, the EKG can demonstrate evidence of myocardial ischemia or infarction causing device malfunction as a result of changes at the electrode-myocardial interface. However, for ICDs, transient ST elevations or depressions can be seen in the postshock period without underlying ischemia.[31]

A chest X-ray study can often be helpful in identifying the type of pacemaker or ICD. The number and location of leads seen on radiograph can provide basic information as to the pacemaker type and function (such as single- or dual-chamber pacing). Moreover, many pacemakers have identification information on the device (such as type and manufacturer) that can be seen radiographically, particularly with digital films that allow magnification and overpenetration. A standard posteroanterior chest radiograph also can demonstrate any lead problems such as fracture, disconnection, dislodgement, or perforation.

Laboratory testing is often necessary to assess for potential causes of pacemaker failure, including electrolyte disturbances or other metabolic abnormalities that may result in device malfunction. Serum cardiac markers may be helpful in assessing for myocardial necrosis or infarction that could have affected or resulted from pacemaker or ICD malfunction. However, shocks from a normally functioning ICD can result in elevated cardiac markers as well.[32] Studies indicate BNP levels may be useful in assessing cardiac function and AV synchrony when considering the possibility of pacemaker syndrome.[33] In addition, looking at the levels of certain drugs known to alter pacing thresholds, such as digoxin, may be of utility.[32]

In many cases, however, advanced testing to assess the function of a pacemaker or ICD device will be required when malfunction is suspected. This device interrogation requires a highly skilled technician using manufacturer-specific equipment to determine whether the pacemaker or ICD is functioning properly or is one that requires adjustment in the device's programming. In addition, most devices log recent events for review during the interrogation to evaluate the function of the device during this period of time.

Disposition

In the setting of hemodynamic compromise, immediate stabilization and resuscitation are the priority. External defibrillation can generally be performed safely in a patient with a pacemaker, so long as the pads are not in close proximity to the pacer generator. Life-threatening pacemaker-mediated tachycardias can often be terminated by placing a magnet over the device to suspend any device sensing. Similarly, placing a magnet over an ICD will deactivate the device and terminate recurrent inappropriate shocks (such as from oversensing) by disabling the tachydysrhythmia detection and treatment, but not its backup bradycardia pacing function. However, this maneuver should be undertaken with caution and only when the ICD shocks are clearly inappropriate or if external defibrillation and resuscitation treatment is readily available.

As noted above, in many cases, pacemaker and ICD evaluation in the ED will require interrogation of the device by a technician either in person or by phone. In some of these cases, no malfunction will be found or small adjustments in the device programming will be required to address the reason for the patient's clinical presentation. Provided no other acute conditions are present, these patients can be discharged home provided close follow-up with their cardiologist is arranged. Similarly, a single ICD shock that appears to be an appropriate response to a malignant rhythm generally does not require admission for further extensive evaluation.[31]

If a major malfunction with the device is found, such as primary device failure, battery depletion, lead fracture, or dislodgement, the patient will require admission for close monitoring and, ultimately, repair or replacement of the device. Other factors to consider when determining the need for admission include the patient's underlying cardiovascular status, the

Table 11-1. NPG code for pacemakers.

I	II	III	IV	V
Chamber(s) Paced	Chamber(s) Sensed	Sensing Response	Rate Modulation	Multisite Pacing
O = none	O = none	O = none	O = none	O = none
A = atrium	A = atrium	T = triggered	R = rate modulation	A = atrium
V = ventricle	V = ventricle	I = inhibited		V = ventricle
D = dual	D = dual	D = dual		D = dual

Table 11-2. NPD code for ICDs.

I	II	III	IV
Shock Chamber	Antitachycardia Pacing Chamber	Tachycardia Detection	Antibradycardia Pacing Chamber
O = none	O = none	E = electrogram	O = none
A = atrium	A = atrium	H = hemodynamic	R = rate modulation
V = ventricle	V = ventricle		
D = dual	D = dual		

dependence on the device (that is, the potential affect on cardiac function should the device malfunction or fail), the frequency of underlying life-threatening dysrhythmias triggering shocks (in the case of ICDs), and whether a significant change is required in the programming of the device based on the initial interrogation.

Section IV: Decision making

- The key to evaluation is knowing what type of device the patient has implanted and understanding the features and functioning of the different pacemakers and ICDs (Tables 11-1 and 11- 2).
- Evaluation of the device includes an EKG, telemetry, chest radiograph, serum electrolytes, and, if indicated, cardiac markers.

Table 11-3. Causes of failure to pace (output failure).

Battery Failure
Lead Fracture, Dislodgement, Disconnection
Oversensing
    Misinterpreted cardiac potentials
    Extracardiac potentials (skeletal myopotentials)
    "Make–Break" signals from lead problems
Electromagnetic Interference
Component Failure (i.e., trauma)

Table 11-4. Causes of failure to capture.

Battery Depletion
Lead Fracture, Insulation Break, Dislodgement
Exit Block
Metabolic Abnormalities
    Electrolyte imbalance (hyperkalemia)
    Hypothyroidism
    Acidemia
Medications (antidysrhythmic agents)
External Defibrillation
Long QT Syndrome

- Placement of a magnet over the device may help diagnostically and therapeutically.
- Pacemaker malfunction can occur from failures to pace, capture, or sense (Tables 11-3, 11-4, 11-5).

Table 11-5. Causes of failure to sense.

Myocardial Infarction
Bundle Branch Block
Dysrhythmias
External Defibrillation
Lead Fracture, Disconnection, Insulation Break
Programming Error
Electrode-Myocardium Interface Inflammation

- Disposition should be predicated on evaluation and interrogation results, dependence of the patient on the device, and underlying cardiovascular status and condition.

References

1 Maisel WH, Moynahan M, Zuckerman BD, et al. Pacemaker and ICD generator malfunctions—analysis of food and drug administration annual reports. *JAMA*. 2006;295:1901–1906.

2 Epstein AE, DiMarco JP, Ellenbogen KA, et al. ACC/AHA/HRS 2008 guidelines of device-based therapy of cardiac rhythm abnormalities: a report of the American College of Cardiology/American Heart Association Task Force on Practice Guidelines (Writing Committee to Revise the ACC/AHA/NASPE 2002 Guideline Update for Implantation of Cardiac Pacemakers and Antiarrhythmia Devices). *J Am Coll Cardiol*. 2008;51:e1–e62.

3 Kusumoto F, Goldschlager N. Implantable cardiac arrhythmia devices—part I: pacemakers. *Clin Cardiol*. 2006;29:189–194.

4 Kusumoto F, Goldschlager N. Implantable cardiac arrhythmia devices—part II: implantable cardioverter defibrillators and implantable loop recorders. *Clin Cardiol*. 2006;29:237–242.

5 Maisel WH, Stevenson WG, Epstein LM. Changing trends in pacemaker and implantable cardioverter-defibrillator generator advisories. *Pacing Clin Electrophysiol*. 2002;25:1670–1678.

6 Bernstein AD, Camm AJ, Fisher JD, et al. North American Society of Pacing and Electrophysiology policy statement. The NASPE/BPEG Defibrillator Code. *Pacing Clin Electrophysiol*. 1993;16:1776–1780.

7 Bernstein AD, Daubert JC, Fletcher RD, et al. The revised NASPE/BPEG generic code for antibradicardia, adaptic-rate, and multisite pacing. North American Society of Pacing and Electrophysiology/British Pacing and Electrophysiology Group. *Pacing Clin Electrophysiol*. 2002;25:260–264.

8 Bernstein AD, Camm AJ, Fisher JD, et al. The NASPE/BPEG defibrillator code. *Pacing Clin Electrophysiol*. 1993;16:1776–1780.

9 Swerdlow CD, Zhang J. Implantable cardioverter defibrillator shocks: a troubleshooting guide. *Rev Cardiovasc Med*. 2001;2:61–72.

10 Maisel WH. Pacemaker and ICD generator reliability. *JAMA*. 2006;295:1929–1934.

11 Brown KR, Carter W Jr, Lombardi GE. Blunt trauma-induced pacemaker failure. *Ann Emerg Med*. 1991;20:905–907.

12 Hayes DL, Vlietstra RE. Pacemaker malfunction. *Ann Intern Med*. 1993;119:828–835.

13 Gross JN, Platt S, Ritacco R, et al. The clinical relevance of electromyopotential oversensing in current unipolar devices. *Pacing Clin Electrophysiol*. 1992;15:2023–2027.

14 Finfer S: Pacemaker failure on induction of anaesthesia. *Br J Anaesth*. 1991;66:509–512.

15 Cardall TY, Brady WK, Chan TC, et al. Permanent cardiac pacemakers: issues relevant to the emergency physician, part I. *J Emerg Med*.1999;17:479–489.

16 Hayes DL, Wang PJ, Reynolds DW, et al. Interference with cardiac pacemakers by cellular telephones. *N Engl J Med*. 1997;336:1473–1479.

17 Goldschlager N, Epstein A, Freidman P, et al. Environmental and drug effects on patients with pacemakers and implantable cardioverter/defibrillators. A practical guide to patient-treatment. *Arch Inter Med*. 2001;161:649–655.

18 Cardall TY, Brady WK, Chan TC, et al. P. Permanent cardiac pacemakers: issues relevant to the emergency physician, part II. *J Emerg Med*.1999;17:697–709.

19 Altamura G, Bianconi L, Lo Bianco F, et al. Transthoracic DC shock may represent a serious hazard in pacemaker-dependent patients. *Pacing Clin Electrophysiol*. 1995;18:194–198.

20 Dohrmann ML, Goldschlager NF. Myocardial stimulation threshold in patients with cardiac pacemakers: effect of physiologic variables, pharmacologic agents, and lead electrodes. *Cardiol Clin*. 1985;3:527–537.

21 Bashour TT. Spectrum of ventricular pacemaker exit block owing to hyperkalemia. *Am J Cardiol*. 1986;57:337–338.

22 Tworek DA, Nazari J, Ezri M, Bauman JL. Interference by anti-arrhythmic agents with function of electrical cardiac devices. *Clin Pharm*. 1992;11:48–56.

23 Sarko JA, Tiffany BR. Cardiac pacemakers: evaluation and management of malfunctions. *Am J Emerg Med*.2000;18:435–440.

24 Snoeck J, Beerkhof M, Claeys M, et al. External vibration interference of activity-based rate-responsive pacemakers. *Pacing Clin Electrophysiol*. 1992;15:1841–1845.

25 Vanderheyden M, Timmermans W, Goethals M. Inappropriate rate response in a VVI-R pacemaker. *Acta Cardiol*. 1996;51:545–550.

26 Mickley H, Andersen C, Nielsen LH. Runaway pacemaker: a still-existing complication and therapeutic guidelines. *Clin Cardiol*. 1989;12:412–414.

27 Glikson M, Hayes DL. Cardiac pacing. A review. *Med Clin North Am*. 2001;85:369.

28 Arya A, Hoghjoo M, Dehghani M, et al. Prevalence and predictors of electrical storm in patients with

implantable cardioverter-defibrillators. *Am J Cardiol.* 2006;97:389–392.

29 Pfeiffer D, Jung W, Fehske W, et al. Complications of pacemaker-defibrillator devices: diagnosis and management. *Am Heart J.* 1994;127:1073–1080.

30 Brady WJ, Lentz B, Barlotta K, Harrigan RA, Chan T. ECG patterns confounding the ECG diagnosis of acute coronary syndrome: left bundle branch block, right ventricular paced rhythms, and left ventricular hypertrophy. *Emerg Med Clin North Am.* 2005;23:999–1025.

31 Stevenson W, Chaitman B, Ellenbogen K, et al. Clinical assessment and management of patients with implanted cardioverter-defibrillators presenting to nonelectrophysiologists. *Circulation.* 2004;110:3866–3869.

32 McMullan J, Valento M, Attari M, Vendkat A. Care of the pacemaker/implantable cardioverter defibrillator patient in the ED. *Am J Emerg Med.*2007;25: 812–822.

33 Sadowski M, Wozakowska-Kaplon B. The influence of permanent cardiac pacing on plasma levels if B-type natriuretic peptide in patients with sick sinus syndrome. *Cardiol J.* 2008;15:39–42.

Non Ischemic Cardiac Disease

12 Acute heart failure

Kevin Reed[1] & Amal Mattu[2]

[1] Assistant Professor of Clinical Emergency Medicine, Georgetown University
School of Medicine, Department of Emergency Medicine, Washington, USA
[2] Professor and Residency Director, Department of Emergency Medicine,
University of Maryland School of Medicine, Baltimore, Maryland, USA

Section I: Case presentation

A 65-year-old man arrived via EMS in the late afternoon with a chief complaint of "trouble breathing." The crew had placed the patient on 100% oxygen, through a non-rebreather mask, with minimal improvement en-route to the Emergency Department (ED).

Upon arrival to the ED, the patient appeared in distress, with increased work breathing. The patient was accompanied by his wife, who gave the majority of the history as the patient could only answer in 2–3 word sentences. He denied chest pain, but did feel like there was a weight on his chest. His symptoms had progressed slowly over the morning, but more rapidly over the prior few hours. The prior night, he had slept sitting up in the living room chair.

His wife stated that he had been in his usual state of health until the prior night when she noticed him "huffing" when he went up the steps to their bedroom, and when taking out the trash. She also noted his legs looked slightly more swollen than usual. The past medical history included a "heart problem," hypertension, and arthritis. She had brought in his medications, which included metoprolol, furosemide, and digoxin. The patient stated that he had been compliant with his medications. He had never smoked, and had only an occasional alcohol drink on special occasions.

The vital signs were: afebrile; pulse 108 beats/min; respirations 32 breaths/min; blood pressure 188/106 mmHg; pulse oximetry 86% on room air, but 94% on 100% oxygen by non-rebreather mask. A finger-stick glucose was 120 mg/dl.

The patient appeared diaphoretic, in moderate distress, but awake and alert. He had jugular venous distention and rales to mid-lung fields bilaterally. The cardiac examination was notable for an S3. The legs had 2+ non-pitting edema without tenderness, warmth, or palpable cords. The pulses were equal in all four extremities.

An EKG demonstrated a sinus tachycardia, voltage criteria for left ventricular hypertrophy, and repolarization changes consistent with a strain pattern in the lateral leads. There were no changes from prior EKGs. A chest X-ray study showed cardiomegaly, prominent vasculature in the upper lung fields, Kerley B lines, and fluid-filled fissures. Laboratory studies including cardiac biomarkers and a BNP (B-type natriuretic peptide) level were sent to the laboratory.

Section II: Case discussion

Dr Peter Rosen: There was a study that suggested a diurnal variation to episodes of acute pulmonary edema. Patients who arrive in the daytime are more

---

Cardiovascular Problems in Emergency Medicine: A discussion-based review, First Edition.
Edited by Shamai A. Grossman and Peter Rosen.
© 2011 John Wiley & Sons, Ltd. Published 2011 by John Wiley & Sons, Ltd.

likely to have a heart attack as the underlying cause of their congestive failure than patients who arrive in the middle of the night. Have you noticed a similar diurnal variation, and what do you believe is the most common trigger in decompensated congestive heart failure?

Dr Edward Ullman: This is somewhat dependent on your patient population and practice environment. When I was in residency training, most of the cases of congestive heart failure (CHF) I encountered were related to medicinal noncompliance and dietary indiscretion. Now I tend to see more ischemia as a trigger. This may reflect a more savvy patient population who tend not to cheat on their diets as much, and are more compliant with their medications. However, I have not noticed a diurnal variation in either of these populations.

PR: When you see a patient like this who is not yet in fulminant pulmonary edema, but who seems well on the way, what makes you decide whether he is sliding in to hypervolemic high resistance failure as opposed to pump failure? I think this is the first distinction we need to make in congestive failure, since the management is very different. Are there any clues, either from the initial appearance or during the evaluation?

Dr William Brady: Patients who have true pump failure most often are having a large myocardial infarction (MI), and usually appear sicker. They often are in shock. They have an ashen appearance. They have cold extremities. They are not perfusing in any shape, manner, or form. When you look at these patients' EKGs and serum cardiac markers, they will be very abnormal with the waveforms of an acute or subacute MI. Sometimes the EKG may show an old infarction, reflecting acute pump failure related to prior cardiac disease. The blood work will show hypoperfusion demonstrated by a low serum bicarbonate level or a significantly elevated lactate level. Nevertheless, patients in volume overload can also be very ill with acute respiratory failure, and also develop shock and all the sequalae of the pump failure. In general, not only are they are less ill, in some ways they are easier to treat. I believe that looking at the patient's history of present illness, their medical history, and your analysis of what is likely going on can point you in the right direction diagnostically and ultimately therapeutically.

PR: One of the early clues is in the blood pressure, as patients who are volume overloaded tend to have high resistance failure and present, as this man did, with hypertension; in patients with pump failure, the initial blood pressures are often normal to low since when these patients are well, their blood pressures are usually elevated. Another clue that the patient's CHF is related to high resistance failure is respiratory distress. When you see a patient with acute onset of respiratory distress, someone who is in the classic bubbling pulmonary edema, do you think that there are any clues as to what's going on in the heart that causes this, or do you think that there is always just volume overload and high resistance?

Dr Amal Mattu: I look at CHF as having two distinct major causes. One of them is fluid overload or volume dysfunction, and the other is vascular dysfunction, or in other words, very high resistance. When people come in with acute onset CHF, it tends to be associated with more of a vascular problem, oftentimes with acute afterload dysfunction. They present with very high blood pressures. Patients who are fluid overloaded tend to present with a more gradual onset of symptoms. When people come in with a more abrupt onset of symptoms, and appear to be doing pretty well but over the course of an hour they go from looking well to looking very sick, then I steer away from diuretics. In this case, I'm not worried about fluid overload. The most important therapy for these patients is to improve their resistance with quick afterload and preload reduction rather than focusing on diuretics and their volume.

PR: There is one finding on physical examination that can really help you in the face of acute rapid decompensation. When you hear a loud murmur in a patient who suddenly presents with acutely decompensated CHF, you must suspect the patient has a rupture of a papillary muscle. It's helpful to pick up this murmur as these patients need acute cardiac surgery more than they need medical manipulation. What would be your initial approach to management of the patient in this case? Which patients need emergent airway management?

SG: Any patient who presents with airway compromise will need some sort of airway management. Generally, we reserve intubation for those patients who cannot tolerate a noninvasive type of ventilation.

A patient who is somnolent or unconscious is not going to be able to tolerate bilevel positive airway pressure (BiPAP) or continuous positive airway pressure (CPAP); these patients will certainly need intubation. If a patient comes in markedly hypotensive or in shock, it is necessary to actively manage the airway. As in all of emergency medicine, first take care of the airway, and then care for breathing and circulation.

PR: I think that's a useful first distinction. In the patient who presents with pump failure, one of the critical first steps in management is to perform intubation to reduce the work of respiration. These patients will not respond to CPAP and to volume manipulation; they're going to need pump assistance.

WB: I would focus on three things: first, make sure the patient is not in extremis. Then, supply some form of high flow oxygen, at least initially a non-rebreather facemask. Lastly, start high dose nitrates, either sublingual, topical, intravenous, or some combination thereof.

SG: I would avoid topical nitrates in this patient as their effect on blood pressure is inconsistent, and their absorption is erratic due to both patient diaphoresis and the nature of a transdermal absorption.

WB: After nitrates, I use noninvasive positive pressure ventilation aggressively. Lastly, I've added ACE inhibitors to my armamentarium, either enalaprilat or sublingual captopril. I have begun to stay away from furosemide, and I try not to use morphine if at all possible. I've recently developed several prehospital protocols for EMS agencies that removed furosemide as a first line drug, and made its use dependent upon a base station medical command. For EMS, we have also significantly deemphasized morphine, and added sublingual captopril.

AM: Maryland has developed similar EMS protocols. Formerly, the paramedics would automatically give morphine and furosemide, but now morphine has been completely excluded from the protocol, and furosemide can only be given upon medical command. Similarly, the state protocols have also incorporated sublingual captopril into prehospital CHF protocols.[1]

PR: Could you explain why this is the case? Most of us grew up in the period where we were told you had to unload the heart, and you had to produce venous

dilatation, as furosemide does, long before it produces diuresis. Morphine also was thought to be a good way to lower peripheral resistance, as well as to interfere with the vicious cycle of hypoxia and adrenalin production by the patient. For years this seemed to work pretty well, so why do we think it's no longer useful?

AM: There are some studies indicating that when you give morphine and furosemide, you get peripheral vasodilatation in the wrist and forearm.[2,3] Based on those studies, people extrapolated and assumed that if you had vasodilatation in the wrist and forearm, then you must also be getting a decrease in right heart filling pressures, but this was only an extrapolation. When they actually studied this using pulmonary artery (PA) catheters, they found that when you give morphine and furosemide peripherally, you often obtain a slight increase in wedge pressures, so patients actually get a little bit worse.[4,5] There are studies indicating that furosemide activates the renin-angiotensin-aldosterone system, which is an endogenous pressor system. This may transiently cause an increase in afterload. It's not until the diuretic effect actually kicks in, which can be an hour or two later, that central preload will drop.[6–8]

To summarize, when giving diuretics, rather than a central improvement there is mild worsening; then, about an hour later, when diuresis begins, there is a drop in the wedge pressure. Similarly, morphine has been found to be a myocardial depressant; the few PA catheter studies show that giving morphine to patients with cardiogenic pulmonary edema worsens the cardiac index.[4,9]

EU: I find afterload reduction with ACE inhibitors particularly useful for the hemodialysis patient who presents in pulmonary edema, as it may buy time until the hemodialysis team comes in for definitive care.

PR: There is one patient who can present like this that we tend to forget about, and that is the patient with cor pulmonale or "blue bloater" rather than the "pink puffer." This is the patient who has chronic obstructive pulmonary disease (COPD), and who presents with an enormous volume overload perhaps triggered by an acute flare-up of bronchitis with worsening hypoxia. This causes the patient not only to have the presentation of someone with acute congestive failure, but the appearance of someone who has acute respiratory failure. How we can distinguish these patients, or does it matter? Can we just lump them together and use a similar therapeutic approach, and only worry about primary lung disease if we hear physical signs of bronchoconstriction?

SG: This is a classic emergency medicine question: the patient presents short of breath, and you don't know if the cause is COPD or CHF. This was part of the controversy when BNP as a marker for CHF was developed. Do you really need to know the whether this is CHF or COPD? Traditionally, the shotgun approach was to treat the patient for both diseases, and then an hour or two later see what was the true etiology of their respiratory difficulty. The issues are several-fold. First, we're using medications that don't clearly have benefit but, at the same time, don't clearly have detriment, such as a beta-agonist in a patient with acute CHF. Although there is some rather old data that suggest that some beta-agonists may have utility in patients with CHF, most studies have not shown benefit, but also have yet to show an adverse affect. At the same time, if you start treating a patient with steroids whom you think is having a COPD exacerbation but who actually has CHF and cardiac ischemia, you may be impairing the cardiac remodeling taking place during the infarction evolution. This is the argument against a shotgun approach and to suggest that there should be some sort of rapid approach to sort out whether the patient really has CHF. Unfortunately, this has led to rampant overutilization of BNP as a marker for CHF.

PR: Often the patient's history can help sort the diagnosis out. I've seen a fair number of patients who were mistreated as COPD patients because they were wheezing, yet there was no prior history of asthma or chronic bronchitis, and they clearly were in acute congestive failure. While I have no problem in using diagnostic tests that help sort things out, I find it the very antithesis of emergency medicine to wait 2 hours for a BNP level while your patient is choking to death and needing emergent therapy. A critical issue in the management of a patient like this who doesn't sound as critically ill as many patients can be, is can we turn him around in the ED? Does he need admission? What should be the follow up once we get his pulmonary overload turned around?

WB: In most cases, you can identify admission candidates when you walk into the room. If someone presents in extremis or having significant respiratory

compromise, I would arrange admission, even with a rapid positive response to intervention. Patients with similar presentations to this case can be treated aggressively, observed over a number of hours, and then reevaluated as to their response to work of breathing and the effectiveness of their perfusion. Diagnostic testing on the front end of the evaluation of congestive heart failure is largely limited to taking an adequate focused history and performing an appropriate physical examination. I do think it's appropriate to consider that, when a patient is in congestive heart failure, why did that patient decompensate? One should always consider acute cardiac ischemia, realizing that shortness of breath can be an anginal equivalent that is present in many patients with acute myocardial infarction. It's very appropriate to perform an EKG. I would check at least two sets of cardiac markers using troponins spaced at least 3 hours apart. I would also consider in the history whether the etiology is related to dietary indiscretion. Was the patient celebrating with a large holiday feast where people ate a lot of salty food that caused the decompensation? Did the patient stop using his routine outpatient therapy? I would also consider respiratory infections, as they can also cause someone with tenuous cardiac function to tip the balance and decompensate.

If the person were not in extremis or exhibiting significant respiratory compromise, and had a positive response to therapy and excellent medical follow-up, then I would consider discharging the patient from the ED. Follow-up is critically important, because many of us forget that congestive heart failure has a very high mortality rate with a large number of people dying in the first year after the diagnosis. For this reason, even if we do turn them around quickly in the ED and they are appropriate discharge candidates, we must assure adequate medical follow-up in the short-term and long-term.

PR: The statistics that I've read are absolutely frightening. I recall data from a couple of years ago that, after the acute onset of congestive failure, well over 80% will be dead within 2 years.

Yet, years ago our cardiac beds were filled with CHF patients who would lie around for 2 or 3 weeks while we diuresed 20 or 30 pounds from them. We didn't have very good diuretics. It seemed as though there were many more patients who were chronically overloaded, and who, to a large degree, fared much better in the hospital, I suppose because they had bed rest, oxygen, and a careful diet. Since that no longer seems to be a possible utilization of a hospital bed, are we just overlooking people like this, or has the quality of congestive failure changed over the years so that we're seeing a different kind of patient?

EU: I think it's a bit of both. There hasn't been a lot of great innovation. In fact, most of the therapies, aside from positive pressure ventilation, are just old school therapies.

SG: I believe we have gotten better at keeping these patients out of the ED. Often dobutamine courses will be done as a day therapy or in observation units. This is more a reflection of improved outpatient clinic care and difficulty sustaining long-term inpatient care then a reflection of therapeutic advances.

PR: Do you think our international diets are becoming more salt-laden?

SG: Congestive heart failure has very high mortality and morbidity, and patients don't seem to realize how sick they really are. Patients want to go out and live the way they enjoy living, and life is so much easier than it was even 10 years ago. Certainly around the world, but especially in the United States, accessibility to any sort of food at any sort of time, in any sort of place, is incredible, and that factors into dietary indiscretion. This is a lifestyle that is very difficult to alter, especially when there is no perception that CHF is as deadly or perhaps more deadly than diseases such as cancer or other major killers.

PR: Do you have difficulty getting your CHF patients admitted?

WB: Most large teaching hospitals today are functioning at or above capacity, so I think my experience is similar to most. Not only housestaff, but admitting physicians in general, look at this patient and say, "Well, they just need a little more furosemide, and I'll see them in a couple of days, or a couple of weeks." There are two scenarios to talk about: One is the patient who does present with significant respiratory compromise. This patient might be underperfused. The emergency physician approaches the problem aggressively, improves the situation, and by the time the admitting physician sees the patient, the situation looks completely different: the patient looks well. Therefore, the admitting physician wants

to know, "Why are you admitting this patient?", not realizing that an hour ago, the patient was on the verge of intubation. The second scenario includes the patients who are much more aggressively managed with loop diuretics than they were even 15 or 20 years ago. Although the loop diuretic is an effective agent in terms of removing fluid, this is often one of the wrong approaches. High-dose furosemide over a very short period of time may make the patient relatively hypovolemic, resulting in acute renal failure. In these patients we have to be quite cautious, but it's very hard to convince many inpatient physicians to admit these patients because they don't see someone who is in extremis; today you have to be quite ill to even qualify for a non-ICU bed.

PR: One of the curses of our crowded hospitals and our crowded EDs is that we often reach for therapies that are suboptimal, because even if we're willing to be the patient's advocate, there just aren't any beds. We can't achieve the same benefit that an inpatient admission would. I think this problem is going to increase over time. We are seeing more and more patients who are having their acute ischemia managed well, but their chronic heart disease is advancing inexorably, and we don't do a very good job managing this. The final issue that I'd like to address is rate disturbance as the trigger of this congestive failure. We have many patients who are in chronic atrial fibrillation. Is there something we can use to slow their rate? Or should we try to convert them to a sinus rhythm? Is there something we should use beyond the treatment for heart failure?

EU: If you have someone who is in CHF with rapid atrial fibrillation, I would be very leery of using a beta-blocker for the theoretical pump disturbance that will go along with it. Instead I find much of the time, just by noninvasive pulmonary management and aggressive nitroglycerin therapy, you're able to improve breathing. Then the atrial fibrillation, or at least the rapid ventricular response, tends to respond appropriately, and you're at a level of heart rate that's not so tenuous. I would tend to avoid chemical or electrical cardioversion as more often than not, these patients have chronic atrial fibrillation, which won't convert anyway, and if they do convert, they would be at high risk for stroke.

PR: What about the patient with valvular heart disease from endocarditis and CHF? When should you start thinking of endocarditis in a patient presenting with symptoms of congestive heart failure?

WB: Endocarditis is a difficult diagnosis to make, very insidious even in the acute forms, such as with a *Staphylococcus aureus* type presentation. The patients will likely present in pulmonary edema, and in a busy and noisy ED in a patient who has significant work of breathing and related respiratory noises, it's often difficult to detect the murmurs that would lead you down that pathway. In someone with a history of IV drug abuse, the diagnosis may be a little easier. Frequently, patients don't admit to drug abuse. I always try to look at the forearms and other prominent vein areas. The IV drug abuser who is relatively young, who presents with signs and symptoms of heart failure, should prompt a consideration of endocarditis. This doesn't mean that you need to pursue the diagnosis with blood cultures, but you should at least consider endocarditis. Transthoracic echocardiography isn't very helpful; if you don't see vegetations, you haven't ruled anything out. While transesophageal echo is a much more helpful study, it's also much more difficult to obtain in the ED.

AM: If you have a patient with endocarditis who now presents with CHF, would you say that almost always the CHF is due to significant valvular dysfunction that perhaps even a transthoracic echocardiogram might be sensitive enough to pick up?

WB: If a patient presents with significant heart failure due to endocarditis, and you can demonstrate valvular dysfunction on a trans-thoracic echocardiogram, you would at least have part of your answer. In terms of making the diagnosis of endocarditis, like many syndromes that are difficult to diagnose, they tend to evolve in front of your eyes over the following 24, 48, 72 hours. In the ED, we do not have the luxury of that kind of serial observation. The emergency physician who is thinking clearly is always asking why; in a young person who may have some drug use history, he needs to ask the question, "Why is this person demonstrating significant mitral dysfunction, or why does this person have significant aortic insufficiency?" If there's really no other explanation for it, consider endocarditis.

PR: One of the things that I was beginning to see more frequently at the start of this century were young people with viral syndromes presenting in congestive

failure, usually with acute pulmonary edema. They would start with a mild flu syndrome, but within 48 hours, were in bubbling pulmonary edema.

AM: We've also seen a few cases of myocarditis presenting as CHF in relatively young people. When you have a young person who is in CHF, you have to consider viral myocarditis.

PR: What about the congestive heart failure of pregnancy? Many of us don't see much of this, as the pregnant patients go to the labor and delivery (L&D) floors. There are many hospitals in this country where there are no L&D floors. Yet, we see many patients who come in short of breath during late pregnancy. Most of us think more of pulmonary embolus than congestive failure, and yet heart failure must be considered in these patients. Do you have any experience with this entity?

SG: What's interesting about the cardiomyopathy of pregnancy is that it can be prepartum (within a month of delivery) or post-partum (within 4–5 months of delivery), and more often than not, left ventricular function will return to normal over the ensuing course of months. It is often missed initially as women who are short of breath prepartum or postpartum are thought to more likely to have pulmonary emboli. Although the etiology of the cardiomyopathy remains unclear, advanced maternal age, multiparity, African descent, pregnancy with multiple fetuses, eclampsia, cocaine abuse, and long term oral tocolytic therapy may help predict which patients will develop this cardiomyopathy. The trick is to recognize that this is in fact congestive heart failure, and once you've recognized it as CHF, then begin much of the same the treatment. The only medications to avoid are ACE inhibitors and ARBs (Angiotensin II Receptor Blockers), as they may be teratogenic.

Case resolution

The patient was felt to be suffering from an acute heart failure syndrome, likely due to acute vascular dysfunction, based on the acute progression of his symptoms, physical examination, and CXR study findings of cardiogenic pulmonary edema. As the patient was alert and well perfused, CPAP at 10 mmHg on 100% oxygen was initiated. Rapid administration and titration of IV nitroglycerin was begun. In addition,

1.25 mg IV enalapril was administered, followed by furosemide 40 mg IV, with an ensuing diuresis of 1.0 liter of urine within 90 minutes of presentation. The patient's respiratory rate, physical appearance, and subjective dyspnea began to improve within the first 15 minutes. Initial laboratory data returned with a normal chemistry profile, a BNP level of 1360 pg/dL, and a normal digoxin level. The patient was admitted to the ICU for close monitoring.

An inpatient echocardiogram showed a worsening EF of 35%, compared with a previous EF of 50%. A nuclear stress test was negative for acute ischemia. The cardiology team optimized the patient's medications, and the patient was discharged home 4 days later in stable condition.

Section III Concepts

Background

Heart failure is a worldwide problem of epidemic proportions, and represents a tremendous cost burden to health care.[10] Recent data from the American Heart Association (AHA) estimates that nearly five million individuals are living in the United States with heart failure (2.3% of the general population), and an additional 550,000 new cases are diagnosed each year.[11] Acute heart failure (AHF) is the most common cause for hospital admission in patients >65 years of age.[12] The ED plays a critical role in the management of acute heart failure syndromes, since approximately 80% of patients hospitalized for the condition are admitted through the ED. There are approximately one million admissions to US hospitals for AHF each year, accounting for more than six million hospital days and $12 billion in charges. Moreover, the prognosis of patients admitted with AHF is dismal, with greater than 20% of patients being readmitted with heart failure (HF) and more than 20% dying during the first year after admission.[13]

Further contributing to the burden of heart failure in the United States is the impact of an aging population, along with hospital and ED crowding.[14] The Institute of Medicine's Report on Emergency Medicine finds that from 1993 to 2003, the number of EDs decreased by 425, and the number of hospital beds decreased by 198,000.[13,15] As many patients are "boarded" in the ED, sometimes for up to 48 hours before an inpatient bed becomes available, emergency physicians are now often required to deliver both acute and ongoing heart failure care.[14]

Definitions and pathophysiology of acute heart failure

The term "acute heart failure syndromes" emerged from meetings of an international workgroup that was convened primarily to establish uniform terminology and definitions in heart failure. The workgroup defined acute heart failure syndromes as the "gradual or rapid deterioration in heart failure signs and symptoms resulting in a need for urgent therapy."[11] The American College of Emergency Physicians (ACEP) Clinical Policies Committee uses the term "acute heart failure syndromes" in their updated guidelines.[11]

Two separate categories of AHF syndromes, first suggested by Cotter, et al. in 2002[16] have been adopted by the European Society of Cardiology in their guidelines on diagnosis and treatment of AHF.[17] The first is termed acute decompensated cardiac failure. These patients suffer from a progressive, relatively slow (days to weeks) deterioration of chronic heart failure. This is typically attributed to noncompliance with medications, dietary indiscretions, or myocardial dysfunction (Figure 12-1). These patients are typically fluid-overloaded and benefit from diuretic therapy, fluid restriction, dietary compliance, improved pharmacotherapy, or other interventions (such as revascularization or resynchronization).[12]

The second is termed acute vascular failure or dysfunction. This is a rapidly progressive condition associated with high blood pressure and severe acute dyspnea, a common ED presentation in patients with acute heart failure syndromes. The acute presentation in these patients is most likely caused by a combination of increased vascular resistance and decreased cardiac contractility (Figure 12-1). This can occur even if the ejection fraction is relatively good. This suggests a largely vascular problem, and not a fluid overload problem. Recent data from registries such as ADHERE suggest that this second category is actually the most common type of AHF in unselected populations.[13] Acute decompensated cardiac failure tends to be overrepresented in studies of patients in academic tertiary care centers, which may be the reason that a majority of the academic teaching has been focused on therapy of fluid overload (diuretics) rather than on therapy of vascular dysfunction (vasoactive agents).

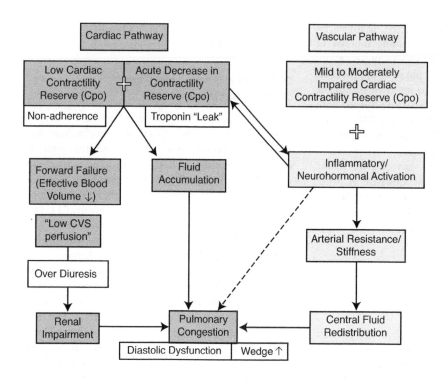

Figure 12.1 Initiation phase of AHF. Reprinted from *Am Heart J*, 155(1), Cotter G, Felker GM, Adams KF, The pathophysiology of acute heart failure–is it all about fluid accumulation?, pages 9–18, Copyright 2008, with permission from Elsevier.

Vascular dysfunction is very important because it may be the most commonly encountered reason for patients presenting in AHF. Steep increases in afterload, combined with poor systolic function, result in an acute increase in left ventricular end-diastolic pressure and a decrease in cardiac output. This model may explain the presence of pulmonary congestion despite (only) modest fluid accumulation.

Standard teaching has been that acute heart failure is mainly due to fluid overload. However, in many cases, an acute increase in afterload is often the precipitant of AHF in many patients, leading to the rapid development of pulmonary congestion even in the absence of fluid overload. More than 50% of patients presenting with cardiogenic pulmonary edema are euvolemic or hypovolemic.[12] Therefore, the key to treatment of AHF in many cases is to focus on afterload reduction and fluid redistribution, rather than aggressive diuresis. (Figures 12-2, 12-3, 12-4, Table 12-1).

Initial CHF workup: history and physical examination

A significant number of patients presenting with AHF syndrome have a prior history of CHF. Common

symptoms reported include dyspnea on exertion progressing to dyspnea at rest, orthopnea, peripheral edema, and paroxysmal nocturnal dyspnea. The progression of symptoms before ED presentation may take hours to days; however, an episode of acute

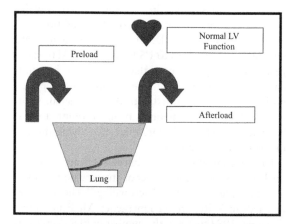

Figure 12.2 Normal physiology. Reprinted from *Am Heart J*, 155(1), Cotter G, Felker GM, Adams KF, The pathophysiology of acute heart failure–is it all about fluid accumulation?, pages 9–18, Copyright 2008, with permission from Elsevier.

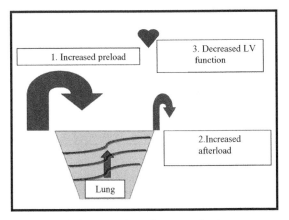

Figure 12.3 Pulmonary edema from 3 mechanisms. Reprinted from *Am Heart J*, 155(1), Cotter G, Felker GM, Adams KF, The pathophysiology of acute heart failure–is it all about fluid accumulation?, pages 9–18, Copyright 2008, with permission from Elsevier.

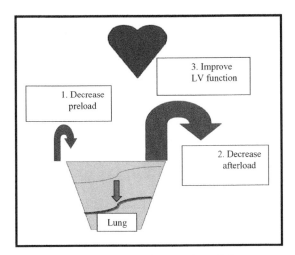

Figure 12.4 Goals of therapy for acute heart failure. Reprinted from *Am Heart J*, 155(1), Cotter G, Felker GM, Adams KF, The pathophysiology of acute heart failure–is it all about fluid accumulation?, pages 9–18, Copyright 2008, with permission from Elsevier.

ischemia or acute valvular dysfunction may cause symptoms to progress much faster. Physical examination findings typically include tachycardia and hypertension (increased catecholamine production), tachypnea, hypoxia, and diaphoresis. Auscultation of the lungs reveals rales or wheezes, and cardiac

Table 12-1. Major etiologies of cardiogenic pulmonary edema.

- Exacerbation of chronic left ventricular failure
- Acute myocardial ischemia/infarction
- Severe systemic hypertension
- Left-sided valvular disorders
- Acute tachydysrhythmias and bradydysrhythmias

Reprinted with permission from Elsevier from: Mattu A, Martinez JP, Kelly BS, Modern management of cardiogenic pulmonary edema. *Emerg Med Clin N Am.* 2005;23(4):1105–1125.

auscultation may be notable for an S3 heart sound. The remainder of the examination may find jugular venous distension (JVD), hepatojugular reflux, and peripheral edema.[18] JVD and a third heart sound (S3) have been reported to have low sensitivities (30% and 24%, respectively) for diagnosing AHF.[19] When AHF is associated with cardiogenic shock, evidence of poor tissue perfusion, including skin mottling or pallor, may be evident. Unfortunately, vital signs and physical examination findings have relatively low sensitivity (70%) for AHF.[20] As many as one-third of patients presenting with dyspnea and similar vital signs have COPD, and many also have risk factors for pulmonary embolism and acute MI.[20,21] This presents a quandary for the clinician, as these alternative diseases can mimic AHF syndrome, thereby complicating one's ability to make an accurate clinical diagnosis.

In some patients, significant mechanical lesions that evolve or deteriorate rapidly can lead to decreased myocardial contractility, leading to subsequent AHF. The most common such mechanical lesion is acute mitral regurgitation. In acute mitral regurgitation, an audible systolic thrill is often present, and the murmur often is harsh.[22] It may be auscultated over the back of the neck, vertebra, or sacrum, and may radiate to the axilla, back, and left sternal border.[22] Other causes of mechanical lesions that may cause an AHF event are ischemic or nonischemic papillary muscle rupture, mechanical valve malfunction due to thrombosis or pannus, infective endocarditis, ventricular septal rupture, and aortic dissection causing severe ischemia or aortic regurgitation. Overall, the prevalence of such mechanical lesions as the primary cause of AHF appears to be low.[12]

Initial testing

Electrocardiogram (EKG)

An electrocardiogram should be performed in all patients presenting with possible AHF syndrome. The EKG should be assessed for acute dysrhythmias, signs of acute coronary syndrome including ST-segment elevation myocardial infarction, and signs of electrolyte abnormalities (i.e., hyperkalemia in renal failure). If the EKG shows evidence of acute myocardial ischemia (acute MI) appropriate anti-ischemia and reperfusion therapies should be pursued. Severe bradyarrhythmias along with normal or elevated right-heart filling can induce elevations in pulmonary capillary hydrostatic pressures, leading to cardiogenic pulmonary edema (CPE). Tachydysrhythmias may lead to CPE caused by poor diastolic filling, which also leads to elevations in pulmonary capillary hydrostatic pressures. Along with initial stabilization measures, treatment of CPE in either case is simply based on correction of the underlying dysrhythmia using standard Advanced Cardiac Life Support protocols.[18] Most registries have reported that atrial fibrillation occurs in 30–42% of patients admitted with AHF.[12] While one study shows that the occurrence of new dysrhythmias, mainly atrial fibrillation, is a strong predictor of recurrent events and death in patients admitted for AHF, the precise role of dysrhythmia in the pathogenesis of AHF remains unknown.[12]

A widened QRS of >120ms has been suggested as a clinical marker of poor prognosis in heart failure and reduced left ventricular ejection fraction (LVEF). It has also been reported to be associated with increased mortality and sudden death in heart failure, as well as an independent predictor of cardiac death in a general medical population.[23–27] However, as these observations were not made in the acutely decompensated patient presenting with an unknown diagnosis, the application of this into routine ED clinical practice is unclear.[28]

Chest radiograph

The classic radiographic findings of CPE are listed in Table 12-2.[29,30] However, these "classic" radiographic findings may not be seen at the time of initial presentation.[18] Up to a 12 hour delay can occur between the abrupt onset of CPE symptoms and the development of significant radiographic abnormalities.[31,32]

Table 12-2. Classic radiographic findings of cardiogenic pulmonary edema.

Cardiomegaly (underlying CHF)
Pulmonary vascular redistribution
Thickening of interlobular septa (Kerley B lines)
Alveolar edema
Pleural effusions
Bilateral infiltrates in a "bat wing" pattern

The presence of cardiomegaly, often considered one of the most reliable radiographic abnormalities associated with systolic dysfunction, may be absent in patients who have rapidly-developing CPE.[33] Radiographs can be difficult to interpret in patients who develop chronic lung abnormalities or may have scarring that impairs image quality or mimics vascular redistribution.[18] Image quality may also be impaired in obese patients and patients with COPD.[34]

Previous research suggest that a combination of medical history, physical examination, and chest radiograph findings can suggest a diagnosis of acute heart failure syndrome.[35–37] Although signs, symptoms, and scoring systems can be highly suggestive of acute heart failure syndromes, they lack sufficient accuracy to serve as a definitive diagnostic strategy.[11] (Table 12-3). Furthermore, these scoring systems have not been extensively validated in the acute setting,

Table 12-3. Test characteristics of heart failure diagnostic scoring systems.

Scoring System	Sensitivity	Specificity
Framingham	63%±4%	94%±1%
Boston*	35%±4%	99%±0%
NHANES**	62%±4%	94%±1%
Gheorghiade	55%±4%	95%±1%

*Test characteristics for a Boston Score greater than 8.

**NHANES, National Health and Nutrition Examination Survey.

Reprinted with permission of Elsevier from: Collins S, Storrow AB, Kirk JD, et al. Beyond pulmonary edema: Diagnostic, risk stratification, and treatment challenges of acute heart failure management in the emergency department. *Ann Emerg Med.* 2008;51(1);45–47.

making their implementation in the ED somewhat limited.[11]

Additional testing in acute heart failure syndromes

As discussed previously, the clinical diagnosis of acute heart failure is estimated to be incorrect in more than 50% of cases, leading to frequent over-diagnosis and underdiagnosis.[21] Because of the limitations of clinical assessment and chest radiography in distinguishing acute heart failure from other causes of acute dyspnea, B-type natriuretic peptide (BNP) testing has emerged as a diagnostic tool in ED practice.[18]

BNP and NT-proBNP

BNP is an endogenous cardiac neurohormone produced by cardiac myocytes in response to increased end-diastolic pressure and volume (increased wall tension), as occurs in the setting of heart failure. Pre-proBNP is synthesized within myocytes and cleaved to proBNP. The latter is released into the circulation and then cleaved to the active BNP and an inactive N-terminal fragment, called NT-proBNP. BNP's main effect is to counteract the renin-angiotensin-aldosterone system by promoting natriuresis, diuresis, and vasodilatation.[18] Plasma BNP levels increase in the setting of acute heart failure and CPE.[18] During the past decade, both BNP and NT-proBNP have been studied as markers for aiding in the diagnosis of acute heart failure syndrome in patients presenting with dyspnea in the acute setting.[11] Elevated levels of BNP have been demonstrated to correlate with the severity of left ventricle filling pressures, clinical status, short-term and long-term mortality, and response to inhospital therapy.[32,38–42]

The largest trial to date is a Class II, industry-sponsored, prospective, multicenter, observational study[38] that enrolled 1586 subjects with a primary complaint of "shortness of breath" and compared a single BNP measurement (Triage; Biosite Inc, San Diego, CA) against a criterion-standard, final diagnosis as determined retrospectively by two cardiologists blinded to BNP levels.[11] The authors suggest a cut point of 100 pg/mL yielding a sensitivity of 90% and specificity of 76%. Higher cut points result in improved specificity, up to 90% at a cut point of 1000 pg/mL but with markedly lower sensitivity.[11] The overall area under the receiver operating characteristic

(ROC) curve for this test is calculated as 0.91.[11,38] In data derived from the same sample population, McCullough, et al.[43] report on 1538 subjects for whom the clinical likelihood of acute heart failure syndromes was recorded by an emergency physician who was blinded to the BNP level.[11] In this study, the area under the curve (AUC) for "estimated congestive heart failure probability" based on clinical evaluation alone is 0.86, as compared to 0.90 for a single BNP measurement and 0.93 for the combination of clinical evaluation and BNP.[11]

Measurement of BNP levels in patients presenting to the ED with acute dyspnea can assist clinicians in distinguishing acute heart failure and CPE from other acute or chronic lung diseases.[44,45] Based on available data, the ACEP guidelines on AHF recommend that the addition of a single BNP or NT-proBNP measurement can improve the diagnostic accuracy, compared to standard clinical judgment alone, in the diagnosis of acute heart failure syndrome among patients presenting to the ED with acute dyspnea (Level B recommendation).[11]

The following are included as cutoffs for ProBNP and NT-proBNP.

1 BNP <100 pg/dL or NT-proBNP <300 pg/dL: acute heart failure syndrome unlikely* (Approximate LR− = 0.1)
2 BNP >500 pg/dL or NT-proBNP >1,000 pg/dL: acute heart failure syndrome likely (Approximate LR+ = 6)

BNP and NT-proBNP measurement have been compared head to head in a number of prospective trials with essentially parallel ROC curves and statistically similar AUCs with respect to the diagnosis of acute heart failure syndrome. Age, sex, body mass index, and renal function may influence BNP and NT-proBNP measurements. Several post hoc analyses show that BNP measurements may retain discriminatory power in various subpopulations, including individuals with systolic and diastolic heart failure, underlying pulmonary disease, advanced renal disease, advanced age, and obesity.[11]

An intermediate "grey zone" BNP level in the range of 100 to 500 pg/mL represents a significant quandary for the ED physician. While an elevated BNP can be caused by acute heart failure, it can also be caused

*BNP conversion: 100 pg/mL = 22 pmol/L; NT-proBNP conversion: 300 pg/mL = 35 pmol/L

by other conditions that induce elevated ventricular wall tension, including cor pulmonale and acute pulmonary embolism.[21] Falsely low BNP levels can occur during the first 1–2 hours after symptom-onset in cases of flash pulmonary edema.[46]

Cardiac troponins

Electrocardiographic changes and troponin release may occur in patients with HF without coronary disease (and may be the result rather than the cause of the AHF syndrome).[12] Available data suggest that the incidence for troponin above the threshold for acute coronary syndrome (ACS) is approximately 20% in patients with AHF. However, the exact incidence of frank myocardial ischemia in AHF remains unknown due to the difficulty of diagnosing ischemia in patients admitted with AHF.[12] Although observational data cited suggest ischemic complications in 20% of AHF admissions, this number may be lower (troponin leak can occur even when ischemic heart disease is not present) or higher (ischemia may occur without significant troponin leakage).[11]

One large study on the incidence and outcome of clinical HF (N > 20,000) in patients with non–ST elevation ACS has concerning findings.[47] Acute HF was observed in 11% of the patients, leading to a 9% 1-month mortality and 16% 6-month mortality—more than triple the mortality observed in patients without HF. Acute HF is correlated with 30% of the overall mortality in the study, being the strongest independent negative prognostic factor in the cohort.[12] Based on this and other studies, patients presenting with the combination of ACS and AHF have a poor prognosis, and should be admitted to the ICU for further management.[12] Patients "ruling in" for cardiac ischemia or non-ST-segment elevation MI (NSTEMI) should have urgent cardiology consultation to help guide further inpatient care, including possible interventional or cardiac revascularization procedures.[18]

Blood chemistries

In patients with chronic HF, the presence of concomitant chronic renal insufficiency (CRI) is a strong risk factor for mortality. Although renal dysfunction predicts all-cause mortality, it is most predictive of death from progressive HF, suggesting that renal dysfunction may be a marker of HF severity. Although the relationship between renal dysfunction and adverse outcomes appears to be linear, several studies have used a threshold of a 0.3-mg/dL rise in serum creatinine over baseline to define this risk level. Changes of this magnitude generally occur in about one-third of patients admitted for AHF and are associated with a prolonged and complicated hospital course, as well as high rates of morbidity and mortality. Worsening renal function may play an important role in the progression and propagation of an AHF episode by leading to greater fluid and sodium retention and neurohormonal activation.[12] Therefore, any significant changes in serum creatinine from baseline or chronic renal insufficiency warrant further evaluation in the inpatient or observation setting.

Management of acute heart failure and cardiogenic pulmonary edema

Rapid triage and initial stabilization

The goals of management of AHF should focus on the suspected etiology of the patient's presentation. Determine if the patient's history and physical examination are consistent with acute decompensated cardiac failure or acute vascular dysfunction. As many patients present to the ED with acute vascular dysfunction, in a majority of cases treatment will need to focus upon decreasing preload and decreasing afterload to improve LV function and to increase cardiac output. Implementation of ionotropic support may be required to improve LV function.

Initial management of patients who experience severe AHF and CPE should focus on the "ABCs" of resuscitation.[18] Large bore IV lines should be inserted to draw needed laboratory tests, and for needed medication administration. Patients should be placed in an upright sitting position, connected to a cardiac monitor and pulse oximeter, and high-flow supplemental oxygen should be provided by way of a facemask with a fraction of inspired oxygen of 1.0.[18]

Patients with AHF should be rapidly triaged to decide on appropriate treatment and diagnostic testing. Immediate stabilization is necessary in patients presenting in extremis, including patients with significant tachypnea, hypoxia, and mental status changes, to prevent further deterioration. Aggressive intervention with noninvasive ventilation or possible endotracheal intubation is recommended to prevent respiratory failure while definitive care is being established; however, patients with significant mental status changes who are unable to cooperate with this modality are not candidates for this intervention. Patients who present with pulmonary edema and concurrent hypotension, along with evidence of end-organ hypoperfusion (altered mental status, reduced urine output, poorly perfused extremities), may require a fluid challenge and aggressive inotropic therapy. This subset of critically ill patients may benefit from right-sided heart catheterization, and need ICU admission for close monitoring and continued treatment.[14]

BiPaP and CPAP

Noninvasive ventilatory assistance may be provided by either continuous positive airway pressure or bilevel positive airway pressure. CPAP provides a constant, positive, end-expiratory airway pressure, whereas BiPAP provides the same constant end-expiratory pressure, as well as added positive pressure at the onset of inspiration to assist ventilation. CPAP and BiPAP devices typically attach to the patient by a nasal or face mask.[11] By improving oxygenation, reducing respiratory work, and decreasing left-ventricular afterload, the positive airway pressure provided by these devices has been thought to improve pulmonary mechanics and hemodynamics, as well as to reduce the need for endotracheal intubation, hospital length of stay, and mortality.[48,49]

Initial studies evaluating CPAP by either nasal or face mask at 5 to 10 mmHg consistently show significant improvements in oxygenation, reductions in heart rate, reductions in respiratory rate, and reductions in blood pressure compared with standard oxygen therapy. Several of these studies also report statistically significant improvements in cardiopulmonary indices (i.e., pulmonary capillary wedge pressure, stroke volume, cardiac output, or cardiac index), as well as a reduction in the rate of intubation.[11]

In a 1997 Class III study, Mehta, et al.[50] report a trial comparing BiPAP, CPAP, and conventional oxygen therapy for patients with acute heart failure syndrome. BiPAP is no more efficacious than CPAP, and is associated with a higher rate of myocardial infarction as defined by elevated cardiac markers.[11] Subsequent studies comparing BiPAP with mask ventilation in patients who present with CPE[51] and BiPAP versus CPAP in acute respiratory failure of heterogeneous causes[52] do not report an increase in MI or mortality in patients receiving BiPAP.[18] Two additional studies directly compare CPAP and BiPAP for patients with acute heart failure syndrome, and neither modality has an advantage over the other.[53,54]

Pharmacologic therapies: preload and afterload reduction

The first goal in pharmacologic treatment of patients with AHF and CPE should be preload reduction. By reducing right heart and pulmonary venous return, and right-heart filling pressures and pulmonary capillary hydrostatic pressures, patients will have early symptomatic improvements in dyspnea.[21] Typical medications utilized for preload reduction are nitroglycerin, morphine sulfate, and loop diuretics. More recently, a recombinant form of beta-natriuretic peptide known as nesiritide has been recommended for preload reduction, but with no clear advantages over conventional therapy.[21]

Utility of nitrates

Nitroglycerin (NTG) is the most effective and rapidly-acting preload-reducing medication.[7,55-58] Multiple studies demonstrate the superiority of NTG over furosemide and morphine sulfate for preload reduction, symptomatic improvement, and patient safety.[5,9,21,48,51,55,59-61] NTG can be administered in sublingual, intravenous, or transdermal form, although the transdermal absorption can be erratic.[21] An additional benefit of NTG is its short half-life. If the patient develops a precipitous fall in blood pressure (generally uncommon in AHF patients), the blood pressure should return to previous values within 5–10 minutes of discontinuation of medication.[21] Preload reduction and subsequent noticeable symptomatic improvements occur within 5 minutes of sublingual administration of NTG, and the dose can be repeated every 3–5 minutes during the first 10–15 minutes of presentation.[21,62,63] Standard anti-anginal dosages of sublingual NTG (400 µg every 5 minutes) with which most physicians are comfortable have the bioequivalence of an IV NTG infusion of 60–80 mg/min.[21] If using IV NTG, an initial dose of 10–20 mg/min should be titrated upwards rapidly until a dose of at least 100 mg/min is achieved.[13] This type of aggressive administration of NTG also produces afterload reduction.[64,65]

Due to concerns for precipitous drops in blood pressure, nitrates should not be used in patients presenting with hypotension, or patients presently taking sidenafil or other similar medications for erectile dysfunction, Furthermore, nitrates should be used with extreme caution (if at all) in patients with aortic stenosis or pulmonary hypertension because of the dependence these conditions place on preload to maintain adequate perfusion.[21]

Utility of morphine

Morphine sulfate (MS) has been administered as a standard preload-reducing medication in patients with suspected AHF, especially in the prehospital setting. However, MS has not been studied in a randomized fashion in these patients to confirm hemodynamic benefits. MS most likely exerts mild indirect hemodynamic benefits through anxiolysis, resulting in a decrease in catecholamine production and indirectly causing vasodilatation.[18] While early studies demonstrate some evidence of vasodilatation and venous pooling in the peripheral circulation, a consistent central preload-reducing effect (i.e., reduction in pulmonary capillary wedge pressures [PCWP]) is not present.[18] In contrast, multiple studies show that MS may be associated with adverse hemodynamic effects, including increases in left and right heart filling pressures and reductions in cardiac index caused by a direct myocardial depressant effect on the already-reduced contractile state of the ischemic heart.[4,9,50,66] The adverse hemodynamic effects have clinical drawbacks. In a prehospital study evaluating the use of various medications in patients with presumed CPE, 38% of patients receiving MS have subjective deterioration (e.g., increased dyspnea) in clinical status, and 46% have objective deterioration (e.g., increased respiratory rate).[18,55]

Morphine sulfate also has an undesirable side effect profile, including nausea, emesis, pruritus, and urticaria. If a patient requires medications for anxiety, low-dose benzodiazepines have a better side-effect profile and are not associated with significant myocardial or respiratory depression.[18] In conclusion, based on available evidence regarding the superiority of NTG over MS to reduce preload and availability of low-dose benzodiazepines for anxiolysis, the routine use of MS is not recommended in acute heart failure (AHF) syndromes.[18]

Utility of diuretics

Furosemide (common loop diuretic) has been used intravenously for years as the cornerstone of treatment in patients who present with CPE. Loop diuretics produce a decrease in preload by inhibiting sodium chloride reabsorption in the ascending loop of Henle, thereby promoting increases in urine volume and excretion.[18] Unfortunately, because patients who develop AHF have elevated systemic vascular resistance (afterload), renal perfusion is markedly diminished.[67] This causes diuretics to have a significantly delayed onset of action, often taking 45–120 minutes to produce effective diuresis.[6–8,52,68] More than half of the patients who present with CPE have intravascular euvolemia or hypovolemia, and diuretic administration in these patients may be associated with adverse effects, including electrolyte abnormalities and hypotension caused by overdiuresis.[55,63,69,70]

Currently, there are no randomized clinical trials evaluating the clinical benefit of furosemide alone in acute heart failure syndromes.[11] Two clinical studies conclude that loop diuretic monotherapy does not improve short-term ED outcomes (i.e., improve hemodynamic status, patient dyspnea, and reduce rate of endotracheal intubation) among patients presenting with moderate-to-severe acute pulmonary edema.[53,55] The adverse hemodynamic changes may be blunted in AHF by administration of preload-reducing (i.e., NTG) and afterload reducing (i.e., angiotensin-converting enzyme inhibitors) medications before furosemide.[18,52]

Potential safety considerations regarding diuretic administration are reported in a multicenter study of 382 patients.[71] Worsening renal function is associated with a greater total dose of furosemide in the preceding 24 hours compared to those patients who don't develop worsening renal function (394 mg versus 262 mg; $P < 0.05$).[63] The possible association of diuretics with worsening renal function is important, given that several recent studies report an association between impaired renal function and increased mortality among acute heart failure syndrome patients.[11] Data from more than 60,000 patients in the ADHERE registry show that in hospital mortality is greater than 20% among patients with an admission blood urea nitrogen level greater than 43 mg/dL, a creatinine level greater than 2.7 mg/dL, and a systolic blood pressure less than 115 mmHg.[72] In a retrospective study of 1681 patients younger than 65 years of age who were admitted for AHF syndromes, an increase in the serum creatinine level of greater than 0.3 mg/dL during the index hospitalization is associated with a nearly three times greater risk of inhospital mortality (OR 2.7, 95% CI 1.6 to 4.6).[73] Furthermore, in a prospective cohort study of 412 hospitalized patients with acute heart failure syndrome, a stepwise increase in 6-month mortality as serum creatinine increases from greater than or equal to 0.1 mg/dL to greater than or equal to 0.5 mg/dl above baseline is reported.[74]

Utility of ACE inhibitors: afterload reduction

Afterload reduction with vasodilator medications produces an increase in cardiac output and reduction in pulmonary interstitial edema. Another benefit is improved renal perfusion, which can lead to substantial improvements in diuresis even before administration of diuretics.[75] High-dose IV NTG effectively reduces afterload, but prolonged infusion can induce tolerance and limit its efficacy. Nitroprusside is a potent afterload-reducing medication used in certain hypertensive emergency states. However, it can induce labile fluctuations in blood pressure, requires intra-arterial hemodynamic monitoring, and cause reflex tachycardia in an already stressed state with AHF.[18]

Angiotensin-converting enzyme inhibitors (ACEIs) interrupt the renin-angiotensin system and lead to decreased preload and decreased afterload.[11] The administration of sublingual (captopril) or IV (captopril, enalapril) forms of ACEIs to patients who develop CPE is associated with reductions in systemic vascular resistance (afterload) and improvements in PCWP (preload), stroke volume, cardiac output, and mitral regurgitation without causing adverse changes in heart rate or mean arterial pressure.[6,21,76-82] Improvements of both hemodynamics and subjective dyspnea are noted within 6–12 minutes. Similar improvements have been shown when ACEIs are administered to patients who have already received other "standard" therapies, including MS, furosemide, and NTG,[83] and in patients who have hemodialysis-dependent renal failure.[18,84] The available data suggest that there are no differences among available ACEIs in their effects on symptoms or survival.[76]

The use of ACEIs in patients with AHF decreases rates of endotracheal intubation, intensive care unit (ICU) admission rates, and ICU length of stay.[70,85] These benefits of ACE inhibition are seen in patients with mild, moderate, or severe symptoms, and in patients with or without coronary artery disease.[86] ACEIs can be used safely in conjunction with NTG to provide combination preload and afterload reduction, or they can be used as an effective single agent in patients who are unable to receive NTG.[18]

Hypotensive patients who may be in or at immediate risk of cardiogenic shock should not initially receive ACEIs or other afterload reducing agents. However, afterload-reducing medications can be administered cautiously after vasopressors therapy is initiated in hypotensive patients, although titrateable afterload-reducers (e.g., nitroprusside) are preferred in this setting. Afterload-reducing agents should also be used with caution in patients who have severe aortic stenosis. In patients with chronic renal insufficiency with markedly increased serum levels of creatinine (greater than 3 mg/dL), known bilateral renal artery stenosis, or elevated levels of serum potassium (greater than 5.5 mmol/liter), repetitive dosing of ACEIs should be avoided; however, a single dose of ACEIs for acute afterload reduction even in the presence of CRI or hyperkalemia should not produce an acute change in renal function or potassium level.[18] Adverse reactions of ACEIs are generally attributable to the two principal pharmacological actions of these drugs: those related to angiotensin suppression (hypotension) and those related to kinin potentiation (angiodema).[76] Patients should not be given an ACEI if they have experienced life-threatening adverse reactions (angioedema or anuric renal failure) during previous exposure to the drug, or if they are pregnant.

Pharmacologic therapies: inotropic support

Inotropic agents can cause tachycardia, dysrhythmias, increased myocardial oxygen demand, myocardial ischemia, and sometimes increased mortality in patients with AHF.[87,88] These medications should be reserved for hypotensive AHF patients who are unable to tolerate the use of first-line preload- and afterload-reducing medications discussed previously.[18] After initiation of inotropic agents and sufficient improvements in blood pressure, IV NTG can then be administered to obtain the desired preload and afterload reduction to relieve pulmonary congestion.[89,90] These critically-ill patients are best managed in the ICU with pulmonary artery catheterization and invasive monitoring to closely track their hemodynamic status and allow precise titration of the medications.[18]

Typical agents fall into two main classifications: catecholamines and phosphodiesterase inhibitors. The catecholamine inotropes include dobutamine, dopamine, and norepinephrine. No studies to date have demonstrated a mortality benefit of these over others in the ED setting. From a hemodynamic standpoint, dobutamine provides the advantage of inducing mild reductions in preload and afterload in addition to inotropic support. Close monitoring is required as may cause a reduction in blood pressure, precluding its continued use.[91] If this occurs, dobutamine should be discontinued, and dopamine or norepinephrine can be administered to support blood pressure. These medications improve blood pressure by increasing systemic vascular resistance, but may at the same time cause a detrimental decrease in cardiac output. In cases when dopamine and norepinephrine are given, preload- and afterload-reducing medications should be added as soon as possible to improve LV performance and relieve pulmonary congestion.

Several limitations of catecholamine inotropes exist. Their activity depends on adrenoreceptor sensitivity. CHF patients have chronically elevated levels of circulating catecholamines that produce adrenoreceptor tolerance, thereby requiring higher inotropic dosages than normal. Additionally, many patients who experience CHF are now treated chronically with beta-adrenergic receptor antagonists (beta-blockers). These medications antagonize the effects of catecholamine inotropes, also leading to higher dosages of the inotropes. Higher dosages are associated with increased adverse effects.[18]

Phosphodiesterase inhibitors (PDEIs) work by increasing intracellular cyclic adenosine monophosphate levels, which produce a positive inotropic effect on the heart, inducing peripheral vasodilatation and reducing pulmonary vascular resistance. Overall, PDEIs induce improvements in preload, afterload, and cardiac output.[92] PDEIs have the advantage over catecholamine inotropes of working independent of adrenoreceptor activity, meaning they are unaffected by circulating catecholamine levels or beta-blocker medications.[93] The most well studied PDEI is milrinone, which has been directly compared with dobutamine in patients with severe acutely decompensated CHF and CPE, and milrinone is consistently noted to produce equal or greater improvements in stroke volume, cardiac output, PCWP, and systemic vascular resistance. Milrinone is well-tolerated, and is associated with fewer episodes of tachycardia and sustained tachydysrhythmias than dobutamine.[94-98] Despite apparent hemodynamic benefits, however, it has not been demonstrated to improve hospital length of stay or mortality.[96,98]

Levosimendan, classified as a "calcium sensitizer," is an inotrope suggested as an alternative to dobutamine for patients presenting with acutely decompensated heart failure.[99,101] One randomized double-blind trial compared 24-hour infusions of this agent with dobutamine in patients who presented with severe low-output heart failure.[100] Levosimendan not only produces more significant improvements in cardiac output and PCWP, but also is associated with a lower 180-day mortality rate (26% versus 38%) compared with patients who receive dobutamine. Further trials are needed to clarify whether levosimendan has a role in the acute ED management of patients who have developed CPE.

Utility of nebulizers (if patient is wheezing)
The use of bronchodilators is common among prehospital providers when caring for patients who have undifferentiated dyspnea.[1] Many patients who have decompensated CHF can present with wheezing, and bronchodilators are commonly administered to these patients.[1] A prehospital study suggests that bronchodilators are safe in all types of patients who have dyspnea regardless of the final diagnosis, finding no increased mortality in patients receiving these medications.[101] However, a nonrandomized, retrospective study suggests otherwise.[102] Over 10,000 patients from the Acute Decompensated Heart Failure National Registry Emergency Module who were provided bronchodilators during acute treatment, in the prehospital setting or in the ED, were evaluated. The use of bronchodilators in patients who do not have a history of COPD is associated with a slightly greater need for "aggressive interventions," including mechanical ventilation. Whether the bronchodilator use is causing adverse outcomes, or is simply a marker of sicker patients, is unclear. Nevertheless, the study does raise concerns regarding the liberal use of bronchodilatators in the management of prehospital and ED patients who have undifferentiated dyspnea, especially if the presumptive diagnosis is decompensated CHF.[1]

Disposition of patients with acute heart failure
Unstable and critically Ill patients with AHF syndromes Patients who require mechanical ventilation, experience acute valvular dysfunction, require inotropic support, and who present with evidence of acute cardiac ischemia or infarction (based on EKG changes or elevated cardiac biomarkers) should be admitted to an ICU setting after initial attempts at stabilization.[103,104] Emergent consultation by a

cardiologist should be obtained if the cause of the acute CHF exacerbation is AMI or acute valvular dysfunction, or if the patient requires inotropic support. Consultation of a cardiac surgeon is also warranted if severe valvular dysfunction is present.

Disposition for the non-critically ill patients Patients who experience mild CHF decompensations that are attributable to dietary indiscretions (excessive salt intake) or medication noncompliance can receive diuretics in the ED for symptomatic improvement, and be discharged safely. This assumes a patient has ready access to close outpatient follow-up, and the ability to continue with medical interventions, either begun or adjusted during the ED evaluation.

Patients who present with active signs of pulmonary edema should be admitted to a cardiac-monitored bed (inpatient or ED observation unit). Several studies have evaluated ED-based risk models for heart failure patients.[105] However, all models fail to identify a truly low-risk patient, and many only assess mortality but not morbidity from treatment failures. Patients with presenting factors that have been shown to be associated with in-hospital mortality include advanced age, renal dysfunction, hypotension, digoxin use, chest pain, and anemia (Table 12-4).[106–110]

Additional data from a large registry (Acute Decompensated Heart Failure National Registry,

Table 12-4. Predictors of inhospital mortality in patients who experience cardiogenic pulmonary edema.

- Need for mechanical ventilation
- Acute valvular dysfunction
- Need for inotropic support
- Elevated cardiac biomarkers
- EKG evidence of ischemia or dysrhythmias
- Advanced age
- Renal dysfunction (serum elevations of blood urea nitrogen or creatinine)
- Hypotension
- Digoxin use
- Chest pain
- Anemia

Reprinted with permission from Elsevier from: Mattu A, Martinez JP, Kelly BS. Modern management of cardiogenic pulmonary edema. *Emerg Med Clin N Am.* 2005;23(4):1105–1125.

ADHERE) of patients hospitalized with decompensated heart failure identifies: (1) high admission blood urea nitrogen (>43 mg/dL), followed by (2) low admission systolic blood pressure (<115 mmHg), followed by (3) high levels of serum creatinine (>2.75 mg/dL) as the best predictors for inhospital mortality.[109] Unfortunately, even a patient presenting with AHF syndrome without any of the above criteria still has a predicted 2.1% "low risk" of mortality.

Patients with any of these criteria, as well as patients unable to complete close outpatient follow-up (poor access or limited financial capabilities), should be admitted to ensure clinical resolution, and to allow for arrangements for longer-term inpatient or outpatient care. The goals of admission should include improvement of a patient's pulmonary edema while simultaneously focusing on discovering and treating the underlying cause.[18] In summary, until a validated risk-stratification tool based on ED data from ED presentations of AHF syndrome is developed, admission to an inpatient or ED observation unit is recommended.

The emergency department observation unit
Observation units allow for continued evaluation and treatment for up to 24 hours, to either discharge based on improved clinical status, or to have an admission for further inpatient care. Preliminary research suggests that an ED observation unit is a safe and efficient alternative for AHF patients with mild symptoms.[111–114] With continued research, the ED observation unit may become part of a viable disposition strategy of low risk patients presenting with AHF syndrome.[18]

Section IV: Decision making

- Acute heart failure and cardiogenic pulmonary edema are at high risk for early morbidity or mortality.
- The diagnosis of AHF is based on history, physical examination, and chest radiography.
- Laboratory testing adds little except in equivocal cases.
- Early management should focus on aggressive preload and afterload reduction.
- Diuresis plays a secondary role in the sickest of patients because of delayed effect and because most

patients with cardiogenic pulmonary edema are not fluid overloaded.

- Early use of noninvasive ventilation can improve oxygenation and may decrease intubation rates and inpatient mortality.
- Almost all patients with AHF require admission for treatment and workup of the underlying condition precipitating the AHF.

References

1 Mattu A, Lawner B. Prehospital management of congestive heart failure. *Heart Failure Clin.* 2009;5: 19–24.

2 Vismara LA, Leaman DM, Zelis R. The effects of morphine on venous tone in patients with acute pulmonary edema. *Circulation.* 1976;54:335–337.

3 Pickkers P, Dormans TP, Russel FG, et al. Direct vascular effects of furosemide in humans. *Circulation.* 1997;96: 1847–1852.

4 Lappas DG, Geha D, Fischer JE, et al. Filling pressures of the heart and pulmonary circulation of the patient with coronary artery disease after large intravenous doses of morphine. *Anesthesiology.* 1975;42: 153–159.

5 Kraus PA, Lipman J, Becker PJ. Acute preload effects of furosemide. *Chest.* 1990;98:124–128.

6 Ikram H, Chan W, Espiner EA, et al. Haemodynamic and hormone responses to acute and chronic furosemide therapy in congestive heart failure. *Clin Sci.* 1980; 59:443–449.

7 Nelson GI, Ahuja RC, Silke B, et al. Haemodynamic advantages of isosorbide dinitrate over furosemide in acute heart-failure following myocardial infarction. *Lancet.* 1983;1(8327):730–733.

8 Francis GS, Siegel RM, Goldsmith SR, et al. Acute vasoconstrictor response to intravenous furosemide in patients with chronic congestive heart failure. *Ann Intern Med.* 1985;103:1–6.

9 Timmis AD, Rothman MT, Henderson MA, et al. Haemodynamic effect of intravenous morphine in patients with acute myocardial infarction complicated by severe left ventricular failure. *Br Med J.* 1980; 280:980–982.

10 Tsao LCG. Heart failure: an epidemic of the 21st century. *Crit Pathways Cardiol.* 2004;3:194–204.

11 Silvers MS (Subcommittee Chair), Howell JM, Kosowsky JM, et al. Clinical Policy: Critical Issues in the Evaluation and Management of Adult Patients Presenting to the Emergency Department with Acute Heart Failure Syndromes. *Ann Emerg Med.* 2007;49(5): 627–669.

12 Cotter G, Felker GM, Adams FA. The pathophysiology of acute heart failure—is it all about fluid accumulation? *Am Heart J.* 2008;155:9–18.

13 Adams KF Jr, Fonarow GC, Emerman CL, et al. ADHERE Scientific Advisory Committee and Investigators. Characteristics and outcomes of patients hospitalized for heart failure in the United States: rationale, design, and preliminary observations from the first 100,000 cases in the Acute Decompensated Heart Failure National Registry (ADHERE). *Am Heart J.* 2005;149:209–216.

14 Collins S, Storrow AB, Kirk JD, et al. Beyond pulmonary edema: diagnostic, risk stratification, and treatment challenges of acute heart failure management in the emergency department. *Ann Emerg Med.* 2008; 51:45–57.

15 Cleland JG, Swedberg K, Follath F, et al. The EuroHeart Failure survey programme—a survey on the quality of care among patients with heart failure in Europe. Part 1: patient characteristics and diagnosis. *Eur Heart J.* 2003;24:442–463.

16 Cotter G, Moshkovitz Y, Milovanov O, et al. Acute heart failure: a novel approach to ts pathogenesis and treatment. *Eur J Heart Fail.* 2002;4:227–234.

17 Nieminen MS, Bohm M, Cowie MR, et al. Executive summary of the guidelines on the diagnosis and treatment of acute heart failure: the Task Force on Acute Heart Failure of the European Society of cardiology. *Eur Heart J.* 2005;26:384–416.

18 Mattu A, Martinez JP, Kelly BS. Modern management of cardiogenic pulmonary edema. *Emerg Med Clin North Am.* 2005;23:1105–1125.

19 Davie AP, Francis Cm, Caruana L, et al. Assessing diagnosis in heart failure: which features are any use? *QJM.* 1997;90(5):335–339.

20 Dao Q, Krishnaswamy P, Kazanegra R, et al. Utility of B-type natriuretic peptide in the diagnosis of congestive heart failure in an urgent-care setting. *J Am Coll Cardiol.* 2001;37:379–385.

21 Gropper MA, Wiener-Kronish JP, Hashimoto S. Acute cardiogenic pulmonary edema. *Clin Chest Med.* 1994;15:501–515.

22 DiSandro D. Mitral regurgitation. *Emedicine* Updated: Aug 13, 2007. Downloaded 3/14/09. Available at: http://*EMedicine*.medscape.com/article/758816-overview. Accessed April 27, 2010.

23 Kearney MT, Zaman A, Eckberg DL, et al. Cardiac size, autonomic function, and 5-year follow-up of chronic heart failure patients with severe prolongation of ventricular activation. *J Card Fail.* 2003;9(2):93–99.

24 De Winter O, Van de Veire N, Van Heuverswijn F, et al. Relationship between QRS duration, left ventricular volumes and prevalence of nonviability in

patients with coronary artery disease and severe left ventricular dysfunction. *E Heart J Fail.* 2006;8(3): 275–277.

25 Selker HP, Griffith JL, D'Agostino RB. A time-insensitive predictive instrument for acute hospital mortality due to congestive heart failure: development, testing, and use for comparing hospitals: a multicenter study. *Med Care.* 1994;32(10):1040–1052.

26 Iuliano S, Fisher SG, Karasik PE, et al. QRS duration and mortality in patients with congestive heart failure. *Am Heart J.* 2002;143(6):1085–1091.

27 Chin MH, Goldman L. Correlates of major complications or death in patients admitted to the hospital with congestive heart failure. *Arch Intern Med.* 1996;156(16):1814–1820.

28 Storrow AB. Diagnosis and risk stratification of acute heart failure syndromes. *Emerg Med Card Res Int Group.* 2007;3:1–10.

29 Sovari AA, Kocheril AG, Bass AS. Pulmonary edema, cardiogenic. *Emedicine* Journal. Available at: http://EMedicine.medscape.com/article/157452-overview. Accessed June 1, 2010.

30 Chait A, Cohen HE, Meltzer LE, et al. The bedside chest radiograph in the evaluation of incipient heart failure. *Radiology.* 1972;105:563–566.

31 Kostuk W, Barr JW, Simon AL, et al. Correlation between the chest film and hemodynamics in acute myocardial infarction. *Circulation.* 1973;48:624–632.

32 Chen JT. Radiographic diagnosis of heart failure. *Heart Dis Stroke.* 1992;1:58–63.

33 Badgett RG, Lucey CR, Mulrow CD. Can the clinical examination diagnose left-sided heart failure in adults? *JAMA.* 1997;277:1712–1719.

34 Omland T. Heart failure in the emergency department: is B-type natriuretic peptide a better prognostic indicator than clinical assessment? *J Am Coll Cardiol.* 2004;44:1334–1336.

35 Ho KK, Anderson KM, Kannel WB, et al. Survival after the onset of congestive heart failure in Framingham Heart Study subjects. *Circulation.* 1993;88:107–115.

36 McKee PA, Castelli WP, McNamara PM, et al. The natural history of congestive heart failure: the Framingham Study. *N Engl J Med.* 1971;285:1441–1446.

37 Fonseca C, Oliveira AG, Mota T, et al. Evaluation of the performance and concordance of clinical questionnaires for the diagnosis of heart failure in primary care. *Eur J Heart Fail.* 2004;6:813–820,821–822.

38 Maisel A, Hollander JE, Guss D, et al. Primary results of the rapid emergency department heart failure outpatient trial (REDHOT). *J Am Coll Cardiol.* 2004;44:1328–1333.

39 Collins SP, Ronan-Bentle S, Storrow AB. Diagnostic and prognostic usefulness of natriuretic peptides in emergency department patients with dyspnea. *Ann Emerg Med.* 2003; 41:532–545.

40 Maisel AS, Krishnaswamy P, Nowak RM, et al. Rapid measurement of B-type natriuretic peptide in the emergency diagnosis of heart failure. *N Engl J Med.* 2002;347:161–166.

41 Ishii J, Nomura M, Nakamura Y, et al. Risk stratification using a combination of cardiac troponin T and brain natriuretic peptide in patients hospitalized for worsening chronic heart failure. *Am J Cardiol.* 2002;89:691–695.

42 Harrison A, Morrison LK, Krishnaswamy P, et al. B-type natriuretic peptide predicts future cardiac events in patients presenting to the emergency department with dyspnea. *Ann Emerg Med.* 2002;39:131–138.

43 McCullough PA, Nowak RM, McCord J, et al. B-type natriuretic peptide and clinical judgment in emergency diagnosis of heart failure: analysis from Breathing Not Properly (BNP) Multinational Study. *Circulation.* 2002;106:416–422.

44 McCullough PA, Hollander JE, Nowak RM, et al. Uncovering heart failure in patients with a history of pulmonary disease: rationale for the early use of B-type natriuretic peptide in the emergency department. *Acad Emerg Med.* 2003;10:198–204.

45 Morrison LK, Harrison A, Krishnaswamy P, et al. Utility of a rapid B-natriuretic peptide assay in differentiating congestive heart failure from lung disease in patients presenting with dyspnea. *J Am Coll Cardiol.* 2002;39:202–209.

46 Silver MA, Maisel A, Yancy CW, et al. BNP consensus panel 2004: a clinical approach for the diagnostic, prognostic, screening, treatment monitoring, and therapeutic roles of natriuretic peptides in cardiovascular diseases. *Congest Heart Fail.* 2004;10(5, Suppl 3):1–30.

47 Khot UN, Jia G, Moliterno DJ, et al. Prognostic importance of physical examination for heart failure in non-ST-elevation acute coronary syndromes: the enduring value of Killip classification. *JAMA.* 2003;290:2174–2181.

48 Collins SP, Mielniczuk LM, Whittingham HA, et al. The use of noninvasive ventilation in emergency department patients with acute cardiogenic pulmonary edema: a systematic review. *Ann Emerg Med.* 2006;48: 260–269.

49 Masip J, Roque M, Sanchez B, et al. Noninvasive ventilation in acute cardiogenic pulmonary edema: systematic review and meta-analysis. *JAMA.* 2005;294:3124–3130.

50 Mehta S, Jay GD, Woolard RH, et al. Randomized, prospective trial of bi-level versus continuous positive airway pressure in acute pulmonary edema. *Crit Care Med.* 1997;25:620–628.

51 Levitt MA. A prospective, randomized trial of BiPAP in severe acute congestive heart failure. *J Emerg Med.*2001;21:363–369.

52 Cross AM, Cameron P, Kierce M, et al. Non-invasive ventilation in acute respiratory failure: a randomized comparison of continuous positive airway pressure and bi-level positive airway pressure. *Emerg Med J.* 2003; 20:531–534.

53 Chadda K, Annane D, Hart N, et al. Cardiac and respiratory effects of continuous positive airway pressure and noninvasive ventilation in acute cardiac pulmonary edema. *Crit Care Med.* 2002;30:2457–2461.

54 Bellone A, Monari A, Cortellaro F, et al. Myocardial infarction rate in acute pulmonary edema: noninvasive pressure support ventilation versus continuous positive airway pressure. *Crit Care Med.* 2004;32:1860–1865.

55 Beltrame JF, Zeitz CJ, Unger SA, et al. Nitrate therapy is an alternative to furosemide/morphine therapy in the management of acute cardiogenic pulmonary edema. *J Card Fail.* 1998;4:271–279.

56 Buseman W, Schupp D. Effect of sublingual nitroglycerin in emergency treatment of severe pulmonary edema. *Am J Cardiol.* 1978;41:931–936.

57 Dupuis J. Nitrates in congestive heart failure. *Cardiovasc Drugs Ther.* 1994;8:501–507.

58 Northridge D. Furosemide or nitrates for acute heart failure? *Lancet.* 1996;347:667–668.

59 Cotter G, Metzkor E, Kaluski E, et al. Randomized trial of high-dose isosorbide dinitrate plus low-dose furosemide versus high-dose furosemide plus low-dose isosorbide dinitrate in severe pulmonary edema. *Lancet.* 1998;351:389–393.

60 Hoffman JR, Reynolds S. Comparison of nitroglycerin, morphine and furosemide in treatment of presumed prehospital pulmonary edema. *Chest.* 1988;92:586–593.

61 Sacchetti A, Ramoska E, Moakes ME, et al. Effect of ED management on ICU use in acute pulmonary edema. *Am J Emerg Med.*1999;17:571–574.

62 Bussmann WD, Kaltenbach M. Sublingual nitroglycerin in the treatment of left ventricular failure and pulmonary edema. *Eur J Cardiol.* 1976;4:327–333.

63 Bussmann WD, Schupp D. Effect of sublingual nitroglycerin in emergency treatment of severe pulmonary edema. *Am J Cardiol.* 1978;41:931–936.

64 Haber HL, Simek CL, Bergin JD, et al. Bolus intravenous nitroglycerin predominantly reduces afterload in patients with severe congestive heart failure. *J Am Coll Cardiol.* 1993;22:251–257.

65 Imhof PR, Ott B, Frankhauser P, et al. Differences in nitroglycerin dose response in the venous and arterial beds. *Eur J Clin Pharmacol.* 1980;18:455–460.

66 Amsterdam EA, Zelis R, Kohfeld DB, et al. Effect of morphine on myocardial contractility: negative inotropic action during hypoxia and reversal by isoproterenol. *Circulation.* 1971;43-44(Suppl II):135.

67 Figueras J, Weil MH. Blood volume prior to and following treatment of acute cardiogenic pulmonary edema. *Circulation.* 1978;57:349–355.

68 Lal S, Murtagh JG, Pollock AM, et al. Acute haemodynamic effects of furosemide in patients with normal and raised left atrial pressures. *Br Heart J.* 1969;31:711–717.

69 Figueras J, Weil MH. Hypovolemia and hypotension complicating management of acute cardiogenic pulmonary edema. *Am J Cardiol.* 1979;44:1349–1355.

70 Henning RJ, Weil MH. Effect of afterload reduction on plasma volume during acute heart failure. *Am J Cardiol.* 1978;42:823–827.

71 Butler J, Forman DE, Abraham WT, et al. Relationship between heart failure treatment and development of worsening renal function among hospitalized patients. *Am Heart J.* 2004;147:331–338.

72 Fonarow GC, Adams KF Jr, Abraham WT, et al, for the ADHERE Scientific Advisory Committee, Study Group, and Investigators. Risk stratification for in-hospital mortality in acutely decompensated heart failure. Classification and regression tree analysis. *JAMA.* 2005;293:572–580.

73 Krumholz HM, Chen YT, Vaccarino V, et al. Correlates and impact on outcomes of worsening renal function in patients >65 years of age with heart failure. *Am J Cardiol.* 2000;85:1110–1113.

74 Smith GL, Vaccarino V, Kosiborod M, et al. Worsening renal function: what is a clinically meaningful change in creatinine during hospitalization with heart failure? *J Card Fail.* 2003;9:13–25.

75 Barnett JC, Zink KM, Touchon RC. Sublingual captopril in the treatment of acute heart failure. *Curr Ther Res.* 1991;49:274–281.

76 Annane D, Bellissat E, Pussard E, et al. Placebo-controlled, randomized, double-blind study of intravenous enalapril at efficacy and safety in acute cardiogenic pulmonary edema. *Circulation.* 1996;94:1316–1324.

77 Haude M, Steffen W, Erbel R, et al. Sublingual administration of captopril versus nitroglycerin in patients with severe congestive heart failure. *Int J Cardiol.* 1990; 27:351–359.

78 Langes K, Siebels J, Kuck KH. Efficacy and safety of intravenous captopril in congestive heart failure. *Curr Ther Res.* 1993;53:167–176.

79 Varriale P, David W, Chryssos BE. Hemodynamic response to intravenous enalapril at in patients with severe congestive heart failure & mitral regurgitation. *Clin Cardiol.* 1993;16:235–238.

80 Southall JC, Bissell DM, Burton JH. ACE inhibitors in acutely decompensated congestive heart failure. *Acad Emerg Med.* 2004;11:503.

81 Brivet F, Delfraissy JF, Giudicelli JF, et al. Immediate effects of captopril in acute left ventricular heart failure secondary to myocardial infarction. *Eur J Clin Invest.* 1981;11:369–73.

82 Tohmo H, Karanko M, Korpilahti K. Haemodynamic effects of enalapril at and preload in acute severe heart failure complicating myocardial infarction. *Eur Heart J.* 1994;15:523–527.

83 Hamilton RJ, Carter WA, Gallagher EJ. Rapid improvement of acute pulmonary edema with sublingual captopril. *Acad Emerg Med.* 1996;3:205–212.

84 Sacchetti A, McCabe J, Torres M, et al. ED management of acute congestive heart failure in renal dialysis patients. *Am J Emerg Med.*1993;11:644–647.

85 Gammage M. Treatment of acute pulmonary edema: diuresis or vasodilatation? *Lancet.* 1998;351:382–383.

86 Hunt SA. ACC/AHA 2005 guideline update for the diagnosis and management of chronic heart failure in the adult: a report of the American College Of Cardiology/American Heart Association task force on practice guidelines (writing committee to update the 2001 guidelines for the evaluation and management of heart failure). *J Am Coll Cardiol.* 2005;46:e1–e82.

87 Felker GM, O'Connor CM. Between Scylla and Charybdis: the choice of inotropic agent for decompensated heart failure. *Am Heart J.* 2001;142:932–933.

88 Ewy GA. Inotropic infusions for chronic congestive heart failure: medical miracles or misguided medicinals? *J Am Coll Cardiol.* 1999;33:572–575.

89 Gagnon RM, Fortin L, Boucher R, et al. Combined hemodynamic effects of dobutamine and IV nitroglycerin in congestive heart failure. *Chest.* 1980;78:694–698.

90 Nohria A, Lewis E, Stevenson LW. Medical management of advanced heart failure. *JAMA.* 2002;287:628–640.

91 Keung EC, Siskind SJ, Sonneblick EH, et al. Dobutamine therapy for acute myocardial infarction. *JAMA.* 1981;245:144–146.

92 Shipley JB, Tolman D, Hastillo A, et al. Milrinone: basic and clinical pharmacology and acute and chronic management. *Am J Med Sci.* 1996;311:286–291.

93 Travill CM, Pugh S, Noble MI. The inotropic and hemodynamic effects of intravenous milrinone when reflex adrenergic stimulation is suppressed by beta-adrenergic blockade. *Clin Ther.* 1994;16:783–792.

94 Anderson JL, Askins JC, Gilbert EM, et al. Occurrence of ventricular arrhythmias in patients receiving acute and chronic infusions of milrinone. *Am Heart J.* 1986;111:466–474.

95 Varriale P, Ramaprasad S. Short-term intravenous milrinone for severe congestive heart failure: the good, bad, and not so good. *Pharmacotherapy.* 1997;17:371–374.

96 Cuffe MS, Califf RM, Adams KF Jr, et al. Short-term intravenous milrinone for acute exacerbation of chronic heart failure: a randomized controlled trial. *JAMA.* 2002;287:1541–1547.

97 Nieminen MS, Akkila J, Hasenfuss G, et al. Hemodynamic and neurohumoral effects of continuous infusion of levosimendan in patients with congestive heart failure. *J Am Coll Cardiol.* 2000;36:1903–1912.

98 Yamani MH, Haji SA, Starling RC, et al. Comparison of dobutamine-based and milrinone-based therapy for advanced decompensated congestive heart failure: hemodynamic efficacy, clinical outcome, and economic impact. *Am Heart J.* 2001;142:998–1002.

99 Slawsky MT, Colucci WS, Gottlieb SS, et al. Acute hemodynamic and clinical effects of levosimendan in patients with severe heart failure. *Circulation.* 2000;102:2222–2227.

100 Follath F, Cleland JG, Just H, et al. Efficacy and safety of intravenous levosimendan compared with dobutamine in severe low-output heart failure (the LIDO study): a randomized double-blind trial. *Lancet.* 2002;360: 196–202.

101 Wuerz RC, Meador SA. Effects of prehospital medications on mortality and length of stay in congestive heart failure. *Ann Emerg Med.* 1992;21:669–674.

102 Singer AJ, Emerman C, Char DM, et al. Bronchodilator therapy in acute decompensated heart failure patients without a history of chronic obstructive pulmonary disease. *Ann Emerg Med.* 2008;51:25–34.

103 Hsieh M, Auble TE, Yealy DM. Predicting the future: can this patient with acute congestive heart failure be safely discharged from the emergency department? *Ann Emerg Med.* 2002;39:181–189.

104 Le Conte P, Coutant V, N'Guyen JM, et al. Prognostic factors in acute cardiogenic pulmonary edema. *Am J Emerg Med.*1999;17:329–332.

105 Hsieh M, Auble TE, Yealy DM. Evidence based medicine. Predicting the future: can this patient with acute congestive heart failure be safely discharged from the emergency department? *Ann Emerg Med.* 2002; 39(2):181–189.

106 Plotnick GD, Kelemen MH, Garrett RB, et al. Acute cardiogenic pulmonary edema in the elderly: factors predicting in-hospital and one-year mortality. *South Med J.* 1982;75:565–569.

107 Chin MH, Goldman L. Correlates of major complications or death in patients admitted to the hospital with congestive heart failure. *Arch Intern Med.* 1996;156:1814–1820.

108 Brophy JM, Deslauriers G, Boucher B, et al. The hospital course and short term prognosis of patients presenting to the emergency room with decompensated congestive heart failure. *Can J Cardiol.* 1993;9:219–224.

109 Fonarow GC, Adams KF Jr, Abraham WT, et al. Risk stratification for in-hospital mortality in acutely decompensated heart failure. *JAMA*. 2005;293:572–580.

110 Felker GM, Gattis WA, Leimberger JD, et al. Usefulness of anemia as a predictor of death and rehospitalization in patients with decompensated heart failure. *Am J Cardiol*. 2003;92:625–628.

111 Storrow AB, Collins SP, Lyons MS, et al. Emergency department observation of heart failure; preliminary analysis of safety and cost. *Congest Heart Fail*. 2005:11(2)68–72.

112 Burkhardt J, Peacock WF, Emerman CL. Predictors of emergency department observation unit outcomes. *Acad Emerg Med*. 2006;12(9):869–874.

113 Peacock WF, Young J, Collins S, et al. Heart failure observation units:optimizing care. *Ann Emerg Med*. 2006;47(1):22–33.

114 Sinclair D, Green R. Emergency department observation unit: can it be funded through reduced inpatient admission? *Ann Emerg Med*. 1998;32(6):670–675.

13

Syncope

Shamai Grossman

Director, Cardiac Emergency Center and Clinical Decision Unit, Beth Israel Deaconess Medical Center, Assistant Professor of Medicine, Harvard Medical School, Boston, Massachusetts, USA

Section I: Case presentation

A 41-year-old woman was brought to the Emergency Department (ED). She had been found unconscious while attending a party. The patient, who was awake on EMS arrival three minutes later, did not remember how long she was unconscious nor the occurrences preceding the event. EMS reported no signs of confusion or lethargy.

In the ED, the patient was sleepy but arousable, and responded appropriately to questions, including name, place, and date. Her husband reported that the patient had been dancing, and subsequently sat down at a table. When he had rejoined her moments later, he found her unresponsive to name or to shaking. This lasted approximately 30 seconds. The patient was otherwise healthy, and not taking any regular medications. There was no clear precipitant nor prodrome prior to the episode. The patient noted no prior episodes. She was a long-distance runner, but had been more easily tired of late, and decided not to compete in any races. She noted her last menstrual period was approximately eight weeks prior, but had a lengthy history of irregular menses. There was no clear precipitate or prodrome prior to the episode. There was no family history of sudden death or cardiac disease. The patient was told previously that her blood pressure ran low.

The initial vital signs were: 90/68 mmHg, heart rate 60 beats/min, respiratory rate 18 breaths/min, temperature 35.6°C (96°F). On further examination, the physician noted a systolic ejection murmur at the cardiac apex radiating to the carotid artery. The patient had no physical findings to suggest trauma. The remainder of the physical examination, and particularly the neurologic examination, was normal. A stool specimen was hemoccult negative. An EKG demonstrated a normal sinus rhythm with normal conduction intervals. A finger-stick test for glucose was normal, and the patient's serum bicarbonate level was normal. Serum electrolytes and a complete blood count were normal. Serum and urine toxicology screens were positive only for an alcohol level of 75 mg/dl. The urine pregnancy test was positive.

Section II: Case discussion

Dr David Brown: An area of great controversy is what to do with a patient with syncope and a normal EKG. Does this patient meet criteria for admission? In addition, if the patient wasn't pregnant would that change your answer?

Dr Amal Mattu: I don't believe pregnancy should change the disposition, particularly in a case like this, where the patient is likely in the first trimester.

Cardiovascular Problems in Emergency Medicine: A discussion-based review, First Edition.
Edited by Shamai A. Grossman and Peter Rosen.
© 2011 John Wiley & Sons, Ltd. Published 2011 by John Wiley & Sons, Ltd.

Nevertheless, I would be inclined to admit this patient to the hospital for a couple of reasons. First, her blood pressure is relatively low, and second, she reported that she's a long distance runner but is now having increasing fatigue. This makes me concerned about whether there may be a cardiac etiology.

Dr William Brady: Would you bring her in to a regular bed or into an observation bed if you had one?

Dr Edward Ullman: I think that the appropriate disposition for this person would be on some sort of telemetry ward as there are multiple issues to consider. Occasionally, a new presentation of pregnancy is in advanced gestation, so late complications of pregnancy need to remain in the back of your mind. It's likely too early to think of cardiac complications of pregnancy, and it's reassuring that she has no cardiac history nor signs of congestive heart failure; therefore, I would place her at low risk for syncope from a cardiac dysrhythmia. However, assuming she has a normal intrauterine pregnancy (IUP), I would be concerned about her murmur; could she have critical aortic stenosis (AS). Lastly, I worry about the low blood pressure. This person may be served just as well being admitted to an observation unit, assuming that there is no critical AS and she doesn't have a low hematocrit. Then, if overnight telemetry is normal, I might discharge her home with an event monitor and appropriate follow up.

Dr Peter Rosen: Although syncope is common in early pregnancy, it can also represent severe anemia, as well as abnormal implantation. While blood pressures are supposed to be low during pregnancy, the murmur may be a flow murmur, which, when associated with symptoms of hypotension and syncope, should make one consider the possibility of an ectopic pregnancy with rupture.

DB: Assuming the patient is early in pregnancy with a relatively normal blood count and has a normal EKG, I would not be concerned about a mild anemia. Critical AS strikes me as being exceedingly unlikely, since one would expect critical AS to develop over a long enough period of time to cause the patient to have some signs of left ventricular hypertrophy (LVH) on the EKG. I think one could make a reasonable case for letting this patient go home, assuming she has reasonable follow up for tests like an echo and possibly a holter monitor. A 41-year-old patient who is pregnant with a normal EKG—so no signs of structural heart disease—whose only abnormality on physical examination is a systolic ejection murmur that may represent AS, or may represent a flow murmur of pregnancy, should be low risk. Although the blood pressure is relatively low, she claims to always have low blood pressure. We could give her a challenge of normal saline and see if she responds. If the emergency physician anticipates trouble with follow up, then it is also reasonable to admit this patient to an ED-based or hospital-based observation unit for a period of telemetry monitoring, and to obtain at least an echocardiogram while in the hospital.

Dr Shamai Grossman: In Boston, we studied markers for adverse outcome in syncope, and she has a number of them.[1] We feel it is prudent to admit patients who have any of these markers, unless the etiology can easily be identified in the ED (Table 13-2). More specifically, this patient has a number of things that should make you a little worried. First, she's a long distance runner, and she had syncope while exerting herself while she was dancing in upright position. This would make dysrhythmia more likely as the etiology of the syncope. Next, she has a blood pressure of 90, yet we're also told that she always runs low blood pressures, so the blood pressure of 90 may actually be her normal blood pressure. It also might represent a normal pregnancy blood pressure. If we can verify that this is really what her blood pressure always runs, then we can take hypotension and its causes out of the equation. Now, we need to address the murmur. Agreed, this is unlikely to be severe aortic stenosis; however, the definition we used of a significant murmur when we studied syncope was that if you actually hear a murmur in the ED, then you have an unusual finding, and you need to be more concerned that there may be a valvular etiology of her syncope. This should be another marker suggesting that this patient will have a worrisome etiology of her syncope, and thus, would warrant admission.

Now, there is no easily defined cause of her syncope, except perhaps pregnancy. The volume issues of pregnancy early on and at eight weeks would be less likely to cause syncope, but it is possible. The primary focus of my workup is: (1) whether she is going to have a dysrhythmia over the course of the next 24 hours, and (2) to better define her valvular abnormality. She deserves to have an echocardiogram in the course of next 24 hours. Assuming I can accomplish both those things from an observation unit, then I would admit her to an observation unit, and have her undergo these two tests. If the telemetry over 24 hours and the echocardiogram do not demonstrate processes that warrant immediate attention, at that point I would be willing to discharge the patient.

DB: Would your answer be different if she were 21 years old instead of 41 years old?

AM: I don't have a definite age cut off to bring somebody into the hospital. If this patient did have aortic stenosis, then the murmur should be heard best at the upper sternal border rather than down at the apex. A systolic murmur heard at the apex has to be concerning for a possibility of hypertrophic cardiomyopathy. If she was 21 years old I'd still be worried about a valvular disorder, and I would still admit her regardless of her age.

WB: Do you think hypertrophic cardiomyopathy is likely in someone who has a normal EKG?

AM: With a completely normal EKG, hypertrophic cardiomyopathy is much less likely. At a minimum there is usually high voltage. In addition, cardiomyopathy is much less common in women.

EU: If you are concerned about hypertrophic cardiomyopathy, you could do some provocative testing such as a valsalva maneuver, and see whether or not the murmur gets louder.

DB: What are the criteria for getting an ECHO on a patient who presents to the ED with syncope? Do you require a murmur, or does the absence of murmur dissuade you from the need for an ECHO? Does a normal EKG change your opinion, and does the age of the patient change your opinion, in terms of the workup of undifferentiated syncope?

SG: The two elements I would use as guidelines for whether or not syncopal patients need an echocardiogram would be: (1) the physical examination, and (2) the EKG. If there is a readily identifiable cause of syncope, for example if the patient was sitting on the toilet and trying to urinate and passed out, had a normal EKG, and otherwise normal ED workup, then I don't think that patient requires an echocardiogram. On the other hand, if the patient has a murmur on examination, regardless of whether or not the patient

passed out on the toilet, then the patient should have an echocardiogram. I don't believe that the echocardiogram always needs to be done emergently if the remainder of the ED workup is normal. I might obtain the ECHO in a more expeditious fashion given that the patient acknowledged a syncopal event, although I do not believe that they are likely to be related if the patient was otherwise asymptomatic. What might prompt me to do an echocardiogram more emergently on this patient is if there were something concerning on the EKG for having additional disease. What I'm thinking is, "Well yes, the patient certainly had micturition syncope, but the reason that the patient was inclined to have micturition syncope was because she didn't have a normal heart to start with."

DB: I believe the echocardiogram would be the one compelling reason to admit this patient, whether to observation or to a hospital bed.

AM: The two strong indications, in my mind, to get an ECHO within the next day would be: exertional syncope and an abnormal murmur. Pregnant patients often times have flow murmurs. If the patient had a fever, she might be in a hyperdynamic state, and you might hear a flow murmur. Yet, this could also go along with congenital or acquired valvular diseases like hypertrophic cardiomyopathy or aortic stenosis. Given these suspicions, I think we should obtain an echocardiogram before discharge.

DB: How many hours of monitoring would satisfy you in the absence of any findings? Is four hours in an emergency department enough, or 12 to 16 hours in an observation area or inpatient unit?

EU: I've rarely had a patient on telemetry for syncope show anything that wasn't initially obvious, such as an EMS capture of large pauses or similar dysrhythmias. Assuming you're holding a patient for an echocardiogram, I think once this test is done, and you have arranged an event or holter monitoring and follow up, they should be able to go.

DB: I think this middle group of patients, without prior known structural heart disease or coronary artery disease with a normal EKG and a non-worrisome physical examination, is the group of patients in whom observation units have really been able to help. The observation unit enables the patient to achieve an expeditious workup, and it helps the emergency physician who therefore doesn't have to fight with the primary care physician to admit the patient. The easiest and safest thing to do for a patient in this age group who has some exertional component to her syncope is to put her in an ED observation unit, to obtain an echo over the first few hours if possible, and monitor her for that period of time that it takes to get the holter monitor set up. If there's no evidence of dysrhythmia and no structural heart disease on ECHO, then allow her to go home. This could be done between 4 and 16 hours in most cases, and I think would speed her overall workup.

SG: There are data that look at the utility of holter monitoring (simple 24 hour monitoring) versus longer term monitoring, like event monitors that can monitor a patient who wears a device for up to 30 days.[2] Clearly, the longer you wear a monitor, the more likely you are to actually discover a dysrhythmia and a possible etiology of the syncopal event. Moreover, the longer you are on telemetry, the more likely you are to discover the etiology. That doesn't mean that we have to admit these patients indefinitely to the hospital in order to determine if the syncope was from a dysrhythmia. If your clinical gestalt is that this patient had a benign etiology for the syncope, if there is nothing worrisome in the workup that you've done in the ED, then it should be safe to discharge that patient.

AM: About 50% of patients who have syncope who present to the ED will end up having a diagnosis during the immediate hospital stay following both the ED and the admission work up. Eighty percent of those will receive an ED diagnosis based on history, physical, EKG and the brief monitoring you do in the ED.[3] Only an additional 20% are going to have a diagnosis made during the remainder of their hospital stay that usually includes the telemetry monitoring. Thus, if your history, physical, and EKG don't tell you that the patient is having a dysrhythmia, subsequent cardiac monitoring, whether in the hospital or even with holter monitoring, is not likely to give you a diagnosis.

Does this particular patient need holter monitoring? I think if the patient didn't have palpitations, wasn't noted to have even brief dysrhythmias on the telemetry monitor in the ED or during the hospital admission, and if the EKG didn't give you some clues to a dysrhythmia, such as delta waves or a prolonged QT,

then I think that the cost effectiveness and utility of subsequent holter monitoring is very, very low. I don't think that holter monitoring in this case is indicated.

DB: Is there any utility in routinely ruling out myocardial infarction or acute coronary syndrome in patients who present with syncope without chest pain or EKG changes?

SG: The patients who need cardiac markers are patients who you think are having myocardial ischemia. Syncope in and of itself is generally not associated with myocardial ischemia. However, if a patient presents with concomitant signs of myocardial ischemia such as chest pressure or dyspnea, or has an EKG that is worrisome for cardiac ischemia, then the patient should get cardiac enzymes. However, if the EKG is not suggestive of myocardial ischemia, and the history is not suggestive of myocardial ischemia, then that patient's risk should be similar to that of the rest of the population, and we generally don't obtain cardiac enzymes on every patient who presents to the ED, although sometimes it feels like we do.

DB: When do you include pulmonary embolus (PE) in your differential diagnosis of a patient with undifferentiated syncope, and do you think that PE needs to be considered in this particular case since she's pregnant?

EU: If the patient is pregnant, she's theoretically hypercoagulable, and she has undifferentiated syncope, I don't think it's unreasonable to evaluate her for PE. The next issue is how to evaluate a pregnant woman in the early part of the first trimester. VQ? MRI? A CTA is a fair amount of radiation for this person. You don't want to empirically start heparin because, then due to teratogencity, she will need to take enoxaparin instead of warfarin for the remainder of the pregnancy.

DB: Would you proceed with a d-dimer in this patient, recognizing that there's a chance for a false positive, but that it may enable you to avoid a radiation-related test, or would you be satisfied that there are other reasons for her syncope?

AM: The patients in whom I work up PE after a syncope presentation, are people who either have chest pain or dyspnea associated with the syncope (either before or after the syncope), or they are hypoxic for an unknown reason, have leg swelling, or a rapid respiratory rate. The respiratory rate is the most unappreciated vital sign. It often seems that everybody has a respiratory rate of 20 at triage, which means nobody ever actually counts the rate. If a patient truly has a normal respiratory rate, no chest pain, no shortness of breath, no unexplained hypoxia before or after the event, I would not obtain a d-dimer, CT scan, VQ, or any other test. In this case the patient had a respiratory rate of 18, which I'm happy about, and no complaints of chest pain or shortness of breath, Therefore, I would not pursue a diagnosis of PE any further.

DB: If the patient has any symptoms or signs of pulmonary embolus, then I would send an Elisa d-dimer, recognizing that it may be positive because of the pregnancy rather than thrombosis. If it were positive, I would probably proceed with a lower extremity non-invasive ultrasound, again trying to avoid radiation to the fetus. If she has a deep vein thrombosis (DVT) in her leg, then that would obligate her to three months of anti-coagulation. If the d-dimer was positive, and the lower extremity ultrasound study was negative, then my practice, after a risk/benefit discussion with the patient, would be to proceed with a VQ scan.

SG: I look at PE the same way I look at myocardial ischemia: if a patient looks like the clinical picture of a PE, regardless of whether there had been a syncopal episode, then it behooves you to do the work up for pulmonary embolus. However if the patient has nothing else suggestive of PE, then we shouldn't be working them up for PE. It's interesting that when they studied the utility of testing in patients with syncope, the only test that had any reasonable yield was an EKG, revealing an etiology in about 5% of patients. Blood testing in patients with syncope was able to make the diagnosis in only about 2% of patients.[4] Thus, blood testing has very limited utility, and you should actually think about what you are testing very carefully before embarking on routine utilization. That said, if a patient did have symptoms that were suggestive of PE, I would do a d-dimer, especially in a first trimester patient. My understanding of the radiation exposure is that a CT angiogram exposes the patient to less radiation than a VQ scan, so that would be the test of choice at that point.

DB: Would you pick an MRI to avoid any radiation at all should you find yourself needing to do confirmatory chest imaging test?

EU: Even though we may be missing small sub-segmental PEs, I would consider an MRI if readily available, as I think these sub-segmental emboli are of limited clinical importance.

PR: To be complete, we should recall that syncope is often seen with aortic aneurysm, but I wouldn't worry about that diagnosis in a woman in this age group. There is also the entity of transient global amnesia that should be distinguished from syncope. It is common in women this age, but lasts longer, and will not have any of the other positive findings such as a murmur or positive pregnancy test, which occurred in this case.

Case resolution

Despite the positive pregnancy test, which may have indicated a benign etiology of the syncope, the ED physician decided to admit the patient for observation based on a concern for valvular heart disease. The patient underwent an echocardiogram, and the presence of a bicuspid aortic valve and mild aortic stenosis were noted. She was informed that the murmur was congenital and, given the current mild nature of her aortic stenosis, that there was no immediate cause for concern. Nevertheless, she needed to be followed up closely by a cardiologist for serial heart examinations and echocardiography. Additionally, the patient was told that the syncopal episode could be explained by increased demands upon cardiac output due to the new onset pregnancy. Physiologic changes during pregnancy affect hemodynamic balance controlled by blood volume and myocardial contractility, and therefore may make the patient more prone to syncope.[5]

Section III: Concepts

Background

Syncope accounts for nearly 3% all ED visits and 1–6% of all hospital admissions.[6] Syncope is defined as a transient loss of consciousness resulting from a brief loss in generalized cerebral blood flow.[7] Syncope produces a brief period of unresponsiveness and a loss of postural tone, and ultimately results in spontaneous recovery requiring no resuscitation measures.

Determining the etiology of a syncopal event is frequently difficult. Often the initiating event is unwitnessed, and not remembered by the patient, making it difficult to uncover the specific circumstances leading up to and occurring during the syncopal episode.[8] Syncopal events are often transient and may resolve independently, without recurrence. It has been estimated that 30–50% of all cases of syncope are not given a definable etiology despite extensive medical evaluation.[9,10] Myocardial ischemia and other conditions that may be responsible for causing syncope may go undiscovered and have potentially life-threatening consequences, such as sudden death.

Concern that potentially life-threatening diseases, such as significant transient dysrhythmia, might be the etiologies, is likely the most significant issue influencing physicians to pursue inpatient evaluations for patients who present to the ED with syncope of unknown origin. The key questions for the emergency physician are then to determine which are the serious etiologies of syncope that need an inpatient workup, what immediate therapy is appropriate, and what follow-up is necessary?

Initial syncope workup: History and physical

The initial task in syncope, as with all ED patients, is to obtain vital signs and determine the need for immediate stabilization. The utility of orthostatic vital signs is controversial, but may be helpful in the elderly or any patient thought to be volume depleted.[11] Measurements of blood pressure in the two arms may be useful to help evaluate for aortic dissection, as most syncope patients are otherwise asymptomatic, and have normal or near normal vital signs. These patients do not need to be stabilized, but do require a thorough history and physical examination. Because syncope is the presentation of a wide variety of diseases, the differential diagnoses must be broad.

Elements within the presenting history can serve to eliminate several causes. In approaching the syncope patient, one must first determine if the event was syncope at all (Table 13-1). Seizures and stroke can cause loss of consciousness, but both can be distinguished from other etiologies of syncope by the history and physical examination. Patients who have had a seizure often exhibit a metabolic acidosis.[12] Seizures classically present with a prodromal aura or "warning" symptoms, and are typically followed by a postictal period, in which the patient is often lethargic, agitated, or confused, with the patient slowly returning to full consciousness.[13] Greater than five minutes of

Table 13-1. Differentiating syncope from a seizure.

Symptom or Sign	Syncope	Seizure
Tongue Biting	Anterior Tongue Biting	Lateral Tongue Biting
Duration	< 5 minutes	> 5 minutes
Aura	No	Yes
Postictal State	Seconds	Minutes or longer
Incontinence	No	Yes
Tonic Clonic Jerks	Occasional	Frequent
Metabolic Acidosis	Occasional	Frequent

loss of consciousness and rhythmic movements can be seen in both seizures and syncope, but are far more common in patients who have had a seizure.[13] Stroke, if associated with a loss of consciousness, will generally not be a self-limited event, but tends to be of extended duration and with focal findings on neurological examination.[14]

Near syncope, defined as the patient "feeling ready to to pass out without actual loss of consciousness," should be treated in the same fashion as syncope.[15]

Critical questions include: What were the precipitating factors (i.e., pain and anxiety, postural or exertional symptoms), or what were the situations in which episodes occurred (e.g., after urination)? Were there associated neurologic symptoms, a history of cardiac disease, or a history of psychiatric illness? What were the medications being used, and is there a family history of sudden death?[16]

When drug intoxication is suspected, careful attention must be paid to EMS reports and "trip sheets," interrogation of accompanying family or companions, or investigation of prior medical records.

The physical examination should include careful auscultation of the carotid arteries, heart and lungs, as well as thorough palpation of the peripheral arteries. Evidence of trauma, such as lacerations from tongue biting, or buccal or other body part contusions, and fractures, should be carefully sought. When appropriate, pupillary size and signs of "track marks" should be recorded. In determining whether the patient experienced a seizure, stroke, or a syncopal episode, several factors should be considered. While lateral tongue lacerations tend to support the existence of tonic-clonic seizures, anterior lacerations can be the result of a fall from syncope.[17] Generalized seizures will often be followed by postictal confusion, while loss of consciousness from a stroke is generally not transient. In our case, the patient did not experience a prodrome, nor were there focal findings on neurological examination. In addition, the event was self-limiting and without postictal confusion or agitation. These aspects support a true syncopal episode. Transient Global Amnesia is unlikely to be confused with syncope, as this is defined by an inability to form new memories. Patients are disoriented in time and often repetitively ask questions about the date or the environment, with an impaired delayed recall.[11] The neurologic examination is otherwise normal. The mean duration of episodes is approximately six hours.[7,8,13] Most last between 1 and 10 hours.

Etiologies of syncope

The causes of syncope are varied, ranging from benign to life threatening. Syncope can best be classified as cardiac and non-cardiac in etiology. In those under 65 years of age, non-cardiac causes make up approximately 40% of syncope cases, while 20% may be attributed to cardiac abnormalities. In those age 65 or greater, cardiac causes may claim up to 40% of cases, while non-cardiac causes comprise only 20%.[18] Syncope is common, but may be debilitating in patients of all age groups. In younger individuals, syncope is most often associated with a single, isolated disease process.[19] Despite thorough evaluation, as mentioned earlier, 30–50% of syncope cases that are seen in the ED are of unexplained etiology.[9,10]

The most commonly identified etiology of syncope is vasovagal or neurocardiogenic syncope. Vasovagal syncope is characterized by a prodrome lasting more than five seconds, and is associated with precipitating events or stresses.[20-22] Common stresses include unexpected pain, fear, or an encounter with an unpleasant sight, sound or smell, after prolonged standing at attention. Situational syncope is also vagally mediated, and is characterized by episodes occurring during or immediately after micturition, defecation, cough, or swallowing.[23] Carotid-sinus syncope is another variety of neurally mediated or vasovagal syncope.

Syncope in younger patients is often due to neurally-mediated hypotension. Women and individuals younger than 55 years of age are more likely to experience neurally-mediated hypotension. These episodes are often greater than five seconds in duration, and occur while standing or when emotionally upset. Symptoms that accompany this form of syncope include palpitations, blurred vision, and nausea.[23]

Hypovolemia, resulting from sources such as dehydration, medication, or hemorrhage from gastrointestinal bleeding, or a leaking aortic aneurysm is also a common cause of syncope.[16] A hypovolemic etiology of syncope is often manifested as orthostatic hypotension, which is defined in adults, as a decrease in systolic blood pressure of 20 mmHg or greater or an increase in heart rate of 15 beats per min within two minutes of standing; in contrast, an isolated tachycardia or hypotension are nonspecific for hemodynamic instability or volume depletion. The presence of orthostatic hypotension may therefore aid in correctly attributing a syncopal episode to volume depletion, autonomic insufficiency, or medications. Orthostatic hypotension is commonly seen in patients who suffer from recurring episodes of syncope or light-headedness, and is a common finding in pregnancy. However, orthostatic hypotension is present in up to 40% of asymptomatic patients older than 70 and 23% of patients who are younger than 60 years.[24]

Medications causing syncope include most antihypertensive and cardiovascular agents such as diuretics and vasodilators. Drugs that prolong the QT interval are associated with life-threatening dysrhythmias. Geriatric patients, who often take multiple medications, are especially at risk for medication-induced syncope.[25] The presence of drug intoxication should be aggressively pursued, particularly if confusion persists following the syncopal event.

Earlier studies suggested that syncope was the initial or predominant clinical feature in 13% of pulmonary emboli, but the absence of frequently occurring signs and symptoms of syncope argue against the presence of pulmonary emboli.[26,27] Recent data suggest pulmonary embolus as the etiology in about 1% of patients presenting with syncope.[28]

Cardiac syncope is characterized by an absent or brief prodrome (less than five seconds), palpitations, and a brief loss of consciousness. Cardiac syncope often occurs while the patient is seated or reclining. However, neurological syncope also may occur in the seated or reclined position.[21]

Syncope of cardiac etiology can be classified into mechanical and dysrhythmic causes. These range from aortic stenosis and cardiac tamponade to paroxysmal ventricular tachycardia and conduction system disease. These types of underlying medical conditions are more easily diagnosed in the presence of associated respiratory or neurological symptoms or chest pain. A patient with a history of cardiac disease will more likely have a cardiac cause of syncope. A history of ventricular dysrhythmia or congestive heart failure is predictive for an adverse outcome.[7,10,13] Patients who experience cardiac syncope who also have poor left ventricular function, have a higher risk of sudden death.[29,30] Syncope following exertion may indicate structural heart disease, such as with obstruction to left ventricular outflow due to fixed (aortic stenosis) or dynamic (hypertrophic cardiomyopathy) causes.[31]

Cardiac syncope patients have 18–33% mortality, as contrasted to 3–4% in non-cardiac or unexplained syncope.[22] In addition, cardiac syncope is an independent predictor of mortality when taking into account baseline cardiac conditions such as past congestive heart failure or myocardial infarction.[32] One prospective cohort study shows that patients older than 60 years and those with any cardiovascular diagnosis, regardless of age, have an increase in sudden death within two years.[19]

Young patients who present with syncope following exercise and who have a family history of syncope, sudden death, or dysrhythmias should be carefully evaluated for a cardiac etiology.[33] Careful attention should be paid to prolonged QT intervals or evidence of hypertrophic cardiomyopathy.[33] Physiologic changes during pregnancy affect hemodynamic balance controlled by blood volume and myocardial contractility, and therefore may make the patient more prone to syncope.[5]

Frequently recurring syncope in young patients with no heart disease may be due to psychiatric disorders; generalized anxiety and panic disorders, as well as major depression, have all been associated with vasovagal syncope.[34] However, fainting is also a known manifestation of somatization disorder.[34]

Syncope in elderly patients is more difficult to diagnose, and is associated with a higher level of morbidity and mortality than in younger patients, particularly as the elderly are both more likely to have associated comorbidities, and are more prone to trauma associated with falls following syncope events.[35] The causes are more complex and often multi-factorial in the elderly.[19] The elderly often have numerous medical conditions requiring multiple medications, many of which can cause syncope. Furthermore, age alone predisposes to syncope, as many of the physiologic changes associated with the aging process result in decreased cerebral perfusion.[19] As one grows older physiologically, there is a decrease in the body's ability to respond to hypotensive challenges, and syncope can commonly ensue.[8]

Thirty percent of non-institutionalized elderly patients over age 75 will experience a repeat syncopal episode within two years.[36] Nevertheless, recent studies have excluded age alone as an independent predictor of adverse outcome in syncope, believing that the morbidity associated with age is by virtue of concomitant risk factors accumulated as one grows old.[35,37]

Testing in syncope

There is no gold standard against which the results of diagnostic tests can be measured in syncope. Hence, it remains difficult to ascertain sensitivity and specificity of routine utilization of these tests.[4,38]

The history and the physical examination may identify a cause of syncope in 45% of patients.[4] The European Society of Cardiology recommends carotid sinus massage in patients over the age of 40 with syncope of unknown etiology, and this should also be considered in patients with spontaneous symptoms suggestive of carotid-sinus syncope, such as syncope while shaving or while turning the head.[39] In patients with a history of carotid artery disease, this test should be avoided.

While the diagnostic yield of an EKG in syncope is only 5%, a standard 12-lead EKG should be used for patients in whom there is a possibility of cardiac disease to help identify myocardial infarction or life-threatening dysrhythmias.[13,35] One study notes that an abnormal EKG is a multivariate predictor for a dysrhythmia or death for one year following an episode of syncope.[40] An EKG is also necessary to identify a prolonged QT interval as the cause of the syncope.[41]

Blood tests are commonly ordered, but are often unnecessary since they do not yield diagnostically useful information.[13,20] In patients in whom seizure rather than syncope is suspected, serum glucose and bicarbonate levels may be helpful.[12] If drug intoxication or overdosage is suspected, then serum and urine toxicologic screens may be useful. Routine cardiac enzymes determinations, particularly in elderly and otherwise asymptomatic patients, have not been shown to be useful in the setting of a normal EKG.[42,43] If blood loss is suspected, examination for the presence of blood in the stool may be more useful than checking hematocrit or hemoglobin, since they may be normal in early stages of blood loss.[44] In addition, women of childbearing age who experience syncope should have a pregnancy test, though a physician should not routinely rely upon pregnancy as the sole cause of a syncopal episode. Rather, a complete evaluation of the patient should be done to fully identify the etiology.[45]

The history, physical examination, and an EKG are often sufficient to identify the presence of heart disease. Only when the presence or absence of underlying cardiac disease cannot be determined clinically is an echocardiogram helpful, as echocardiograms rarely reveal unsuspected abnormalities and generally do not lead to the diagnosis of a cause.[46] If the presence of a significant dysrhythmia is suspected, prolonged cardiac monitoring of up to 72 hours or longer may be warranted on ED discharge.[32]

Table 13-2. Risk factors and disposition in syncope.

The Boston Syncope Guidelines suggest that if a patient has any of these risk factors, he should be admitted:
Syncope Risk Factors for Adverse Outcome

I. Signs and Symptoms of Acute Coronary Syndrome
    1. Complaint of chest pain
    2. Ischemic ECG changes (ST elevation or deep ST depression)
    3. Other ECG changes (any abnormal atrial heart rhythm) or new STT wave change
    4. Complaint of shortness of breath

II. Worrisome Cardiac History
    5. History of CAD, hypertrophic, or dilated cardiomyopathy
    6. History of congestive heart failure or LV dysfunction
    7. History of or current Ventricular Tachycardia, Ventricular Fibrillation
    8. Pacemaker
    9. ICD
    10. Antidysrhythmic medication not including digoxin, b blockers or cc blockers
    11. Significant Heart Murmur by history or heard in the ED

III. Family History of Sudden Death
    12. Family history (first-degree relative) with sudden death, HOCM, Brugada's syndrome, or long QT syndrome

IV. Signs of Conduction Disease
    13. Multiple syncopal episodes within the last 6 months
    14. Rapid palpitations
    15. Syncope during exercise
    16. QT interval > 500 ms
    17. High grade or complete heart block

V. Volume Depletion
    18. Gastrointestinal bleeding
    19. Hematocrit < 30
    20. Dehydration not corrected in the ED

VI. Persistent Abnormal Vital Signs in the Emergency Department
    21. Respiratory Rate > 24
    22. O2 saturation < 90
    23. Sinus rate < 50 or Sinus rate > 100
    24. Blood Pressure < 90

VII. CNS
    25. Primary CNS event (i.e., SAH, stroke)

Neurologic testing is useful only in patients who have focal neurologic findings or a history consistent with a seizure.[4,38] An electroencephalogram provides diagnostic information in fewer than 2% of cases of syncope.[47] Routine use of a head CT scan should not be performed on patients with syncope, but should be limited to those with signs of trauma, neurologic deficit, or neurologic complaints.[48,49] Psychiatric evaluation should be considered in patients with known psychiatric illness, no organic heart disease, and recurrent syncope.[16]

Disposition of patients with syncope

Syncope accounts for up to 6% of all hospital admissions nationwide. The cost of care per hospital admission for syncope has been estimated at roughly $5300 per stay, for a total cost of over $1 billion per year nationally.[6,38] The American College of Emergency Physicians suggests criteria for patient admission should include those patients with a history of congestive heart failure or ventricular dysrhythmias, associated chest pain or other symptoms compatible with an acute coronary syndrome, valvular heart disease on physical examination, or EKG findings of ischemia, dysrhythmia, prolonged QT interval, or bundle branch block.[45]

Despite these guidelines, there is little data available concerning the short-term outcome of syncope patients following discharge from the ED. Most literature has studied outcomes of patients at six-month and one-year intervals.[35,45] However, one study determines four predictors of adverse outcomes in 72 hours; these factors include a history of ventricular dysrhythmia, an abnormal EKG in the ED, age older than 45 years, and a history of congestive heart failure.[40] In patients with none of these risk factors, there is no risk of cardiac mortality, but a 0.7% risk of dysrhythmia.[40]

The San Francisco Syncope Rule was hoped to be promising tool to predict which patients would have serious outcomes at one week.[37] However, multiple recent studies have been unable to validate this rule.[50–52]

More recently, the Boston Syncope Guidelines accurately identify ED patients at risk for adverse outcomes at 30 days.[35] Utilizing risk factors to screen syncope patients yields a sensitivity of 97%, and a specificity of 62%, with a negative predictive value of 99%. In this population, admitting only those

Table 13-3. Management of syncope: What every patient needs.

Test or Diagnostic Modality	Utility in Diagnosis	Appropriate Population
History	45%	All
ECG	5%	All
Finger Stick Glucose	Unknown	All
CBC, Electrolytes	2%	Tailored to presenting complaints
Head CT	4%	Patients with neurological complaints, trauma, on warfarin
Pregnancy Test	Unknown	Women of child-bearing age
Cardiac Enzymes	5% in appropriate population	History, ECG concerning for ischemia, or unable to communicate
Carotid Massage	Unknown	Age > 40 or syncope while shaving or turning head
Stool for Occult Blood	Unknown	All

patients identified by these guidelines would lead to a 48% reduction in hospital admissions (Table 13-2).

Section IV: Decision making

Please see Table 13-3.

References

1 Grossman SA, Fischer C, Lipsitz L, et al. Predicting adverse outcomes in syncope. *J Emerg Med.* 2007;33:233–239.
2 Linzer M, Pritchett ELC, Pontinen M, McCarthy E, Divine GW. Incremental diagnostic yield of loop electrocardiographic recorders in unexplained syncope. *Am J Cardiol.* 1990;66:214–219.
3 Linzer M, Yang EH, Estes NA III, Wang P, Vorperian VR, Kapoor WN. Diagnosing syncope. 1. Value of history, physical examination, and electrocardiography: Clinical Efficacy Assessment Project of the American College of Physicians. *Ann Intern Med.* 1997;126:989–996.
4 Huff JS, Decker WW, Quinn JV, et al. Clinical policy: Critical issues in the evaluation and management of

adult patients presenting to the emergency department with syncope. *Ann Emerg Med*. 2007;49:431–444.

5 Gei AF, Hankins GD. Cardiac disease and pregnancy. *Obstet Gynecol Clin North Am*. 2001;28:465–512.

6 Lipsitz LA. Syncope in the elderly. *Ann Intern Med*. 1983;99:92–105.

7 Kapoor W, Snustad D, Peterson J, et al. Syncope in the elderly. *Am J Med*. 1998;80:419–428.

8 Lipsitz LA, Pluchino FC, Wei JY, Rowe JW. Syncope in institutionalized elderly: The impact of multiple pathological conditions and situational stress. *J Chronic Dis*. 1986;39:619–630.

9 Getchell WS, Larsen GC, Morris CD, McAnulty JH. Epidemiology of syncope in hospitalized patients. *J Gen Intern Med*. 1999;14:677–687.

10 Kapoor W, Hanusa B. Is syncope a risk factor for poor outcomes? Comparison of patients with and without syncope. *Am J Med*. 1996;100:647–655

11 Ooi WL, Hossain M, Lipsitz LA. The association between orthostatic hypotension and recurrent falls in nursing home residents. *Am J Med*. 2000;108:106–111.

12 Harwood-Nuss AL, Linden CH, Luten RC, Shepherd SM, Wolfson AB, eds. *The Clinical Practice of Emergency Medicine*. 2nd ed. Philadelphia: Lippincott-Raven; 996:891.

13 Kapoor WN, Karpf M, Wieand S, et al. A prospective evaluation and follow-up of patients with syncope. *N Engl J Med*. 1983;309:197–204.

14 Marx JA, Hockberger RS, Walls RM, Adams *J. Rosen's Emergency Medicine: Concepts and Clinical Practice*. 5th ed. St. Louis; Mosby, Inc.; 2002:172–176.

15 Grossman SA, Babineau M, Mottley L. Outcomes of near syncope parallel syncope patients in the emergency department. *Acad Emerg Med*. 2009;16:S66–67.

16 Kapoor WN. Syncope. *N Engl J Med*. 2000;343:1856–1862.

17 Benbadis S, Wolgamuth B, Goren H, et al. Value of tongue biting in the diagnosis of seizures. *Arch Intern Med*. 1995;155:2346–2349.

18 Kapoor WN. Evaluation and management of the patient with syncope. *JAMA*. 1992;268:2553–2560.

19 Kapoor WN. Evaluation of syncope in the elderly. *J Am Geriatr Soc*. 1987;35:826–828.

20 Martin G, Adams S, Martin H, et al. Prospective evaluation of syncope. *Ann Emerg Med*. 1984;13:499–504.

21 Calkins H, Shyr Y, Frumin H, et al. The value of the clinical history in the differentiation of syncope due to ventricular tachycardia, atrioventricular block, and neurocardiogenic syncope. *Am J Med*. 1995;98:365–373.

22 Day S, Cook E, Funkenstein H, et al. Evaluation and outcome of emergency room patients with transient loss of consciousness. *Am J Med*. 1982;73:15–23.

23 Braunwald E, ed. *Heart Disease: A Textbook of Cardiovascular Medicine*. 5th ed. Philadelphia, WB Saunders; 1997:868–935.

24 Atkins D, Hanusa B, Sefcik T, et al. Syncope and orthostatic hypotension. *Am J Med*. 1990;91:179–185.

25 Hanlon J, Linzer M, MacMillan J, et al. Syncope and presyncope associated with probable adverse drug reactions. *Arch Intern Med*. 1990;150:2309–2312.

26 Thames MD, Alpert JS, Dalen J. Syncope in patients with pulmonary embolism. *JAMA*. 1977; 238:2509–2511.

27 Sarasin FP, Louis-Simonet M, Carballo D et al. Prospective evaluation of patients with syncope: A population-based study. *Am J Med*. 2001;111:177–184.

28 Bell WR, Simon TL, DeMets DL. The clinical features of submassive and massive pulmonary emboli. *Am J Med*. 1977;62:355–360.

29 Middlekauff H, Stevenson W, Saxon L. Prognosis after syncope: Impact of left ventricular function. *Am Heart J*. 1993;125:121–127.

30 Middlekauff H, Stevenson W, Stevenson L, et al. Syncope in advanced heart failure: High risk of sudden death regardless of origin of syncope. *J Am Coll Cardiol*. 1993;21:110–116.

31 Manolis AS. The clinical spectrum and diagnosis of syncope. *Herz*. 1993;18:143–154.

32 Bass E, Curtiss E, Arena V, et al. The duration of Holter monitoring in patients with syncope. *Arch Intern Med*. 1990;150:1073–1078.

33 Driscoll D, Jacobsen S, Porter C, et al. Syncope in children and adolescents. *J Am Coll Cardiol*. 1997;29:1039–1045.

34 Kapoor WN, Fortunato M, Hanusa BH, et al. Psychiatric illnesses in patients with syncope. *Am J Med*. 1995;99:505–512.

35 Kapoor WN. Diagnostic evaluation of syncope. *Am J Med*. 1991;90:91–106.

36 Kapoor WN. Evaluation and outcome of patients with syncope. *Medicine*. 1990;69:160–175.

37 Quinn JV, Stiell IG, McDermott DA, et al. Derivation of the San Francisco syncope rule to predict patients with short-term serious outcomes. *Ann Emerg Med*. 2004;43:224–232.

38 Linzer M, Yang EH, Estes NA III, et al. Diagnosing syncope. 2. Unexplained syncope: Clinical Efficacy Assessment Project of the American College of Physicians. *Ann Intern Med*. 1997;127:76–86

39 Brignole M, Alboni P, Benditt D, et al. Guidelines on management of syncope. *Eur Heart J*. 2001;22:1256–1306.

40 Martin TP, Hanusa BH, Kapoor WN. Risk stratification of patients with syncope. *Ann Emerg Med*. 1997;29:459–466.

41 Klitzner TS. Sudden cardiac death in children. *Circulation*. 1990;82:629–632.

42 Grossman SA, Van Epp S, Arnold R, et al. The value of cardiac enzymes in elderly patients presenting to the emergency department with syncope. *J Gerontol A Biol Sci Med Sci.* 2003;58:1055–1058.

43 Link MS, Lauer EP, Homoud MK, et al. Low yield of rule-out myocardial infarction protocol in patients presenting with syncope. *Am J Card.* 2001;88;706–707.

44 Shotan A, Ostrzega E, Mehra A, et al. Incidence of arrhythmias in normal pregnancy and relation to palpitations, dizziness, and syncope. *Am J Cardiol.* 1997;79:1061–1064.

45 ACEP Board of Directors. Clinical policy: Critical issues in the evaluation and management of patients presenting with syncope. *Ann Emerg Med.* 2001;37:771–776.

46 Recchia D, Barzilai B. Echocardiography in the evaluation of patients with syncope. *J Gen Intern Med.* 1995;10:649–655.

47 Davis TL, Freemon FR. Electroencephalography should not be routine in the evaluation of syncope in adults. *Arch Intern Med.* 1990;150:2027–2029.

48 Goyal N, Donnino MW, Vachhani R, et al. The utility of head computed tomography in the emergency department evaluation of syncope. *Intern Emerg Med.* 2006;1:148–150.

49 Grossman SA, Fischer C, Bar JL, et al. The yield of head CT in syncope. *Intern Emerg Med.* 2007;2:46–49.

50 Fischer CM, Shapiro NI, Lipsitz L, et al. External validation of the San Francisco Syncope Rule. *Acad Emerg Med.* 2005;12:S127.

51 Sun BC, Mangione CM, Merchant G, et al. External validation of the San Francisco Syncope Rule. *Ann Emerg Med.* 2007;49:420–427.

52 Birnbaum A, Esses D, Biju P, et al. Failure to validate the San Francisco Syncope Rule in an independent emergency department population. *Ann Emerg Med.* 2008;52:151–159.

14 Valvular heart disease

Jeffrey Soderman[1] & Edward Ullman[2]

[1] *Attending Physician, Department of Emergency Medicine, Beverly Hospital, Beverly, MA, USA*
[2] *Assistant Professor of Medicine, Harvard Medical School, Director of Medical Student Education, Division of Emergency Medicine, Beth Israel Deaconess Medical Center, Boston, Massachusetts, USA*

Section I: Case presentation

A 76-year-old man was brought by ems to the emergency department (ED) for chest pain after walking to get the mail. The patient reported progressive difficulty in daily activities due to chest pain and shortness of breath. The patient also noted the chest pain was increasing in frequency and duration. It was described as a dull ache that radiated to the left shoulder. He denied associated abdominal pain. Over the prior week, it had taken increasing time for the pain and dyspnea to resolve. This current episode lasted 30 minutes, which prompted the call to 911. On ED arrival, he did not have chest pain. The patient denied any fever, chills, or cough. He noted occasional dizziness with the recent chest pain episodes without a loss of consciousness.

The past medical history included hypertension, hyperlipidemia, and chronic obstructive pulmonary disease (COPD). His current medications included atorvastatin., furosemide, metoprolol, and albuterol and fluticasone /salmeterol inhalers. The patient reported a 40 pack/year smoking history. He drank one to two glasses of wine with dinner. He was a retired stockbroker who occasionally played golf, but otherwise did not perform any exercise.

Initial vital signs were: temperature 37°C (98.6°F), blood pressure 167/98 mmHg, heart rate 68 beats/min, respiratory rate 16 breaths/min, and an oxygen saturation of 98% on room air. On further examination, the patient was resting comfortably in no distress. Pertinent positive findings included a delayed carotid upstroke, a 3/6 crescendo-decrescendo systolic ejection murmur best heard at the upper right sternal border, and lungs clear to auscultation. The remainder of the physical examination was unremarkable. An EKG showed left ventricular hypertrophy with nonspecific ST and T abnormalities. Laboratory values were unremarkable. A chest film showed an enlarged cardiac silhouette.

Section II: Case discussion

Dr Peter Rosen: What concerns me particularly in this case is not the angina or heart failure, but the concomitant possibility of valvular heart disease. What kind of cardiac complications are we likely to encounter with this cardiac disease? What kind of complications cause emergency visits in patients who have valvular disease? Let's start with the problem that this man likely presents with: aortic valve disease.

Dr David Brown: The physical examination does sound like the patient has aortic stenosis (AS), and with an EKG showing left ventricular hypertrophy, this seems even more likely. So we have a patient presenting with one of the classical presentations of critical aortic stenosis, namely chest pain. The three classic presentations of patients with critical aortic stenosis are: chest pain,

Cardiovascular Problems in Emergency Medicine: A discussion-based review, First Edition.
Edited by Shamai A. Grossman and Peter Rosen.
© 2011 John Wiley & Sons, Ltd. Published 2011 by John Wiley & Sons, Ltd.

congestive heart failure, and syncope. A fourth presentation that perhaps hasn't been publicized as much, at least by the physicians in our specialty, is sudden death. Patients may present with anginal-sounding chest pain, as this man does, and it can be progressive and seem much like coronary artery disease. They can present with an exacerbation of congestive heart failure. They can present with syncope, or they can present with some of these symptoms in combination. Aortic stenosis can also present with the findings of endocarditis, such as with a subacute illness that includes fever, rash, malaise and loss of energy, symptoms that may have gone on for days to weeks before presentation.

PR: We'd like to know what his echocardiogram shows, but we're not going to have that readily available. Are there any physical findings that you find particularly helpful in making a clinical diagnosis of aortic stenosis?

Dr Amal Mattu: There are only a couple of systolic murmurs that I think emergency physicians need to readily recall, and they are aortic stenosis and mitral regurgitation. They are usually easy to distinguish based on where they are heard at maximal intensity, and where they radiate. Mitral regurgitation is generally heard at the apex, radiating to the axilla; aortic stenosis, in contrast, is generally heard at the right upper sternal border, radiating north to the carotids and the axilla.

Dr Shamai Grossman: The most common signs of aortic stenosis include a pulse of small amplitude and a laterally displaced apex. Pulsus parvus et tardus is also associated with aortic stenosis; this is an arterial pulse with a delayed and plateaued peak, decreased amplitude, and gradual downslope. A blowing, diastolic murmur may be present if the patient has associated aortic regurgitation.

PR: This patient is likely to have a movement of his point of maximal impact (PMI) to his axilla, since these patients usually tend to have fairly large-sized hearts. Is he likely to have a palpable thrill in his neck, or is he likely to have a thrill when you feel his chest?

SG: A systolic thrill may be palpable at the base of the heart, in the jugular notch, and along the carotid arteries. In addition, as aortic stenosis becomes more severe, often the murmur will become less prominent because of heart failure, so a patient with critical aortic stenosis may have a quieter murmur when compared to a patient with more moderate aortic

stenosis. It's generally an ominous sign when you have a patient who you know has aortic stenosis and you cannot hear the murmur.

PR: What causes the angina?

DB: A lot of these patients have concomitant coronary artery disease, so it's important to continue to consider that diagnosis, even in patients who have known aortic stenosis. If one doesn't have concomitant coronary artery disease, it is thought that the left ventricle has hypertrophied to the point where it can't relax enough during diastole to allow sufficient flow to some portion of the myocardium, and patients become ischemic based on that, independent of coronary artery disease.

SG: Rising left ventricular end-diastolic pressure eventually will lead to a sustained pressure overload, giving way to myocardial decompensation, loss of contractility of the myocardium, and ultimately a decrease in cardiac output. This manifests itself in all three symptoms of critical aortic stenosis: angina, syncope, and heart failure.

PR: One of my favorite medical quotes is from John Hunter, an anatomist and surgeon in the 1700s in England who developed syphilitic aortitis with aortic stenosis, which he claimed was from cutting his hand doing an autopsy. When he developed angina, he said, "Now, I'm at the mercy of any fool who chooses to annoy me." In fact, I think that's a pretty good description of angina. Angina can come on with exercise, or it can come on with aggravation. Is there a difference in precipitation of aortic stenosis angina from the different kinds of physical exercise that is performed? With coronary artery disease, angina is more likely to come with isometric exercises like snow shoveling, and with changes in weather, walking in a cold wind, or walking up a hill.

SG: Given that most anginas associated with aortic stenosis are secondary to underlying atherosclerotic heart disease, I would suspect that the precipitants would be very similar.

PR: Endocarditis can be a precipitant of increased symptoms from a stenotic valve, but this man does not appear to have this problem. Given that he is functionally more diminished, are there indications for admitting such a patient? In other words, with this story, would we run some enzymes and try to make sure that this wasn't concomitant ischemic coronary artery disease? However, the chances are that the time has come for this patient to receive a valve replacement, and that's unlikely to be done on an emergent basis, unless he has endocarditis. With this in mind what would be your indications for admission for a patient like this?

DB: To avoid admission, I would need to feel confident that he did not have concomitant coronary artery disease. In a patient who I didn't know from a previous interface with our healthcare system, this kind of presentation, regardless of the sound of the murmur, is going to require admission for evaluation of coronary artery disease. In a patient who was known to our system with known critical AS and without coronary artery disease, surgery doesn't necessarily need to be done on an emergent basis. Nevertheless, the progressive nature of his symptoms are concerning to me, and I might admit him anyway.

PR: Is the angina of aortic stenosis relievable by nitroglycerin?

AM: Aortic stenosis patients are preload sensitive, so when nitrates are used, they have to be used with extreme caution, if at all, especially in the patient with a critically stenotic aortic valve. Sublingual nitroglycerins can bottom out the blood pressure. You're stuck between a rock and a hard place with standard angina treatments, because these therapies can also be very harmful in these patients.

SG: If one chooses to use nitroglycerin, it may relieve the angina, but one must use it judiciously; if you have a patient who says when I have discomfort I use nitroglycerin, and it relieves the angina, then there is less of a risk in giving it in that case compared to a patient who is nitroglycerin-naive. In that particular case, I would try to avoid giving nitroglycerin.

PR: If this patient presented in heart failure would you use diuretics?

SG: Managing these patients is particularly tricky. Firstly, if we use nitroglycerin for afterload reduction, it will also decrease preload; secondly, diuretics may also significantly reduce preload, causing the patient to deteriorate further. In these patients, I may end up using a diuretic very judiciously, and would give any of these medications in conjunction with discussions with my cardiothoracic surgeon and cardiologist, with the idea that if the patient deteriorates further after administering these

therapies, the patient may require an emergent intervention, such as an immediate trip to the cardiac catheterization laboratory for an intraaortic balloon pump and a full pre-op evaluation prior to a more emergent trip to the operating room for a valve replacement.

PR: Should this patient have an echocardiogram (ECHO) in the ED?

SG: This would depend on how sick the patient was. Given the presentation that we have thus far, this patient does not need an emergent echocardiogram in the ED. Instead, this patient will likely have an echocardiogram during his admission to better evaluate the current status of his aortic valve and his cardiac function. Generally, when patients begin to develop symptoms, that's when their coronary function begins to deteriorate, so not only are the measurements of his aortic valve and the measurements of velocity across the valve important, but the degree of left ventricular malfunction now needs to be measured to assess how quickly the patient needs to go to the operating room. Were this patient to have presented with signs of heart failure, I might be more eager to get the ECHO in the ED.

PR: If you had some evidence that there was concomitant coronary artery disease, such as a mildly elevated troponin level, would that move you more towards sending him for cardiac surgery as opposed to the catheterization laboratory?

DB: The patient would still need to go to the catheterization laboratory to have his coronary anatomy further elucidated, and also to understand to what degree he has aortic stenosis so that operative planning could be most optimally arranged, only now on an emergency basis. In a more stable patient, this could be done electively as part of that hospital admission.

SG: When we think about admission, we must consider that we're not good at listening to heart murmurs in the ED. Generally, we're impatient and pressured and usually don't hear murmurs because there is so much background noise; if we hear something, we're often surprised, and think that there must be something wrong. In patients with valvular emergencies, particularly in patients who have had valve replacements, one must be meticulous and try to listen for their heart sounds, because if you don't hear them, or if they are muffled, that is an ominous sign.

PR: I think that one of the reasons that we are poor at physical examination is that we don't do it. Housestaff are used to obtaining imaging studies rather than doing a physical examination because they don't trust their physical examination; because they don't trust it, they don't do it; and the less often they do it, the less they trust it, so it is a vicious cycle. One thing that I have found extraordinarily helpful is an electronic stethoscope. I am amazed at how much more I can hear now that I have this stethoscope. Perhaps this is something that should be part of the armamentarium of every emergency physician, because there is an enormous amount of background noise in every ED.

SG: I might add that obtaining a good history from these patients in terms of the type of valve replacement that has been placed, if they present after surgery, is important, because you will hear different things from a patient who has a porcine valve or a mechanical valve. The likelihood that they are going to have valve failure is also somewhat different depending on the kind of valve that they have. Porcine valves generally deteriorate more quickly, and mechanical valves have longer life expectancies. That said, porcine valves or bovine valves in the aortic position often don't require anticoagulation, so you often don't see complications from warfarin therapy, whereas, patients with mechanical valves must be on warfarin, so you will often see the complications associated with valve failure and the lack of anticoagulation in these patients.

PR: Let's change the case. Let's say that we're seeing this patient 6 months to a year postoperatively. We know that he has both diseases; we know that both diseases have supposedly been fixed. What kind of problems do we need to be alert to over time? We have already discussed endocarditis, given an artificial valve, but do we often see valve failure early on in these patients, or does it take so long to develop that we're probably not going to have to deal with it?

DB: The complications of a prosthetic valve that we might see in the ED, in such a short interval, are likely related to either infection or thrombosis of the valve. It's not likely that we'll see patients with gradual restenosis or valve failure of some sort if it's subacute. Occasionally, valve failure can be acute (mechanical valves can get stuck in the opened position, leading to wide-open aortic regurgitation), but that's going to be rare and very dramatic. More likely we'll see patients who aren't sufficiently anticoagulated and have developed thrombosis of their valve, and present with signs of heart failure and valve failure.

AM: Inadequate anticoagulation, from either too little or excessive warfarin dosing and bleeding complications may be the most likely complications.

PR: Warfarin is a hard drug to live with. I remember a study that came out of Denmark that stunned me; the Danes used to anticoagulate their post-myocardial infarction (MI) patients who had survived for more than two years. This study found that after patients had been on the drug for more than one year, 100% had some sort of bleeding complication from warfarin. This suggests that we're going to see a lot of complications on warfarin therapy.

This kind of patient is going to be admitted in most EDs. What else do we need to know before admitting him? Are there any special studies that we might consider ordering in addition to a routine EKG and cardiac enzymes?

SG: Given his current presentation, that's all I would do. Unless he rapidly deteriorates in the ED, we shouldn't need to do an emergent echocardiogram, but clearly, when admitted, he will need a full evaluation and preparation for an aortic valve repair. I think he is showing that if he does not get his aortic valve replaced, his short-term mortality over the course of the next months to year or two is very high. Admitting him to the hospital, if only to expedite his evaluation and preparation for surgery, becomes a priority.

PR: It seems to me that we don't see as much rheumatic heart valve disease anymore, and that the predominant valvular disorder that comes our way is aortic stenosis. How often do you see other valve pathologies in the ED?

DB: This depends on what population one serves. The incidence of rheumatic heart disease has definitely dropped significantly in the United States over the past 30 to 40 years. If one practices in Europe, or in parts of the developing world, rheumatic heart disease may not be a vanishing disease. We may be more likely, as emergency physicians, to see valvular emergencies that are related to myxomatous degeneration of the mitral valve, such as mitral valve prolapse leading to mitral regurgitation. If a chordae tendonae ruptures in that setting, then acute mitral regurgitation can be dramatic with acute congestive heart failure. The other valvular related emergencies we're likely to see are related to ischemia, such as an infarcted papillary muscle, which may rupture after an acute MI. This can also lead to acute, wide-open mitral regurgitation that can present as dramatic congestive heart failure.

AM: In Baltimore, we often see right-sided endocarditis related to intravenous drug abuse. We also see a lot of patients who have tricuspid and mitral valve replacements following endocarditis, and occasionally these patients will have subacute bacterial endocarditis, and ultimately present after they've ruptured their valve. These patients are in fulminant heart failure, hypotensive, and very dramatic in presentation.

PR: When I was in San Diego, we had a fairly large population of IV drug abusers, and we didn't see that much valvular disease; perhaps it varies with what kind of drug they are injecting. What impressed me the most about these patients was how hard it was to make the diagnosis; rarely did we find classical murmurs. This forced us to work up every patient who came in with a fever and a heart murmur for endocarditis. We were often surprised which valve was involved when we found the diagnosis.

PR: Is mitral valve prolapse associated with endocarditis?

DB: I believe that there is risk of endocarditis when mitral valve prolapse is associated with mitral regurgitation, which would just be a subset of patients with myxomatous degeneration of the valve.

SG: The American Heart Association (AHA) does not recommend prophylaxis with antibiotics before procedures for patients who simply have mitral valve prolapse unless they have concomitant mitral valve regurgitation.

PR: Let's say that this man comes back after his valve replacement and he had an abscess on his leg; would you want to give him some antibiotic coverage as you drain that abscess, and what sort of antibiotic prophylaxis is he going to require?

SG: I probably would give him antibiotics even though that's not clearly the scenario described in the AHA guidelines; the prophylaxis I would give him would be staphlococcal and streptococcal prophylaxis, with probably a first-generation cephalosporin, like cephalexin or dicloxacillin.

PR: I am rather underwhelmed on the data on the success of prophylaxis for valvular heart disease. It sounds like a great idea, but there are so many places in life where one has bacterial showers that the patient doesn't get prophylaxed and doesn't develop endocarditis that I'm not convinced that there's value in prophylactic treatment of patients with valvular disease.

DB: I think that most clinicians follow the guidelines that are published by the AHA in terms of when to give prophylaxis, and most of these procedures are not done in the ED, so they don't impact us much. Instead, we see patients afterwards with complications, but we don't see the large numbers of patients who don't have complications.

PR: Are you using prophylaxis for valvular patients who have laceration repair?

AM: I would prophylax for laceration repair, as well as for incision and drainage of abscesses. The most recent guidelines are a little less liberal in terms of routine prophylaxis. It used to be that just about anybody with any kind of valvular disorder would get prophylaxis. Prophylaxis is now recommended only with an acquired or prosthetic valve disorder. We use prophylaxis for patients who have an acquired valvular disorder, like aortic stenosis or aortic regurgitation, if they've had previous valvular surgery or a prior history of endocarditis. In line with the most recent AHA recommendations, we are not prophylaxing for urinary types of procedures, such as Foleys, intubations, laryngoscopies, or gastrointestinal procedures.

PR: We used to believe that we could prevent infections with antibiotics, and I think that over time we've come to realize that all we do is select for resistant bacteria. Perhaps the only true antibiotic prophylaxis is bowel prep before colon surgery, and I am very underwhelmed by prophylaxis elsewhere. I would like to see us stop using it for places where we routinely use it, like some of the less dirty open fractures, because here, I think, that we are just selecting for resistant bacteria.

Case resolution

The patient was given an aspirin and admitted to the hospital. The combination of the history, physical examination, and EKG prompted an echocardiogram that showed severe aortic stenosis and an ejection fraction of 45%. With the patient's anginal complaints, there was significant concern for underlying coronary artery disease. He underwent a cardiac catheterization that showed significant three-vessel coronary disease, and verified the aortic stenosis. On hospital day two the patient underwent a three-vessel coronary artery bypass graft surgery with aortic valve replacement. His postoperative course was uneventful, and he was discharged from the hospital on post-op day ten.

Section III: Concepts

Background

The spectrum of valvular heart disease that the emergency physician encounters in practice ranges from the relatively benign, such as asymptomatic mitral valve prolapse, to the acutely life threatening. This chapter focuses on the acute and life threatening etiologies of valvular disease, including acute mitral and aortic regurgitation, endocarditis, and chronic aortic stenosis, in the setting of acute heart failure.

The epidemiology of valvular heart disease has been changing in recent years. As acute rheumatic fever becomes less common, there has been an increase in the incidence of degenerative valvular disease. This, in turn, has changed the epidemiology of acute valvular pathology, as elderly patients tend to have more structural damage to their valves.

Most valvular disease results from either direct or indirect degeneration of the native valve. The spectrum of etiologies for this damage includes senile degeneration, infection (specifically endocarditis), congenital anomalies of valves that make the native valve more susceptible to wear and tear damage, and, less commonly, rheumatic disease.

Intravenous drug abuse (IVDA) is also a major risk factor for valvular disease, particularly endocarditis. Population-wide rates of endocarditis have been shown to be higher with higher rates of IVDA.

With the emergence of methicillin-resistant *Staphylococcus aureus* (MRSA) infections, its prevalence in endocarditis is also increasing. MRSA needs to be entertained in any patient with a history of prior MRSA, IVDA, or multiple treatment failures for endocarditis.

Initial workup: history and physical examination

Endocarditis

Patients who present with endocarditis can present with a multitude of symptoms, and the presentation may differ depending on whether it is acute or subacute infective endocarditis (IE.) Acute IE is a fulminant illness that presents with high fevers and rigors, whereas subacute IE has a more indolent course. One common thread, however, is the presence of a valve lesion, which may be unknown at presentation. A history of recent bacteremia should prompt concern for IE, and past medical history and social history can be very useful in suggesting the presence of infective endocarditis. The major risk factors for developing IE include structural heart disease, intravenous drug abuse, and prior valve replacement. Structural heart disease includes any valvular abnormality, such as aortic stenosis, mitral regurgitation, or a bicuspid aortic valve. Mitral valve prolapse must not be overlooked, as these patients have been estimated to have an up to five times greater risk of developing IE than the general population. Patients should be asked about any history of congenital heart disease, as any of these abnormalities provide an unnatural surface in which vegetations can develop. Patients who are status post-valve replacement or repair are also at risk, as the prosthetic valve or ring is foreign material that may become colonized by bacteria. The last major risk factor is intravenous drug abuse. Patients with a history of IVDA are most likely to have mitral or aortic valve endocarditis; nevertheless, right-sided endocarditis (pulmonic and tricuspid valve lesions) are almost exclusively seen in IVDA. One must consider IE in any patient who is at risk for bacteremia, as this is all that is necessary for seeding of a previously undetected damaged valve. Patients most at risk are those with chronic vascular access devices or people with poor dentition.

Although the physical examination often can be of limited utility, there are findings that are suggestive of IE. Fever is the most common vital sign abnormality. Cardiac auscultation must be thorough, as a new or changing murmur is suggestive of valve damage; however, this is frequently challenging for the emergency physician to diagnose, as the sound of patient's specific murmur is rarely known, and patients frequently do not know if they even have a murmur at baseline. Specific physical signs of endocarditis include Roth spots (round or oval white spots seen on the retina in SBE), Janeway lesions (small hemorrhagic spots on the palms and soles seen in SBE), and splinter hemorrhages, all of which are secondary to emboli from the endocarditis lesion and appear in the retina, palms, and fingernails, respectively. These findings are only present in a minority of patients, and their absence does not exclude endocarditis. The patient may have complaints or findings that are relatable to embolic disease, such as neurologic deficits or renal infarcts. Portions of the vegetation can break off and embolize to other parts of the body. Any patient who appears to have a cerebrovascular accident or other neurological symptoms and fever should also be worked up for endocarditis. Other types of vaso-occlusive symptoms can be found as well, such as limb ischemia, renal infarcts, or mesenteric ischemia.

Actue valvular regurgitation

The hallmark in the history of patients with acute valvular insufficiency is the rapid onset of symptoms. Patients will report acute onset of shortness of breath, and will often also report chest pain, secondary to cardiac ischemia or aortic dissection. Past medical history often is revealing in these patients; recent admission for myocardial infarction is important, as ischemia can be an important cause of mitral dysfunction. A history of endocarditis, mitral valve prolapse, Marfan's syndrome, prior valve replacement, or rheumatic heart disease are useful to the clinician, as these conditions predispose to valvular pathology. On examination, these patients are usually in extremis, with evidence of cardiogenic shock and associated pulmonary edema. Intubation is essential, especially if the patient is to be transferred to a higher level of care, as these patients have a high potential to deteriorate en route. Invasive monitoring (arterial and central venous lines) should be strongly considered given the tenuous hemodynamic nature of the patients.

In both acute aortic insufficiency and acute mitral regurgitation lesions, the signs of congestive heart failure (CHF) will be seen on examination, including pulmonary edema and elevated jugular venous pressure. The vital signs will likely be unstable, with tachycardia being very common as the heart attempts to compensate for decreasing cardiac output with increasing heart rate. The pulse pressure will likely be low as well, as the systolic pressure falls in both mitral and aortic disease. Respiratory distress is common, and the chest examination will invariably reveal crackles from fluid overload.

The cardiac examination is very important in acute valve regurgitation. Palpation of the chest will usually show a PMI in roughly the spot of a normal-sized heart, as the heart has not had a chance to hypertrophy in response to the increased ventricular and atrial volumes. Auscultation is of primary importance in determining which valve is causative. In acute mitral regurgitation (MR) one can hear the usual holosystolic murmur of MR; however, the murmur may not be completely holosystolic in its acute phase, and in some cases a murmur may not be present at all. An S3 can often be heard as well. In acute aortic regurgitation (AI), one can hear the typical diastolic murmur of AI, but since there is no large pressure difference between the proximal aorta and the left ventricle, the sound may be softer than expected. All of these variations can make definitive diagnosis confusing.

Etiologies and differential diagnosis of acute valvular disease

The patient at risk for endocarditis will frequently have a known valvular lesion, and a history of, or at least predisposition to, bacteremia (i.e., chronic vascular access or IVDA). As rheumatic heart disease becomes less prevalent, endocarditis is becoming more a disease of the elderly, as they are more likely to have indwelling vascular access, dialysis, and age-related degenerative disease of the valves. The microbiology of IE is very important, as it will guide empiric antibiotic therapy until a definite pathogen is known. Most authors report that *Staphylococcus* and *Streptococcus* species will account for about 80% of cases of IE. Also possible are the HACEK organisms (*Haemophilus*, *Actinobacillus actinomycetemcomitans*, *Cardiobacterium hominis*, *Eikenella corrodens*, *Kingella*), fungi, and various gram-negative organisms, and each of these account for approximately 2% of cases. Additionally, culture negative endocarditis, where the clinical picture is that of endocarditis but with persistently negative blood cultures, accounts for approximately 10% of cases.[1] Enterococcus is an important pathogen when there is a history of genitourinary or gastrointestinal tract surgery or procedures.[2]

Complete valvular dysfunction has various etiologies, depending on the affected valve. The aortic valve can be affected by an aortic dissection extending proximally into the valve and rupturing of one of the leaflets of the valve itself, or as a consequence of endocarditis. Acute mitral regurgitation has multiple causes, including damage to the tethering structures like the chordae tendineae or papillary muscles. The rupture of either of these structures can be caused by ischemia, secondary to an endocarditic lesion, or idiopathic rupture. Similar to aortic disease, the leaflets of the mitral valve can rupture as well. Those patients with a history of valvular surgery are predisposed to acute valvular failure.[3-5]

The pathophysiology of both acute aortic and mitral failure is similar. When the valve becomes acutely incompetent, the resultant regurgitant flow overloads the unprepared ventricle or atrium, forcing the end-diastolic volume to rise (increasing left ventricular filling pressure) or the end-systolic volume to fall (causing an increase in left atrial pressure). This forces the affected chamber to function on a much more rightward point (i.e., the downward sloping portion) of the Frank-Starling curve. Once the chamber is overloaded and unable to effectively pump forward, pulmonary vascular congestion results, giving the clinical picture of CHF. This is in contrast to chronic valve incompetence, where the heart has time to remodel to the slowly increasing chamber size, making the onset of symptoms more insidious.

Testing in valvular disease

Echocardiography is the gold standard for the evaluation of valvular disease. The hemodynamically unstable patient with a suspected blowout valve lesion requires emergent echocardiography to confirm the diagnosis. The stable patient with suspected endocarditis, for example, can usually be admitted to the hospital and receive the ECHO on a less urgent basis.

Choice of ECHO modality is important as well. Trans-thoracic echocardiography (TTE) has the advantage of being faster, portable, and does not require sedation like trans-esophageal echocardiography (TEE). Additionally, it may not require specialized physician operators who can be difficult to obtain during off hours. All of these advantages make TTE an attractive choice for the hemodynamically unstable emergency department patient with a suspected valve lesion. Transesophageal echocardiography has the advantage of increased sensitivity and specificity over TTE; some series show sensitivities for endocarditic vegetations of 95% for TEE vs. 60% for TTE.[6-9] However, TEE suffers from logistical difficulties, such as not being readily available in many centers and the danger of sedation in the unstable patient. However, in the stable patient, TEE can provide much greater detail of the valve structure and presence of vegetations on the valve

leaflets, and as such may be the preferred test in the patient with suspected endocarditis. TEE can usually be delayed to the inpatient setting in the stable patient.

Chest radiography is useful in the patient with acute valvular disease as well, and should be obtained in all patients. Helpful signs that can be seen in acute valve failure can include pulmonary edema and radiographic signs of aortic dissection, such as a widened mediastinum or aortic knob. In endocarditis, septic pulmonary emboli may be seen as well.

An EKG also should be obtained on all patients with suspected valvular disease. While there are no pathognomic EKG findings, evidence of infarction or ischemia (particularly with an anterolateral distribution) may be seen when this is the etiology of acute mitral regurgitation due to papillary muscle dysfunction.

Blood cultures are of paramount importance in the patient with suspected endocarditis. Patients should have at least three blood cultures drawn at initial presentation; ideally, they should be temporally separated by an hour to expose intermittent bacteremia. It is also important that blood cultures be obtained prior to the initiation of antibiotics, and all efforts should be made to ensure this, although the patient's stability should always be taken into account. While the specific microbiology will not be available to the emergency physician, it may be invaluable information during hospitalization. Meticulous care must be taken in obtaining these cultures, as culture contamination can lead to clinical confusion, especially since *Staphylococcus aureus* is both a common skin contaminant and a cause of endocarditis.

Baseline complete blood count and chemistry panels may be useful as well. Blood testing is of limited value in acute valvular incompetence, as the diagnosis is usually made clinically or with an echocardiogram. Obtain cardiac markers if ischemia maybe the underlying cause of valve failure.

Since infective endocarditis is a disease that presents with varying signs and symptoms, various classification and diagnostic criteria have been developed, the most widely used is the Duke criteria and its variations (Table 14-1). Since the Duke criteria rely heavily on the echocardiographic and blood culture findings, it is difficult to prove the diagnosis of endocarditis while in the ED.

Table 14-1. Duke criteria for diagnosing endocarditis.

Major Criteria

1. Blood cultures
   A. 2 blood cultures positive for IE-causing organisms (*Strep bovis*, HACEK group, *Staph aureus*, or *Viridans streptococci*, or *enterococci* without another source)
   B. Persistently positive blood cultures: at least 2 cultures drawn 12 hrs apart
2. Evidence of endocardial involvement
3. Echocardiographic evidence
   A. Intracardiac mass on valve or associated structures
   B. Abscess
   C. Partial dehisance of prosthetic valve
4. New valvular regurgitation
   A. Not just worsening of preexisting murmur

Minor Criteria

1. Historical factors: predisposing heart condition or intravenous drug abuse (IVDA)
2. Fever greater than 38°C (100.4°F)
3. Embolic phenomenon
   A. Cerebrovascular accident (CVA), septic lung emboli on chest *x*-ray (CXR), Janeway's lesions
4. Immunologic evidence
   A. Osler's nodes, Roth's spots
5. Microbiologic evidence
   A. Positive blood cultures that do not meet the major criteria

For a definitive diagnosis one must have 2 major criteria OR 1 major and 3 minor criteria OR 5 minor criteria

A diagnosis of possible infective endocarditis requires 1 major criteria and 1 minor criteria OR 3 minor criteria

The diagnosis of infective endocarditis is rejected if an alternative diagnosis is much more likely OR resolution of syndrome with < 4 days of antibiotics OR no evidence of endocarditis at surgery or autopsy OR does not meet above criteria

Treatment of patients with acute valvular heart disease

Due to the nature of acute valvular disease, the emergency physician will rarely provide definitive care for these patients. Nevertheless, in many cases of acute valvular disease, the patient will have life-threatening illness, and the emergency physician will be called upon to provide potentially life-saving diagnosis and stabilization.

The treatment of patients with valvular heart disease starts, as does every emergency department encounter, with assessment of the ABCs. The patient with acute valve regurgitation or acute valve dysfunction from endocarditis is frequently in extremis, and will require prompt control of the airway. Rapid sequence intubation medications that drop blood pressure should be used with caution, as the hemodynamics of these patients are frequently tenuous at best. Along these lines, hemodynamic support may be necessary. Dobutamine is a good first choice, as it will help augment forward flow by increasing inotropy. Dopamine can also be used; however, many patients will have compensatory tachycardia already, and dopamine may worsen this. Nitroprusside has also been used. Although this appears counterintuitive, this medication can lower afterload and facilitate forward blood flow, thereby limiting retrograde flow via the mitral valve and reducing pulmonary congestion.[10] Aortic balloon counterpulsation can be very useful in the case of mitral regurgitation, as it can help reduce preload, and help augment forward flow.[11] It is contraindicated with aortic valve pathology, as it will worsen valvular regurgitation. Ultimately, the patient with acute valvular incompetence requires surgical repair (Figure 14-1).

Treatment of the patient with severe AS will depend upon presentation. Syncope, CHF, atrial fibrillation, or ischemic symptoms in the presence of severe AS portend a poor long-term survival rate, usually on the order of 2–3 years.[10] The patient may present asymptomatically with a previously undetected systolic ejection murmur. Frequently, these patients' first symptomatic presentation will be in the ED, such as after their first syncopal episode. Many cardiologists and cardiac surgeons will consider valve replacement once a patient with known stenosis becomes symptomatic. Thus, it is important to communicate this information to the patient's cardiac team once discovered by the emergency physician. If a new systolic ejection murmur is found in a patient, even one presenting for an unrelated complaint, this patient needs echocardiography to evaluate the valve lesion and to acquire information about a surgical replacement.

The patient with known critical aortic stenosis who presents in acute CHF must be handled differently than the usual CHF patient. These patients are extremely preload-dependant, as their ventricles have to operate on a fairly rightward portion of the Frank-Starling curve to contract with enough force to overcome the resistance of a tightly stenoic valve. As such, the usual treatment for heart failure (nitrates, diuretics, blood pressure reduction) can be quite dangerous,

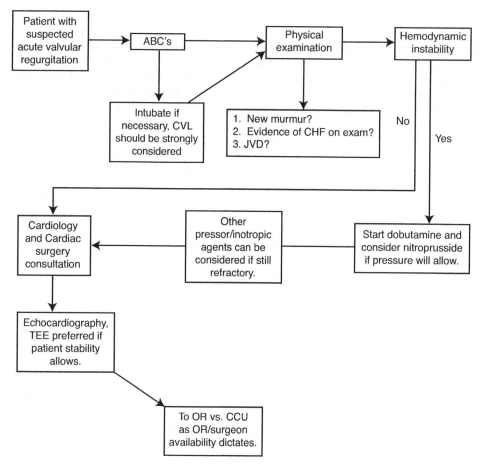

Figure 14.1 Flowchart for acute valvular regurgitation.

and can precipitously drop the blood pressure. Frequently, these patients need inotropic support with a drip medication such as dobutamine or dopamine. Perhaps somewhat counterintuitively, these patients may actually need IV fluid if they are hypotensive, similar to how a patient suffering a right-sided MI may need fluid resuscitation. In spite of traditional thinking, Khot et al. report that in 25 patients with severe CHF and tight AS, nitroprusside increases the cardiac index at 6 and 24 hours with minimal side effects.[12] However, these patients were highly selected, and nitroprusside therapy is probably not appropriate for all AS patients with CHF. Nitrate therapy can be initiated in close consultation with the cardiologist who will be caring for the patient, and should preferably be done in a patient who has appropriate monitoring devices in place (arterial and central venous lines,

perhaps a pulmonary artery catheter). Aortic balloon counterpulsation can be considered as a bridge to surgery, but is contraindicated in patients with aortic insufficiency. Once heart failure has developed in the patient with critical AS, aortic valve replacement must be undertaken quickly, as the outcomes for non-operative patients are very poor.

In the patient with endocarditis, the most important ED treatment, after hemodynamic stabilization and obtaining blood cultures, is starting an appropriate antibiotic regimen. Broad-spectrum antibiotics are necessary, and most empiric regimens suggest *antistaphylococcal* and *streptococcal* coverage, such as oxacillin or nafcillin 2g IV plus gentamycin 1mg/kg plus ampicillin 2g IV daily. Alternately, one gram of vancomycin can replace the penicillin derivatives if MRSA is suspected based on local resistance patterns. In the case of IVDA, vancomycin should be substituted, as the rate of MRSA in this population is very high.[13,14] Once culture results become available, antibiotic coverage can be tailored, but this will be after the patient is admitted. The medical record should also be reviewed for evidence of recent cultures, and may provide a clue to the specific causative agent; however, antibiotics should not be narrowed until definitive culture data is obtained (Figure 14-2).

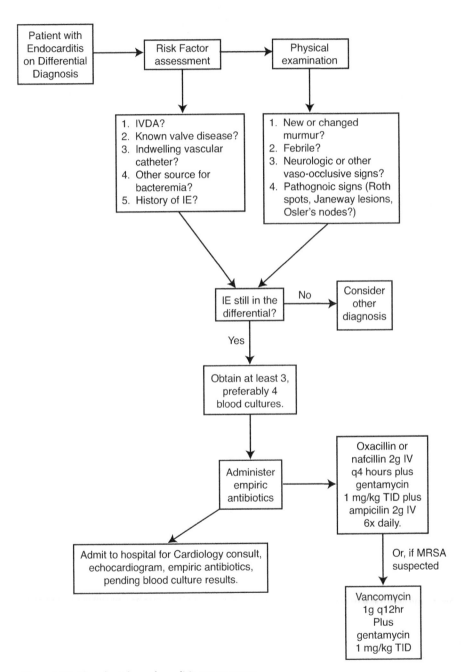

Figure 14.2 Flowchart for endocarditis management.

Disposition of patients with valvular disease

All patients with suspected acute valvular disease need admission to the hospital, often to very high levels of care. The patient with acute valvular blow-out will frequently be brought directly to the operating room for emergent valve repair or replacement. In the case that an operating room or cardiothoracic surgeon is not immediately available, these patients should be admitted to a cardiac or cardiac surgery intensive care unit while awaiting the surgery. For the community emergency physician, this will frequently require transfer to a tertiary care center. Because of the extreme instability of the blowout patient, one should consider aeromedical transport, or at minimum a ground unit with experience with vasoactive/cardioactive drip medication, as they are frequently required in the care of these patients. When transferring these patients via EMS services, central venous access, arterial cannulation, and intubation should be placed, if possible, prior to departure.

In the case of the endocarditis patient, the usual decision-making process for level of care applies. Patients may be admitted to a floor service if hemodynamically stable and no deterioration in their status is expected; otherwise ICU or step down level of care is appropriate.

Section IV: Decision making

See Figure 14-1 and Figure 14-2.

References

1 Nishimura, RA, Carabello, BA, Faxon, DP, et al. ACC/AHA 2008 guideline update on valvular heart disease: focused update on infective endocarditis: a report of the American College of Cardiology/American Heart Association Task Force on Practice Guidelines: endorsed by the Society of Cardiovascular Anesthesiologists, Society for Cardiovascular Angiography and Interventions, and Society of Thoracic Surgeons. *Circulation.* 2008;118:887–896.

2 Brook I. Infective endocarditis caused by anaerobic bacteria. *Arch Cardiovasc Dis.* 2008;101(10):665–676.

3 DePace, NL, Nestico, PF, Morganroth J. Acute severe mitral regurgitation, pathophysiology, clinical recognition, and management. *Am J Med.* 1985;78:293–306.

4 Walsh RA O'Rourke RA. The diagnosis and management of acute left–sided valvular regurgitation. *Curr Probl Cardiol.* 1979;4(9):1–34.

5 Janz TG. Valvular heart disease: clinical approach to acute decompensation of left–sided lesions. *Ann Emerg Med.* 1988;17:201–208.

6 Schoepf UJ, Yucel EK, Bettmann MA, et al. Expert Panel on Cardiovascular Imaging. Suspected bacterial endocarditis. [online publication]. Reston (VA): American College of Radiology (ACR); 2006. Available at: http://www.acr.org/SecondaryMainMenuCategories/quality_safety/app_criteria/pdf/ExpertPanelonCardiovascularImaging/SuspectedBacterialEndocarditisDoc17.aspx. Accessed on July 28, 2011.

7 Mugge A, Daniel WG, Frank G, Lichtlen PR. Echocardiography in infective endocarditis: reassessment of prognostic implications of vegetation size determined by the transthoracic and the transesophageal approach. *J Am Coll Cardiol.* 1989;14:631–638.

8 Cicioni C, Di Luzio V, Di Emidio L, et al. Limitations and discrepancies of transthoracic and transoesophageal echocardiography compared with surgical findings in patients submitted to surgery for complications of infective endocarditis. *J Cardiovasc Med.* 2006;7:660–666.

9 Reynolds HR, Jagen MA, Tunick PA, Kronzon I. Sensitivity of transthoracic versus transesophageal echocardiography for the detection of native valve vegetations in the modern era. *J Am Soc Echocardiogr.* 2003;16:67–70.

10 Bonow RO, Carabello BA, Chatterjee K, et al. ACC/AHA VHD Guidelines: 2008. *J Am Coll Cardiol.* 2008;52:1–142

11 Folland ED, Kemper AJ, Khuri SF, Josa M, Parisi AF. Intraaortic balloon counterpulsation as a temporary support measure in decompensated critical aortic stenosis. *J Am Coll Cardiol.* 1985;5:711–716.

12 Khot UN, Novaro GM, Popovi ZB, et al. Nitroprusside in critically ill patients with left ventricular dysfunction and aortic stenosis. *N Engl J Med.* 2003;348:1756–1763.

13 Miro JM, Anguera I, Cabell CH, et al. Staphylococcus aureus native valve infective endocarditis: report of 566 episodes from the International Collaboration on Endocarditis Merged Database. *Clin Infect Dis.* 2005;41:507–514.

14 Millar, BC, Prendergast, BD, Moore, JE. Community–associated MRSA (CA–MRSA): an emerging pathogen in infective endocarditis. *J Antimicrob Chemother.* 2008;61(1):1–7.

15 Myocarditis

Jehangir Meer[1] & Amal Mattu[2]
[1] *Director of Emergency Ultrasound, St Agnes Hospital Center, Baltimore, Maryland*
[2] *Professor and Residency Director, Department of Emergency Medicine, University of Maryland School of Medicine, Baltimore, Maryland, USA*

Section I: Case presentation

A 36-year-old man presented to the emergency department (ED) for evaluation of progressive chest heaviness and dyspnea experienced over the prior 4 days. The patient denied a history of the same symptoms and any prior past medical history of cardiac or respiratory problems.

He had been in good health with the exception of "the flu" 2 weeks earlier. At that time, he experienced fevers, upper respiratory symptoms, myalgias, and malaise. All of his symptoms had resolved with the exception of malaise, which had worsened in association with the chest heaviness and dyspnea. He reported progressive dyspnea on exertion to the point now that he felt very out-of-breath walking up a flight of stairs. He added that he had difficulty laying flat in bed the night before because of dyspnea. He reported mild subjective fevers throughout the day, though he had not taken his temperature.

He had no abdominal or back pain, lower extremity edema, nausea, diarrhea, anorexia, or headaches. The patient took no medications except for multivitamins, and had no family history of early cardiac disease. He did not smoke cigarettes or use illicit drugs. He customarily jogged 4 miles per day 3 times per week, and had never had any of these symptoms during his workouts. Notably, he had been too fatigued to exercise over the past 2 to 3 weeks.

The vital signs were: temperature 38°C (100.4°F), pulse 145 beats/min, respirations 28 breaths/min, blood pressure 87/40 mmHg, pulse oximetry 96%. A finger-stick glucose level was 100 mg/dl.

The physical examination revealed basilar rales in both lung fields, and mild jugular venous distension. The cardiac, abdomen, back, and extremity examinations were normal, and the pulses were symmetric bilaterally, though slightly weak. The skin was cool and slightly moist.

The patient was placed on a cardiac monitor and supplemental oxygen was provided. An EKG demonstrated sinus tachycardia, an intraventricular conduction delay (QRS 100 ms), and nonspecific ST-segment abnormalities. The patient reported that he had never had an EKG before. A chest X-ray study demonstrated cardiomegaly and pulmonary vascular prominence in the upper lung fields, consistent with mild heart failure. Laboratory studies were normal with the exception of a troponin-I level of 3.5 mcg/L (normal <1.0 mcg/L).

Section II: Case discussion

Dr Peter Rosen: This patient sounds like he was well-conditioned; he ran frequently, and has now undergone a change in his ability to perform exercise that

Cardiovascular Problems in Emergency Medicine: A discussion-based review, First Edition.
Edited by Shamai A. Grossman and Peter Rosen.

he was conditioned to do. This prior conditioning may not protect him from having coronary artery disease. I think that it's rare to see patients suddenly change their exercise pattern without having underlying coronary artery disease. He's in the right age group, and certainly it's prudent to do the kind of work up that was done here. Are there any clues in the history or in the physical examination that could help trigger the thought of myocarditis, and to help you distinguish it from coronary artery disease?

Dr Shamai Grossman: In this particular patient, there are some very specific clues that may be applicable to any patient in which you might consider the diagnosis of myocarditis. First, this is a young man, and although young men can have coronary artery disease, it is less likely. He has never had disease before, of cardiac or any other etiology. He presents with a fever, and in particular, he presents with a fever and symptoms that sound like he's having congestive heart failure (CHF) or left ventricle (LV) dysfunction. All of those things are very suggestive, almost classic, for a patient who has myocarditis. Patients who just have coronary artery disease usually do not present febrile, they will often have some symptoms suggestive of ischemia aside from dyspnea, although dyspnea itself can be a manifestation of angina, and they generally are older.

PR: Is it rare to see myocarditis without an element of pericarditis?

Dr Amal Mattu: It seems that many of the patients diagnosed with myocarditis have both myocarditis and pericarditis, and often times it is referred to as "myopericarditis." There may be some selection bias in my statement because pericarditis tends to be a little bit easier to diagnose based on the classic EKG changes with diffuse ST elevation and PR depression, whereas myocarditis by itself may be more frequently missed because there's no specific EKG finding associated with pure myocarditis.

PR: Pericarditis can be very hard to diagnose before it develops specific changes and classical findings may not be present early on. A pericardial friction rub is a useful clue for pericarditis, although it shouldn't be relied on for that diagnosis. I recall that a pericardial friction rub can be heard in up to 40% of patients with acute myocardial infarction (MI), depending on how often and where you listen, so clearly it isn't diagnostic

for pericarditis, but can help if you hear it. As for PR depression, I don't think that I've seen that in any other condition except pericarditis. Usually there are also clues in the history favoring pericarditis, such as a positional component with chest pain, and classic relief with sitting up and leaning forward; however, I haven't found these very helpful. I have noticed that most patients with pericarditis get relief with changing positions, some sitting up and leaning forward, some by lying down, some by lying on their side. Fever alone doesn't distinguish coronary artery disease from myocarditis or pericarditis, because, up to 30% of acute MI patients can run a low-grade fever as they necrose heart muscle. Higher fevers would be more suggestive of a viral infection, but this is a picture that could also be compatible with acute endocarditis even without a drug abuse history. I've seen a number of patients who were not IV drug abusers and without underlying valvular disease, yet who had acute endocarditis. Would you get blood cultures on this patient or an echocardiogram?

AM: I would obtain blood cultures on this patient to evaluate him for possible endocarditis, and an echocardiogram to look for evidence of this diagnosis. We always think about using echocardiograms to look for vegetations on the valves, but with myocarditis it would be useful to demonstrate diffuse wall motion abnormalities or a pericardial effusion, which may be found in either pericarditis or myocarditis. For these reasons, I would obtain an echocardiogram urgently, if not emergently.

PR: This patient has already declared himself as needing admission, given that whatever his underlying problem is, he's presenting with acute heart failure and a large heart. An echocardiogram could help us sort out whether there was a pericardial effusion, a regional wall abnormality, or a cardiomyopathy. What if the patient appeared to be less ill? What about the patient who presents more with positional chest pain, a pericardial friction rub, or perhaps an EKG suggestive of pericarditis? What should you use as your indications for admission, as not all patients with pericarditis need admission, and some patients who have myocarditis initially look more like pericarditis?

SG: If I have a patient who has a history of positional chest discomfort without a history of coronary artery disease; without a history of similar symptoms associated with coronary artery disease; a friction rub on physical examination; an EKG not concerning for ischemia, but consistent with pericarditis; and I've convinced myself that this is pericarditis, then I would do a bedside ultrasound to feel comfortable with sending the patient home. I think most emergency medicine physicians should be able to determine whether there is a pericardial effusion. If there is no pericardial effusion in a patient who very clearly has pericarditis, and who is hemodynamically stable, then that patient should be able to be discharged home with follow-up within 48 hours. These patients mostly do very well. Myocarditis, isolated from pericarditis, is a somewhat different entity, and without a classic history it can be very difficult to make this particular diagnosis in the first place. These patients often end up admitted to the hospital simply because it's hard to figure out what's going on, or what is the etiology of their presentation.

PR: The patient who looks predominantly like pericarditis, perhaps with a concomitant viral syndrome, in the absence of an effusion, is safe to manage as an outpatient. I would not start such a patient on steroids, but I usually do start nonsteroidal antiinflammatory medication, and I'm quick to add steroids.

I had a patient a couple of summers ago who was a middle-aged woman who, while picking up her son from hockey practice, slipped on the walkway in the ice rink and fell against a post. She presented a few days later with severe, ischemic sounding pain, chest wall tenderness, a very audible pericardial friction rub, and an EKG with nonspecific ST-T wave changes without the PR depressions typical of pericarditis. She was referred to our hospital for admission for ischemic heart disease because the troponin was slightly elevated, but I chose not to admit her because I thought she had traumatic pericarditis. How can you differentiate between traumatic and ischemic pericarditis? What can the physician expect to happen to the troponin and other cardiac enzymes with both pericarditis and myocarditis, and how do you distinguish them from ischemic changes?

AM: Based on the history you provided, it doesn't sound like ischemia was the etiology. I am unaware of a case of acute coronary syndrome (ACS) being precipitated by acute trauma. I would make sure the trauma was not just a red herring, and that she wasn't having these symptoms before the trauma. Based on the history that you presented, I would also call it traumatic pericarditis. Slipping and falling does not sound like a severe enough event to be a cardiac contusion. However, it's often very difficult, when patients present to an ED with chest pain and an elevated troponin, to distinguish between myopericarditis and a true acute coronary syndrome. Often we have to assume the worst, admit them to the hospital, and perhaps even require a cardiac catheterization. If you're lucky, you see classic pericarditis findings with ST elevations and PR depressions, but without a diagnostic EKG, the only other way to be certain about the diagnosis is to follow the progression of cardiac enzymes.

In an acute coronary syndrome, the patient's troponin levels should follow the classic rise and fall: with a rise within 24 hours and elevations for typically about a week. In pericarditis and myocarditis, the rise does not go very high; usually it's a relatively small elevation in troponin, which usually falls to normal levels within 24–48 hours. I am unaware of studies that differentiate myopericarditis from an acute coronary syndrome based purely on troponins. As a result, a lot of these patients end up in the catheterization laboratory and are diagnosed with myopericarditis only after the angiogram is clean for coronary artery disease.

PR: My patient did respond very well to steroids. Within 48 hours she was pain-free, but in follow-up, her physician, worried about the troponin rise, sent her off for a cardiac catheterization, which was negative. Subsequently, as the symptoms subsided, she's done quite well.

SG: To complicate matters, growing data suggest that elevated troponins can be found in patients with sepsis, in patients with pulmonary emboli, or in other patients who truly are very sick, but are not having an acute coronary syndrome. This is contrary to what is generally thought about troponin, namely that troponin is myocardial specific, or is specific for an acute coronary syndrome.

AM: There are a large number of diseases that are now known to produce some elevation in troponin; not necessarily huge increases in troponin, but it's really thrown a huge monkey wrench into the concept that we can simply diagnose acute MI based on an elevated troponin. Importantly, we're also learning now that when somebody has a non-ACS cause of a troponin rise, in most cases you need to still worry about that elevation in troponin because even if it's not ACS, the elevation in troponin in most cases is still a good predictor of short-term and long-term adverse events. That applies for pulmonary emboli, sepsis, neurologic abnormalities, CHF, and likely for myopericarditis as well.

PR: I suspect that it does represent some damage to the myocardial cell, which is causing it to leak enzymes. Returning to our case, we have a patient with myocarditis deteriorating into heart failure. He does not appear to be failing because of peripheral resistance, but appears to be failing due to pump failure, with the disease affecting his ability to produce a normal cardiac output. What sort of therapeutic considerations should the emergency physician undertake as he prepares to get this patient admitted?

AM: The emergency physician needs to keep one word in his mind as he approaches this patient and that is, "supportive." One must be supportive in every possible way, because there's no other effective therapy for myopericarditis except supportive therapy. In regards to pump failure, probably dobutamine would be the best choice of medication if the patient continues to be hypotensive and has worsening heart failure. Diuretics might be useful as well. I would not use preload or afterload reducing medications, given that the patient is already hypotensive. I would consult cardiology as quickly as possible. There are some studies indicating that with very aggressive supportive therapy with pressors, or with an intraaortic balloon pump, these patients can survive with reasonable outcomes. If all else fails, some of these patients may benefit from cardiac transplantation, but there is no simple drug or combination of drugs that fixes these people. One can only try very aggressive supportive therapy, supporting the pump and supporting the oxygenation, and getting cardiology involved early.

PR: Is there any way of distinguishing infectious myocarditis from patients with a different etiology of myocarditis? The etiology appears to be infectious in this patient, probably viral, but what about the patients who have amyloidosis, or patients who present this way who have malignancies in their heart?

SG: The echocardiogram in this patient is potentially very useful in differentiating the etiology of the myocarditis. An echocardiogram may be useful for looking for valvular disease, or endocarditis as perhaps the

precipitant, which may take you out of the myocarditis category. An echocardiogram may demonstrate an atrial myxoma, lymphoma, or other tumors that may be a precipitant of acute LV dysfunction. A patient who presents without any evidence of an infectious process, without any other signs suggesting ischemia as its etiology, or some of the other more atypical causes of myocarditis, such as cocaine abuse, but with sudden onset of LV dysfunction, may need a biopsy. To review, the elements that would help me discern an etiology would be a careful history, an echocardiogram, and occasionally, when you have exhausted all else, some patients may require a myocardial biopsy to make a definitive diagnosis.

PR: Are there any metabolic causes of patients presenting like this? For example, we know older patients don't always present with all of the signs of acute thyrotoxicosis, but instead, present with cardiac disease.

AM: I'm not aware of thyroid disorders causing myocarditis. From a metabolic standpoint, there are some rheumatologic disorders that can produce myocarditis, as well as medications and hypersensitivity reactions, but by far the majority of patients have infectious causes.

SG: Sarcoidosis and lupus are associated with myocarditis, but I am also not aware of any thyroid etiologies.

PR: To switch directions, I find that patients with high resistance pulmonary edema often don't need intubation, and usually respond to lowering peripheral resistance and unloading the heart, and can recover pretty quickly, whereas the patients who have pump failure from coronary artery disease fare better if you intubate them early because the work of breathing is more than their failing heart can sustain. Would we be prudent to go ahead and intubate this patient with myocarditis? This is another form of pump failure. This patient is relatively stable now, but it seems likely that he's going to get worse before he gets better.

AM: We can probably expect that he will get worse, and he's already working hard to breathe. He's a 36-year-old healthy man, and so that might be why he appears to be somewhat "stable." He has a heart rate of 145 beats per minute, a classic tachycardia out of proportion to fever. He's tachypnic to 28 breaths per minute, already slightly hypotensive, and he's early in the time course of his disease. Taking some of the stress off the heart would probably be a good idea in this patient, and again, that would be a form of aggressive supportive therapy. Thus, it would be reasonable to intubate him. However, one, must be careful that when you intubate this hypotensive patient and increase intrathoracic pressure, you may drop the preload, dropping the blood pressure more. Hopefully that would be offset by giving concomitant inotropes.

SG: Once you determine this is more likely to be myocarditis in etiology rather than ischemic in etiology, then your likelihood of turning the patient around rapidly in the ED diminishes significantly, so even non-invasive ventilation, which is usually very effective for heart failure patients, is not going to be an appropriate solution in this patient; this makes intubation in a more emergent fashion particularly appropriate.

PR: Are there any precautions that we need to be concerned about for this patient's caregivers, as we would if he had, let's say, meningitis? He has a viral disease. What precautions, if any, are there?

SG: I'm not sure that he has a viral disease. I think that he has an infectious disease, but the infectious causes of myocarditis are myriad. There are bacterial etiologies, there are viral etiologies, and there are tapeworms that cause it. Chagas disease is one of the well-known etiologies of myocarditis. I think that you first have to get a better idea of what's the most likely infectious etiology. Does this patient come from a place where tuberculosis (TB) is endemic? Does this patient have a history of a positive purified protein derivative (PPD) test? If yes, you must worry that this may be the etiology of the myocarditis, and if that's the case, then the patient needs isolation, and very careful care on the part of the healthcare workers. If the patient describes having been exposed to people who are having similar, but benign viral syndrome symptoms, you might be able to be less cautions, and putting the patient in isolation may not be necessary.

AM: I would emphasize TB; immigrants from Africa and HIV-positive patients are at higher risk of having tuberculosis as the cause of myopericarditis. Within the past month, we've had a patient with methicillin-resistant *Staphylococcus aureus* (MRSA) myopericarditis with a large MRSA pericardial effusion and tamponade. I'm not sure it should change our ED management, but it is important to keep in mind that although viruses are the most common causes, there are some other diseases that may be associated with myocarditis. Thus, you may need to take respiratory or contact precautions.

Case resolutions

The patient was admitted to the coronary care unit and underwent urgent echocardiography, which demonstrated diffuse myocardial hypokinesis. An urgent cardiac catheterization was performed to rule out an acute coronary syndrome, given the positive troponin level. The catheterization demonstrated no coronary lesions, and so the patient continued supportive therapy for a presumed diagnosis of myocarditis. The patient's congestive heart failure and hemodynamic status worsened, requiring mechanical ventilation and the use of vasopressors on hospital day two, but he made a gradual recovery and was discharged from the hospital after 10 days.

Section III: Concepts

Background

Myocarditis is generally defined as an inflammation of the myocardium from a nonischemic cause. It is an acute infectious or immunological emergency that is uncommon, but which can have devastating or fatal consequences if untreated or misdiagnosed. Its initial presentation can be variable, and some patients present in severe distress and cardiogenic shock. Their initial presentation may be with acute chest pain, dyspnea or profound weakness. On the other hand, other patients may have milder symptoms and variable cardiac dysfunction. Yet another group of patients have predominately infectious symptoms (gastrointestinal or respiratory), and the clinician may ignore or overlook subtle cardiac symptoms, to the patients' peril. Long-term cardiac dysfunction and cardiomyopathy are not uncommon. Many patients exhibit a full recovery, while some go on to develop chronic cardiomyopathy; a small minority, however, progress to death or require cardiac transplantation. Histopathologically, myocarditis is characterized by diffuse or focal myocardial inflammation. In the industrialized world, it is a major cause of dilated cardiomyopathy and the need for cardiac transplantation.[1]

Epidemiology

Histological evidence of myocarditis has been found in up to 10% of general autopsies, but clinical myocarditis was not suspected in the majority of these patients.[2] The overall incidence of disease in the general population is unknown, in part due to the wide spectrum of clinical presentations, which ranges from asymptomatic patients to patients exhibiting severe hemodynamic instability and death. In the group of patients diagnosed clinically with myocarditis, and having had an endomyocardial biopsy, one-third have histologic evidence consistent with myocarditis. Of those patients who go on to develop dilated cardiomyopathy, 40% have microscopic confirmation.

The natural history of myocarditis in large populations is unknown, because there is no established noninvasive diagnostic test for confirmation, clinical manifestations are variable, the diagnosis can be challenging, and invasive endomyocardial biopsy is utilized in a minority of patients.[3] Men are slightly more predisposed to the development of myocarditis than women, and a fulminant presentation is seen more often in infants and children. Additionally, up to 20% of young patients with sudden cardiac death have been found to have histologic evidence of myocarditis.[4]

Etiologies of myocarditis

Acute myocarditis can be categorized into two broad categories (Table 15-1): infectious and noninfectious.[5,6] The infectious category is further broken down into viral, bacterial, fungal, and parasitic agents, while the non-infectious group can be subdivided into immunologic, post-irradiation, medication/chemical, and idiopathic. One study finds half the patients admitted to a European hospital have an infectious etiology, while the other half is idiopathic.[7] Of the infectious agents, viruses are the most common (Coxsackie's, adenovirus, Epstein-Barr, influenza A and B, parainfluenza, mumps). Additionally, bacteria (*mycoplasma, chlamydia* and *streptococcus*), postvaccination status, and medications are implicated as causative factors. Other infectious agents include other viruses (*cytomegalovirus*; rubella; rubeola; hepatitis A, B, and C; human immunodeficiency virus; varicella zoster; echovirus; and poliovirus)[8]

In the industrialized world, viruses are the most common cause of myocarditis when an etiology can be found, of which the enteroviruses (Coxsackie A and B) are the most frequently encountered. Coxsackie B virus is ubiquitous, with at least half of the general population thought to be seropositive.[9] Seroepidemiologic studies suggest the majority of cases of Coxsackie B virus infection are subclinical; have a benign, self-limited course; and have seasonal peaks in the summer and fall.

Bacterial causes of myocarditis include Lyme disease, *legionella, mycoplasma, diphtheriae,* tuberculosis, *chlamydia,* and *streptococcus.* In Lyme disease, a tick-borne infection transmitting the spirochete *Borrelia burgdorferi,* patients commonly present with an erythema chronicum migrans rash and rheumatologic symptoms; fewer than 10% of patients develop myocarditis, which can be manifested with atrioventricular blocks and other conduction abnormalities. Diphtheria myocarditis occurs in two thirds of patients infected with *Corynebacterium diphtheria,* but is clinically significant in only 10% of patients.

Immunocompromised patients, whether secondary to HIV, cancer, or postcardiac transplant, show a higher rate of clinical and subclinical myocarditis; the infectious agents most often seen include *Toxoplasma gondii* and *cytomegalovirus.* Travelers returning from overseas can develop myocarditis secondary to parasites causing Chagas disease, trichinosis, and echinococcosis. Worldwide, Chagas disease is the leading cause of myocarditis and dilatated cardiomyopathy. Trichinosis can occur after ingestion of the nematode *Trichinella spiralis,* found in undercooked meat, especially pork. Echinococcosis develops after ingestion of the tapeworm *Echinococcus granulosus.*

Noninfectious etiologies or secondary causes of myocarditis, such as cardiotoxins and collagen vascular disorders, usually occur in older patients taking multiple medications. Immunologic etiologies can be subdivided into postviral and postmyocardial injury syndromes, connective tissue diseases, and inflammatory bowel disease. Connective tissue diseases implicated in myocarditis include systemic lupus erythematosis, rheumatoid arthritis, sarcoidosis, churgstrauss syndrome, acute rheumatic fever, sjogren's syndrome, and kawasaki disease in children.

Several medications and chemicals have also been associated with development of myocarditis. Cocaine, an illicit cardiotoxin, can cause myocyte damage by different mechanisms. The chemotherapeutic drug doxorubicin has been implicated in left ventricular dysfunction and myocarditis.

Table 15-1. Causative agents of myocarditis

INFECTIOUS			

Virus

Coxsackie	Parainfluenza	Herpesvirus	Rabies
Adenovirus	Human Immunodeficiency	Varicella zoster	Echovirus
Epstein-Barr	Virus	Rubella	Polio
Influenza	Mumps	Rubeola	Hepatitis A, B, C, and D
	Cytomegalovirus		

Bacteria

Borrelia burgdorferi (Lyme disease)	*Mycobacterium tuberculosis*
Legionella pneumophila	*Chlamydia pneumoniae*
Mycoplasma pneumoniae	*Streptococcus*
Corynebacterium diphtheriae	

Parasite

Toxoplasmosis	Trichinosis
Chagas disease	Echinococcosis

Fungal

NONINFECTIOUS			

Immunological

Vasculitis/Connective Tissue	**Inflammatory Bowel Disease**	**Postmyocardial injury**	**Postviral**
Systemic lupus erythematosis	Crohn's disease	Churg-Strauss syndrome	Acute rheumatic fever
Rheumatoid arthritis	Ulcerative colitis	Sarcoidosis	Sjogren's syndrome
			Kawasaki disease

Postirradiation

Medication/chemical
Cocaine
Doxorubicin
Idiopathic

Pathophysiology

It is believed that myocardial injury from myocarditis occurs via three main mechanisms. In the beginning, in the acute phase (0–3 days), cellular injury occurs from direct invasion of the virus and its replication. Myocyte antigens are released and cytokine induction follows with the release of tumor necrosis factor-alpha, interferons, and interleukins.[10] The body's immune response can limit the degree of viremia, but if the response is insufficient, the virus may not be eliminated, and further damage to myocardium can occur.[11-13] Next, in the subacute phase (4–14 days), destruction of cardiac tissue occurs due to host immune response to the infectious agent. Molecular mimicry plays a big role here, with the similarity of the antigens on viral pathogen and myocytes; an immune response to the former would cause damage to the latter. Viral-induced myocyte damage can provoke release of intracellular proteins and trigger a host immune cascade in a genetically predisposed individual.[14] Lastly, in the chronic phase, toxicity occurs from exogenous chemicals or endotoxins produced by the agent.[15] In neonates, damage is thought to be related to direct cytotoxicity from the offending virus, whereas in adults, an exaggerated host response plays a larger role.[8]

Myocarditis has been linked to the development of chronic dilatated cardiomyopathy, and autoantigens are often seen at this stage. This has led to the hypothesis that cardiomyopathy postmyocarditis is due to an abnormal host immune response, resulting from either shared antigens or molecular mimicry.[16]

The microscopic/pathologic diagnosis of myocarditis requires evidence of myocyte degeneration or death with a surrounding inflammatory response, such as myocyte fiber necrosis with an infiltrate of neutrophils and monocytes. Gross examination of the heart often reveals myocardial hemorrhage with degeneration or necrosis, and the subendocardium and valves are spared. Biventricular dilatation is often seen, with the left greater than right. Scar tissue is produced after the acute injury, and this reduces cardiac contractility and ejection fraction. The conduction system may be involved, with resulting brady- and tachydysrhythmias.[17,18]

Initial presentation: History and physical

In the early stages of viral myocarditis, the majority of patients often have nonspecific flu-like complaints.[19] Half of the patients will note a recent upper respiratory or gastrointestinal infection.[20] Many cases are probably subclinical and asymptomatic, and the cardiac symptoms and signs are overshadowed by the systemic manifestations of the viral infection (i.e., cough, dyspnea, dizziness, weakness, fever, emesis, diarrhea, and myalgias). In general, onset of cardiorespiratory symptoms usually appear 7–10 days after infectious complaints develop, and include dyspnea, orthopnea, paroxysmal nocturnal dyspnea, palpitations, syncope, and pedal edema. Congestive heart failure and dysrhythmia are the most frequent presentations in admitted patients. Pleuritic chest pain is common when there is pericardial involvement, and patients may additionally complain of fatigue, decreased exercise capacity, and palpitations secondary to tachydysrhythmias or heart block.[20] Some patients may describe a substernal chest pressure or ache, similar to patients with an acute coronary syndrome.[21] Myocarditis is frequently a diagnosis of exclusion.[15]

On physical examination, careful note of vital signs should be made. Abnormal vital signs include fever (found in half of the cases), tachycardia, tachypnea, and hypotension.[3] Traditional teaching is that tachycardia disproportionate to the temperature or toxicity should be a clinical clue to the diagnosis. The cardiac examination may be normal, or exhibit rales, an S3 gallop, or a pericardial friction rub.[22] Failure is a common manifestation of myocarditis, as are dysrhythmias, and some patients will present in cardiogenic shock.

In children, physical examination findings include grunting respirations and intercostal retractions. Some will have wheezing. On cardiac examination, an S3 gallop and rales may be heard. Infants often have a fulminant course characterized by fever, cyanosis, respiratory distress, tachycardia, and cardiac failure.[22] New-onset wheezing in a child should prompt the clinician to obtain a chest radiograph to exclude either foreign body in the airway or pulmonary edema.

Special presentations

A history of a recent tick bite, arthritis, the classic rash (erythema chronicum migrans), or fever, especially when seen together with conduction abnormalities (atrioventricular blocks), should make one consider a Lyme myocarditis.[23] Myocarditis usually develops within 2–4 weeks of onset of symptoms.

Mucocutaneous lymph node syndrome, also known as Kawasaki disease, is an illness that affects young children. Four out of five features are required for diagnosis: (1) fever greater than five days duration, (2) conjunctivitis without exudate, (3) lymphadenopathy (4) erythematous exanthem with subsequent desquamation, and (5) changes in lips and oral mucous membranes. It is thought to be caused by an autoimmune response to an infectious agent or toxin. Patients can develop myocarditis as well as other complications, including myocardial infarction, dysrthymias, CHF, and coronary artery aneurysm formation. Look for the diagnosis in children with prolonged fever, rash and conjunctivitis.

Testing in myocarditis

Diagnostic studies can assist in confirming a diagnosis of myocarditis (Table 15-2). Commonly ordered tests include an electrocardiogram (EKG), chest radiograph, and laboratory tests, including serum cardiac markers and echocardiography. Additional specialized testing studies are nuclear medicine imaging, MRI, viral titers, coronary angiography, and endomyocardial biopsy.

Table 15-2. Diagnostic studies for evaluation of myocarditis

Diagnostic Study	Findings
Basic Tests	
EKG	Sinus tachycardia, atrioventricular and intraventricular blocks, ventricular tachycardia, nonspecific ST-segment/T-wave changes, prolonged QT interval
	ST-segment elevation and depression
Chest radiograph	Normal
	Cardiomegaly with clear lung fields
	Pulmonary edema
	Redistribution of blood flow (cephalization)
	Interstitial edema
	Alveolar edema
	Pleural and pericardial effusions
	Right ventricular failure
	Right atrial enlargement
	Prominent azygos vein
	Superior vena cava enlargement
Serum cardiac markers (troponin and CPK)	Elevation
Other laboratory tests	Inflammation (ESR, CRP, platelet count, WBC), multiorgan failure (AST/ALT, creatinine), poor systemic perfusion (lactate)
Echocardiogram	Multichamber dilatation, reduced left ventricular ejection fraction, pericardial fluid, wall motion hypokinesis (focal or global)
Additional Tests	
Cardiac MRI	Diffuse inflammation, involves epicardial surface preferentially, can distinguish myocarditis from AMI
Nuclear medicine imaging	Indium-111: detects diffuse myocardial necrosis. Used with resting stress thallium showing normal perfusion, can rule out AMI in favor of myocarditis
Viral/serologic testing	Low yield, not helpful in the ED
Coronary angiography	Normal coronary vessels
Endomyocardial biopsy	Dallas Criteria: lymphocytic infiltration with myocyte injury or death

Abbreviations: AST/ALT, aspartate aminotransferase/alanine aminotransferase; CPK, creatine phosphokinase; CRP, C-reactive protein; ESR, erythrocyte sedimentation rate; WBC, white blood cell count; ED, emergency department.

Common EKG abnormalities include sinus tachycardia (Figure 15-1) and low voltage. Other dysrhythmias seen include atrial fibrillation with bundle branch block, complete atrioventricular block with narrow (Figure 15-2) or wide QRS complex escape rhythm, and ventricular tachycardia. Additional changes can include a prolonged QT interval or a pseudoinfarction pattern with the following abnormalities: ST-segment elevation or depression, T-wave inversions, and pathologic Q-waves.[24] Twenty percent of patients develop a left bundle branch block.

When present, ST-elevations are convex (dome-shaped) mimicking acute myocardial infarction, though generally the magnitude of the ST-elevations is less than 5 mm. There can sometimes be reciprocal changes. Additionally, new Q waves may appear, and there may be PR depression. Prolongation of the PR interval may also occur. Cardiac dysrhythmias are common (up to 60%), and more often ventricular than supraventricular.[3] Heart block is also common, but usually transient, and rarely requires permanent pacemaker placement.

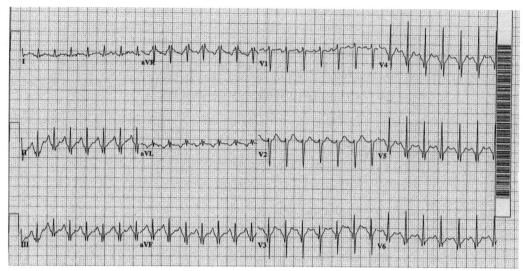

Figure 15.1 Extreme sinus tachycardia.

When patients present with myopericarditis, their EKGs are more typical of acute pericarditis, and evolve through four stages. Stage One is notable for generalized ST-segment elevation and PR depression (Figure 15-3), followed by resolution of these changes and T-wave flattening in Stage Two. Stage Three is characterized by T-wave inversion (usually in the same leads in which ST-elevations had been present in Stage One), followed by normalization of inversions and return to baseline in Stage Four. The progression through the various stages is variable and unpredictable, taking days to weeks. One may also see low voltage and electrical alternans if a large pericardial effusion is present.

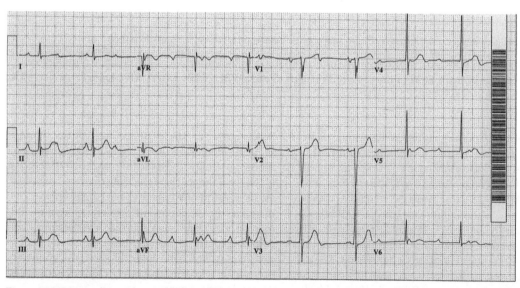

Figure 15.2 Myocarditis with complete heart block.

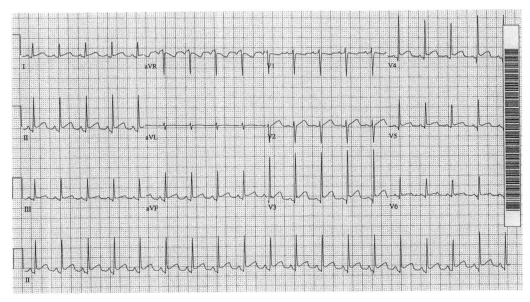

Figure 15.3 Myopericarditis.

Chest radiography in myocarditis patients may be entirely normal or show cardiac enlargement, pulmonary venous blood flow redistribution, interstitial and alveolar edema, and pleural and pericardial effusions.[25] The chest radiograph may show a normal cardiac silhouette with pulmonary edema. The X-ray findings of right ventricular failure include right atrial enlargement, prominent azygos vein, and superior vena cava enlargement. A normal chest radiograph, however, does not exclude the diagnosis.[26]

Laboratory abnormalities include elevations of cardiac enzymes, which have been reported in both myocarditis and pericarditis. Elevations in cardiac troponin are more common than CK-MB in biopsy-proven myocarditis.[27,28] The degree of troponin elevation seems to be related to the extent of myocardial inflammation, and does not carry an adverse prognosis as it does in ACS.[29,30] Despite this, troponin levels may be normal in half of the patients with biopsy-proven myocarditis.[27,28] The white blood cell count, platelet count, Erythrocyte Sedimentation Rate (ESR), and C-Reactive Protein (CRP) are non-specific markers of inflammation, and are often elevated. An elevated serum lactate can confirm poor perfusion in a patient in cardiogenic shock, and elevated transaminases and serum creatinine are found in multiple organ failure.

Echocardiography can be helpful, but is often neither specific nor diagnostic. It can be used to document the presence of a pericardial effusion (uncommon in acute myocarditis, more common in pericarditis), ventricular systolic dysfunction (generally global, but may be segmental), decreased ejection fraction, and multichamber enlargement. Specific findings on echo include increased echogenicity/brightness of the pericardium due to fibrin deposition and inflammation of the pericardial layers.[3] Left ventricular thrombi are often seen. Additionally, right ventricle (RV) systolic dysfunction is an independent predictor of death or need for cardiac transplantation in acute myocarditis.[31] This test is becoming increasingly available in EDs as more emergency physicians perform bedside echocardiograms. A limited or focused bedside echocardiogram can assess the presence or absence of a pericardial effusion, as well as global left ventricular function.[32-34]

An additional imaging modality, cardiac MRI, has the advantage of being able to distinguish a myocardial infarction from myocarditis. The myocardial infarction pattern involves enhancement of the subendocardium, which becomes transmural in severe cases, since necrosis begins in the subendocardium and extends towards the epicardium. It is also limited to coronary perfusion territory. Acute myocarditis, on the other hand, involves the epicardium, the mid-wall of the left ventricular free wall, and the intraventricular septum.[35,36] The MRI abnormalities can persist for at least 1 month after the onset of symptoms. Overall diagnostic sensitivity is 86% with 95% specificity in one study.[37] An MRI may be difficult to obtain through the ED, and is not suitable in the unstable patient or in a patient with ferromagnetic contraindications.

Nuclear medicine imaging is another specialized diagnostic modality. Gallium-67, one type of nuclear medicine imaging, is considered to be an excellent imaging study for chronic inflammation, but is not specific for an acute myocarditis.[5] However, its use has decreased over time due to a lack of specificity. With Indium-111, antimyosin antibodies bind specifically to exposed myosin in damaged myocytes, and in one study this test has a sensitivity of 100% and specificity of 58%.[38] It can be used to detect ongoing myocardial necrosis in myocarditis, acute MI, dilatated cardiomyopathy, and cardiac transplantation rejection.[39] Antimyosin scans, used together with resting thallium imaging, can distinguish myocarditis from acute MI. Acute myocarditis is suggested when antimyosin scans show myocardial inflammation in the presence of normal perfusion on thallium scans.[40]

Viral titers can be helpful, but the yield is low, and not helpful to the emergency physician in the acute phase of illness.[41] A small proportion of patients show a significant rise in titers for Coxsackie B virus, and a fourfold rise in enteroviral IgG titers over a 4-week period helps identify an acute viral infection.[42]

In clinical cases where ACS is a major differential or strong consideration, coronary angiography can be useful to exclude ACS, as the young acute myocarditis patient would be expected to have no clinically significant occlusions. Endomyocardial biopsy has been considered to be the "gold standard," but even it has variable specificity and sensitivity and is available only at specialized centers.[43] It was pioneered by Richardson at King's College Hospital (London) in 1974.[44] The Dallas Criteria for the histological diagnosis of myocarditis were introduced in 1986, and the biopsy specimen criteria specifies lymphocytic infiltration associated with myocyte injury in the absence of ischemia.[45] Unfortunately, it underestimates the incidence of myocarditis because of patchy involvement of the myocardium and large intraobserver variability.[45,46] Histologic criteria for myocarditis are

present in only 5–30% of patients with a clinically suspected myocarditis, 41% of patients with an acute dilatated cardiomyopathy, and up to 63% of patients with a chronic dilatated cardiomyopathy. Patients who have virus present on biopsy tissue have a much worse prognosis.[47]

Molecular genetic probes, such as polymerase chain reaction (PCR), are used to supplement endomyocardial biopsy. The preferred biopsy method is a transvenous endomyocardial biopsy of the right ventricular septum, which carries a 1/250 risk of perforation, and 1/1000 risk of death when performed with experienced hands.[48] Given the risks of biopsy and limited benefits, it tends to be used selectively in patients with significant myocardial involvement and severe left ventricular dysfunction who are not responsive to conventional medical management, for example prior to cardiac transplantation.[49,50]

Treatment of myocarditis

The treatment of acute myocarditis in the ED is generally supportive, and includes stabilization of abnormal vital signs and the treatment of acute congestive heart failure. There is general consensus for bed rest, and avoidance of physical activity for these patients since exercise can worsen dysrthymias.[8] These patients should all be placed in a monitored bed where aggressive resuscitation can be carried out, as nontoxic patients may deteriorate rapidly. Additionally, myocarditis patients show more ectopy at rest, and are at high risk for dysrhythmias. Immediate interventions required may range from providing supplemental oxygenation to securing an airway with endotracheal intubation and mechanical ventilation. Perfusion status needs to be evaluated, and if inadequate, increasing preload with small fluid boluses of normal saline, and the use of vasopressors and inotropic support may be required. Acute pulmonary edema should be treated in the standard manner, assuming the patient is not hypotensive. Use of preload agents such as nitroglycerin (oral, topical, or parenteral) and intravenous furosemide is encouraged. Afterload reducers may be used if the patient is hypertensive: angiotensin converting enzyme inhibitors (orally or parenterally). The bedside echocardiogram looking for the presence of a pericardial effusion may be invaluable in certain cases, as a large pericardial effusion or signs of tamponade on echocardiography can signal the need for acute intervention with pericardiocentesis. Additional measures, such as correcting anemia, treating dysrhythmias, and reducing fevers, can help by decreasing myocardial oxygen demand.

For those patients presenting in extremis and cardiogenic shock, aggressive cardiac and pulmonary resuscitation measures can be life saving. In addition to the measures mentioned above, these patients may require ventricular assist devices, intraaortic balloon counterpulsation and even cardiopulmonary bypass as a bridge while awaiting recovery or cardiac transplantation. These devices have been used successfully over extended periods of time (up to 70 days), allowing time for some patients to recover without the need for cardiac transplantation.[51] The decision to initiate heparin therapy is controversial, needs to be individualized to each patient, and is usually made by the consultant cardiologist following the results of a bedside echocardiogram. On the one hand, myocarditis patients have compromised left ventricular function and are at higher risk for thromboembolic complications. On the other hand, they are also at risk for hemopericardium with cardiac tamponade.

High dose gamma globulin (IVIG) therapy

Additional therapies may be utilized in patients once they have been admitted; they generally do not have a role in the acute resuscitation in the ED. These include immunologic agents (including antiviral agents), immunosuppressants, and immunoglobulin. Antiviral agents have been utilized in the early stage of acute myocarditis following studies showing replicating enterovirus RNA in the myocardium.[52,53] There is some evidence of benefit in uncontrolled studies using immunosuppressive therapy in the later stages of myocarditis, but the National Institutes of Health (NIH)-sponsored multicenter trial for myocarditis treatment does not establish benefit in using immunosuppressive therapy; however, using cyclosporine or azathioprine has been studied in a pediatric population, and is associated with improvement in LV function and increased survival after a year.[20,53–55] Nevertheless, a systematic review concludes there is insufficient data to recommend routine IVIG therapy in patients with acute myocarditis, and another systemic review shows no benefit to immunosuppresive therapy in children.[56,57]

The use of corticosteroids in the setting of viral myocarditis has been found to be an independent risk factor for recurrences, since they promote viral replication, and therefore, they are not generally recommended.[58,59] A Cochrane review shows no evidence of benefit from use of corticosteroids for viral myocarditis.[60] Nevertheless, there are case reports that show a benefit in postvaccinal myocarditis and inflammatory myopathy-related myocarditis, which are both thought to be autoimmune mediated.[61–64]

Specific therapies in certain populations

Patients with Lyme myocarditis may require atropine, isoproterenol, and cardiac pacing for treatment of conduction abnormalities. Antibiotic therapy is also indicated (ceftriaxone, tetracycline, or erythromycin). A tapering course of corticosteroids is also recommended. Children with Kawasaki disease will require high-dose aspirin therapy, as well as treatment with intravenous gamma globulin.

Prognosis

The clinical course of myocarditis is variable, and the prognosis is difficult to determine upon initial presentation. The majority of patients recover within weeks to months following diagnosis.[8,65] Most of the survivors are symptom-free, and do not require further medical care; some need ongoing medical therapy, and a proportion of those will require cardiac transplantation.

An initial presentation involving acute CHF or dysrhythmias portends a higher mortality. In these patients, the 1-year mortality ranges between 15 and 20%; at 4 years, mortality rates of 50% are found despite optimal management in the NIH myocarditis trial.[66] The ejection fraction and RV function 1 year after presentation may be the best predictor of subsequent survival.[54] Some patients develop a fulminant, rapidly progressing form of myocarditis. Prognostic factors associated with a fulminant course of myocarditis include prolongation of QRS complex and depressed left ventricular ejection fraction. These factors predict inhospital mortality of 45%.[67]

A clinicopathologic classification was developed by Lieberman et al.[68] subdividing patients into different disease course categories and prognosis based on the biopsy and clinical presentation. Four categories are described: fulminant, acute, chronic active, and chronic persistent.

1 Fulminant: these patients have abrupt onset of symptoms and usually present with cardiogenic shock and pulmonary edema. Disease progression is rapid, with either a full recovery or death within 30 days. Endomyocardial biopsy typically shows widespread inflammation with necrosis.

2 Active: these patients have a less distinct onset of symptoms, with gradual progression and slow recovery. They often have persistent left ventricular dysfunction, and some patients develop dilatated cardiomyopathy. Biopsy shows inflammation with scattered necrosis.

3 Chronic active: onset of symptoms is indistinct and there is a slow progressive course leading to dilatated cardiomyopathy and LV dysfunction. Biopsy typically shows a lesser degree of inflammation.

4 Chronic persistent: these patients have atypical or few symptoms, and minimal or no LV dysfunction. Biopsy shows a mild persistent inflammation.

Disposition of patients with myocarditis

All patients with suspected myocarditis should be admitted to a monitored hospital bed; in most cases, this should be a critical care unit. Invasive monitoring with central venous catheters, arterial line catheters, and pulmonary artery catheters may be required, depending on the clinical status of the patient and whether vasopressors and inotropic medications are required. A multispecialty approach to these patients is often needed, and consultations from critical care, cardiology, cardiovascular surgery, and infectious disease physicians should be obtained at the discretion of the admitting physician. Complications of myocarditis include ventricular dysrhythmia, LV dysfunction, and cardiac failure.

Summary

The first major challenge is to consider myocarditis in the differential diagnosis of these patients, especially if the patient is young and previously healthy. These patients will be seen intermixed with the large numbers of patients being evaluated for chest pain or viral syndrome, and it is easy to overlook the possibility of myocarditis in the differential diagnosis. Additionally, these patients often have pronounced infectious respiratory or gastrointestinal symptoms, and it takes an astute clinician to tease out historical features of CHF (exertional dyspnea, nonproductive cough, weakness). Abnormal vital signs, especially tachycardia, are red flags, and patients (especially infants and children) with tachycardia out of proportion to fever should be suspected of having myocarditis.

The differential diagnosis in these patients includes acute coronary syndrome (unstable angina or acute MI), acute pulmonary edema, pulmonary embolism, pneumonia, aortic dissection, and esophageal rupture. Even if the diagnosis is correctly and appropriately considered, the next challenge in these patients is to differentiate myocarditis from ACS, as both sets of patients may have severe chest pain, EKG changes, elevated cardiac biomarkers, and congestive heart failure. Features that may distinguish myocarditis from ischemia include younger age and an absence of risk factors for coronary artery disease. The EKG abnormalities in myocarditis are often diffuse, rather than limited to coronary anatomy. They should also not evolve with ongoing chest pain, as one may expect with ACS. Echocardiographic abnormalities are often global, rather than segmental as seen in ACS.[69] Nevertheless, the EKG findings in myocarditis may be localized to coronary artery anatomy, and the echocardiography may show segmental wall-motion abnormalities, making differentiation of myocarditis from ACS very difficult clinically.[70]

Normal coronary angiography in the presence of an elevated cardiac troponin should prompt consideration of myocarditis rather than coronary vasospasm. Up to 78% of patients who present with possible ACS, and who have a normal coronary angiogram, have evidence of myocarditis on further imaging.[40] Antimyosin scintigraphy (Indium-111 scanning) can be employed. Myocarditis is characterized by a faint, diffuse uptake of antimyosin antibody caused by widespread myocardial necrosis. In contrast, acute MI is seen as an intense, localized uptake of antibody in the region of the occluded artery. A normal antimyosin scan excludes both acute MI and myocarditis.[71] When used with the results of a normal resting perfusion scan, a positive antimyosin scan is diagnostic of acute myocarditis. If there is still clinical doubt, a cardiac MRI and an endomyocardial biopsy may be employed.

Section IV: Decision making

There are three major pitfalls clinicians should try to avoid:

- Failure to seek the diagnosis in a patient presenting with mainly infectious symptoms or new onset CHF in an otherwise young or healthy patient in the setting of a viral syndrome.
- Failure to admit to the hospital a well-appearing patient with suspected myocarditis, instead arranging an outpatient follow-up and testing. This occurs when the clinician does not appreciate the rapid downhill course some myocarditis patients can take when complications develop, which can include dysrhythmias, thromboembolism, and cardiogenic shock.
- Administering the wrong therapy: giving a myocarditis patient thrombolytics for an EKG with a pseudoinfarction pattern. This could be potentially catastrophic, as these patients are at higher risk for hemopericardium and tamponade.

References

1 Hosenpud J, Novick R, Bennet L. The registry of the International Society for Heart and Lung Transplantation: thirteenth official report. *J Heart Lung Transplant.* 1996;15:655–674.

2 Ledford D. Immunologic aspects of cardiovascular disease. *JAMA.* 1992;268:2923–2929.

3 Imazio M, Trinchero R. Myopericarditis: etiology, management and prognosis. *Int J Cardiol.* 2008;127:17–26.

4 Herskowitz A, Ansari A. Myocarditis. In Braunwald E, ed: *Atlas of Heart Diseases.* Philadephia; Current Medicine: 1995:9.2–9.24.

5 O'Connell J. Diagnosis and medical treatment of inflammatory cardiomyopathy. In: Topol E, ed. *Textbook of Cardiovascular Medicine.* Philadelphia; Lippincott–Raven: 1998:2309–2336.

6 Baughman K, Hruban R. Treatment of myocarditis. In Smith T, ed. *Cardiovascular Therapeutics: A Companion to Braunwald's Heart Disease.* Philadelphia; W.B. Saunders: 1996:243–253.

7 Karjalainen J, Heikkila J, Nieminen M, et al. Viral myocarditis. *Rev Infect Dis.* 1991;13:951–956.

8 See D, Tilles J. Viral myocarditis. *Rev Infect Dis.* 1991;13:951–956.

9 O'Connell J, Henkin R, Robinson J, et al. Gallium–67 imaging in patients with dilated cardiomyopathy and biopsy–proven myocarditis. *Circulation.* 1984;70:58–62.

10 Kawai C. From myocarditis to cardiomyopathy: mechanisms for inflammation and cell death—learning from the past for the future. *Circulation.* 1999;99:1091–1100.

11 Klingel K, Hohenadl C, Canu A, et al. Ongoing enterovirus–induced myocarditis is associated with persistent heart muscle infection: quantitative analysis of virus replication, tissue damage, and inflammation. *Proc Natl Acad Sci USA.* 1992;89:314–318.

12 Wessely R, Henke A, Zell R, Kandolf R, Knowlton K. Low–level expression of a mutant coxsackie viral cDNA induces a myocytopathic effect in culture: An approach to the study of enteroviral persistence in cardiac myocytes. *Circulation.* 1998;98:450–457.

13 Wessely R, Klingel K, Santana L, et al. Transgenic expression of replication–restricted enteroviral genomes in heart muscle induces defective excitation–contraction coupling and dilated cardiomyopathy. *J Clin Invest.* 1998;102:1444–1453.

14 Caforio A, Goldman J, Haven A, et al. Circulating cardiac–specific auto–antibodies as markers of autoimmunity in clinical and biopsy–proven myocarditis. *Eur Heart J.* 1997;18:270–275.

15 Olinde K, O'Connell J. Inflammatory heart disease: pathogenesis, clinical manifestations, and treatment of myocarditis. *Ann Rev Med.* 1994;45:481–490.

16 Sole M, Liu P. Viral myocarditis: a paradigm for understanding the pathogenesis and treatment of dilated cardiomyopathy. *J Am Coll Cardiol.* 1993;22:99A–105A.

17 Woodruff J. Viral myocarditis: a review. *Am J Pathol.* 1980;101:425–484.

18 Wegner N, Abelmann W, Roberts W. Myocarditis. In: Hurst J, ed. *The Heart.* 6th edition. New York: McGraw–Hill; 1986.

19 Kearney M, Cotton J, Richardson P, Shah A. Viral myocarditis and dilated cardiomyopathy: mechanisms, manifestations, and management. *Postgrad Med J.* 2001;77:4–10.

20 Mason J, O'Connell J, Herskowitz A. A clinical trial of immunosuppressive therapy for myocarditis. *N Engl J Med.* 1995;333:269–275.

21 Matias D, Luis L, Felix Z, et al. Acute myocarditis: retrospective analysis in 28 patients. First Virtual Congress of Cardiology 2000. Available at: http://pcvc.sminter.ar/cvirtual/tlibres/tnn2741/tnn2741.htm. Accessed July 28, 2011.

22 Singer J, Isaacman D, Bell L. The wheezer that wasn't. *Pediatr Emerg Care.* 1992;8:107–109.

23 Sobera C, Rubin D, Baum S, et al. Diagnosis and treatment of Lyme carditis. *Primary Cardiol.* 1991;17:28–33.

24 Wiles HB, Gillette PC, Harley RA. Cardiomyopathy and myocarditis in children with ventricular ectopic rhythm. *J Am Coll Cardiol.* 1992;20:359–362.

25 Brady W, Ferguson J, Ullman E, Perron A. Myocarditis: emergency department recognition and management. *Emerg Med Clin North Am.* 2004;22:865–885.

26 Brady W, Aufderheide T, Kaplan P. Cardiovascular chest radiography. In: Reisdorff E, Schwartz D, Williamson B, eds. *Emergency Radiology.* New York: McGraw–Hill; 1999: 479–508.

27 Smith S, Ladenson J, Mason J, Jaffe A. Elevations of cardiac troponin I associated with myocarditis. Experimental and clinical correlates. *Circulation.* 1997;95:163–168.

28 Lauer B, Niederau C, Kuhl U, et al. Cardiac troponin T in patients with clinically suspected myocarditis. *J Am Coll Cardiol.* 1997;30:1354–1359.

29 Imazio M, Cecchi E, Demichelis B, et al. Myopericarditis versus viral or idiopathic acute pericarditis. Frequency, clinical clues to diagnosis, and prognosis. *Heart.* 2008;94(4):498–501.

30 Imazio M, Demichelis B, Cecchi E, et al. Cardiac troponin I in acute pericarditis. *J Am Coll Cardiol.* 2001;87:1326–1328.

31 Mendes L, Dec G, Picard M, et al. Right ventricular dysfunction: an independent predictor of adverse outcome in patients with myocarditis. *Am Heart J.* 1994;128:301–307.

32 Moore C, Rose G, Tayal V, et al. Determination of left ventricular function by emergency physician echocardiography of hypotensive patients. *Acad Emerg Med.* 2002;9(3):186–193.

33 Randazzo M, Snoey E, Levitt M, Binder K. Accuracy of emergency physician assessment of left ventricular ejection fraction and central venous pressure using echocardiography. *Acad Emerg Med.* 2003;10(9):973–977.

34 Ciccone T, Grossman S. Cardiac Ultrasound. *Emerg Med Clin North Am.* 2004;22:621–640.

35 Mahrholdt H, Wagner A, Deluigi C, et al. Presentation, patterns of myocardial damage, and clinical course of viral myocarditis. *Circulation.* 2006;114:1581–1590.

36 Kuhl U, Lauer B, Souvatzoglu M, Vosberg H, Schultheiss H. Antimyosin scintigraphy and immunohistologic analysis of endomyocardial biopsy in patients with clinically myocarditis–evidence of myocardial cell damage and inflammation in the absence of histologic signs of myocarditis. *J Am Coll Cardiol.* 1998;32:1371–1376.

37 Liu P, Yan A. Cardiovascular magnetic resonance for the diagnosis of acute myocarditis. Prospects for detecting myocardial inflammation. *J Am Coll Cardiol.* 2005;45:1823–1825.

38 Yasuda T, Palacios I, Dec G, et al. Indium 111–monoclonal antimyosin antibody imaging in the diagnosis of acute myocarditis. *Circulation.* 1987;76:306–311.

39 Matsuura H, Palacios IF, Dec GW, et al. Intraventricular conduction abnormalities in patients with clinically

suspected myocarditis are associated with myocardial necrosis. *Am Heart J.* 1994;127:1290–1297.

40 Sarda L, Colin P, Boccara F, et al. Myocarditis in patients with clinical presentation of myocardial infarction and normal coronary angiograms. *J Am Coll Cardiol.* 1992;20:85–89.

41 Ramamurthy S, Talwar K, Goswami K, et al. Clinical profile of biopsy proven idiopathic myocarditis. *Int J Cardiol.* 1993;41:225–232.

42 Jouriles NJ. Pericardial and Myocardial Disease. In *Rosen's Emergency Medicine: Concepts and Clinical Practice.* 5th edition. Mosby, Inc. St Louis; 2002:1138–1140.

43 Lambert K, Isaac D, Hendel R. Myocarditis masquerading as ischemic heart disease: the diagnostic utility of antimyosin imaging. *Cardiology.* 1993;82:415–422.

44 Richardson P. King's endomyocardial bioptome. *Lancet.* 1974;i:660–661.

45 Aretz H, Billingham M, Edwards W, et al. Myocarditis: a histopathologic definition and classification. *Am J Cardiovasc Pathol.* 1987;1:3–14.

46 Shanes J, Gahli J, Billingham M, et al. Interobserver variability in the pathologic interpretation of endomyocardial biopsy results. *Circulation.* 1987;75:401–405.

47 Why HJ, Meany BT, Richardson PJ, et al. Clinical and prognostic significance of detection of enteroviral RNA in the myocardium of patients with myocarditis of dilated cardiomyopathy. *Circulation.* 1994;89:2582–2589.

48 Wu L, Lapeyre A, Cooper L. Current role of endomyocardial biopsy in the management of patients with dilated cardiomyopathy and myocarditis. *Mayo Clin Proc.* 2001;76:1030–1038.

49 Cassimatis D, Atwood J, Engler R, et al. Smallpox vaccination and myopericarditis: a clinical review. *J Am Coll Cardiol.* 2004;43:1503–1510.

50 Magnani J, Dec G. Myocarditis: current trends in diagnosis and treatment. *Circulation.* 2006;113:876–890.

51 Morishima I, Sassa H, Sone T, et al. A case of fulminant myocarditis rescued by long–term percutaneous cardiopulmonary support. *Jpn Circ J.* 1994;58:433–438.

52 Kandolf R, Klingel K, Mertsching H, et al. Molecular studies on enteroviral heart disease patterns of acute and persistent infections. *Eur Heart J.* 1991;12:49–55.

53 Rose N, Neumann D, Herskowitz A. Autoimmune myocarditis: concepts and questions. *Immunol Today.* 1991;12:253–255.

54 Talwar K, Goswami K, Chopra P. Immunosuppressive therapy in inflammatory myocarditis: long–term follow–up. *Int J Cardiol.* 1992;34:157–166.

55 Drucker NA, Colan DS, Lewis AB, et al. Gamma globulin treatment of acute myocarditis in the pediatric population. *Circulation.* 1994;89:252–257.

56 Robinson J, Hartling L, Crumley E, Vandermeer B, Klassen T. A systematic review of intravenous of intravenous gamma globulin for therapy of acute myocarditis. *BMC Cardiovasc Disord.* 2005;5:12.

57 Hia C, Yp W, Tai B, Quek S. Immunosuppressive therapy in acute myocarditis; an 18 year systematic review. *Arch Dis Child.* 2004;89:580–584.

58 Imazio M, Demichelis B, Parrini I, et al. Management, risk factors, and outcomes in recurrent pericarditis. *Am J Cardiol.* 2005;96:736–739.

59 Imazio M, Bobbie M, Cache E, et al. Colchicines in additional to conventional therapy for acute pericarditis. *Circulation.* 2005;112:2012–2016.

60 Chen H, Liu J, Yang M. Corticosteroids for viral myocarditis. *Cochrane Database Syst Rev.* 2006;4:CD004471.

61 Baldini G, Bani E. Cardiac complications in Jennerian vaccination. Clinical and echocardiographic studies. *Minerva Pediatr.* 1979;31:35–39.

62 Matthews A, Griffiths I. Post–vaccinal pericarditis and myocarditis. *Br Heart J.* 1974;36:1043–1045.

63 Murphy J, Wright R, Bruce G, et al. Eosinophilic–lymphocytic myocarditis following immunization for smallpox in a previously healthy 29–year–old man. *Lancet.* 2003;363:1378–1380.

64 Allanore Y, Vignaux O, Arnaud L, et al. Effects of corticosteroids and immunosuppressors on idiopathic inflammatory myopathy related myocarditis evaluated by magnetic resonance imaging. *Ann Rheum Dis.* 2006;65:249–252.

65 Friman G Fohlman J. The epidemiology of viral heart disease. *Scand J Infect Dis.* 1993;88:7–10.

66 Mason JW, O'Connell JB, Herskowitz A, et al. A clinical trial of immunosuppressive therapy for myocarditis. The Myocarditis Treatment Trial Investigators. *N Engl J Med.* 1995;333(5):269–75.

67 Lee C, Tsai W, Hsu C, et al. Predictive factors of a fulminant course in acute myocarditis. *Int J Cardiol.* 2006;190:142–145.

68 Lieberman E, Herskowitz A, Rose N, Baughman K. A clinicopathologic description of myocarditis. *Clin Immunol Immunopathol.* 1993;68:191–196.

69 Dec G, Waldman H, Southern J, et al. Viral myocarditis mimicking acute myocardial infarction. *J Am Coll Cardiol.* 1992;20:85–89.

70 ACC/AHA guidelines for the clinical application of echocardiography: a report of the American College of Cardiology/American Heart Association Task Force on Assessment of Diagnostic and Therapeutic Cardiovascular Procedures. *J Am Coll Cardiol.* 1990;16:1505–1528.

71 Narula J, Khaw BA, Dec GW Jr. et al. Brief report: recognition of acute myocarditis masquerading as acute myocardial infarction. *N Engl J Med.* 1993;328:100–104.

Pericarditis

Theodore Chan

Medical Director, Department of Emergency Medicine, University of California,
San Diego Medical Center, Professor of Clinical Medicine, University of California,
San Diego, San Diego, California, USA

Section I: Case presentation

A 42-year-old man with no prior cardiac history presented to the emergency department (ED) complaining of left-sided chest pain of 2 days duration. He described the pain as sharp and intermittent, with radiation to his left shoulder, and worsening with deep inspiration or upper extremity movement. The patient stated the pain was worse when lying down to go to sleep. He denied shortness of breath, lightheadedness, palpitations, nausea, or abdominal pain.

The week prior, the patient had an upper respiratory tract infection with cough and congestion for which he took over-the-counter medications for symptomatic relief. He exercised regularly, but had been unable to do so for the last week because of his illness. The past medical history was significant for hypertension, for which he was not taking any medication. The family history was notable in that his father had suffered a myocardial infarction (MI) at the age of 62.

The triage vital signs were: blood pressure 147/86 mmHg, pulse rate 98 beats/min, respiratory rate 16 breaths/min, and temperature 38.2°C (100.7°F). On initial evaluation, the patient was in mild distress, slightly diaphoretic in appearance, and sitting up on the gurney. The physical findings were notable for clear breath sounds on lung examination, and a regular rate with no murmurs on cardiac auscultation. The remainder of the examination was unremarkable.

The patient was placed on a cardiac monitor, and a 12-lead EKG showed a normal sinus rhythm with slight ST elevation in the inferior and lateral leads (Figure 16-1). There was no prior EKG available for comparison. A complete blood count showed a mild increase in white blood cell count (12.3k/mm³), but was otherwise normal. Serum electrolytes were normal and the cardiac troponin-I level was < 0.02 ng/ml. A chest radiograph was noted to have no significant disease.

Section II: Case discussion

Dr Peter Rosen: Is there anything in particular on this EKG that you would find diagnostic?

Dr Shamai Grossman: There is marked diffuse PR depression that is very unusual, with the exception of one disease entity, and that's pericarditis. There is also a hint of diffuse ST elevation, which is nonspecific, but more consistent with pericarditis than with cardiac ischemia.

PR: This patient has a history of hypertension that is untreated, a family history of coronary artery disease, and a presentation that is compatible either with an ischemic coronary syndrome or with pericarditis. What are the clues you use to distinguish the two, assuming that you can? Or how do you safely manage the patient for both?

Cardiovascular Problems in Emergency Medicine: A discussion-based review, First Edition.
Edited by Shamai A. Grossman and Peter Rosen.
© 2011 John Wiley & Sons, Ltd. Published 2011 by John Wiley & Sons, Ltd.

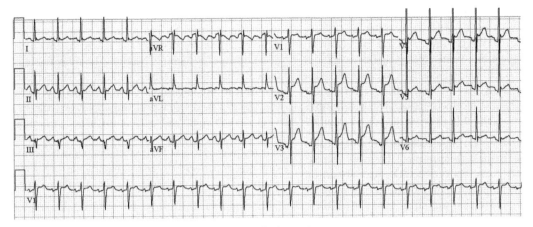

Figure 16.1 12-lead EKG for case patient presenting with chest pain.

Dr David Brown: The clinical approach has become more complicated in the last several years as we are now very focused on shortening door-to-balloon time for patients with a ST-segment elevation myocardial infarction (STEMI). This in turn means markedly reducing the ED time for patients who present with a presumed STEMI. Nevertheless, this patient does not present with the findings of acute heart failure as one might see if this were an active transmural infarction. There are no other historical features or examination features particularly reassuring in this case to exclude STEMI, because the spectrum of people presenting with ST elevation MI includes patients with positional chest pain, pleuritic chest pain, and sharp chest pain. The physical examination of a STEMI patient is usually unremarkable unless there is a complication of the STEMI, such as heart failure or a valvular problem, which doesn't seem to be the case here. This patient doesn't have a rub on physical examination, which if present might further suggest pericarditis. However, rubs are usually absent and even when present are very hard to hear in a busy, noisy ED. Patients with pericarditis or suspected pericarditis often have findings on the EKG like this one that are consistent with an ST elevation MI. However, the PR depressions are striking here, and there is PR elevation in aVR, also striking; both findings are much more consistent with pericarditis than ST elevation MI. In addition, the EKG has diffuse ST elevation in the precordial leads and in II, III and aVF, and it is hard to imagine an anatomic distribution of atherosclerosis in the coronary arteries that would create these widespread findings

on EKG. While all of these findings point to pericarditis, they're not enough to exclude the diagnosis of cardiac ischemia.

PR: This leaves me with the impression that in some of these cases the only way that we will be able to distinguish between these two diseases is in the catheterization laboratory, which may be appropriate, even though we will probably receive a fair amount of scorn from our cardiology colleagues once they discover that it is pericarditis. They will want to know why we couldn't figure it out after doing all the studies that we did. Nevertheless, I think this case sounds more like pericarditis. I have noticed that our colleagues in Italy are much quicker to obtain cardiac echocardiogram (ECHO) imaging studies on patients than we seem to be. Perhaps they are just more adept at doing them personally, or it is just their practice style, but a cardiac echocardiogram can be a very important study in pericarditis.

Dr Ted Chan: An echocardiogram could help pick up any wall motion abnormality associated with an ischemic episode, in addition to the more common complications of pericarditis, such as pericardial effusion. An echocardiogram can also be very helpful in terms of determining whether this patient can be treated as a straightforward pericarditis on an outpatient basis, or whether an admission will be necessary with concerns for either ischemia or impending cardiac tamponade.

SG: I would make the argument that there is a time where door-to-balloon time is a reasonable and worthy goal. This is in a patient who has a clear cut ST elevation MI. However, in a patient whose presentation is less clear, and which may be suggestive of pericarditis, I think it behooves us to be as thorough as possible and investigate all other causes. If you can obtain an echocardiogram in a relatively expeditious fashion in the ED, then I think you should. One ethically must say, "My priority here is to take the best care of the patient." There is morbidity associated with cardiac catheterization, and if I can avoid this, then I should.

PR: I think that is fair. Nevertheless, there will be cases that we rush to the catheterization laboratory because we can't sort it out easily in the ED, and if we err on the side of caution and go to the catheterization laboratory too quickly, that is preferable to getting there too late. On the other hand, an inadvertent trip to the catheterization laboratory is also expensive, time consuming, and may deprive a deserving ischemic patient of a procedure needed expeditiously.

DB: I am not advocating that strategy, as from a public health standpoint I think it makes no sense. The problem is that we are being held to a sensitivity marker without a specificity marker. We can take every single patient that comes through the ED to the catheterization laboratory, and have a door-to-balloon time of 60 minutes or less on every patient without being criticized. Yet, if we take our time and do an echocardiogram on these patients, 1 in 50 might have a STEMI and we are going to get penalized for these cases.

SG: Our real job is giving appropriate care to a patient, and sending a patient to the catheterization laboratory who doesn't belong there is not good care. Every time we take a patient to the catheterization laboratory, there is morbidity and mortality.

PR: The pragmatic reality is that we do things ideally that don't happen in the real world, and I think it is much more probable that the emergency physician is going to abdicate responsibility for making the distinction in consultation with the cardiologist. This is not because he should do so, but is because he is more likely to do so, as the personal benefit/reward relationship is better with shared responsibility. I still think we should be teaching responsibility, and trying to imbue a sense of empowerment in our trainees that they have the right to do what's best for the patient.

We also appear to have no trust in our physical diagnosis examinations, probably because we become reluctant to use them, but I think that auscultating a pericardial friction rub can be very helpful in these

patients. I wonder if we listen closely enough before we conclude there is no friction rub present. I switched to an electronic stethoscope as I started to go a little deaf with age, and started hearing a lot more findings than I remembered hearing without it. Perhaps we all ought to use an electronic stethoscope or at least upgrade to a better quality stethoscope. Nevertheless, a rub doesn't completely rule out ischemic syndrome as about 25% of patients with acute MIs have a rub at some point. Do you have a feeling for when the rub develops in pericarditis, and any particular clues for where to listen for it besides directly over the heart?

DB: I find that if a rub is present, it is very helpful in supporting the diagnosis of pericarditis, but when absent it is not useful to exclude the diagnosis of pericarditis. The rub can be fleeting, can be intermittent, and therefore examining the patient more than once and in a quiet room away from all the noises and monitor beeps can be very helpful. The easiest way to hear a friction rub is to sit the patient up, and have them lean forward. Occasionally I have only heard the rub in the back. Doing a more complete cardiac examination than you would routinely do on a patient with chest pain is useful and may increase the likelihood that one will hear a rub.

SG: If you can hear a three-component rub you are almost certainly dealing with pericarditis.

PR: I know classically we find positional change helpful in differentiating pericarditis from an ischemic syndrome, but this is probably like any other physical finding—if it's there it may be helpful, but if it's not there it doesn't exclude anything.

What are your indications for admission in a patient with pericarditis?

DB: If I'm convinced the diagnosis is pericarditis, and I'm able to establish clinically either by a formal or bedside echocardiogram that there is no significant pericardial effusion, then I would feel comfortable discharging such a patient to be treated with non-steroidal antinflammatory agents (NSAIDS) and to have close follow-up. Having said that, this assumes that I was satisfied with my history, physical examination, and EKG in excluding myocardial infarction, and didn't feel that the patient needed to be evaluated any further for cardiac ischemia. It also assumes that I could obtain at least a bedside ECHO in a timely fashion in the ED or as an outpatient. In the absence of those two conditions, it would be reasonable to admit a patient like this to an observation unit for serial cardiac markers and EKGs, and to obtain an ECHO study in the morning, assuming this is the middle of the night.

PR: Most of us agree that the presence of an effusion is worrisome and would warrant putting the patient into the hospital. How accurate are chest X-ray and ultrasound studies in revealing an effusion?

TC: An echocardiogram is much better than a chest radiograph. I believe the cutoff for detecting a significant effusion on X-ray study would be somewhere between 200 and 250 cc of fluid, but an ultrasound study should be able to pick up 50 cc of fluid. Therefore, you cannot rely on a chest X-ray study to detect a pericardial effusion; you would have to obtain an echocardiogram.

SG: I might add that we may not need a formal echocardiogram on all these patients, as we have become very adept at bedside ultrasound in the ED. I think most of us would put a probe on a patient, and if we see an effusion, then we arrange a formal echocardiogram. If we don't see an effusion, we would likely be satisfied that the patient didn't have any of the complications of pericarditis.

PR: The conventional wisdom is to start therapy with NSAIDs, but I am underwhelmed by their effectiveness in pericarditis. Would you ever keep a patient in the ED to see if he or she is going to respond to NSAIDs before discharge?

SG: I usually start these patients on ketorolac in the ED because it is a rapid-acting antiinflammatory agent, and I've had good success with it. Using ketorolac offers me an opportunity to look at the patient after they have had time to respond. Assuming the patient improves, I'm convinced that the patient indeed has pericarditis, and I am no longer concerned with myocardial ischemia or other etiologies of the symptoms, then I would be comfortable sending that patient home on an oral antiinflammatory such as ibuprofen or naproxen. I cannot recall a pericarditis patient who did not respond to ketorolac in the ED.

PR: What are your indications for steroids and when would you start them?

TC: The literature on the benefit of steroids in pericarditis is equivocal, to be honest, and I'm not sure I would ever use them unless my consultant strongly desired them. There is some recent literature in Europe that talks about combining NSAIDs with colchicine, and I think that some of those studies also looked at steroids, but did not find them much more helpful.

PR: I think steroids are more likely to be useful in traumatic pericarditis, where I haven't found much benefit from NSAIDs. Most of the patients I see with fresh pericarditis in the ED I never see again, so I don't know if they have benefited from NSAIDs. But, I have seen a number of patients who came back to the ED with traumatic pericarditis who had been started on NSAIDs, and they did seem to benefit from adding steroids.

Is there a difference between pericarditis that develops from a viral infection, such as from coxsackie virus, which is the most common viral agent, and a traumatic pericarditis from striking your chest wall?

TC: Traumatic pericarditis is more likely to need admission for observation and concern for an underlying myocardial contusion or other injuries.

PR: What are the complications of pericarditis, other than tamponade from the effusion?

DB: Tamponade is clearly the most concerning complication. The development of tamponade can be insidious, or it can be more rapid if there is hemorrhagic conversion and the patients bleed into their pericardium. Unless there is an associated myocarditis, there is not much risk of dysrhythmia or of other complications of heart muscle disease.

SG: Although rare, constrictive pericarditis should be in the back of your mind as a complication. This is only seen in patients who have recurrent pericarditis where ultimately there is an encasement of the heart with fibrous tissue from the pericarditis. With constrictive pericarditis, one would see patients who have the clinical presentation or an EKG suggestive of pericarditis, but might have concomitant signs of congestive heart failure. Calcifications on the chest X-ray study or pericardial thickening on echocardiogram are also suggestive of constrictive pericarditis. Management will be somewhat different, as these patients will need to have the pericardium resected or a pericardial window created.

PR: Do you have a sense for how quickly the effusion can develop? In other words, if we are using effusion as one of the criteria for admission, and we don't see one on a patient, how rapidly is the patient likely to develop one at home that would make us concerned about follow up?

SG: This would depend on the etiology of the pericarditis. A viral pericarditis would be more likely to have a rapid onset; pericarditis from tuberculosis or the many noninfectious etiologies, such as malignancy, uremia, or post-radiation, would be more likely to develop an effusion slowly, as you gradually develop the effects of the primary disease process.

PR: Would you look for other causes of pericarditis, perhaps new renal failure as the etiology of the pericarditis, or are you comfortable with trying to distinguish between viral and bacterial etiologies?

TC: In this particular case, the patient has a clear precipitating infectious history. He had congestion and a cough in the 2 weeks preceding the onset of his chest pain, and he's otherwise healthy. Although hypertension will put him at risk for renal failure and uremia, I would expect to see other signs and symptoms consistent with uremia before I tried to attribute his pericarditis to renal failure. On the other hand, there is probably some additional history that we should obtain from this patient. Is he in the military, for example? Did he get a smallpox vaccination, as there is an association between acute pericarditis and that vaccination? By obtaining more history, we might be better able to focus or limit our considerations to a viral etiology, which is most likely in this case.

PR: Is there any benefit to giving an antiviral agent?

TC: I am unaware of a literature suggesting antivirals to be effective in viral pericarditis.

PR: I think pericarditis is a lot more common than we sometimes expect, and given our propensity to worry about ischemic coronary syndromes, we often fail to think of the diagnosis, and so fail to look for and recognize the EKG changes.

Case resolutions

The patient was admitted with a preliminary diagnosis of new onset angina. Serial cardiac markers were normal. An echocardiogram revealed a small pericardial effusion, but was otherwise normal. During hospitalization, repeat cardiac examinations revealed a faint three-phase friction rub with the patient in the left lateral position. With a presumptive diagnosis of acute pericarditis, the patient was subsequently treated with antiinflammatory medications and discharged. He recovered uneventfully with full resolution of symptoms. Six months later, a repeat EKG revealed resolution of the ST-segment findings seen on the ED presentation.

Section III: Concepts

Background/Epidemiology

The normal pericardium is a double-layered fibroserous sac that envelops the heart and base of the great vessels within the middle mediastinum. The inner visceral pericardium and outer parietal pericardium are each approximately 1–2 mm thick, and are separated by the pericardial cavity, which contains 15–50 ml of serous pericardial fluid in a healthy individual. The pericardium protects the heart, as well as constrains the motion of the heart, and is an important determinant of cardiac filling.[1]

Acute pericarditis, or inflammation of the pericardium, can present in many clinical settings including the ED, and has a wide range of causes (Table 16-1). The disease is often accompanied by some degree of underlying myocarditis, or inflammation of the superficial myocardium adjacent to the inflamed pericardium.[2] The term "myopericarditis" has been used to describe a primary pericarditis with lesser degree of related myocardial inflammation, whereas the term "perimyocarditis" indicates a primary myocarditis with accompanying overlying pericarditis, though the terms are used interchangeably.[3]

The true incidence and prevalence of percarditis are unknown. Autopsy studies, however, indicate a prevalence of approximately 1%, suggesting the potential for subclinical cases.[1] Clinically, approximately 5% of all chest pain patients who are not diagnosed with an acute myocardial infarction may have pericarditis as the etiology for their presentation.[4] However, the underlying causes of acute pericarditis are changing. For example, the rising incidences of HIV infection, invasive cardiac procedures, and radiation therapy have all resulted in an increase in acute pericarditis associated with these underlying etiologies. Acute

Table 16-1. Causes of Acute Pericarditis

Infectious	Viral	Coxsackie A and B, hepatitis viruses, HIV, EBV, CMV, varicella, rubella, mumps, rubeola, poliomyelitis, rhinoviruses, vaccinia, parvovirus B19, others
	Bacterial	*Streptococcus (pneumococcus, meningococcus, gonococcus), hemophilus, treponema pallidum, borreliosis, chlamydia, listeria, rickettsial, M. tuberculosis,* others
	Fungal	*Candida, histoplasma, blastomyces,* others
	Parasitic	*Entamoeba histolytica, echinococcus, toxoplasma,* others
Autoimmune Disorders		Lupus, rheumatoid arthritis, sarcoidosis, scleroderma, Sjogren's syndrome, Reiter's syndrome, ankylosing spondylitis, Wegener's granulomatosis, giant-cell arteritis, polymyositis, dermatomyositis, familial Mediterranean fever, Churg-Strauss syndrome, Periarteritis nodosa, acute rheumatic fever, Stevens-Johnson syndrome, TTP, leukoclastic vasculitis, others
Metabolic and Endocrine		Renal failure/uremia, dialysis-related Addison's disease, DKA, hypothyroidism, gout, scurvy, cholesterol pericarditis, pregnancy
Malignancy-related	Primary or metastatic	Mesothelioma, sarcoma, melanoma Breast and lung cancers Lymphoma, leukemia GI cancers, carcinoid, others
	Secondary	Postradiation therapy
Adjacent structures and other organ system	Cardiac and vascular	Myocarditis Acute myocardial infarction Postmyocardial infarction, Dressler's syndrome, aortic dissection, aortic aneurysm
	Postcardiac or thoracic procedure	Postpericardiotomy, cardiac surgery Postcatheterization, pacemaker placement, ablation
	Pulmonary	Pneumonia, pulmonary embolism, empyema, pulmonary infarction
	GI	Pancreatitis, inflammatory bowel disease, esophageal diseases Perforation (esophageal or gastric)
Trauma		Penetrating injury Blunt chest/cardiac trauma
Medications and drugs		Hydralazine, penicillin, phenytoin, procainamide, INH, rifampin, dantrolene, doxorubicin, methyldopa, methysergide, sulfonamides, cocaine, others
Idiopathic		

pericarditis from *mycobacterium tuberculosis* is now less common in developed countries, but remains an important infectious etiology of the disease in developing parts of the world.

Most cases of acute pericarditis resolve without major long-term sequelae. However, depending on the underlying etiology, certain patients may be at risk for significant complications, including recurrent pericarditis, chronic or constrictive pericarditis, pericardial effusions, and cardiac tamponade.

Initial workup history and physical examination

The classic presentation for acute pericarditis is chest pain, central or retrosternal in location, sharp and pleuritic in nature, and often sudden in onset and severe. The pain is worse with recumbency or in the supine position, and accordingly the patient is often sitting up and leaning forward in an effort to relieve the symptoms. The pain can radiate to the neck, arms, or shoulders, making it difficult to differentiate from acute cardiac ischemia, particularly given the likelihood of some degree of associated myocarditis. However, pain radiation to the trapezius muscle ridge, which is innervated by the phrenic nerve and stimulated by pericardial inflammation, makes acute pericarditis more likely.[5]

Clinical presentation of the disease, however, can be quite variable, likely reflecting the underlying etiology, degree of myocardial involvement, and presence of complications. Many cases may be subtle or subclinical, with little evidence of cardiac or systemic signs or symptoms. On the other hand, the clinical presentation may reflect the underlying cause of the acute pericarditis. A history of febrile illness has been reported in half of all cases of myopericarditis of suspected viral etiology.[6] Similarly, patients may present with other symptoms consistent with a viral infection, including myalgias, malaise, and respiratory and gastrointestinal complaints. A history of recent cardiac surgery or intervention should raise the possibility of a postprocedure pericarditis.

With significant myocardial involvement, patients may complain of fatigue, decreased exercise capacity, shortness of breath, and palpitations in addition to chest pain. These presenting complaints should raise concern for diminished cardiac function potentially resulting from a large pericardial effusion or cardiac tamponade.

The initial physical examination should first focus on vital signs and an assessment of cardiac function. Hypotension and tachycardia may be the result of decreased cardiac output from accumulated pericardial fluid and increased pressure, reducing filling of the right heart chambers. The neck veins should be examined for any distension indicating decreased cardiac filling. The presence of a pulsus paradoxus, a decrease in systolic arterial pressure greater than 10 mmHg with inspiration, may herald cardiac tamponade physiology; this is more common with certain etiologies, including acute pericarditis from neoplastic, tuberculosis, and purulent (bacterial) causes.[7] The best way to determine a pulsus paradoxus is to inflate the sphynomanometer above systolic pressure. While auscultating over the brachial artery, determine the difference between the onset of the first Korotkoff sound and when it becomes steady. If this difference is greater than 12 mmHg, a pulsus paradoxus is present. It is very difficult to try to measure this difference in conjunction with a patient inspiration. If tamponade

is present, the radial pulse may disappear with inspiration, but this is a late finding. The pathophysiologic response to tamponade is a tachycardia, but for poorly understood reasons, immediately prior to the patient arresting, a bradycardia will suddenly develop. The removal of even a small volume of fluid can restore life-sustaining cardiac function. Acute tamponade will often develop with 200–300 cc of fluid, but chronic effusions that have developed more slowly can sometimes contain up to a liter or more of serosanguinous fluid. Viral-induced effusions are easy to aspirate; however, those associated with bacterial pericarditis can be very viscous, and may require surgical removal as they cannot easily be aspirated through a needle.

The classic finding on examination that indicates an acute pericarditis is the pericardial friction rub, typically described as a high-pitched "scratchy," "raspy," "creaky," or "squeaky" sound best heard along the left sternal border at end expiration with the patient leaning forward. This rub was previously thought to be caused by inflamed visceral and parietal pericardial surfaces rubbing against one another, but it is also present when there are large effusions separating these surfaces. The rub is described as having three components, corresponding to atrial systole, ventricular systole, and early rapid ventricular filling. However, the rub is often heard as a biphasic or monophasic, as well as a triphasic, sound. Unlike a pleural rub from pleuritis, the pericardial friction rub is audible and does not vary throughout the respiratory cycle. The presence of a pericardial friction rub is virtually pathognomonic with near 100% specificity for pericarditis, but has low sensitivity because it tends to be transient, and intermittently comes and goes over hours.[5,8] Accordingly, repeated and frequent auscultations over time will increase the sensitivity and likelihood of detecting this finding.

The remainder of the physical examination should focus on assessing overall cardiac function, and detecting the underlying etiology of the acute pericarditis.

Etiologies/Differential diagnosis

A wide variety of etiologic conditions can cause acute inflammation of the pericardium, producing serous, purulent, or dense fibrinous material within the pericardial sac. These conditions include infectious etiologies, most commonly of viral origin; systemic autoimmune, metabolic, or endocrinologic disorders;

traumatic injury such as esophageal perforation or invasive cardiac procedures; extension of other local inflammatory processes; malignancy and neoplasm spread; medications and drugs; and, most commonly, idiopathic causes (see Table 16-1).

Advances in pericardial fluid collection and analysis, as well as immunohistochemistry and PCR techniques, have allowed more comprehensive determination of the etiologies of acute pericarditis; even with this, however, the cause of pericarditis still cannot be determined in up to 30% of patients.[1] Of those where a cause can be determined, infection remains the most common. Viral agents account for the large majority of cases, particularly enteroviruses such as coxsackie, adenoviruses, and influenza. HIV-related pericardial disease is common, and immunosuppressed patients are at risk for a variety of opportunistic pathogens such as *cytomegalovirus*.[9] An unusual viral-mediated pericarditis has been reported following smallpox vaccination with vaccinia virus.[10]

Though less common than viral pathogens, bacterial pericarditis typically causes a purulent pericarditis that has greater risk of complications. Bacterial infection can spread to the pericardium hematogenously, or by direct extension from nearby organs, particularly the lungs. *Mycobacterium tuberculosis* remains an important cause of the disease in developing countries, as well as in immunosuppressed patients. Risk of rapid pericardial fluid formation and tamponade is high in with these infections.

Acute pericarditis and myopericarditis have been associated with both early and late acute myocardial infarction. Dressler's syndrome is an acute pericarditis that develops late, more than one week after an acute infarction. Acute inflammation of the pericardium is common after cardiac surgery as part of the postpericardiotomy syndrome. While less common, patients undergoing percutaneous cardiac procedures, including pacemaker placement, ablation or angioplasty, and coronary artery stenting, are also at risk for acute pericarditis.[11]

Neoplastic-related pericarditis can arise from a number of pathophysiologic mechanisms, including primary malignancy (rare), direct tumor invasion, lymphatic or hematogenous spread, or as a complication of therapy. Lung tumors, breast cancer, and lymphomas are the most common cancers that may metastasize to the pericardium.[12] Radiation therapy, particularly for breast cancer, as well as certain chemotherapeutic agents such as doxorubicin, may also cause acute pericarditis. Cancer-related pericarditis has a high rate of complications, including the development of large pleural and pericardial effusions.

A wide variety of other noninfectious diseases, including endocrinologic, metabolic, and autoimmune diseases, can all result in acute pericarditis or myopericarditis. Common causes in these categories include systemic lupus erythematosus, end-stage renal failure and uremia, and a variety of connective tissue and rheumatologic disorders.

Testing

The 12-lead electrocardiogram can provide useful information in the diagnosis of acute pericarditis. Typical electrocardiographic abnormalities result from the degree of subepicardial inflammation and myocardial involvement. Classically, the EKG in acute pericarditis evolves through 4 stages, occurring over a period of several weeks. Stage I, occurring in the first hours or days, is characterized by diffuse ST elevations, concave upward in morphology, most prominent in the anterior and inferior leads.[12] Reciprocal ST depressions may be seen in leads aVR and V1. There are also PR segment deviations from the normal P wave polarity with depressions diffusely, most prominent in leads V5 and V6, as well as elevation in lead aVR and possible. The PR segment changes may precede the ST-segment findings. In stage II, which occurs over several days to 3 weeks, the PR- and ST-segment changes resolve. There may also be T wave flattening with decreased amplitude. In stage III, diffuse T wave inversions are seen. Finally, in stage IV, the T waves normalize and the EKG returns to baseline after several weeks.

This typical evolution on EKG, particularly the rapid early stage I findings, may be missed or not recorded electrocardiographically. In addition, atypical findings are common depending on the underlying myocardial tissue involvement and inflammation. In the setting of myopericarditis, ST-segment changes, particularly of a local or regional nature, earlier T wave inversions, and various cardiac dysrhythmias are more common than with simple acute pericarditis.[6]

Accordingly, findings associated with acute pericarditis can be difficult to differentiate from acute ischemia electrocardiographically. Morphologically, the ST-segment elevation in ischemia is more commonly convex (dome-shaped) than concave, localized rather than diffuse, and T wave inversions may occur at nearly the same time, unlike those associated with acute pericarditis. PR-segment depression is also not seen with ischemia. In addition, the evolution of electrocardiographic findings occurs over a much shorter time frame with an ischemic infarction (hours to days), than with acute pericarditis (days to weeks). Studies also suggest that an ST-segment elevation-to-T wave apex (ST/T ratio) of greater than 0.25, particularly in lead V6, is more suggestive of acute pericarditis.[2,6,13]

On laboratory testing, the cardiac enzymes, including troponin and CK-MB, are often elevated in acute pericarditis, and are thought to result from epicardial inflammation rather than myocyte necrosis.[7] The level of troponin elevation correlates with the magnitude of ST-segment elevation and usually resolves after 1–2 weeks, but prolonged elevations may indicate a significant myocarditis. Troponin elevations seen with acute pericarditis do not necessarily portend a poor outcome from the disease.[14,15]

Other serologic tests including markers of acute inflammation, such as CBC, CRP, and ESR, are often elevated in the setting of acute pericarditis, but the clinical utility of these findings remains unclear.[7] In general, additional laboratory tests should be guided by clinical presentation and possible etiologies, and may include other, more specific, tests, such as HIV serologies and various autoimmune disease markers.

Imaging should begin with a chest radiograph. While frequently normal, the radiograph may reveal an enlarged cardiac silhouette as a result of a large pericardial effusion, with greater than 250 mL of accumulated fluid in the sac.

Transthoracic echocardiography has been recommended in the evaluation of patients with pericardial disease, and in particular, to find the complications associated with acute pericarditis.[16] Echocardiography is useful for detecting the presence of a pericardial effusion, including small fluid collections, and also provides information on cardiac function, which may aid in the diagnosis of constrictive pericarditis. Newer modalities, including doppler imaging and intracardiac echo, may increase its use in the future. However, in straightforward unequivocal cases of acute pericarditis with no evidence of complications and no poor prognostic indicators, emergent echocardiography may be unnecessary.[7] MRI, CT and radionuclide scanning have been shown to provide excellent visualization of the pericardial sac,

inflammation and complications, but the exact clinical role for each has yet to be determined.[1,3]

Pericardiocentesis and fluid drainage may be diagnostically or therapeutically indicated in patients with large pericardial effusions, and for those with suspected or confirmed purulent or neoplastic pericarditis. Depending on the clinical presentation and etiologies considered, fluid may require analysis with a variety of studies, including cell count, Gram's stain, culture, PCR assays (for suspected viral causes), adenosine deaminase activity (which may indicate *M. tuberculosis*), triglycerides (for chylous effusions), cytology studies, and pH, LDH, protein and glucose levels (to determine the nature of the fluid collection), as well as other more advanced tests. Pericardial biopsy may be indicated for recurrent pericarditis or pericardial fluid collections of unknown etiology.

Disposition

Most cases of acute pericarditis have a benign course and are self-limited, with management that is largely supportive and focused on pain relief, and on potential complications. In uncomplicated cases, primarily viral and idiopathic, the mainstay of initial therapy is treatment with the NSAIDs. Therapy may be required for weeks to relieve symptoms. Indomethacin should be avoided in patients with coronary artery disease because of an association with diminished coronary blood flow.[17] Aspirin can be used as alternative, and may be preferable for patients who have suffered a recent myocardial infarction. Colchicine has been shown to be a useful adjuvant to conventional therapy, significantly reducing the recurrence rate for patients with first-time acute pericarditis.[18] Corticosteroid treatment is controversial because of evidence suggesting the potential for increased risk of recurrence.[3,19] Steroids have been recommended for use only after patients fail conventional therapies, and also may have some utility in tuberculosis pericarditis.[1] Therapy should otherwise focus on the specific etiology of the acute pericarditis, if identified and treatable.

Hospitalization is not always necessary, and patients may potentially be managed as outpatients in unequivocal and uncomplicated cases. Follow-up care should be assured in these cases to monitor resolution, and to check for the development of complications. Recurrence of the disease is common, and may occur in up to 30% of patients.

Table 16-2. Differentiating acute pericarditis and Acute Coronary Syndromes (ACS)

	Acute Pericarditis	ACS
Chest pain history		
• Quality	Sharp, stabbing, intermittent	Dull, pressure-like, squeezing
• Duration	Hours to days	Minutes to hours
• Positional	Yes, worse with supine position	No
• Radiation	Patient often sitting up, leaning forward; trapezius ridge specifically, also neck, jaw, shoulder/arms	Neck, jaw, shoulder/arms
Examination		
• Friction rub	Present—no respiratory variation	Usually not present
Electrocardiogram		
• ST elevation	Diffuse, concave upward	Regional, convex
• PR depression	Diffuse (elevated in aVR)	Absent
• T-wave inversion	After ST elevations resolve	Present with ST elevations
• Q waves	Absent	May be present

Table 16-3. Indications for hospitalization for patients with acute pericarditis

Cardiac Tamponade
Large Pericardial Effusion
Anticoagulation Therapy
Immunocompromised State
HIV
Extensive Myocardial Involvement
Elevated Troponin
Traumatic Etiology
Fever
Subacute Onset
Conventional Treatment Failure

- Cardiac tamponade is the most worrisome complication, as evidenced by hypotension, elevated jugular venous pressure, and pulsus paradoxus, and must be treated emergently with pericardiocentesis and drainage.
- Most cases of acute pericarditis are self-limited and can be managed with supportive care, including NSAIDs, aspirin, and colchicine.
- Several factors are associated with potential risk for complications and poor outcome and are indications for inpatient hospitalization (Table 16-3).

Patients with significant complications, such as large pericardial effusions with or without tamponade physiology, may require emergent drainage and hospitalization. Similarly, patients may present with cardiac decompensation as a result of constrictive pericarditis, and require inpatient care. Other poor prognostic signs and indications for admission include fever above 38°C (100.4°F), subacute onset (over several weeks), anticoagulant therapy, immunocompromised state, evidence of myocardial involvement (myopericarditis), elevated troponin levels, conventional treatment failure, and a traumatic etiology for the acute pericarditis.

Section IV: Decision making

- The patient's presentation must be differentiated from other causes of chest pain, such as acute coronary syndromes.
- Careful history and examination and a 12-lead EKG can be of great utility in making the diagnosis (Table 16-2).

References

1 Troughton RW, Asher CR, Klein AL. Pericarditis. *Lancet.* 2004;363:717–727.
2 Chan TC, Brady WJ, Pollack M. Electrocardiographic manifestations: acute myopericarditis. *J Emerg Med.* 1999;17:865–872.
3 Imazio M, Trinchero R. Myopericarditis: etiology, management, and prognosis. *Internat J Cardiol.* 2008;127:17–26.
4 Launbjerg J, Fruergaard P, Hesse B, et al. Long-term risk of death, cardiac events and recurrent chest pain in patients with acute chest pain of different origin. *Cardiology.* 1996;87:60–66.
5 Spodick DH. Acute pericarditis—current concepts and practice. *JAMA.* 2003;289:1150–1153.
6 Imazio M, Cecchi E, Demichelis B, et al. Myopericarditis versus viral or idiopathic acute pericarditis *Heart* 2008;94:498–501.
7 Lange RA, Hillis LD. Acute pericarditis. *N Engl J Med.* 2004;351:2195–2202.
8 Tingle LE, Monia D, Calvert CW. Acute pericarditis. *Am Fam Physician.* 2007;76:1509–1514.

9 Barbaro G, Klatt EC. HIV infection and the cardiovascular system. *AIDS Rev.* 2002;4:93–103.

10 Cassimatis DC, Atwood JE, Engler RM, et al. Smallpox vaccination and myopericarditis: a clinical review. *J Am Coll Cardiol.* 2004;43:1503–1510.

11 Vasquez A, Butman SM. Pathophysiologic mechanisms in pericardial disease. *Curr Cardiol Rep.* 2002;4:26–32.

12 Maisch B, Seferovic PM, Ristic AD, et al. Guidelines on the diagnosis and management of pericardial disease—executive summary of the task force on the diagnosis and management of pericardial disease of the European Society of Cardiology. *Eur Heart J.* 2004;25:587–610.

13 Ginzton LE, Laks MM. The differential diagnosis of acute myopericarditis from the normal variant: new electrocardiographic criteria. *Circulation.* 1982;65:1004–1009.

14 Bonnefoy E, Godon P, Kirkorian G, et al. Serum cardiac troponin I and ST segment elevation in patients with acute pericarditis. *Eur Heart J.* 2000;21:832–836.

15 Imazio M, Demichelis B, Cecchi E, et al. Cardiac troponin I in acute pericarditis. *J Am Coll Cardiol.* 2003;42:2144–2148.

16 Cheitlin MD, Armstrong WF, Aurigemma GP, et al. ACC/AHA/ASE 2003 guideline update for the clinical application of echocardiography: summary article: a report of the ACC/AHA Task Force on Practice Guidelines. *Circulation.* 2003;108:1146–1162.

17 Schifferdecker B, Spodick DH. Nonsteroidal anti–inflammatory drugs in the treatment of pericarditis. *Cardiol Rev.* 2003;11:211–217.

18 Imazio M, Bobbio M, Cecchi E, et al. Colchicine in addition to conventional therapy for acute pericarditis—results of the colchicine for acute pericarditis trial. *Circulation.* 2005;112:2012–2016.

19 Imazio M, Demichelis B, Parrini I, et al. Management, risk factors, and outcomes in recurrent pericarditis. *Am J Cardiol.* 2005;96:736–739.

17 Cardiac toxins and drug-induced heart disease

Jeffrey Green[1] & Richard Harrigan[2]

[1] Associate Professor of Emergency Medicine, U.C. Davis School of Medicine, Sacramento, CA, USA
[2] Professor of Emergency Medicine, Temple University School of Medicine, Philadelphia, PA, USA

Section I: Case presentation

A 66-year-old woman presented to the emergency department (ED) with worsening dyspnea and orthopnea over several days. She denied chest pain, abdominal pain, nausea, or emesis. She also had a mild intermittent global headache. She reported a dry, non-productive cough, but denied fever and chills. She was compliant with her medications.

The past medical history included congestive heart failure (CHF), with an ejection fraction of 10–20%, hypertension, diabetes mellitus type II, chronic obstructive pulmonary disease (COPD), and a cholecystectomy. Medications included aspirin, nitroglycerin tablets, furosemide, digoxin, metoprolol, pantoprazole, citalopram, albuterol/ipratropium, and fluticasone/salmeterol. She was allergic to clarithromycin and azithromycin. She smoked cigarettes, and did not use alcohol or illicit drugs.

On physical examination, the vital signs were: temperature 36.1°C (96.9°F), pulse 60 beats/min, respirations 24 breaths/min, blood pressure 154/82 mmHg, and O_2 saturation 98%. The skin was nondiaphoretic. The eyes had no conjunctival pallor. The neck had jugular venous distention. The lungs had bilateral rales and expiratory wheezes. Cardiovascular examination showed a regular rate and rhythm with a III/VI holosystolic murmur radiating to the axilla. The abdomen was soft, nontender, without masses or bruits. The extremities had equal pulses with symmetric peripheral edema.

Laboratory studies were: BUN 63 mg/dL, creatinine 2.4 mg/dL, a hematocrit at her baseline of 30.1%, BNP 2370 pg/mL, and troponin I <0.05 ng/mL. A chest X-ray study showed mild-to-moderate pulmonary edema. The EKG is shown in Figure 17-1.

While awaiting admission to an inpatient bed, a bradycardic rhythm was noted on the telemetry monitor, and a rhythm tracing was obtained (Figure 17-2). The patient's clinical status remained stable, with no change in blood pressure.

Section II: Case discussion

Dr Peter Rosen: This patient appears to have a variety of causes for her congestive heart failure, including hypertension and probably some degree of mitral regurgitation. It seems her heart is not doing very well at baseline with an ejection fraction of 20%, and it also sounds like she is beginning to fail in terms of being unable to cope with her daily living requirements. I'm a little puzzled as to why a BNP was ordered on this patient; I don't know what a BNP would tell you that you don't already know. Was this part of an ED protocol or the universal poor practice of ordering laboratory tests because they are available?

Cardiovascular Problems in Emergency Medicine: A discussion-based review, First Edition.
Edited by Shamai A. Grossman and Peter Rosen.
© 2011 John Wiley & Sons, Ltd. Published 2011 by John Wiley & Sons, Ltd.

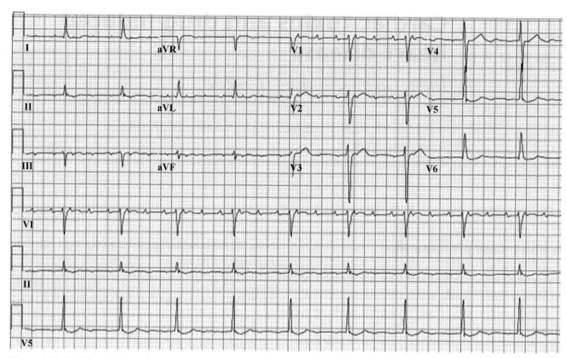

Figure 17.1 Cardiotoxic drugs (1).

Dr Richard Harrigan: The BNP was likely ordered for both reasons. The early working diagnoses were COPD and CHF; if the X-ray study were nondiagnostic, or if there were a delay in obtaining the X-ray study, the BNP could help. Invariably, it does seem that the X-ray is finished in a timely

fashion, you also have the clinical diagnosis, and the BNP results arrive later and aren't useful in many cases.

PR: They also fell into a common trap thinking that because a patient has asthma, COPD must be present. While there is some overlap between the two diseases,

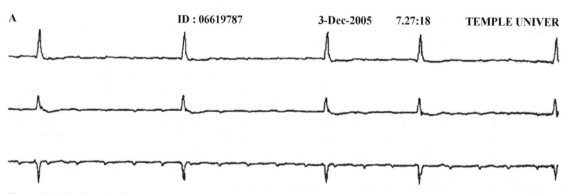

Figure 17.2 Cardiotoxic drugs (2).

it's unlikely that this patient's heart failure is related to cor pulmonale. Were the examining physicians aware of an abnormal heart beat, or was this only noted on cardiac monitoring?

RH: They thought she was in a regular rhythm, which she did have initially on the EKG. They did notice a slow heart rate. This was thought to be related to the metoprolol and digoxin, and to her age as well. At 65 years old, perhaps her conduction system had begun to degenerate.

PR: I noticed she is taking a powerful diuretic, furosemide, without taking a potassium supplement. I'm somewhat surprised that her potassium was normal, but it may be an alternate explanation for her ultimate illness. There was a time when all patients with hypertension were treated with diuretics without potassium. Many of them also had heart failure, and were being treated with a form of digitalis. The most common reason for dig toxicity in those days was hypokalemia. Digoxin was a relatively late-comer to digitalis therapy. For years we used digitalis leaf, and then we used digitoxin, which was thought to be preferable because it was longer acting. This meant that when you became dig-toxic, you could expect to be dig-toxic for a month. Today we use less "dig," and when we do, we use the shorter-acting digoxin so we are not as sensitized to the potential for dig toxicity. I'm not sure the long-acting agents are even available, yet it's still unwise to use digoxin and a diuretic without accompanying potassium replacement.

Dr Shamai Grossman: I suspect that the patient had some known renal failure. In the setting of someone who has chronic renal insufficiency, giving potassium may not be ideal.

PR: Taking furosemide isn't ideal in renal failure either. This patient may be between a rock and a hard place; perhaps worsening renal failure, rather than potassium changes with furosemide, led to digoxin toxicity. In any event, I can see why the clinicians were not particularly alert to digoxin toxicity. I was also surprised that she didn't manifest some other symptoms of dig toxicity, such as nausea and vomiting or optical complaints such as color changes. Often patients feel dizzy and become more aware of irregularities in their heart beat.

RH: The principal symptoms of digoxin toxicity are gastrointestinal, including nausea, vomiting, abdominal cramping, and diarrhea. Neurologic symptoms can include headache, confusion, hallucinations, or delirium at higher levels. The classic visual complaints are less common.

PR: When you see an EKG like this, should you start with dig toxicity? As I recall, the most common abnormality with dig toxicity is premature ventricular contraction. Is there any other explanation for this kind of block?

RH: There is a clue on this EKG that suggests digoxin. There is a mixture of excitability and atrioventricular (AV) nodal suppression with an accelerated atrial beat at about 150 beats per minute—an atrial tachycardia—with a delayed ventricular rate at the same time. There is also evidence of digoxin effect: scooping- or coving-type ST-segment depression that is best seen in leads V5 and V6 on this EKG, and on the V5 rhythm strip on the bottom. I would assume this was digoxin toxicity if I knew the patient was taking digoxin.

SG: If digoxin were not on the patient's medication list, either the patient managed to find a digoxin source and take it without a prescription or the dysrhythmia must have another etiology. Electrolyte abnormalities cause many abnormal rhythms. Hyperkalemia, in particular, is notorious for causing a variety of abnormal rhythms, and although this is not a classic hyperkalemic dysrhythmia, this could have resulted from intrinsic conduction disease as well. Part of discovering the etiology in this case may require a better knowledge of the medical history.

RH: Nevertheless, seeing dig effect should make you think that the patient is taking this medication even when the patient isn't forthcoming with a complete medication list. This doesn't predict toxicity, however.

PR: Dig effect does not mean dig toxicity, but paroxysmal atrial tachycardia (PAT) with block almost always does. With good evidence that she is on dig, and that she is digitoxic, what are your indications for using Digibind fragments to reverse the toxicity?

RH: There are a number of different views about when to administer Digibind. It is easy to administer the Fab fragments when the patient is at or near cardiac arrest from a ventricular dysrhythmia; otherwise, the indications seem to be less agreed upon, and somewhat subjective. This patient didn't receive Digibind, although I believe she should have. Digibind may be appropriate for ventricular dysrhythmias, AV nodal conduction disease such as a Mobitz II second-degree AV block, or a third-degree AV block, especially with a very slow escape rhythm. Hyperkalemia (K+ >5) in a patient who has taken an acute digoxin overdose, with the high potassium signaling poisoning of the sodium-potassium-ATPase pump, is another possible indication for Digibind. Lastly, a digoxin level of 10 or above, regardless of the clinical status, or if the amount of digoxin ingested is >10 mg for adults or >4 mg in a child, are all indications for the administration of Digibind.

SG: There is a well-established view that if you have a patient who can be safely and effectively paced without giving them Fab fragments, you should. The thinking behind this is that the random use of Fab fragments is too expensive a cost for our healthcare system to sustain. This view always bothered me because I think that subjecting someone to the discomfort of pacing or the danger of transvenous pacing when we have a drug that can reduce its effect raises some difficult ethical issues.

PR: Given this patient has chronic renal failure, and we don't know whether it is acutely worsening, would that change your thinking about reversing the digoxin with Fab fragments?

Dr Edward Ullman: Renal failure doesn't equate to a need for Fab fragments.

PR: Given that this also could be beta-blocker toxicity, would you entertain giving this patient some glucagon, despite the fact that the patient's glucose was not bad at 176 mg/dL?

SG: If I decided to treat the patient for digoxin toxicity because I thought that's probably what it was, I wouldn't start glucagon. If Fab fragments didn't work, and it wasn't clear that this was dig toxicity, and the patient had a subsequent digoxin level that was zero or near zero, then I'd seriously consider glucagon, but I wouldn't use it empirically in this case.

PR: Since we are moving away from using digoxin for heart failure, do you think that is a reason to stop this patient's digitalis?

SG: Digoxin doesn't work acutely, and in the short-term there are other medicines that are effective and should be used for rate control in atrial fibrillation. Therefore, I have no problem with suppressing digoxin, particularly when it's causing conduction problems. Long term, digoxin remains unique as an effective cardiac inotrope, and could always be restarted later.

PR: Before we had easy access to digoxin levels, we used clinical parameters to decide whether a patient was sufficiently digitalized. If a patient's rate were slow, we felt we were where we needed to be. One of the clinical tests for adequate digitalization was to give a dose of atropine, and if the heart speeded up, we thought we needed more digoxin. Given the fact that this patient's heart rate is already slow, would you expect to see a very high level even before the laboratory value comes back?

EU: A high digoxin level wouldn't surprise me in this case, more so because of the EKG findings of atrial tachycardia with AV block. The vague neurologic complaints would have also clued me in.

PR: Is there a role for hemodialysis in digoxin toxicity, particularly in a patient with concomitant renal failure?

RH: Dialysis doesn't play a role in removing digoxin or the digoxin bound with Fab fragments. Hemodialysis does not enhance elimination due to the large volume of distribution of digoxin. Nevertheless, most patients recover well after receiving Digibind. If days later they do deteriorate, there may be a role for plasma exchange to rid the body of the digoxin-Fab fragments, particularly if there is a concern that the complex may come apart and cause a high rebound digoxin level.

PR: I thought the problem with giving Fab fragments was that it removes all of digoxin's effectiveness, and may worsen the patient's heart failure. This patient's CHF already seems to be worsening, and I wonder if that's why they chose not to use the Fab fragments.

RH: I agree. Although this patient was oxygenating, her reserve with an ejection fraction of 10–20% is limited. She is already in CHF, with impaired kidney function.

PR: This is a tough patient: she doesn't fit criteria for dialysis, but it's an ominous picture. I don't know if she fits criteria for replacing her mitral valve, as we don't have any detailed information about her valve, but we have a patient who is in pulmonary edema with mitral regurgitation, with diabetes and renal failure, who has digoxin toxicity. What can you do for her heart failure short of dialysis?

SG: You can try high-dose diuretics. High-dose diuretics are more likely to work in patients who still make urine, and may be useful. Preload reduction with intravenous nitroglycerin or afterload reduction with an ACE inhibitor may also be useful. There are a number of case reports of using an ACE inhibitor as a bridge to dialysis, and this might be that scenario.

PR: Would it worry you that she already has a dry nonproductive cough, which is supposedly associated with ACE inhibitors?

SG: No, simply because you have a cough from what is likely an intrinsic respiratory illness or perhaps as a manifestation of her heart failure, I wouldn't assume that the patient is at risk for a worsened cough from an ACE inhibitor. The cough from an ACE inhibitor is a unique side effect from the drug and associated with a delayed sensitization.

PR: Would you consider changing the diuretics?

EU: If you are going to continue her on the digoxin, then you have to be very careful about further worsening the renal function with more or higher doses of diuretics. ACE inhibitors might help to optimize the renal function in house, but it's not clear that another diuretic will lessen the risk of renal failure.

RH: Although we are not prescribing a lot of digoxin, we do cross paths with it, and we have to be careful what drugs we add that may precipitate toxicity down the road. While digoxin is not in the same tier of complications as is warfarin, where you have to look up almost any drug that you add for concerns regarding effect on the international normalized ratio (INR), there are a lot of drug interactions with digoxin, including quinidine, verapamil, tetracycline, erythromycin, and cyclosporine. All of these

can increase the dig level. We don't use all of these agents very frequently in the ED, but we do frequently use nonsteroidal antiinflammatory drugs (NSAIDS). There is literature suggesting a rising dig level with indomethacin, as well as other NSAIDS. You may be in a dangerous situation where a patient's renal perfusion may be compromised, and you impair it further with an NSAID, ultimately causing a dig toxic rhythm in the face of worsening renal failure.

PR: Is the use of Fab fragments a contraindication for surgery, assuming she has some degree of mitral regurgitation that someone may want to fix?

RH: I agree that when the heart is irritated, as it is here with digoxin, that that situation has to be quelled before any surgical stress on the heart can be superimposed on the clinical situation.

PR: I think she has a failing heart in the sense that the medications that we are giving her aren't going to improve her cardiac output that much. I wouldn't have had the nerve to hold off on the Fab; I haven't all that much faith in dig levels. I would have thought hers would be higher given the toxicity, and I'm not sure that the dig level is a reflection of dig activity anyway. This is a tough case and I think that it is a very interesting one, but I'm not sure what we have to offer this patient in long-term therapy.

SG: Digoxin is only one of the many medications we give that has potential for adverse outcomes, and needs careful monitoring of many different metabolic parameters. As we use less digoxin, we encounter more issues with other cardiac medications, such as calcium channel blocker and beta-blocker toxicity. I think that although we may not have to fight at the digitalis front as much as we used to, there are many new battles to be fought.

Case resolution

The patient was observed on telemetry; digoxin and metoprolol were held. Digoxin levels were monitored serially, and fell from an initial level of 2.1 ng/ml to 0.8 ng/mL by the second hospital day. She had no worsening of her dysrhythmias, and her heart failure improved with treatment. The EKG improved to atrial tachycardia with 2:1 block, and then reverted to atrial fibrillation; rate control was achieved with oral metoprolol. She was discharged home on metoprolol but without digoxin.

Section III: Concepts

Recreational toxins

Cocaine

Cocaine is the second most commonly used illicit drug, after marijuana, in the United States. More than 20% of Americans have tried cocaine, and 5.5% of Americans abused cocaine at least once in 2002. Men are twice as likely as women to abuse cocaine.[1] Cocaine-related complaints accounted for approximately 450,000 ED visits in 2005, more than any other illicit drug, and 40% of cocaine-related ED visits were for chest pain.[2]

Cocaine is an alkaloid extracted from the leaves of the *Erythroxylon coca* bush, which is found mostly in South America. It is ingested in one of two forms: as a hydrochloride salt or as freebase. The hydrochloride salt is water-soluble and is usually taken intranasally (snorting) or intravenously (mainlining). Cocaine ingestion causes catecholamine release and increased sympathetic tone, which leads to a faster heart rate, increased myocardial muscle contractility, and oxygen consumption. Cocaine reduces myocardial oxygen supply by causing coronary artery vasoconstriction via increased alpha-adrenergic smooth muscle contraction and decreased nitric oxide production.[3–5] It induces a prothrombotic state by increasing platelet production and aggregation, and it causes systemic hypertension by increasing both the cardiac index and arterial smooth muscle vasoconstriction.[6–8]

Cocaine ingestion is known to cause several cardiovascular complications, including angina, myocardial ischemia and infarction, hypertensive emergency, cardiomyopathy, dysrhythmias, and endocarditis.[9] The incidence of acute myocardial infarction (MI) among ED patients with cocaine-associated chest pain is approximately 1–6%, and another 15% of patients have an acute ischemic coronary syndrome (AICS).[10] The adjusted risk of MI is 24 times greater in the first hour after cocaine use; however, cocaine has been implicated as a causative factor in an AICS as much as a week after use.[11] It is thought that the metabolites of cocaine (benzoylecgonine and ecgonine methyl ester), which have a much longer half

life than cocaine itself, can cause coronary artery vasospasm and a delayed AICS.[9] Additionally, there is some evidence that cocaine withdrawal is related to the development of myocardial ischemia.[12] The toxic effect cocaine has on the cardiovascular system appears to be disproportionately increased by concomitant use of both tobacco and alcohol. Alcohol ingestion with cocaine leads to the development of cocaethylene, a unique metabolite that causes direct myocardial depression and increased coronary atherosclerosis, independent of the coronary artery spasm caused by cocaine.[13,14] Tobacco appears to increase the degree of coronary artery spasm caused by cocaine, and it independently decreases microvascular blood flow.[3]

Patients with a cocaine-related AICS tend to develop complications earlier than patients with a non-cocaine-related AICS. In one study, more than 90% of complications for cocaine-related acute MI (including CHF, dysrhythmias, and cardiogenic shock) occurred within 24 hours of presentation.[15] On the other hand, short-term mortality appears to be lower, and the likelihood of surviving a sudden cardiac arrest is higher, in patients with cocaine-related AICS.[16] The better prognosis for patients with a cocaine-associated AICS is believed to be related to their overall younger age and therefore lower level of underlying coronary atherosclerosis. Patients who have had chest pain and then abstain from further cocaine use have significantly better long-term outcomes than patients who continue to abuse cocaine.[17]

The presentation of a cocaine-related AICS is variable. Cocaine has been implicated as a cause in up to 25% of acute MI in patients aged 18–45 years, but it has also been known to cause an AICS in patients more than 60 years of age.[18,19] A detailed social history, including drug habits, frequency of use, and most recent use, should be elicited from all patients with symptoms consistent with a possible AICS. Urine screening for cocaine metabolites should be considered in any young person with chest pain, as underreporting is common, and confirmed cocaine use could affect short-term management strategies. About 45% of patients with a cocaine-associated AICS present with chest pain; the pain is most commonly described as substernal (71%) and pressure-like (47%). Other common presenting symptoms of acute MI among cocaine abusers are dyspnea (60%), diaphoresis (44%), and less commonly palpitations, dizziness, nausea, and anxiety.[10] Patients may present with symptoms of anxiety and restlessness related to the sympathomimetic stimulation of cocaine, but these symptoms are variable. In fact, "speedballing" (concomitant use of heroin and cocaine) may cause an initially depressed sensorium.[20]

The initial electrocardiogram (EKG) is abnormal in 55–80% of patients with a cocaine-associated AICS, but the findings are nonspecific. Benign early repolarization is a common finding that is not caused by the cocaine, and very few patients with J-point elevation and cocaine use have an acute MI.[21] Other common findings are left ventricular hypertrophy, nonspecific T-wave abnormality, and ST-segment elevation or depression. In one study, the EKG is 36% sensitive and 89% specific for an AICS in cocaine users.[10] A chest X-ray study should be performed on all patients with cardiopulmonary symptoms following cocaine abuse. Crack cocaine use can lead to the development of a pneumothorax and "crack lung," which is a syndrome of hypoxia, hemoptysis, and eventual respiratory failure associated with bilateral pulmonary infiltrates on the chest X-ray study. It occurs after the ingestion of freebase cocaine.[22]

Patients who abuse cocaine are at increased risk of developing rhabdomyolysis, which makes interpretation of serum myoglobin and total creatine kinase levels unreliable for risk stratification of a possible AICS; as such, serum troponin T and I levels are the most accurate markers for an AICS in patients abusing cocaine.[23,24] Patients with cocaine-associated chest pain who are considered a low risk for an AICS based on clinical presentation and EKG findings have a low rate (<3%) of fixed or reversible defects on myocardial perfusion imaging.[25] Cocaine use is associated with concentric left ventricular hypertrophy, which can mask localized wall-motion abnormalities, making echocardiography an insensitive test for detection of a cocaine AICS.[26] The majority of cocaine users (55–80%) with proven acute MI have evidence of underlying coronary artery disease on cardiac catheterization.[27]

Patients with a possible cocaine-associated AICS should be treated similarly to those with a non-cocaine-associated AICS, with a few notable exceptions. Patients with EKG evidence of an acute MI should be treated with emergent cardiac catheterization. There is evidence that patients who abuse cocaine who receive IV fibrinolytics are more likely to have intracranial bleeding and other complications than nonabusers; fibrinolytics should be given only to those patients suffering an acute ST elevation myocardial infarction when early percutaneous intervention is not possible.[28] Drug-eluting coronary stents should be considered for only the patients with a high probability of complying with long-term antiplatelet therapy.[2]

Patients with a possible cocaine-associated AICS should be treated with benzodiazepines early in their management. Benzodiazepines relieve chest pain, decrease heart rate, systolic blood pressure, and cardiac index in patients with cocaine-associated chest pain.[29] Hypertension associated with cocaine abuse should be treated initially with benzodiazepines, but if sympathomimetic symptoms are controlled with IV benzodiazepines and the patient remains hypertensive, treatment with phentolamine (a direct alpha-adrenergic blocker), sodium nitroprusside, or nitroglycerin can be utilized.[30]

Beta-adrenergic blockers increase the rate of coronary vasospasm in animal models exposed to cocaine, likely due to the effects of unopposed alpha-sympathetic stimulation on coronary smooth muscle cells.[31] Labetalol (a combined alpha- and beta-adrenergic antagonist, which has theoretical advantages over pure beta-adrenergic blocking agents) has been shown to increase the rate of seizure and death in cocaine animal models, and should be avoided in the acute setting. The current ACC/AHA guidelines recommend withholding all beta-adrenergic blockers from patients with a cocaine-associated AICS due to the increased risk of coronary vasoconstriction.[32]

Nitroglycerin reduces cocaine-associated chest pain, reverses coronary vasoconstriction and effectively treats hypertension.[29] Phentolamine reverses cocaine-associated hypertension and coronary vasoconstriction and, as mentioned previously, it can be used in patients not responding to benzodiazepine and nitroglycerin therapy.[30] Calcium channel blockers have no proven efficacy in patients with a cocaine-associated AICS, and are harmful in patients with heart failure. Antiplatelet and antithrombotic agents are indicated for a cocaine-associated AICS due to the direct prothombotic effects of cocaine.[2]

Patients with a high probability for a cocaine-induced AICS should be admitted to a monitored bed; low-to-moderate risk patients without other coronary risk factors can be safely evaluated in an observation unit. In one study, patients with cocaine-associated chest pain stratified as low-to-moderate risk for AICS were monitored with serial cardiac enzymes for 9 hours from initial presentation and then discharged. Fewer than 1% of patients discharged have had a postobservation MI at one-year follow-up.[33] Other studies of 9–12 hour observation periods for low-risk patients have similar results.[34]

Cocaine use can cause significant myocardial dysfunction, caused by direct myocardial toxicity and coronary artery vascoconstriction. Adulterants and virulent organisms administered with the cocaine can also cause myocarditis or endocarditis. Treatment for myocardial dysfunction includes abstinence from the drug in addition to standard therapy.[35]

Cocaine can cause atrial dysrhythmias, most commonly supraventricular tachycardia and atrial fibrillation, with intravenous fluids and benzodiazepines generally being effective for reversal. Beta-adrenergic blockers should be avoided in this population. Ventricular dysrhythmias can occur due to increased sympathetic tone and direct sodium channel blockade, with intravenous sodium bicarbonate, 1 to 2 mEq/kg, being the treatment of choice.[36] There has been some concern that lidocaine might increase dysrhythmic complications, but the clinical experience finds it to be efficacious; it should be considered second-line therapy for any wide complex dysrhythmia not responsive to sodium bicarbonate.[37]

Intravenous cocaine use can cause endocarditis, usually of left-sided valves, in contradistinction to other intravenous drug-associated endocarditis, which preferentially affects the right-sided valves. Cocaine use has also been associated with aortic dissection and rupture. One study of 38 patients with aortic dissection finds that 37% of the cases are related to cocaine use, most within 12 hours of ingestion.[38] Cocaine use is associated with an increased risk of ruptured intracerebral aneurysms, likely due to increased systemic blood pressure.

Alcohol

There are approximately 18 million alcoholics in the United States, and 8% of ED visits are related to alcoholism or inappropriate drinking.[39] Cardiovascular complications of heavy drinking and alcoholism include alcoholic cardiomyopathy, the "holiday heart" syndrome, and atrial fibrillation/flutter. Alcoholic cardiomyopathy typically presents in patients with a history of excessive drinking for more than 10 years, though subclinical decreased left ventricular function can occur with as little as 5 years of heavy drinking. Most cases occur during the fourth to sixth decades of life.[9] Men make up more than 85% of cases, but this difference can largely be attributed to the prevalence of alcoholism by gender, although they constitute a minority of cases, women appear to develop cardiac dysfunction at a lower cumulative alcohol dose than men.[40,41] Patients may present with symptoms as mild as a limited exercise tolerance, or as severe as decompensated heart failure. Symptoms include fatigue, dyspnea, orthopnea, and paroxysmal nocturnal dyspnea.

All patients presenting with symptoms of heart failure should be queried for acute and chronic alcohol consumption habits, with appropriate referral for counseling whenever possible. Counseling and group therapy are the only effective methods for decreasing drinking habits, which is the most successful treatment for alcoholic cardiomyopathy.[42] Patients with alcoholic cardiomyopathy may suffer from other stigmata of alcohol-related syndromes, including hepatic cirrhosis, malnourishment, alcoholic ketoacidosis, electrolyte abnormalities, and delirium tremens. Alcoholics with hepatic cirrhosis frequently have asymptomatic ventricular dysfunction, which should be considered in their acute management.[43,44]

Physical examination findings of alcoholic cardiomyopathy closely resemble those of idiopathic dilatated cardiomyopathy. Patients may have a narrow pulse pressure because systemic vasoconstriction causes an elevated diastolic pressure. Other findings include a presystolic gallop, displaced apical impulse, and a murmur of mitral regurgitation, auscultated best at the apex. Peripheral edema and an elevated jugular venous pressure may occur due to fluid retention.[9] There appears to be a relationship between the malnourishment common among alcoholics and the development of alcoholic cardiomyopathy.[44-46] The physical examination should include an assessment for malnourishment, which commonly presents in alcoholics as atrophy and skeletal myopathy of the shoulders and pelvic girdle.[47,48] An irregular pulse or tachycardia may be present, which would be consistent with an alcohol-induced dysrhythmia.

The etiology of alcoholic cardiomyopathy is not fully understood, but it appears that several mechanisms are involved. Alcohol has a direct toxic effect on cardiac myocytes by interfering with myocardial protein synthesis, limiting calcium efflux from the sarcoplasmic reticulum, and causing cellular apoptosis.[49–51] It appears that some individuals have a genetic susceptibility to the effects of alcohol abuse, as patients with certain genotypes of the angiotensin-converting enzyme are more likely to develop alcoholic cardiomyopathy.[52]

Thiamine deficiency is a known cause of congestive cardiomyopathy (termed wet beriberi), and alcoholics may be thiamine-deficient; however, alcoholic cardiomyopathy cannot be fully explained by thiamine deficiency, as chronic alcoholics are at risk of developing a cardiomyopathy regardless of nutritional status.[53,54] It is not clear what proportion of cardiac dysfunction in alcoholics is due to thiamine deficiency. Nevertheless, thiamine supplementation should be used in alcoholics with evidence of cardiac dysfunction, as vitamin supplementation has been shown to improve cardiac performance and quality of life in patients at risk of malnourishment, including alcoholics.[55]

Alcoholic cardiomyopathy presents similarly to idiopathic cardiomyopathy. Cardiomegaly, pulmonary vascular congestion and pleural effusions are frequent chest X-ray study findings. The EKG may show evidence of left ventricular hypertrophy, but should not be consistent with coronary artery ischemia. Other findings include first-degree heart block, bundle branch block, poor precordial R-wave progression, and atrio-ventricular conduction blocks. Cessation of alcohol consumption can, in just a few days, lead to normalized ST segments and T waves in some cases. Dysrhythmias, such as atrial fibrillation, atrial flutter, or multiple premature ventricular contractions, may be present, and are consistent with the "holiday heart syndrome." Hypomagnesemia should be sought in alcoholics, and has been linked to EKG changes such as a prolonged QT interval, U waves, ST-segment depression, widened QRS complexes, and atrial and ventricular dysrhythmias, usually with concomitantly low calcium or potassium stores. Alcoholic cardiomyopathy is typically characterized by a dilatated left ventricle, normal or reduced ventricular wall thickness, and increased left ventricular mass on echocardiography, findings that are indistinguishable from other dilatated cardiomyopathies.

Symptoms consistent with tachydysrhythmias in heavy binge drinkers, such as palpitations, weakness, dizziness, or syncope, may be a manifestation of the "holiday heart syndrome." This syndrome, as defined by Ettinger et al., refers to an "acute cardiac rhythm or conduction disturbance associated with heavy ethanol consumption in a person without other clinical evidence of heart disease, and disappearing, without evident residual, with abstinence."[56] Patients typically present with a sinus tachycardia or reentrant tachycardia after an episode of heavy drinking. The episodes are transient and respond to supportive care, hydration, and electrolyte repletion. Chronic, heavy alcohol use is a significant risk factor for the development of atrial fibrillation or flutter.[57] These dysrhythmias may in some cases be caused by an underlying alcoholic cardiomyopathy, but more commonly occur in heavy drinkers with structurally normal hearts. There is some evidence that patients with atrial abnormalities identified by P-wave averaging on EKGs are at increased risk of developing alcohol-induced atrial fibrillation.[58]

Patients should be admitted to a monitored setting if they demonstrate evidence of decompensated heart failure or potentially unstable dysrhythmias like rapid atrial fibrillation or persistent ventricular dysrhythmias. No specific therapies for alcohol-induced cardiomyopathy or dysrhythmias have been identified; these patients should be treated according to accepted guidelines for the care of heart failure and cardiac dysrhythmias.[59,60] In addition, thiamine should be administered to any chronic alcohol user with evidence of decompensated heart failure. Hypokalemia and hypomagnesemia should be sought, and appropriately treated if identified. Abstention significantly decreases the frequency of recurrences. Vitamin K antagonists are generally not indicated for patients less than 75 years of age with alcohol-induced atrial fibrillation or flutter, unless significant risk factors for coronary atherosclerosis are present; daily aspirin therapy should be initiated for these patients to decrease the risk of thrombotic complications.[61]

Alcoholic cardiomyopathy portends a lower relative mortality rate and need for cardiac transplantation than other cardiomyopathies (when adjusted for presenting heart failure class), especially when habitual, heavy drinkers abstain from further drinking.[62] Abstention has been shown to decrease mortality and the need for cardiac transplantation in patients, but reduction in drinking to even moderate alcohol consumption (up to two drinks per day) appears to decrease the risk of CHF.[63,64] Some studies show a slightly lower risk of CHF in patients who drink a light to moderate amount of alcohol (no more than two standard drinks per day) when compared to non-drinkers.[65] Similarly, there is evidence for a decreased incidence of coronary atherosclerosis in patients with light to moderate drinking, and it appears that this benefit is most striking in patients who preferentially consume wine.[66–69] It is unclear whether moderate consumption of beer has a beneficial effect, but ingestion of hard liquor does not appear to provide any benefit.[66] Recent studies suggest that resveratrol, a potent antioxidant found in red wine, may impart much of the cardioprotective effects of moderate wine consumption. Resveratrol decreases arterial damage, plasma LDL levels and cardiac myocyte cell death.[70,71] Animal studies show a decreased rate of coronary atherosclerosis in rabbits fed nonalcoholic resveratrol compounds.[72]

Amphetamines

Amphetamine abuse continues to increase in the United States, and now rivals cocaine as the most common cause of ED visits for illicit drug abuse.[73] Cardiovascular complications of amphetamine use include angina, MI, palpitations, dysrhythmias, cardiomyopathy, myocarditis, hypertension, and sudden death. Amphetamines have historically been used as an inhalant for the treatment of rhinitis and asthma, as a stimulant to improve concentration and physical performance, and as a dietary supplement.[74] Large quantities of amphetamines were produced in the United States until the mid 1950s, mostly as a treatment for obesity.[75] Amphetamine derivatives, including methamphetamine, propylhexedrine, aminorex fumarate, fenfluramine, and methylphenidate (Ritalin), have varying abuse potentials and limited medical utility. Methylphenidate is commonly used for the treatment of attention deficit hyperactivity disorder, and has a toxicity profile similar to other amphetamines.

Patients presenting with acute amphetamine toxicity demonstrate the cardiovascular signs and symptoms typical of other sympathomimetic ingestions, including chest pain, palpitations, diaphoresis, hypertension, and tachycardia.[76] Hypertension is common and should be treated initially with aggressive sedation and minimization of external stimuli. Patients who are persistently hypertensive after adequate sedation may require specific antihypertensive therapy; intravenous

nitroprusside or IV calcium channel blockers such as nifedipine or nicardipine can be used, as well as IV alpha-antagonists such as phentolamine. Beta-adrenergic blockers should be avoided due to the risk that unopposed alpha stimulation might cause paradoxical vasospasm and hypertension.[77]

Amphetamines increase the risk for angina and acute MI. The cause of the myocardial ischemia is multifactorial. Amphetamines cause a dose-related vasospasm of the coronary arteries similar to cocaine, and they also appear to cause myocarditis secondary to direct cardiac toxicity, and to increase the risk of coronary artery thrombosis. Myocardial ischemia secondary to amphetamine toxicity has been reported in all age groups, even adolescents.[78] Treatment includes vasodilatators such as nitrates, analgesia, and emergent reperfusion strategies for infarction, including thrombolytics and cardiac catheterization.

Patients with acute amphetamine toxicity frequently present in sinus tachycardia. Fluids, supportive care, and sedation typically normalize the heart rate; temperature elevation may coexist and contribute to the tachycardia. Amphetamine abuse is also associated with ventricular and supraventricular dysrhythmias, with the direct catecholamine effects of amphetamines and the ischemia caused by coronary artery vasospasm thought to be the cause of these dysrhythmias. Supraventricular tachycardias (other than sinus tachycardia) can be treated with adenosine, calcium channel blockers, and electrical cardioversion as indicated. Beta-adrenergic blockers should generally be avoided, but if required, esmolol should be used due to its short half-life. Fortunately, ventricular dysrhythmias are uncommon, and can be treated with conventional therapy. Massive amphetamine ingestion can lead to bradycardia, profound hypotension, and metabolic acidosis due to relative catecholamine depletion. Treatment includes aggressive intravenous hydration and vasopressors, such as norepinephrine and phenylephrine. Dopamine may not be effective in this catecholamine-depleted state. Amphetamine abuse is also a risk factor for sudden death.

Amphetamines can be responsible for either an acute or chronic cardiomyopathy, caused by direct myocardial toxicity and chronic hypertension.[79] Treatment is generally supportive, with avoidance of further amphetamine use being essential to recovery. Sodium nitroprusside and IV diuretics may be needed for treatment of acute episodes. Long-term care typically includes ACE inhibitors for afterload reduction and diuretics. Certain amphetamine derivatives that were developed as appetite suppressants, such as fenfluramine and dexfenfluramine, have been implicated in the development of cardiac valvular insufficiency. Chronic use of fenfluramine with phentermine, a phenylethylamine derivative (Fen-phen), has been associated with the development of mitral and aortic valvular regurgitation. The mechanism is unknown, but cessation of use has been associated with some improvement in valvular function. Fenfluramine has been removed from the market due to this toxic effect.[80]

Amphetamine abuse is associated with several other cardiovascular diseases. Intravenous amphetamine use can cause bacterial endocarditis, which can lead to a dilatated cardiomyopathy and stroke.[81] Localized extravasation of intravenous amphetamines causes tissue ischemia; immediate injection of alpha-antagonists such as phentolamine can reverse this vasospastic phenomenon. Idiopathic pulmonary hypertension is more likely to occur in patients who previously used amphetamines or cocaine, but the mechanism is not known.[82] Amphetamine abuse has also been associated with visceral and cerebral artery aneurysms, acute aortic dissection, and coronary artery rupture.[83–85] Treatment for these entities includes sedation, blood pressure control, and surgical management as indicated.

Environmental toxins

Cobalt
Certain additives to alcoholic beverages have been implicated in cardiac toxicity. Several cases of "beer drinker's cardiomyopathy" occurred in North America during the mid-1960s. It was soon found that cobalt, used as a foam stabilizer in many beers, accumulated in the hearts of these patients. When cobalt was subsequently removed from beer, no further cases occurred from domestic beer consumption, though nonregulated beer remains a potential source of cobalt ingestion and cardiomyopathy. Patients present with symptoms typical of cardiomyopathy, but cobalt exposure can also cause hypothyroidism, which can complicate the clinical course.[86] There have been cases of cobalt toxicity during occupational exposures, usually from cutting cobalt-laced metals with heavy equipment, but these episodes are

primarily characterized by dermatitis and pulmonary symptoms. Calcium disodium EDTA chelation therapy has been used with some success in treatment.[87]

Lead
Typically, lead poisoning presents with neurologic and gastrointestinal symptoms, but there is some risk for cardiovascular complications. Hypertension can occur with chronic lead poisoning; in fact, the triad of hypertension, gout, and chronic renal failure should prompt an investigation for subclinical lead poisoning.[88] Chronic lead poisoning can also cause a cardiomyopathy and congestive heart failure. There is some evidence that calcium disodium EDTA chelation therapy can improve cardiac function in these patients.[89]

Mercury
Acute mercury toxicity most commonly causes pulmonary, neurologic, and renal pathology, but metallic mercuric vapors can occasionally cause MI and systemic hypertension.[90] Chronic mercury accumulation in humans is largely caused by seafood ingestion, and there is some concern that mercury accumulation from seafood ingestion may counteract the beneficial effects of omega-3 fatty acids on the risk of coronary artery disease.[91] However, other studies do not support this concern.[92]

Antimony
A toxic gas or silver-gray metal depending on ion composition, antimony is used in glass manufacturing, as an alloy for copper and tin, for lead hardening, and in the textile industry. Occupational exposures can occur during welding and metallurgy. Conjugated forms of antimony are used as antibiotics in the treatment of leishmaniasis and schistosomiasis. Toxicity occurs via inhibition of thiol-containing enzymes.[93]

Symptoms of acute exposure include vomiting, diarrhea and abdominal pain. Noncardiogenic pulmonary edema, prolonged QT syndrome, and T-wave inversion can occur. Other occasional symptoms include chest pain, hypotension, bradycardia, ventricular dysrhythmias, and sudden death. Chronic occupational exposure can present as epistaxis, pneumoconiosis, and cardiomyopathy. Death is typically due to multisystem organ failure. Diagnosis is based on identification of the element in a 24-hour urine sample, and a chest X-ray study, EKG, and pulmonary function tests should also be obtained. The treatment is largely supportive, with activated charcoal recommended, though it does not appear to cause significant absorption. Chelation therapy with dimercaprol is effective if initiated early.[93]

Arsenic

Elemental arsenic is found concentrated in mineral belts in various parts of the world. It accumulates in food, especially shellfish, and contaminated water supplies, leading to chronic toxic exposures. It is used medicinally for the treatment of African sleeping sickness and as a chemotherapeutic agent for acute promyelocytic leukemia. Until quite recently, arsenic was used as a component of the outdoor wood sealant CCA (copper chromium arsenate), but concerns about arsenic leaching from CCA-treated wood, especially at children's playgrounds, led to the FDA banning its use in 2004; however, large quantities of treated wood are still present in American playgrounds.[94] CCA-treated wood used as firewood has also caused several acute exposures in recent years. The mechanism of arsenic toxicity is via inhibition of pyruvate dehydrogenase, limiting acetyl-coenzyme-A availability for the Krebs cycle.[95]

Acute ingestion causes mucosal irritation, vomiting, and severe diarrhea. Increased vascular permeability leads to third spacing and hypotension, followed by severe peripheral neuropathy. A clue to heavy metal poisoning is the presence of transverse white lines on the fingernails (Mee's lines). A prolonged QT interval is common on the EKG, and dysrhythmias such as torsades de pointes and ventricular fibrillation may occur.[96] Bradycardia, profound hypotension, and sudden death have also been reported. The diagnosis is based on clinical presentation; potential exposure, which can be confirmed with a 24-hour urine sample; and also by measurement of arsenic levels in hair and fingernails. Treatment is supportive, with aggressive crystalloid fluid resuscitation, and vasopressors as needed. Ventricular dysrhythmias should be treated using standard AHA protocols. Gastric lavage should be performed for acute ingestions when radiopaque material is seen on abdominal radiography. Continuous nasogastric suction is recommended to remove arsenic resecreted in gastric secretions. Chelation therapy with DMPS, or 2,3-dimercaptopropanol-sulfonic acid, is the antidote for arsenic poisoning, and should be started as soon as poisoning or accidental ingestion is suspected.[97]

Thallium

Salts of thallium are used in optical, electronic, and chemical research. Acute ingestion causes gastrointestinal and neurologic symptoms. Thallium is similar to potassium in structure and interferes with performance of the sodium-potassium pump. Flattened or inverted T waves may be seen on the EKG. Patients are at risk for cardiac dysrhythmia and sudden death up to several weeks after the initial exposure.[9] Treatment includes gastrointestical decontamination with activated charcoal and administration of Prussian blue to increase fecal elimination. Potassium supplementation may be useful, but chelation therapy is not recommended.[98]

Organic solvents

Children and adolescents sometimes abuse solvents via inhalation. Toluene (airplane glue), nail polish remover, shoe polish, typewriter correction fluid, adhesives, lighter fluid, kerosene, gasoline, and acrylic paint sprays have been reported in cases of intentional inhalations, and solvent inhalation leading to sudden death.[99] Typically in these cases, after inhalation, the child becomes panicky, engages in frantic exertion, and suddenly collapses, and witnessed cases have been found to be in ventricular fibrillation.[100] Animal studies show that inhalational solvents potentiate myocardial sensitivity to epinephrine; it is believed that agitation and exertion following solvent inhalation increases epinephrine release, which leads to ventricular dysrhythmias. Patients presenting following solvent inhalation should be sedated, and placed in a quiet environment with minimal stimulation to minimize catecholamine release.[101] Solvent abuse has also been associated with myocarditis and myocardial infarction.[9] Chronic abusers also develop renal tubular acidosis.

Medicinal toxins

Phosphodiesterase 5 inhibitors

Sildenafil (Viagra), tadalafil (Cialis), and vardenafil (Levitra) are selective cyclic GMP inhibitors used in the treatment of erectile dysfunction. They potentiate the effects of nitroglycerin and other nitrates on smooth muscle dilatation and, when taken with nitrates, can cause severe hypotension.[102] It is recommended that these agents not be taken within 24 hours of nitrate ingestion, and that nitrates should be withheld for at least 48 hours after tadalafil use; a safe time period to delay nitrates after vardenafil use has yet to be determined.[103] However, there is some evidence that nitroglycerin can be safely administered to patients with recent sildenafil ingestion if given intravenously and slowly titrated.[104]

Medication-induced QT prolongation

Long QT syndrome, which is frequently caused by complications of medication use, increases the risk of torsades de pointes and sudden death. Antidysrhythmics are the most common cause of prolonged QT-related dysrhythmias, but some antihistamines, antibiotics, antipsychotics, gastrointestinal medicines, cardiac medicines, and drugs of abuse have been implicated.[105] The website www.torsades.org maintains a complete, updated list of drugs that cause prolonged QT syndrome. Many of these drugs are cleared by the cytochrome p450 system. Co-administration of medicines that block this system can cause a dangerous accumulation of drugs that prolong the QT, with a resultant increased risk for dysrhythmia. The QT interval is measured from the beginning of the QRS complex to the end of the T wave, or U wave if the U wave is prominent and continuous with the T wave. The QT interval should be measured and averaged from 3–5 beats of the EKG lead with the longest recognizable QT interval (most commonly leads V3 or V4).[106] The QT interval shortens with tachycardia and lengthens with bradycardia. The formula most commonly used for rate correction (QTc) is to divide the QT interval by the square root of the RR interval.[107] QTc intervals less than 440 milliseconds are normal, and intervals of greater than 460 milliseconds in men and greater than 470 milliseconds in women are abnormal, while intervals in between are borderline.[105] For patients with atrial fibrillation, the QT interval should be measured over 10 beats and averaged.[107] There is no accepted definition for prolonged QT intervals in patients with a wide QRS complex.

Drug-induced QT prolongation is caused by delayed repolarization secondary to drug-induced blockade of the potassium efflux channels of the myocardial cells. The likelihood of a drug causing premature ventricular contractions and sudden death is directly related to the strength with which it blocks these channels.[108] This delayed repolarization leaves the myocardium vulnerable to depolarizations late in the T wave. As the T wave lengthens, the risk of depolarization

during the vulnerable phase increases. There is repolarization heterogeneity amongst ventricular cells, so if some cells depolarize early while others do not, a feedback loop and ventricular reentry can occur, potentially leading to torsades de pointes or sudden death.[109]

QT prolongation increases the risk for torsades de pointes, but most patients with prolonged QT do not develop dysrhythmias. In fact, the majority of patients with drug-induced QT prolongation that results in torsades de pointes have other identifiable risk factors, including hypokalemia, hypomagnesemia, coronary artery disease, female gender, excessive medication use, bradycardia, drug interactions, and a family history of a prolonged QT.[110] Some patients with drug-induced prolonged QT and ventricular dysrhythmias actually have underlying genetic mutations that predispose to the condition. It is believed in these cases that the medication unmasks the underlying tendency to prolonged repolarization.[111]

The majority of patients with a prolonged QT syndrome are asymptomatic, but patients can present with symptoms of dysrhythmias, including palpitations, chest pain, dizziness, and syncope. All patients with symptoms possibly due to dysrhythmias should have an EKG with measurement of the QTc. Patients with a possible causative drug should discontinue the medicine whenever possible, especially in patients with any of the above risk factors for torsades. Electrolyte abnormalities should be corrected, and potential drug-drug interactions investigated. Symptomatic patients should be monitored until the QT interval normalizes.[103]

Torsades de pointes can occur at any time in these patients. It tends to initiate and terminate spontaneously, and can be asymptomatic or cause dizziness, palpitations, or syncope, with possible degeneration into ventricular fibrillation and death. Stable patients presenting with polymorphic ventricular tachycardia should be treated with immediate intravenous magnesium sulfate (2 g bolus followed by 2–4 mg/minute) regardless of the serum magnesium level. The serum potassium should be maintained at a high normal range (4.5–5 mmol/L). Patients who become unstable, or who develop ventricular fibrillation, should undergo immediate nonsynchronized cardioversion. Overdrive transvenous pacing (rate 90–110 beats/min) may be necessary for patients with recurrent episodes, or those not responding to intravenous magnesium.

The QT interval narrows as the heart rate becomes faster, so maintaining a rapid heart decreases the likelihood of a depolarization during the vulnerable phase and recurrent torsades. Isoproterenol can be used to maintain the heart rate if pacing is unavailable, but it is contraindicated in patients with congenital prolonged QT syndrome or ischemic heart disease. Long-term care includes discontinuing the causative agent, possibly permanent pacing, and using an implantable defibrillator for recurrent symptoms.[105]

Cardiac agents

Recognizing that overdose (accidental or intentional) with any antihypertensive medication can cause hypotension, several agents deserve special mention when considering the cardiotoxicity of cardiac drugs.

Digitalis

Various drugs (principally digoxin, but also digitoxin in some countries) and related compounds (e.g., foxglove, oleander, squill, lily of the valley, ouabain), collectively referred to as digitalis preparations, exert both toxic and therapeutic effects on the heart.[112] Pharmacotherapeutic applications include atrioventricular (AV) nodal blockade, the treatment of supraventricular tachydysrhythmias (e.g., atrial fibrillation), and a positive inotropic effect employed at times in the treatment of CHF. The cardiotoxicity varies depending upon whether toxic levels of the drug, generally felt to occur above a serum level of approximately 2.0 ng/mL, recognizing individual variation, occurs by acute ingestion or chronic poisoning, and it is exacerbated in the sick or elderly patient.

Digitalis inhibits the sodium-potassium adenosine triphosphatase (ATPase) enzyme, resulting in an intracellular increase in calcium and thus augmenting myocardial contractility. The effect on conduction is mediated by a central vagotonic pathway as well as a direct, depressive effect on the AV node.[113,114] Toxicity occurs as a result of a narrow therapeutic window, numerous drug-drug interactions (salient examples include warfarin, paroxetine, quinidine, verapamil, cyclosporine, and amiodarone), electrolyte effects, and a dependency on renal clearance for digoxin, which can lead to toxicity in the presence of renal insufficiency.[113] Symptoms of digitalis toxicity are principally gastrointestinal (anorexia, nausea, vomiting, diarrhea) and neurologic (confusion, headache, dizziness,

delirium), but the paramount toxicologic manifestations are cardiac.[113-115] The EKG is the principal tool used to investigate cardiotoxicity, and complements both clinical findings and serum drug levels.

Digitalis effect on the EKG should be differentiated from digitalis toxicity. The former includes PR-segment prolongation; QT-interval shortening; a characteristic diffuse, coved/concave-upward ST-segment depression best seen in those leads with prominent R waves, and T wave changes; a U wave may also emerge.[114] These occur with therapeutic (as well as toxic) serum levels of the drug, and are not indicative of cardiotoxicity. The EKG manifestations of digitalis toxicity can be broadly split into rhythms that are too slow, because of depressed conduction velocity, and too fast, secondary to increased automaticity and excitability; also, the two may coexist (e.g., paroxysmal atrial tachycardia with high-grade AV block). Premature ventricular and atrial contractions are a common manifestation, as are bradyarrhythmias (sinus bradycardia, sinoatrial block, sinus pause/arrest, and all degrees of AV block). Typical tachydysrhythmias include paroxysmal atrial tachycardia (with AV block, at times high-grade), accelerated junctional rhythm, and ventricular tachycardia (including the pathognomonic bidirectional ventricular tachycardia).[114,115] Hyperkalemia is a poor prognostic factor in the setting of acute digitalis poisoning. Hypokalemia should be cautiously corrected in cases of chronic toxicity, as it may potentiate the cardiotoxic effects of the drug.[113,116]

Symptomatic bradyarrhythmias are treated first with atropine; although transvenous cardiac pacing may be effective, isoproterenol should be avoided. The cornerstone of treatment for profound digitalis poisoning is the administration of digoxin-specific antibody (Fab) fragments; its use as first-line monotherapy (i.e., with or without atropine but before other antidysrhythmics) carries a low mortality rate with proven efficacy.[113,117]

Beta-adrenergic blockers

Belonging to the Vaughan Williams antidysrhythmic Class II, beta-adrenergic blockers may manifest profound cardiotoxicity that is an extension of their therapeutic effect. Beta-1 selective antagonists decrease automaticity of cardiac pacemaker cells (sinus bradycardia), decrease conduction velocity through the AV node (AV block), and diminish myocardial contractility (decreased cardiac output and blood pressure). Beta-2 blockade causes bronchoconstriction (wheezing) and peripheral vasoconstriction.[118] These beta-1 actions are the principal cardiotoxic effects; they may occur in the diseased heart during therapeutic use, or in any individual with toxic levels, such as in overdose. However, beta-adrenergic blockers vary as to their degree of beta-1 selectivity, and must be considered individually in this regard; for example, atenolol and metoprolol are relatively beta-1 selective, whereas carvedilol, sotalol (which also is a Class III antidysrhythmic), and propranolol are not. Serum levels are not readily available, as they are in digoxin therapy, to guide therapy or management in poisoning scenarios.

The leading factor associated with the development of cardiovascular morbidity in beta-adrenergic blocker ingestion is the co-ingestion of another cardioactive agent, principally calcium channel blockers, cyclic antidepressants, or neuroleptics. When co-ingestion is controlled for, exposure to a beta-adrenergic blocker with membrane stabilizing activity is the next most important issue linked to an increased cardiovascular risk.[118,119] Those agents with significant membrane stabilizing activity include acebutalol and propranolol, as well as, to a lesser degree, betaxolol, oxprenolol, and carvedilol; QRS-complex widening and a prodysrhythmic effect may develop in poisoning.[120,121] Beyond sinus bradycardia, the most common EKG finding with beta-adrenergic blocker poisoning has been found to be first-degree AV block. Acebutalol may cause QTc prolongation, as well as behave like a sodium channel blocker (R wave in lead aVR > 3mm, widening of the QRS, see below).[120] With a propensity for bradycardia, hypotension, and EKG abnormalities in poisoning, beta-adrenergic blockers present similarly to digitalis toxicity (when digitalis-toxic patients are bradycardic, although they are not typically hypotensive), but even more closely resemble calcium channel blockers and clonidine (a central-acting alpha-2-agonist) in overdose. Other clues to beta-adrenergic blocker ingestion may include hypoglycemia (more common in children), mental status alteration, seizure, and bronchospasm. If the patient remains asymptomatic for 6 hours, significant toxicity is unlikely to occur, with the notable exception of sotalol, which can present in a delayed fashion.[118]

Initial treatment of the cardiovascular toxicity of beta-adrenergic blockers includes intravenous fluids for hypotension and atropine for symptomatic bradycardia. Bradycardia and hypotension refractory to these measures should stimulate the use of glucagon (first-line), calcium, vasopressor support, and perhaps high-dose insulin/glucose infusions. Amrinone should be considered for situations of refractory decrease in cardiac output. As with other sodium channel blockers, sodium bicarbonate is used to treat the wide-complex dysrhythmias associated with membrane stabilizing agents such as acebutalol and propranolol. Other non-pharmacologic considerations include cardiac pacing, hemodialysis (for agents such as atenolol or sotalol with low-lipophilicity and minimal protein binding), intra-aortic balloon counterpulsation, and extracorporeal support.[122]

Calcium channel blockers

These agents exert a cardiotoxic effect similar to that of the beta-adrenergic blockers, with some notable exceptions. Their toxicologic behavior is linked to their chemical structure; they can be classified as phenylalkylamines (verapamil), benzothiazepines (diltiazem), dihydropyridines (amlodipine, felodipine, nicardipine, isradipine, nifedipine, nimodipine, nisoldipine), diarylaminopropylethers (bepridil), and tetraline derivatives (mibefradil).[123] To varying degrees, these agents, depending upon their pharmacology, cause cardiac effects (negative inotropy and chronotropy) and peripheral vascular smooth muscle relaxation with coronary vascular dilatation, and are used principally for blood pressure and heart rate control.[123, 124] The dihydropyridines are potent peripheral vasodilators with relatively little effect on cardiac inotropy and chronotropy; diltiazem, and, to a greater degree, verapamil, are weak vasodilatators, yet potent negative inotropes/chronotropes.[123] As with beta-adrenergic blockers, there are long-acting preparations in use; verapamil, especially, has numerous drug interactions (e.g., digoxin, propranolol, cyclosporine, prazosin) and may have strong additive effects on heart rate when co-administered with other agents (e.g., beta-adrenergic blockers, digoxin, halothane, amiodarone).[123]

As with beta-adrenergic blockers, the hallmark of cardiotoxicity is hypotension and bradycardia for potentially all classes of calcium channel blockers, with the bradycardia being more common and profound with verapamil and diltiazem.[124] A telltale difference from beta-adrenergic blocker poisoning is an increased likelihood to cause hyperglycemia, rather than hypoglycemia; noncardiogenic pulmonary edema may also occur.[125] Bepridil causes QT-interval prolongation with the attendant risks of ventricular dysrhythmia.[123]

Treatment of calcium channel blocker poisoning is similar to that of beta-adrenergic blocker toxicity.[122] Drug levels are not readily available. Whole bowel irrigation is recommended with sustained-release preparations.[123]

Class IA antidysrhythmic agents (sodium channel blockers)

This drug class includes quinidine, disopyramide, and procainamide, which are classic in their association with cardiotoxicity, but seen far less in clinical practice today. They are known to cause QT-interval prolongation (potassium efflux antagonism) and multiple dysrhythmias, including sodium channel blockade-mediated ventricular dysrhythmias. They are best considered as members of the sodium channel blocker class for toxicologic purposes (they are also referred to as membrane stabilizing drug, as discussed in the beta-adrenergic blockers section), and join a long list of drugs with similar pharmacology, including type IC antidysrhythmics, tricyclic antidepressants, some phenothiazines, carbamazepine, diphenhydramine, propoxyphene, and cocaine, to name a few. Coincident toxicologic features across these agents vary, as they share some, but not all, pharmacologic characteristics (e.g, anticholinergic effects).[126]

Cardiotoxicity includes a variety of dysrhythmias, more commonly ventricular (ventricular fibrillation, ventricular tachycardia, and torsades de pointes) in origin rather than supraventricular (atrial tachycardia), and AV block. The electrocardiographic hallmark of sodium channel blocker toxicity is widening of the QRS complex, at times resembling a bundle branch block and often occurring with an anticholinergic-mediated tachycardia.[126] Rightward deviation of the terminal 40 msec of the frontal plane QRS axis, resulting in a tall ($\geq$3 mm) R wave in lead aVR, is predictive of cardiotoxicity in tricyclic antidepressant poisoning, but its predictive value in all sodium channel blockers is unclear.[126–128]

Treatment of wide-complex dysrhythmias with suspected sodium channel blocker toxicity begins with sodium bicarbonate. Bradycardia and hypotension

are treated initially with atropine and intravenous fluids, respectively. If torsades de pointes occurs, magnesium sulfate by intravenous bolus (2 gm) is the initial agent, and followed by continuous infusion (1–2 gm/hr); overdrive pacing can also be used.[129]

Anti-cancer chemotherapeutic agents

A number of drugs used in cancer chemotherapy can cause cardiotoxicity, but rarely will the emergency physician deal with acute toxicity from these drugs. A chart of the different agents and their cardiotoxic effects is presented below (Table 17-1). The effects are usually cumulative and dose-dependent.[130,131]

Table 17-1. Chemotherapeutic cardiac toxins.

Drug	Pharmacologic Class	Cardiotoxic Effect
Doxorubicin Daunorubicin Epirubicin	Anthracycline	Cardiomyopathy Congestive heart failure
Mitoxantrone	Anthraquinone	Cardiomyopathy Congestive heart failure
Fluorouracil	Antimetabolite	Cardiac ischemia Dysrhythmias
Capecitabine	Fluoropyrimidine	Cardiac ischemia Dysrhythmias
Fludarabine Pentostatin Cladribine	Purine antagonists	Cardiac ischemia Congestive heart failure
Vinblastine Vincristine Vinorelbine	Vinca alkaloids	Cardiac ischemia Hypertension
Paclitaxel Docetaxel	Taxane	Conduction delays Bradycardia
Cyclophosphamide	Alkylating agent	Acute cardiomyopathy Hemorrhagic pericarditis
Ifosfamide Cisplatin	Alkylating agents	Dysrhythmias Cardiac ischemia Cardiomyopathy
Mitomycin	Antitumor antibiotic	Congestive heart failure
Bleomycin	Antitumor antibiotic	Cardiac ischemia Pericarditis

Section IV: Decision making

- Cocaine and other sympathomimetic drugs such as amphetamines may cause cardiac ischemia; treatment includes conventional medications (e.g., nitroglycerin, aspirin, heparin) as needed as well as non-conventional medications (e.g., benzodiazepines).
- Avoid beta-adrenergic blockers when treating acute coronary syndrome in patients acutely intoxicated with cocaine or amphetamine because of the possibility of unopposed alpha-adrenergic stimulation.
- The differential diagnosis for bradycardia mediated by cardiac medications includes digitalis, calcium channel blockers, beta-adrenergic blockers, and clonidine.
- Digitalis toxicity may induce almost any dysrhythmia (tachydysrhythmia or bradyarrhythmia), except atrial fibrillation with a rapid ventricular response.

References

1 Fryar CD, Hirsch R, Porter KS, et al. Drug use and sexual behaviors reported by adults: United States, 1999-2002. *Adv Data*. 2007;384:1–14.

2 McCord J, Jneid H, Hollander JE, et al. Management of cocaine-associated chest pain and myocardial infarction: a scientific statement from the American Heart Association Acute Cardiac Care Committee of the Council on Clinical Cardiology. *Circulation*. 2008;117:1897-1907.

3 Moliterno DJ, Willard JE, Lange RA, et al. Coronary-artery vasoconstriction induced by cocaine, cigarette smoking, or both. *N Engl J Med*. 1994;330:454-459.

4 Wilbert-Lampen U, Seliger C, Zilker T, Arendt RM. Cocaine increases the endothelial release of immunoreactive endothelin and its concentrations in human plasma and urine: reversal by coincubation with sigma-receptor antagonists. *Circulation*. 1998;98:385–390.

5 Mo W, Singh AK, Arruda JA, Dunea G. Role of nitric oxide in cocaine-induced acute hypertension. *Am J Hypertens*. 1998;11:708–714.

6 Moliterno DJ, Lange RA, Gerard RD, et al. Influence of intranasal cocaine on plasma constituents associated with endogenous thrombosis and thrombolysis. *Am J Med*. 1994;96:492–496.

7 Rinder HM, Ault KA, Jatlow PI, Kosten, TR, Smith BR. Platelet alpha-granule release in cocaine users. *Circulation*. 1994;90:1162–1167.

8 Kugelmass AD, Oda A, Monahan K, Cabral C, Ware JA. Activation of human platelets by cocaine. *Circulation*. 1993;88:876–883.

9 Lange RA, Hillis DA. Toxins and the heart. In: Libby P, ed. *Braunwald's heart disease: a Textbook of Cardiovascular Medicine*. 8th ed. Saunders/Elsevier; Philadelphia: 2008;1805–1814.

10 Hollander JE, Hoffman RS, Gennis P, et al. Prospective multicenter evaluation of cocaine-associated chest pain. Cocaine Associated Chest Pain (COCHPA) Study Group. *Acad Emerg Med*. 1994;1:330–339.

11 Mittleman MA, Mintzer D, Maclure M, et al. Triggering of myocardial infarction by cocaine. *Circulation*. 1999;99:2737–2741.

12 Nademanee K, Gorelick DA, Josephson MA, et al. Myocardial ischemia during cocaine withdrawal. *Ann Intern Med*. 1989;111:876–880.

13 Henning RJ, Wilson LD, Glauser JM. Cocaine plus ethanol is more cardiotoxic than cocaine or ethanol alone. *Crit Care Med*. 1994;22:1896–1906.

14 Pirwitz MJ, Willard JE, Landau C, et al. Influence of cocaine, ethanol, or their combination on epicardial coronary arterial dimensions in humans. *Arch Intern Med*. 1995;155:1186–1191.

15 Hollander JE, Hoffman RS, Burstein JL, Shih RD, Thode HC. Cocaine-associated myocardial infarction. Mortality and complications. Cocaine-Associated Myocardial Infarction Study Group. *Arch Intern Med*. 1995;155:1081–1086.

16 Hsue PY, McManus D, Selby V, et al. Cardiac arrest in patients who smoke crack cocaine. *Am J Cardiol*. 2007;99:822–824.

17 Hollander JE, Hoffman RS, Gennis P, et al. Cocaine-associated chest pain: one-year follow-up. *Acad Emerg Med*. 1995;2:179–184.

18 Qureshi AI, Suri MF, Guterman LR, Hopkins LN. Cocaine use and the likelihood of nonfatal myocardial infarction and stroke: data from the Third National Health and Nutrition Examination Survey. *Circulation*. 2001;103:502–506.

19 Weber JE, Chudnofsky CR, Boczar M, et al. Cocaine-associated chest pain: how common is myocardial infarction? *Acad Emerg Med*. 2000;7:873–877.

20 Rao RB, Hoffman RS. Cocaine and other sympathomimetics. In: Marx JA, ed. *Rosen's Emergency Medicine: Concepts and Clinical Practice*. 6th ed. Philadelphia: Mosby/Elsevier; 2006:2386–2393.

21 Hollander JE, Lozano M, Fairweather P, et al. "Abnormal" electrocardiograms in patients with

cocaine-associated chest pain are due to "normal" variants. *J Emerg Med*.1994;12:199–205.

22 Forrester JM, Steele AW, Waldron JA, Parsons PE. Crack lung: an acute pulmonary syndrome with a spectrum of clinical and histopathologic findings. *Am Rev Respir Dis*. 1990;142:462–467.

23 Gitter MJ, Goldsmith SR, Dunbar DN, Sharkey SW. Cocaine and chest pain: clinical features and outcome of patients hospitalized to rule out myocardial infarction. *Ann Intern Med*. 1991;115:277–282.

24 Hollander JE, Levitt MA, Young GP, et al. Effect of recent cocaine use on the specificity of cardiac markers for diagnosis of acute myocardial infarction. *Am Heart J*. 1998;135:245–252.

25 Kontos MC, Schmidt KL, Nicholson CS, et al. Myocardial perfusion imaging with technetium-99m sestamibi in patients with cocaine-associated chest pain. *Ann Emerg Med*. 1999;33:639–645.

26 Neuman Y, Cercek B, Aragon J, et al. Comparison of frequency of left ventricular wall motion abnormalities in patients with a first acute myocardial infarction with versus without left ventricular hypertrophy. *Am J Cardiol*. 2004;94:763–766.

27 Kontos MC, Jesse RL, Tatum JL, Ornato JP. Coronary angiographic findings in patients with cocaine-associated chest pain. *J Emerg Med*.2003;24:9–13.

28 Bush HS. Cocaine-associated myocardial infarction. A word of caution about thrombolytic therapy. *Chest* 1988;94:878.

29 Baumann BM, Perrone J, Hornig SE, Shofer FS, Hollander JE. Randomized, double-blind, placebo-controlled trial of diazepam, nitroglycerin, or both for treatment of patients with potential cocaine-associated acute coronary syndromes. *Acad Emerg Med*. 2000;7:878–885.

30 Lange RA, Cigarroa RG, Yancy CW, Jr., et al. Cocaine-induced coronary-artery vasoconstriction. *N Engl J Med*. 1989;321:1557–1562.

31 Smith M, Garner D, Niemann JT. Pharmacologic interventions after an LD50 cocaine insult in a chronically instrumented rat model: are beta-blockers contraindicated? *Ann Emerg Med*. 1991;20:768–771.

32 2005 American Heart Association Guidelines for Cardiopulmonary Resuscitation and Emergency Cardiovascular Care. *Circulation*. 2005;112:IV1–203.

33 Cunningham R, Walton MA, Weber JE, et al. One-year medical outcomes and emergency department recidivism after emergency department observation for cocaine-associated chest pain. *Ann Emerg Med*. 2009;53:310–320.

34 Kushman SO, Storrow AB, Liu T, Gibler WB. Cocaine-associated chest pain in a chest pain center. *Am J Cardiol*. 2000;85:394–396, A10.

35 Zaca V, Lunghetti S, Ballo P, et al. Recovery from cardiomyopathy after abstinence from cocaine. *Lancet*. 2007;369:1574.

36 Kerns W, 2nd, Garvey L, Owens J. Cocaine-induced wide complex dysrhythmia. *J Emerg Med*.1997;15:321–329.

37 Shih RD, Hollander JE, Burstein JL, et al. Clinical safety of lidocaine in patients with cocaine-associated myocardial infarction. *Ann Emerg Med*. 1995;26:702–706.

38 Hsue PY, Salinas CL, Bolger AF, Benowitz NL, Watters DD. Acute aortic dissection related to crack cocaine. *Circulation*. 2002;105:1592–1595.

39 McDonald AJ, 3rd, Wang N, Camargo CA, Jr. US emergency department visits for alcohol-related diseases and injuries between 1992 and 2000. *Arch Intern Med*. 2004;164:531–537.

40 Fernandez-Sola J, Estruch R, Nicolas JM, et al. Comparison of alcoholic cardiomyopathy in women versus men. *Am J Cardiol*. 1997;80:481–485.

41 Urbano-Marquez A, Estruch R, Fernandez-Sola J, et al. The greater risk of alcoholic cardiomyopathy and myopathy in women compared with men. *JAMA*. 1995; 274:149–154.

42 Ahmed M. Towards evidence based emergency medicine: best BETs from the Manchester Royal Infirmary. Is emergency department based brief intervention worthwhile in adults presenting with alcohol related events? *Emerg Med J*. 2007;24:785–788.

43 Estruch R, Fernandez-Sola J, Sacanella E, et al. Relationship between cardiomyopathy and liver disease in chronic alcoholism. *Hepatology*. 1995;22: 532–538.

44 Sacanella E, Fernandez-Sola J, Cofan M, et al. Chronic alcoholic myopathy: diagnostic clues and relationship with other ethanol-related diseases. *QJM*. 1995;88: 811–817.

45 Nicolas JM, Estruch R, Antunez E, Sacanella E, Urbano-Marquez A. Nutritional status in chronically alcoholic men from the middle socioeconomic class and its relation to ethanol intake. *Alcohol*. 1993;28:551–558.

46 Nicolas JM, Garcia G, Fatjo F, et al. Influence of nutritional status on alcoholic myopathy. *Am J Clin Nutr*. 2003;78:326–333.

47 Urbano-Marquez A, Estruch R, Grau JM, Vernet M, Casademont J. Skeletal muscle changes in chronic alcoholic patients. *Acta Neurol Scand*. 1985;72:72–73.

48 Estruch R, Nicolas JM, Villegas E, Junqué, A, Urbano-Marquèz, A. Relationship between ethanol-related diseases and nutritional status in chronically alcoholic men. *Alcohol*. 1993;28:543–550.

49 Vary TC, Deiter G. Long-term alcohol administration inhibits synthesis of both myofibrillar and sarcoplasmic proteins in heart. *Metabolism*. 2005;54:212–219.

50 Fernandez-Sola J, Fatjo F, Sacanella E, et al. Evidence of apoptosis in alcoholic cardiomyopathy. *Hum Pathol.* 2006;37:1100–1110.

51 Aistrup GL, Kelly JE, Piano MR, Wasserstrom JA. Biphasic changes in cardiac excitation-contraction coupling early in chronic alcohol exposure. *Am J Physiol Heart Circ Physiol.* 2006;291:H1047–H1057.

52 Fernandez-Sola J, Nicolas JM, Oriola J, et al. Angiotensin-converting enzyme gene polymorphism is associated with vulnerability to alcoholic cardiomyopathy. *Ann Intern Med.* 2002;137:321–326.

53 Wooley JA. Characteristics of thiamin and its relevance to the management of heart failure. *Nutr Clin Pract.* 2008;23:487–493.

54 Dancy M, Bland JM, Leech G, Gaitonde MK, Maxwell JD. Preclinical left ventricular abnormalities in alcoholics are independent of nutritional status, cirrhosis, and cigarette smoking. *Lancet.* 1985;1:1122–1125.

55 Witte KK, Nikitin NP, Parker AC, et al. The effect of micronutrient supplementation on quality-of-life and left ventricular function in elderly patients with chronic heart failure. *Eur Heart J.* 2005;26:2238–2244.

56 Ettinger PO, Wu CF, De La Cruz C, et al. Arrhythmias and the "holiday heart": alcohol-associated cardiac rhythm disorders. *Am Heart J.* 1978;95:555–562.

57 Mukamal KJ, Tolstrup JS, Friberg J, Jensen G, Gronbaek M. Alcohol consumption and risk of atrial fibrillation in men and women: the Copenhagen City Heart Study. *Circulation.* 2005;112:1736–1742.

58 Steinbigler P, Haberl R, Konig B, Steinbeck G. P-wave signal averaging identifies patients prone to alcohol-induced paroxysmal atrial fibrillation. *Am J Cardiol.* 2003;91:491–494.

59 Fuster V, Ryden LE, Cannom DS, et al. ACC/AHA/ESC 2006 Guidelines for the management of patients with atrial fibrillation: A report of the American College of Cardiology/American Heart Association Task Force on Practice Guidelines and the European Society of Cardiology Committee for Practice Guidelines. *Circulation.* 2006;114:e257–e354.

60 Carley S, Ali B, Mackway-Jones K. Towards evidence based emergency medicine: best BETs from the Manchester Royal Infirmary. Acute myocardial infarction in cocaine induced chest pain presenting as an emergency. *Emerg Med J.* 2003;20:174–175.

61 Singer DE, Albers GW, Dalen JE, et al. Antithrombotic therapy in atrial fibrillation: American College of Chest Physicians Evidence-Based Clinical Practice Guidelines (8th Edition). *Chest.* 2008;133:546S–592S.

62 Prazak P, Pfisterer M, Osswald S, Buser P, Burkart F. Differences of disease progression in congestive heart failure due to alcoholic as compared to idiopathic dilated cardiomyopathy. *Eur Heart J.* 1996;17:251–257.

63 Gavazzi A, De Maria R, Parolini M, Porcu M. Alcohol abuse and dilated cardiomyopathy in men. *Am J Cardiol.* 2000;85:1114–1118.

64 Salisbury AC, House JA, Conard MW, Krumholz HM, Spertus JA. Low-to-moderate alcohol intake and health status in heart failure patients. *J Card Fail.* 2005;11:323–328.

65 Abramson JL, Williams SA, Krumholz HM, Vacarrino V. Moderate alcohol consumption and risk of heart failure among older persons. *JAMA.* 2001;285:1971–1977.

66 Tolstrup J, Gronbaek M. Alcohol and atherosclerosis: recent insights. *Curr Atheroscler Rep.* 2007;9:116–124.

67 Femia R, Natali A, L'Abbate A, Ferrannini E. Coronary atherosclerosis and alcohol consumption: angiographic and mortality data. *Arterioscler Thromb Vasc Biol.* 2006;26:1607–1612.

68 Janszky I, Mukamal KJ, Orth-Gomer K, et al. Alcohol consumption and coronary atherosclerosis progression—the Stockholm Female Coronary Risk Angiographic Study. *Atherosclerosis.* 2004;176:311–319.

69 da Luz PL, Coimbra SR. Wine, alcohol and atherosclerosis: clinical evidences and mechanisms. *Braz J Med Biol Res.* 2004;37:1275–1295.

70 Penumathsa SV, Maulik N. Resveratrol: a promising agent in promoting cardioprotection against coronary heart disease. *Can J Physiol Pharmacol.* 2009;87:275–286.

71 Wu JM, Wang ZR, Hsieh TC, et al. Mechanism of cardioprotection by resveratrol, a phenolic antioxidant present in red wine (Review). *Int J Mol Med.* 2001;8:3–17.

72 Wang Z, Zou J, Cao K, et al. Dealcoholized red wine containing known amounts of resveratrol suppresses atherosclerosis in hypercholesterolemic rabbits without affecting plasma lipid levels. *Int J Mol Med.* 2005;16:533–540.

73 Maxwell JC, Rutkowski BA. The prevalence of methamphetamine and amphetamine abuse in North America: a review of the indicators, 1992–2007. *Drug Alcohol Rev.* 2008;27:229–325.

74 Rasmussen N. America's first amphetamine epidemic 1929–1971: a quantitative and qualitative retrospective with implications for the present. *Am J Public Health.* 2008;98:974–985.

75 Albertson TE, Kenyon NJ, Morrissey B. Amphetamines and derivatives. In: Shannon MW, ed. *Haddad and Winchester's Clinical Management of Poisoning and Drug Overdose.* 4th ed. Philadelphia: Saunders/Elsevier; 2007:781–790.

76 Derlet RW, Albertson TE. Emergency department presentation of cocaine intoxication. *Ann Emerg Med.* 1989;18:182–186.

77 Bashour TT. Acute myocardial infarction resulting from amphetamine abuse: a spasm-thrombus interplay? *Am Heart J.* 1994;128:1237–1239.

78 Westover AN, Nakonezny PA, Haley RW. Acute myocardial infarction in young adults who abuse amphetamines. *Drug Alcohol Depend.* 2008;96:49–56.

79 Ayres PR. Amphetamine cardiomyopathy. *Ann Intern Med.* 1983;98:110.

80 Rasmussen S, Corya BC, Glassman RD. Valvular heart disease associated with fenfluramine-phentermine. *N Engl J Med.* 1997;337:1773.

81 Kaku DA, Lowenstein DH. Emergence of recreational drug abuse as a major risk factor for stroke in young adults. *Ann Intern Med.* 1990;113:821–827.

82 Chin KM, Channick RN, Rubin LJ. Is methamphetamine use associated with idiopathic pulmonary arterial hypertension? *Chest.* 2006;130:1657–63.

83 Welling TH, Williams DM, Stanley JC. Excessive oral amphetamine use as a possible cause of renal and splanchnic arterial aneurysms: a report of two cases. *J Vasc Surg.* 1998;28:727–731.

84 Dihmis WC, Ridley P, Dhasmana JP, Wisheart JD. Acute dissection of the aorta with amphetamine misuse. *BMJ.*1997;314:1665.

85 Brennan K, Shurmur S, Elhendy A. Coronary artery rupture associated with amphetamine abuse. *Cardiol Rev.* 2004;12:282–283.

86 Alexander CS. Cobalt-beer cardiomyopathy. A clinical and pathologic study of twenty-eight cases. *Am J Med.* 1972;53:395–417.

87 Morin Y, Daniel P. Quebec beer-drinkers' cardiomyopathy: etiological considerations. *Can Med Assoc J.* 1967;97:926–928.

88 Shannon MW. Lead. In: Shannon MW, ed. *Haddad and Winchester's Clinical Management of Poisoning and Drug Overdose.* 4th ed. Philadelphia: Saunders/Elsevier; 2007:781–790.

89 Balestra DJ. Adult chronic lead intoxication. A clinical review. *Arch Intern Med.* 1991;151:1718–1720.

90 Baum CR. Mercury, Heavy metals and inorganic agents. In: Shannon MW, ed. *Haddad and Winchester's Clinical Management of Poisoning and Drug Overdose.* 4th ed. Philadelphia: Saunders/Elsevier; 2007: 1111–1116.

91 Guallar E, Sanz-Gallardo MI, van't Veer P, et al. Mercury, fish oils, and the risk of myocardial infarction. *N Engl J Med.* 2002;347:1747–1754.

92 Yoshizawa K, Rimm EB, Morris JS, et al. Mercury and the risk of coronary heart disease in men. *N Engl J Med.* 2002;347:1755–1760.

93 Lauwers LF, Roelants A, Rosseel PM, Heyndrickx B, Baute L. Oral antimony intoxications in man. *Crit Care Med.* 1990;18:324–326.

94 Peters HA, Croft WA, Woolson EA, Darcey BA, Olson MA. Seasonal arsenic exposure from burning chromium-copper-arsenate-treated wood. *JAMA.* 1984;251:2393–2396.

95 Pigott DC, Liebelt EL. Arsenic and arsine. In: Shannon MW, ed. *Haddad and Winchester's Clinical Management of Poisoning and Drug Overdose.* 4th ed. Philadelphia: Saunders/Elsevier; 2007:781.

96 Beckman KJ, Bauman JL, Pimental PA, Garrard C, Hariman RJ. Arsenic-induced torsade de pointes. *Crit Care Med.* 1991;19:290–292.

97 Aposhian HV. Mobilization of mercury and arsenic in humans by sodium 2,3-dimercapto-1-propane sulfonate (DMPS). *Environ Health Perspect.* 1998;106 Suppl 4:1017–1025.

98 Insley BM, Grufferman S, Ayliffe HE. Thallium poisoning in cocaine abusers. *Am J Emerg Med.*1986;4:545–548.

99 Lorenc JD. Inhalant abuse in the pediatric population: a persistent challenge. *Curr Opin Pediatr.* 2003;15: 204–209.

100 Williams DR, Cole SJ. Ventricular fibrillation following butane gas inhalation. *Resuscitation.* 1998;37:43–45.

101 Murphy NG, Benowitz NL, Goldschlager N. Cardiovascular toxicology. In: Shannon MW, ed. *Haddad and Winchester's Clinical Management of Poisoning and Drug Overdose.* 4th ed. Philadelphia: Saunders/Elsevier; 2007:133–156.

102 Webb DJ, Muirhead GJ, Wulff M, et al. Sildenafil citrate potentiates the hypotensive effects of nitric oxide donor drugs in male patients with stable angina. *J Am Coll Cardiol.* 2000;36:25–31.

103 Anderson JL, Adams CD, Antman EM, et al. ACC/AHA 2007 guidelines for the management of patients with unstable angina/non-ST-elevation myocardial infarction: a report of the American College of Cardiology/American Heart Association Task Force on Practice Guidelines. *J Am Coll Cardiol.* 2007;50:e1–e157.

104 Parker JD, Bart BA, Webb DJ, et al. Safety of intravenous nitroglycerin after administration of sildenafil citrate to men with coronary artery disease: a double-blind, placebo-controlled, randomized, crossover trial. *Crit Care Med.* 2007;35:1863–1868.

105 Gupta A, Lawrence AT, Krishnan K, Kavinsky CJ, Trohman RG. Current concepts in the mechanisms and management of drug-induced QT prolongation and torsade de pointes. *Am Heart J.* 2007;153:891–899.

106 Indik JH, Pearson EC, Fried K, Woosley RL. Bazett and Fridericia QT correction formulas interfere with

measurement of drug-induced changes in QT interval. *Heart Rhythm*. 2006;3:1003–1007.

107 Al-Khatib SM, LaPointe NM, Kramer JM, Califf RM. What clinicians should know about the QT interval. *JAMA*. 2003;289:2120–2127.

108 De Bruin ML, Pettersson M, Meyboom RH, Hoes AW, Leufkens HG. Anti-HERG activity and the risk of drug-induced arrhythmias and sudden death. *Eur Heart J*. 2005;26:590–597.

109 Roden DM, Lazzara R, Rosen M, et al. Multiple mechanisms in the long-QT syndrome. Current knowledge, gaps, and future directions. The SADS Foundation Task Force on LQTS. *Circulation*. 1996;94:1996–2012.

110 Zeltser D, Justo D, Halkin A, et al. Torsade de pointes due to noncardiac drugs: most patients have easily identifiable risk factors. *Medicine* (Baltimore). 2003;82:282–290.

111 Roden DM. Taking the "idio" out of "idiosyncratic": predicting torsades de pointes. *Pacing Clin Electrophysiol*. 1998;21:1029–1034.

112 Newman LS, Feinberg MW, LeWine HE. A bitter tale. *N Engl J Med*. 2004;351:594–599.

113 Lapostolle F, Borron SW. Digitalis. In: Shannon MW, Borron SW, Burns MJ, eds. *Haddad and Winchester's Clinical Management of Poisoning and Drug Overdose*. 4th ed. Philadelphia: Saunders/Elsevier; 2007: 1001.

114 Holstege CP, Kirk MA. Digitalis. In: Chan TC, Brady WJ, Harrigan RA, et al, eds. *ECG in Emergency Medicine and Acute Care*. Philadelphia: Elsevier Mosby; 2006:255–260.

115 Williamson KM, Thrasher KA, Fulton KB, et al. Digoxin toxicity: An evaluation in current clinical practice. *Arch Intern Med*. 1998;158:2444–2449.

116 Bismuth C, Gaultier M, Conso F, Efthymiou ML. Hyperkalemia in acute digitalis poisoning: Prognostic significance and therapeutic implications. *Clin Toxicol*. 1973;6:153–162.

117 Lapostolle F, Borron SW, Verdier C, et al. Digoxin-specific Fab fragments as single first-line therapy in digitalis poisoning. *Crit Care Med*. 2008;36:3014–3018.

118 Love JN, Howell, JM, Litovitz TL, Klein–Schwartz W. Acute beta blocker overdose: factors associated with the development of cardiovascular mortality. *J Toxicol Clin Toxicol*. 2000;38:275–281.

119 Taboulet P, Cariou A, Berdeaux A, Bismuth C. Pathophysiology and management of self-poisoning with beta-blockers. *J Toxicol Clin Toxicol*. 1993;31: 531–551

120 Love JN. Acebutalol overdose resulting in fatalities. *J Emerg Med*.2000;18:341–344.

121 Love JN, Enlow B, Howell JM, Klein-Schwartz W, Litovitz TL. Electrocardiographic changes associated with beta-blocker toxicity. *Ann Emerg Med*. 2003;42:156–157.

122 Baud FJ, Megarbane B, Deye N, Leprince P. Clinical review: Aggressive management and extracorporeal support for drug-induced cardiotoxicity. *Crit Care*. 2007;11:207–215.

123 Salhanick SD. Calcium channel antagonists. In: Shannon MW, Borron SW, Burns MJ, eds. *Haddad and Winchester's Clinical Management of Poisoning and Drug Overdose*. 4th ed. Philadelphia: Saunders/ Elsevier; 2007: Available at: "UrlBlockedError.aspx" www.mdconsult..com/das/book/body. Accessed September 18, 2009.

124 Proano L, Chiang WK, Wang RY. Calcium channel blocker overdose. *Am J Emerg Med*.1995;13:444–450.

125 Brass BJ, Winchester-Penny S, Lipper BL. Massive verapamil overdose complicated by noncardiogenic pulmonary edema. *Am J Emerg Med*.1996;14:459–461.

126 Holstege CP, Baer AB. Other sodium channel blocking agents. In: Chan TC, Brady WJ, Harrigan RA, et al., eds. *ECG in Emergency Medicine and Acute Care*. Philadelphia: Elsevier Mosby; 2006:274–278.

127 Nieman JT, Bessen HA, Rothstein RJ, Laks MM. Electrocardiographic criteria for tricyclic antidepressant cardiotoxicity. *Am J Cardiol*. 1986;57:1154–1159.

128 Liebelt EL, Francis PD, Woolf AD. ECG lead aVR versus QRS interval in predicting seizures and arrhythmias in acute tricyclic antidepressant toxicity. *Ann Emerg Med*. 1995;26:195–201.

129 Nanagas KA, Furbee RB. Class IA antiarrhythmics: Quinidine, procainamide, and disopyramide. In: Shannon MW, Borron SW, Burns MJ, eds. *Haddad and Winchester's Clinical Management of Poisoning and Drug Overdose*. 4th ed. Philadelphia: Saunders/Elsevier; 2007: Available at: "UrlBlockedError.aspx" www. mdconsult..com/das/book/body. Accessed September 18, 2009

130 Floyd J, Morgan JP, Perry MC. Cardiotoxicity of anthracycline-like chemotherapy. 2009 Available at; www.utdol.com. Accessed June 8, 2010.

131 Floyd J, Morgan JP, Perry MC. Cardiotoxicity of nonanthracycline cancer chemotherapeutic agents. 2009. Available at; www.utdol.com. Accessed June 8, 2010.

Cardiomyopathy

Alden Landry[1] & Shamai Grossman[2]

[1] Instructor in Medicine, Harvard Medical School, Beth Israel Deaconess Medical Center, Fellow, Commonwealth Fund/Harvard University, Minority Health Policy Fellowship, Boston, Massachusetts, USA
[2] Director, Cardiac Emergency Center and Clinical Decision Unit, Beth Israel Deaconess Medical Center, Assistant Professor of Medicine, Harvard Medical School, Boston, Massachusetts, USA

Section I: Case presentation

A 35-year-old woman was brought to the emergency department (ED) with complaints of shortness of breath for the past 2 weeks, which worsened over the prior day. She had experienced the symptoms even with simple tasks such as washing dishes or walking up stairs. She denied chest pain with the shortness of breath, but did think that her legs were more swollen than before. She stated that she did not feel her heart beat fast intermittently. Her husband noted that his wife had been breathing more heavily at night, and had also complained of decreased energy.

The past medical history was unremarkable except for a prior appendectomy and tonsillectomy as a child. The patient was 5 weeks postpartum after an uncomplicated first pregnancy that was carried to term. She did not associate her symptoms with the recent pregnancy nor with new motherhood.

The initial vital signs were: blood pressure 112/76 mmHg, heart rate 72 beats/min, respiratory rate 22 breaths/min, and temperature 36.8°C (98.2°F). The patient was mildly obese, and was sitting upright in mild respiratory distress. The physician noted a mild 2/6 systolic ejection murmur with no rubs or gallops. There was moderate jugular venous distention in the external jugular veins. There were crackles at the base of both lungs. There was trace-pitting edema in the ankles to the mid-calves. The remainder of the examination was unremarkable.

The physician ordered a battery of laboratory tests. A complete blood count and serum electrolytes were all normal. The patient was noted to have an elevated beta-naturetic pepide (BNP) level. An EKG was done, and was notable for a left axis deviation, but was otherwise normal. A chest X-ray study was performed that showed an enlarged cardiac silhouette and mild vascular congestion, most prominent in the lung bases. The cardiology and obstetric services were consulted.

Section II: Case discussion

Dr Peter Rosen: In looking at the presenting complaints of this patient, I would not immediately think that this patient had a cardiac problem. We have a patient who is 5 weeks postpartum; it's not unusual for patients to have weakness and fatigue and leg swelling postpartum, even this far out, and swelling may have been present all along the pregnancy. One of the things I would be concerned about here is pulmonary embolus (PE), which has a higher incidence not just toward the end of pregnancy, but also in the first 2 months thereafter(1A). I think that part of the initial workup should include a workup for PE. Nevertheless, there are a number of heart diseases that

Cardiovascular Problems in Emergency Medicine: A discussion-based review, First Edition.
Edited by Shamai A. Grossman and Peter Rosen.
© 2011 John Wiley & Sons, Ltd. Published 2011 by John Wiley & Sons, Ltd.

seem to present during pregnancy. While we don't see as many of them as often as we once did, it is not uncommon for valvular heart disease to worsen during pregnancy, and sometimes have pregnancy as the first manifestation of it. Do you have any experience along those lines? How do these patients present?

Dr Shamai Grossman: In patients who are pregnant, like with any patient who presents to the ED, you always need to consider the worst possible diagnosis, which may be rare, as well as the more common ones; only once you've decided there is no catastrophe, and you've ruled out any of the more ominous causes of their problem, can you begin to attribute their current presentation to some of the more benign etiologies. For instance, if a pregnant patient comes in with leg swelling and nonspecific symptoms such as feeling more weak or overwhelmed, or just unable to function with the daily activities of living, you can only assume that those symptoms are related to the pregnancy itself and not some other etiology only after you've thoroughly evaluated the patient. Given that our postpartum patient presents acutely dyspneic with leg swelling, you must consider that this patient has some other disease than pregnancy or the postpartum physiology. The diseases that I would be concerned about would be unmasked valvular heart disease, pulmonary embolus, and perhaps a cardiomyopathy. All of these can present with acute shortness of breath, and all of these diseases can present with edema. However, if you are considering pulmonary embolus, then you would think the etiology was from a deep venous thrombosis, and expect unilateral, rather than bilateral, lower extremity edema. If you were thinking about cardiomyopathy or valvular heart disease, you would expect the patient to present volume-overloaded, and with valvular heart disease you would expect a very noticeable murmur as well. These diseases may be the most ominous that occur in pregnancy, but a pregnant woman can also present just like any other patient, and the disease may be simply coincidental to the pregnancy.

PR: I remember a number of women with mitral valve disease whose murmurs were not very loud, probably because they were diastolic. The systolic flow murmur of pregnancy can last for at least a month postpartum, since some women diurese the expanded volume of pregnancy more slowly than others. Edema of pregnancy can also represent eclampsia,

and you can have eclampsia even after delivery, even though one of the therapies for severe eclampsia is delivery, to terminate the pregnancy. This diagnosis may be missed because you don't think of it; after all, the patient is no longer pregnant. Similarly, rheumatic heart disease can be subtle when you can't hear the murmur, and since we don't see much rheumatic fever, we may stop thinking about it as a complication of pregnancy. Congenital valve disease can also be well-tolerated until pregnancy, but here I would suspect that the murmurs would be louder, and the patient would probably be aware of that murmur for years, and may have had a cardiac workup prior to the pregnancy. Are there any symptoms or signs that quickly point you towards a cardiomyopathy, or is it a diagnosis of exclusion?

SG: First, I would think about the stage of the pregnancy; if the patient is third trimester or postpartum, cardiomyopathy is within the differential, especially in late third trimester. If we're earlier in pregnancy, the likelihood of cardiomyopathy is minimal. Next I would consider the past medical history, including a history of similar symptoms. If a patient has no history of a murmur, and suddenly has one, that would make me think that it was brought on specifically by the pregnancy. If the patient has a history of a coagulopathy, then I might consider a thrombotic disease rather than a cardiomyopathy. If on physical examination there are findings of volume overload, I don't think I could differentiate between a cardiomyopathy and another cardiac or even noncardiac etiology. Ultimately, this is going to depend on some diagnostic testing to better decide whether this is cardiomyopathy or something else.

PR: My understanding is that, by definition, it can't be cardiomyopathy if it occurs earlier than the last 5 weeks of pregnancy, but it can occur as long as 5 months after delivery. I think that whenever I see an artificial definition of time-constraint, I always wonder why it's so important to have that time-constraint, and since the etiology isn't well-known, but has been suggested to be postviral myocarditis, it would seem that it could develop at any point in pregnancy, and not just in the last trimester. Perhaps it takes the volume overload and the work of carrying the heavy fetus to decompensate.

SG: The etiologies of peripartum cardiomyopathy even today are still unclear. Therefore, because we don't really know the etiology, in terms of classifying this as a disease entity, all we are left with is its timing.

PR: There have been a number of different suggested etiologies, none of which have been proven, in part because this is still a pretty rare disease, and in part because some of the suggestions were too farfetched. For example, it is hard to understand physiologically the use of tocolytics during labor as a cause of cardiomyopathy. Infectious etiologies are also hard to prove, as most of these patients don't have an infection history, and this infection doesn't appear to affect the fetus the way that other third-trimester infections often do. It's hard to imagine a viral infection that can affect the mother's heart but not affect the fetus. I think that we have to accept that we don't know the cause of this disease, but when you see pregnant patients with symptoms of heart failure, weakness and swelling, then, at this point, this becomes a disease entity that needs to cross your mind. One of the things that strikes me as I read this presentation is that there are a number of other disease entities that are rare in late pregnancy and early puerperium that one also is reluctant to think about, but may have similar symptomatology as well. One of these is postpartum depression. Not every patient who has this appears depressed. They can complain of poor appetite and some of the vegetative symptoms of depression more than the psychiatric symptoms; it's something that I would think about in a patient who may be losing weight, can't eat, has fatigue, and complains of inability to do simple tasks, such as housework or caring for a new baby. Another is metabolic failure. We've all seen patients who appear to be stable, but gradually develop symptoms that don't fit any single disease complex. Whenever I hear symptoms from a patient that I can't add together, one of the entities that enters my mind is metabolic disease, such as adrenal failure, such as diabetes or thyroid failure, and I think that these also can be triggered by pregnancy. Having said that, let's move down the path of cardiomyopathy. What kind of workup is going to help us to confirm or reject that diagnosis?

SG: There are a number of things that we do routinely on many patients in the ED that may be reasonable in this case, such as an EKG looking for ventricular hypertrophy and conduction disease, and a chest X-ray study. Although you may not see overt signs of congestive heart failure, you may see cardiomegaly, which, in a 35-year-old woman, would be unusual. Even if this patient were still pregnant, in the third trimester, I would have no concern about doing a chest X-ray study, given that this study has very minimal amounts of radiation exposure to the patient, and could give you some very useful information. These are the two tests that I would start with in the ED, coupled with a standard metabolic work up including a complete blood count, serum electrolytes, and renal function.

PR: One can obtain a decent chest X-ray study and even shield the fetus, so the presence of a third-trimester pregnancy certainly wouldn't stop me from ordering that test.

SG: My understanding as well is that the radiation from a chest X-ray study is the equivalent of what one gets when one goes on an airplane. Although third-trimester women are concerned about going on an airplane because of the possibility of going into labor on the airplane, the radiation does not preclude them from flying.

PR: What about an echocardiogram? Is that at all useful in this entity?

SG: An echocardiogram would be the test of choice. Although an echocardiogram is not always easily available in the ED, it does need to be included in this patient's work up. Regardless of whether the EKG or chest X-ray study suggest a possible cardiomyopathy, I would want an echocardiogram to better evaluate this patient. However, there is nothing in this patient's medical history to suggest that I must do the echocardiogram in the ED. If this patient is admitted, I would get the echocardiogram while this patient is in the hospital, to better understand the etiology of her symptoms.

PR: What would make you admit this patient? Is it the new onset cardiac disease, or is it the possibility of cardiomyopathy? Is it that these patients may do very well, but can also do very poorly, and it's hard to predict which patient is going to fall into which group?

SG: I believe it is a mixture of all of those things. First, as with any patient, when we evaluate them in the ED, we have to decide whether they are sick or not sick. Does this patient look to be in decompensated heart failure, or does the patient have ongoing symptoms that look unchanged over the course of the week or longer? Were it to be the latter, I would be less concerned that the patient needs an emergent hospitalization. That would not preclude a need for an evaluation in an expeditious fashion, but the patient may not need it in the hospital. However, I think that your concerns are well-founded in that some of these patients, despite looking well and having had relatively slow onset symptoms, can develop acute worsening fairly rapidly, and, more often than we'd like, end up with a poor outcome.

PR: It's always hard to take a new mother away from her infant, and I think that some of our admission decisions are distorted by the reality that we want to preserve the mother's ability to care for her baby. Yet this is one instance in which you need to unhesitatingly call for admission once you think that you are dealing with a cardiomyopathy.

Could you quickly review for us the cardiomyopathies, and how we decide which one is which, and what are the concerns we need to focus upon for the individual entities?

SG: There are a number of classifications of cardiomyopathies; one of the more common classifications divides the cardiomyopathies into "dilatated" and "restrictive" cardiomyopathies. The dilatated cardiomyopathies include ischemic cardiomyopathy, valvular cardiomyopathy, viral cardiomyopathy, which you alluded to as a possible etiology within our postpartum and peripartum patients, and then there are genetic cardiomyopathies. The restrictive cardiomyopathies include infiltrative diseases like amyloid and sarcoidosis, and noninfiltrative such as idiopathic hypertrophic subaortic stenosis or hypertrophic cardiomyopathy, and the more obscure storage diseases like hemochromatosis and Fabry's disease.

PR: What are some of the early therapeutic concerns that we should be thinking about and undertaking in the ED?

SG: You may differentiate somewhat between the pregnant patient with peripartum cardiomyopathy and the postpartum patient, as once you've delivered the baby, you may not need to worry about the fetal effects of your medication. In all patients, we should be able administer some of the standard medications used for any other patient presenting with congestive heart failure, which would be the most likely set of complaints to be found on their presentation in the ED. So if this 35-year-old woman presents with shortness of breath, lower extremity swelling, and increased fluid on examination or chest X-ray study, it would be appropriate to give this patient a diuretic to try to achieve a diuresis. Diuretics would be an appropriate therapy in both the pre-partum and postpartum patient.

PR: We don't need to be concerned about the fetus in this patient, because she has delivered. Is there a role for beta-blockade?

SG: In the acute setting, I would not use beta-blockers in this patient. Beta-blockers should not be used in a patient who is currently in congestive heart failure, even if that patient presents in rapid atrial fibrillation. Instead, if the patient remains with a rapid ventricular response, despite diuresis, I would use a calcium channel blocker for rate control. In the long term she may benefit from beta-blockade therapy for congestive heart failure, but not in the acute setting.

PR: What about afterload reduction? What would you use for that?

SG: I would stay away from angiotensin-converting enzyme inhibitors (ACE) inhibitors and angiotensin II receptor blockers in the prepartum patient as they are contraindicated any time in pregnancy due to the high risk of adverse fetal effects. Nitrates, however, reduce both preload and afterload, and are considered safe. Given that this patient has already delivered, you might want to use an ACE inhibitor as well. I don't think that this case mentioned whether this patient was breastfeeding, but ACE inhibitors, or at least captopril, are not recommended by the manufacturer while nursing because it crosses into the mother's milk; the data is less clear with lisinopril. Given that, I would also stay away from ACE inhibitors if the mother were nursing.

PR: Given her current congestive failure, she's likely going to have to come up with a substitute feeding pattern for her child anyway, so maybe that's a decision that can be predicated on how she appears clinically, and whether or not she needs to be admitted. I'm not sure that we would want to put her child into the hospital as well if we could avoid it. The long-term prognosis for postpartum cardiomyopathy seems to be biphasic, with a rather high initial mortality rate, but with the majority recovering almost completely. I don't know that we can determine which direction this patient will take in the ED, but clearly it's a significant disease that we need to take very seriously. As emergency physicians, we may be inclined to do less since we don't see this frequently, and thus may not realize how rapidly these patients can deteriorate. This patient doesn't sound like she's particularly sick given this presentation. Would you admit this patient?

SG: I probably would admit her for a number of reasons. First, although the mother doesn't want to be taken away from her child, sometimes the only way to really treat the mother is by arranging for someone else to care for the child. This may be the only way to get a patient to be compliant, and to obtain the appropriate workup. In addition, this patient also has a number of symptoms that have been worsening over the course of the prior day, although she has had several weeks of symptoms. Lastly, she's not able to function with the daily tasks of living, such as taking care of her newborn, which amplifies her daily tasks enormously. Hopefully by admitting her we would enable the workup to take place in a more expeditious fashion, and get her on the road to recovery quickly.

PR: If the patient were still pregnant, presenting during the third trimester of her pregnancy, then clearly she would need to be admitted to the obstetrics service. Is there any value to the early delivery of these patients?

SG: Many of the patients seem to go to caesarean section for other reasons, but I don't believe there is clear data to suggest emergent delivery as therapeutic for this maternal disease. Perhaps this lack of data is because this cardiomyopathy is found more often in the postpartum patient.

PR: Other than trying to unload the heart, is there a role for early digitalization of these patients in the ED?

SG: I believe digoxin, in general, doesn't really have a role in the ED. Basically this goes back to the definition of what we term an emergency department. Starting any medication in which you can't see the effect in the ED is hard to justify. That said, we give antibiotics for a wide variety of infections, and we don't see the benefit. The problem is that digoxin takes many hours in order to produce a benefit. At a minimum, it will take 2–3 hours to have an adequate amount of medication

onboard to achieve any effect, and on average, it will take much longer. In addition, digoxin isn't particularly effective in patients who have increased sympathetic tone, which is true of most patients we see in the ED. With this in mind, I would say there is no need to start digoxin in the ED; rather, I would start it after the patient is admitted to a hospital bed, and had a chance to quiet down. You may then see some benefit in the long term.

PR: I take it from your comments that this kind of patient would not be a good candidate for an emergency observation unit or chest pain center holding unit.

SG: I would agree with that. Generally, the role of observation units should be limited to patients who you think will be able to have a very rapid turnaround, with a likelihood of 85% or better that they will be adequately improved enough to be discharged within 24 hours. I don't think it that likely that 85% of the time a patient like this will be ready for discharge within 24 hours.

PR: Are there any dysrhythmias that this condition induces that we need to be alert for, or are there any drugs that we could commence that would lower their likelihood of onset?

SG: I believe these patients are like any patients with cardiomyopathy. They are at a higher risk for having both atrial and ventricular dysrhythmias. However, I don't know of any data that has shown that prophylactic medications for dysrhythmias are useful. The data from the CASS study in the 1970s, where they tried suppressing ventricular dysrhythmias during myocardial infarctions, found that rather than help people, it increased mortality. With this study, the use of prophylactic dysrhythmics fell by the wayside.

PR: How about intubation? Are these patients likely to require it, and if so, is it prudent to undertake that in the ED, where we are used to emergency airway management, rather than letting the patient get up to a unit where they have to call for help from the anesthesiology service?

SG: I think that again depends on the individual patient, and the clinical appearance in the ED. A patient who is in respiratory distress should be intubated in the ED, because we are the experts in emergency intubation. However, a patient who presents, such as the one in this case, with a satisfactory respiratory status probably shouldn't require intubation, hopefully at all, during the hospitalization. Although, unfortunately, there is no good way to predict which patient is going to end up deteriorating unless she has already begun to deteriorate while in the ED.

PR: What kind of bed would you want to request for this patient? Can they go to a step-down unit or can they go to a regular floor bed?

SG: I think that is a very good question, because part of that depends on whose service this patient should go to. Obstetricians have much expertise in dealing with obstetrical patients and many of the complications of postpartum, but on the other hand, obstetricians are not cardiologists and don't deal regularly with cardiomyopathies, and therefore depending on the institution that you're in, the patient might go to either service. The first thing that you need to weigh is the comfort of the physician taking care of the patient. In my mind, I think that a cardiology service might be the most appropriate service to take care of this patient regardless of whether she is pregnant or not, with obstetrics consulting particularly for the peripartum issues or the postpartum issues. I know that in many institutions, obstetrics cannot admit to a step-down or intensive care unit whatsoever, so that may easily take them out of the loop in that scenario. My preference in this patient would be to admit her to a cardiology floor, probably one such as a step-down unit or at least dedicated to cardiology patients, where they can get the expertise of both nursing and physicians, in dealing with the most pressing issue for this patient.

PR: I would guess that if the patient was still pregnant, she would be admitted to an obstetric service during the third trimester with a cardiac consult, but postpartum, I would not see a need for admission to the obstetric service. As it turns out, this patient was admitted without much of a workup.

Is this a place where BNP can play a useful role?

SG: That's a good question. I am unaware of any studies looking at BNP in postpartum cardiomyopathy patients. In general, if a patient has a markedly elevated BNP, not 500, but in the thousands, it is very likely that that patient is volume overloaded. This should help solidify a diagnosis of cardiomyopathy. I can't think of a good reason why BNP would not be useful in this particular patient population, as long

as she does not have concomitant sepsis or renal failure, and so I don't see what should preclude one from ordering it.

PR: How do you feel about doing a CT scan on this patient as opposed to just a simple chest X-ray study?

SG: It depends on what you are looking for. If you are looking for a cardiomyopathy, then the study of choice is an echocardiogram. If you are looking for a pulmonary embolus, then a CT scan would be a better choice. I think that this is where you might go back to our earlier question and say, well, what test does this patient actually need in the ED? We talked about whether the patient actually needed an emergent echocardiogram; if that echocardiogram is going to preclude the patient from going for a CT scan, and she is still pregnant, then it might be very useful to get that echocardiogram emergently. I may not need to know whether this is a cardiomyopathy definitively in the ED just to treat the patient, but it would be useful to know if this is truly a cardiomyopathy to avoid doing a potentially dangerous test on this patient and exposing a fetus to CT scan radiation. In our patient, as she is postpartum, if you had a reasonable concern that this is a pulmonary embolus and not a cardiomyopathy, then a CT scan would be a reasonable test to do. Given her presentation, pulmonary embolus is lower down on my differential diagnosis tree, and I probably wouldn't pursue a CT scan on this patient.

PR: I'm not sure that I would have diagnosed her immediately with a cardiomyopathy, and I suspect that I would have initially obtained a CT scan looking for a pulmonary embolus.

Case resolution

The patient was admitted to the obstetrics service for monitoring and workup. The patient also underwent a CT angiogram of the chest to evaluate for pulmonary embolism, which was negative for clot, but did show pulmonary edema and vascular congestion. An echocardiogram was obtained, and showed normal valve structure and function. Nevertheless, mild diastolic dysfunction was noted as well as slight left ventricular enlargement. The ejection fraction was measured at 55%. The patient was started on furosemide for a short course of diuresis, and on an ACE inhibitor that was continued as an outpatient. The patient remained in the hospital for 3 days and left after an uneventful course.

Section III: Concepts

Background

Cardiomyopathy is a disease of heart muscle, important because it can lead to heart failure, dysrhythmia, or even death. It is unusual for a cardiomyopathy to present initially to the ED; it is more likely to be identified on a routine health check up. However, recognition of certain characteristics of the illness assists in making the correct diagnosis, regardless of the locale of presentation.

Cardiomyopathy is an umbrella term that covers a number of cardiac diseases. There are three traditional categories of cardiomyopathy: dilatated, hypertrophic and restrictive, with dilatated and hypertrophic cardiomyopathies occurring more frequently than the restrictive forms.[1] Determining the underlying cause of the cardiomyopathy is heavily dependent on the history of the patient, including the progression of the symptoms, past medical history, and physical examination findings. Asking key questions can direct the physician to the etiology of the disease. Appropriate laboratory data and imaging studies further aid in the ultimate diagnosis.

Initial cardiomyopathy workup: history and physical

The initial workup, as with all ED patients, begins with obtaining vital signs, identifying patients in extremis, and initiating immediate resuscitation of the unstable patient. Patients may present with tachycardia or hypotension, and the administration of intravenous fluids may be enough to stabilize the patient while more information is collected.

The history of a patient presenting with cardiomyopathy often overlaps with other illnesses, but attention to detail allows the physician to make the right diagnosis. Symptoms of the disease include fatigue, dyspnea (made worse with exertion), orthopnea, increased edema, ascites, and weight gain. Angina is an uncommon symptom, but should angina be a part of the chief complaint, an EKG should be done immediately to rule out other life-threatening diseases such as a myocardial infarction.[2]

The past medical history can be helpful in the workup of cardiomyopathy. Obtaining a history of a recent viral illness, use of certain medications, pregnancy, exposures either environmental or self-inflicted (alcohol or cocaine), or chronic medical problems can help with identifying the underlying cause of the patient's symptoms. Syncope can be the only presenting symptom of a cardiomyopathy, which can be ominous and requires further workup.

The physical examination should focus on the cardiovascular and pulmonary systems; however, vigilance for extracardiac abnormalities may help to discover the underlying cause. Key cardiovascular findings include distant heart sounds, jugular venous distention, S3 gallop, enlargement of the liver, or presence of a hepatojugular reflux. Peripheral edema is likely to be present as well. No change in blood pressure as in pulsus paradoxus occurs with the restrictive forms of the disease. Other symptoms that may be identified include a goiter or proptosis and exophthalmos indicating thyrotoxicosis. Skin changes, such as increased pigmentation, can help to identify underlying illnesses such as hemochromatosis.

Etiologies of cardiomyopathy

There are numerous causes of cardiomyopathy, ranging from genetic and exposure to infectious and autoimmune.[3,4] (Table 18-1)

Testing in cardiomyopathy

Initial testing for all patients in which cardiomyopathy is part of the differential diagnosis list should include a chest X-ray study and an EKG. Atrial fibrillation or left ventricular hypertrophy may be the only findings on the initial EKG. A chest X-ray study is helpful in two ways. First, it can help to identify cardiomegaly or an enlarged cardiac silhouette. Second, it can help to reveal fluid overload and venous congestion. Radiologic findings of fluid overload include pleural effusions, Kerley B lines, interstitial edema, and cephalization of vessels.[5]

Laboratory data can be helpful in the workup of cardiomyopathy as well. Cardiac markers are helpful in differentiating between ischemic disease and cardiomyopathy. However, a grossly elevated troponin may be evidence for a more severe case and increased mortality.[2] Other helpful laboratory data include a beta-naturetic peptide that may indicate fluid overload.[6] Thyroid function tests, drug screens, and pregnancy testing may help to indentify more rare causes of the disease as well.

Table 18-1. Etiologies of cardiomyopathy.

Congenital
- Autosomal dominant, X-linked

Infectious
- Viral: coxsackivirus, cytomegalovirus, or human immunodeficiency virus (HIV)
- *Mycobacteria, Staphylococcus* species
- Parasites (Chagas disease, toxoplasmosis, trichinosis)

Metabolic diseases
- Diabetes mellitus, hypothyroidism, thyrotoxicosis, acromegaly, Cushings disease, pheochromocytoma
- Nutritional deficits

Systemic disorders
- Systemic lupus erythematosus, hemochromatosis, amyloidosis, sarcoidosis

Cardiac disorders
- Myocardial ischemia, valvular diseases, hypertension

Neuromuscular dystrophies
- Duchenne muscular dystrophy, Friedreich's ataxia, myotonic dystrophy, X-linked cardioskeletal myopathy

Pregnancy

Autoimmune
- Kawasaki disease

Idiopathic

Toxic
- Alcohol, cocaine, doxirubicin, antiretrovirals, steroids, heavy metals

The test of choice in the workup of cardiomyopathy is an echocardiogram (ECHO). An ECHO can be used to differentiate between the types of cardiomyopathy, as well as other cardiac diseases. An ECHO showing dilatated chambers and diffuse hypokinetic muscle is consistent with a dilatated cardiomyopathy. Focal hypokinesis is found in ischemic cardiomyopathy. Hypertrophy of cardiac muscles, incomplete emptying of the ventricle, and outflow tract obstruction can be seen in hypertrophic cardiomyopathy.[7]

Disposition of patients with cardiomyopathy

The decision to admit or discharge a patient with cardiomyopathy depends on the severity of the symptoms, concern for deterioration, and ability of the patient to obtain adequate follow up. If the patient is in extremis, the ideal location for admitting the patient is to an ICU with a cardiologist involved in the patient's care. Stable patients should be admitted to the hospital with telemetry and close monitoring. If a patient is to be discharged, close follow up with a cardiologist should be arranged prior to the patient leaving the ED.

Section IV: Decision making

- The greatest challenge of working up and treating a cardiomyopathy is to include it in the differential diagnosis list and then to make the proper disposition for the patient.
- To sort out the etiology in the ED, obtain the best history possible and a thorough physical examination.
- EKG and chest X-ray studies are appropriate ED tests, while an echocardiogram can usually can wait until after ED evaluation.
- Disposition should be predicated on the initial evaluation and risk factors for an adverse outcome. Close interaction with a cardiologist or internist who can follow the patient can aid in the disposition.

References

1 *Heart Disease and Stroke Facts*. Dallas: American Heart Association; 2006.
2 La Vecchia L, Mezzena G, Zanolla L, et al. Cardiac troponin I as diagnostic and prognostic marker in severe heart failure. *J Heart Lung Transplant*. 2000;19:644–652.

3 Sasson Z. Hypertrophic cardiomyopathy *Cardiol Clin.* 1988;6:233–288.

4 Arbustini E, Morbini P, Pilotto A, Gavazzi A, Tavazzi L. Genetics of idiopathic dilated cardiomyopathy. *Herz.* 2000;25:156–160.

5 Wang CS, FitzGerald JM, Schulzer M, Mak E, Ayas NT. Does this dyspneic patient in the emergency department have congestive heart failure? *JAMA.* 2005;294:1944–1956.

6 Azevedo VM, Albanesi Filho FM, Santos MA, Castier MB, Tura BR. How can the echocardiogram be useful for predicting death in children with idiopathic dilated cardiomyopathy? *Arq Bras Cardiol.* 2004;82: 505–514.

7 Egan D, Bisanzo M, Hutson H. Emergency department evaluation and management of peripartum cardiomyopathy. *J Emerg Med.*2009;36:141–147.

Vascular Emergencies

SECTION FOUR

Vascular Emergencies

19 Aortic dissection

Keith A. Marill[1] & David F. M. Brown[2]

[1] *Assistant Professor, Division of Emergency Medicine, Harvard Medical School, Attending Physician, Department of Emergency Medicine, Massachusetts General Hospital, Boston Massachusetts, USA*
[2] *Vice Chair, Department of Emergency Medicine, Massachusetts General Hospital, Associate Professor, Harvard Medical School, Boston, Massachusetts, USA*

Section I: Case presentation

A 76-year-old woman came to the emergency department (ED) complaining of anterior chest pain that radiated to the back. She had a multiyear history of hypertension. The pain began abruptly while watching television, and she reported it as 10/10 on a pain scale. She also reported left flank pain, diaphoresis, and nausea. She had one episode of vomiting when the pain first came on. There was no dyspnea. The pain was nonpositional and nonpleuritic. There was no fever, cough, or sputum. In addition to hypertension, she had mild chronic obstructive pulmonary disease (COPD). She was a one pack per day smoker for the prior 40 years, and drank alcohol occasionally.

On physical examination, she was diaphoretic and in moderate distress. She was moving around on the stretcher, and appeared unable to get comfortable. The vital signs were: blood pressure 180/110 mmHg, heart rate 100 beats/min, respirations 20 breaths/min, temperature 37°C (98.6°F), oxygen saturation 95% on room air. The head was normal, the neck was without bruits, and the carotid pulses were normal. The chest was clear to auscultation, and there was no chest wall tenderness. The cardiac examination revealed a normal S1 and S2 with an S4. There were no systolic or diastolic murmurs and no rubs or heaves. The abdomen was soft and nontender; there were no masses or bruits. The back had no tenderness

over the spine, but there was left costovertebral angle tenderness. The extremities were notable for 1+ bilateral ankle edema and symmetric pulses. The capillary refill was brisk. The neurological examination was without any focal findings.

The patient was treated with fentanyl for pain, and intravenous labetalol was started. The blood pressure improved to 150/90 mmHg, and then declined to 120/70 mmHg. The pulse rate dropped to 80 beats/min. She was taken to radiology for a CT scan. While in the CT scanner, the blood pressure further dropped to 60 mmHg by palpation. The CT revealed a Type A thoracic aortic dissection and a pericardial effusion was seen. She was taken directly to the operating room, and underwent emergent surgical repair.

Section II: Case discussion

Dr Peter Rosen: Did this patent describe ever having chest pain before?

Dr David Brown: She had no prior history of a chest pain syndrome, and no known coronary artery disease.

PR: Was she diabetic?

DB: No

Dr Shamai Grossman: Was the pain truly sudden in onset, or did it begin abruptly and gradually worsen?

Cardiovascular Problems in Emergency Medicine: A discussion-based review, First Edition.
Edited by Shamai A. Grossman and Peter Rosen.
© 2011 John Wiley & Sons, Ltd. Published 2011 by John Wiley & Sons, Ltd.

DB: The pain began suddenly while she was watching TV. It was immediately at its most intense point.

PR: How well controlled was her hypertension?

DB: She took one medication daily, and was moderately compliant.

PR: Had there been any episodes of hypertensive urgency or clear lack of blood pressure control?

DB: No.

PR: Did she also complain of a headache or weakness in either of her arms or legs?

DB: No, the only other complaint was left flank pain.

PR: Aortic dissection is a disease process that if you don't think about its possibility, you'll never find it. What would lead you away from considering that chest pain is from coronary artery disease, and lead you to start thinking about dissection?

SG: There are a couple of clues that push me away from coronary artery disease and more toward other diagnoses. First, I would assess the description of the pain. Sudden onset of symptoms in a patient who has never had any pain before, and as well as sudden onset pain that is already at its worst and radiates to the back, all would make me think that perhaps that this isn't coronary ischemia in etiology. Next, I'd consider how the patient appears. Is the patient in extremis? Is there an appearance of serious illness? If not, then I start to think that perhaps this may be something more ordinary. If the patient starts to look sick, then I would have to start looking for something that would explain this. If the EKG is normal, then aortic dissection would jump to the top of my differential list.

PR: The cases that I've encountered of aortic dissection, in which the patient wasn't in extremis, all had significant pain. However, in these cases it was impossible to distinguish that pain from the pain of a myocardial infarction (MI). Helpfully, their EKGs were relatively normal. When the patient presents with the sequelae of aortic dissection, with symptoms of a stroke or an abdominal process, it can be an even more subtle diagnosis. Do you have any other clues that you use to trigger the concern about dissection?

DB: Again, pain that is most severe at its onset is much less typical of acute myocardial ischemia, and more suggestive of aortic dissection, or for that matter, pulmonary embolus. Acute myocardial ischemic pain tends to increase over time whereas, in my experience, patients with aortic dissection can often tell you exactly what they were doing when the chest pain started because it was so intense. In addition, the pain is often sharp or tearing, rather than pressure-like. However, in acute myocardial ischemia the chest pain can also be sharp or tearing, and still represent MI rather than dissection. Next, I look for a history of hypertension, which is the principal risk factor for aortic dissection, and is frequently present in those patients who present with dissection, unless the patient has a connective tissue disorder.

PR: I think those are the less difficult-to-diagnose dissections, as these patients tend to be younger and have some of the physical stigmata of a Marfan's syndrome, such as height and a family history. Seventy-six-year-old patients, or even patients a little younger with a history of hypertension, are the cases in which it is the most difficult to diagnose a dissection.

DB: Another clue is the presence of two separate vascular lesions separated by distance in the body. For example, an MI or chest pain with a stroke, chest pain with a cold foot, chest pain with what might be interpreted as flank pain or renal colic, or concomitant abdominal pain with mesenteric ischemia would be much more suggestive of aortic dissection than of myocardial ischemia.

PR: We were always taught to look for differential blood pressures, but I honestly don't know anyone who does. Is there value in trying a left versus right arm pressure routinely? I think that most of us accept the pressures that are given to us by the nursing staff, and they are almost always unilateral.

DB: I find that blood pressure asymmetry is not very helpful, especially in a population that has had long-standing hypertension, and is likely to have atherosclerosis outside of their coronary arteries. A differential blood pressure in two extremities may be related to a fixed obstructive atherosclerotic lesion, which has nothing to do with the patient's presentation. Similarly, patients could have a dissection without impairment of flow to an extremity. Therefore, one should be cautious of being falsely reassured by symmetric blood pressures.

SG: On the other hand, I find that the one of the simplest way to almost immediately make this diagnosis is by feeling a patient's pulses. If they are asymmetric, I have invariably found that the patient is having a dissection. This is a very simple thing to do, particularly in a case when symptoms don't make sense. Here, aortic dissection should be in the back of your mind, and you should be checking for symmetry of pulses, which you can often do while you are talking to the patient.

DB: I think pulse asymmetry is important when it is present, but doesn't appear often enough to be very helpful when it is not present.

PR: I encountered a case recently that horrified me because I was sure that I would have missed it. It was a young man who presented with a seizure without having a prior history of epilepsy, and then became comatose with obvious signs of a one-sided stroke. He did not have a history of IV drug abuse, so these symptoms were unlikely to be induced by cocaine or crystal methamphetamine. I assumed that he had some sort of acute cerebral crisis. As he was comatose, after he was intubated, a CT scan was obtained, but it was normal. I am hard pressed to think of an acute onset cerebral catastrophe, in a young patient, that would have a normal acute CT scan. As it turns out, this unfortunate young man's symptoms were related to a huge carotid and aortic dissection beginning in the proximal aorta and extending to the internal carotid artery. Do you think that this entity needs to be on our differential diagnosis list for acute seizures?

DB: I would limit my concern for dissection to those patients with seizures that are followed by acute localizing neurologic deficits. Most of the time, these patients simply have a Todd's paralysis and recover, becoming asymptomatic; nevertheless, I think it's important to exclude acute stroke in patients who have a localizing neurologic deficit after a seizure. This is an example of when a CT angiogram of the head and neck is very helpful in patients presenting with an acute stroke. In our institution, a patient like this would initially have a head CT without contrast, which would be negative. To be considered a candidate for thrombolytic therapy in our institution, he would then have a CT angiogram (CTA) of the head and neck. In this case, we would have discovered the dissection, and consequently avoided the catastrophic mistake of giving thrombolytics to a Type A aortic dissection. The CTA can be performed on a patient on the same trip to the CT scanner, avoiding delays in the time to thrombolytic therapy in those

patients who do truly have thromboembolic stroke. It helps to identify the smaller group of patients who have other entities causing the neurologic deficits, but who could be injured by thrombolytic therapy.

PR: Is there an association between dissection and drugs of abuse? Can methamphetamine cause a hypertensive burst that triggers a dissection? When we see stroke in those patients, is it more likely to be vasospasm in the cerebral area?

SG: Clearly, amphetamines can give you hypertension, and profound hypertension potentially could trigger a dissection in someone who has underlying disease. A number of case reports have similarly suggested that the use of amphetamines, like cocaine, enhance noradrenaline release, and that by causing surges in blood pressure, the amphetamine participates in the pathogenesis of aortic dissection.[1]

PR: Are there other physical findings beyond pulse differential and multiorgan involvement that would help you think of aortic dissection? What about the presence of cardiac murmurs?

DB: For a Type A or for Debakey Type 1 or 2 dissections, patients may present with acute aortic regurgitation, but those patients are usually in so much heart failure that it is difficult to hear the diastolic murmur. If I did hear a diastolic murmur consistent with aortic regurgitation, it would increase my concern for aortic dissection. However, I don't think there's any particular pathognomonic finding on cardiac examination that would be extremely helpful.

PR: We used to think that you had to do angiography to find the exact anatomic location of the lesion for the surgeon, but this is rarely done today as CT angiography has become the diagnostic method of choice. Is there any utility in bedside ultrasound in the ED to help you with this diagnosis?

SG: A transthoracic echocardiogram will show a dissection about 60% of the time. A transthoracic ECHO is relatively easily available, depending on the time of day and depending on the institution, but still not as universally available as a CTA. If you're going to use ultrasound to look for a dissection, ideally you should use a transesophageal echocardiogram (TEE). A TEE has a sensitivity very similar to that of a CTA. The issue with TEE is that it is difficult to obtain in a timely fashion, while the less sensitive transthoracic echocardiogram is more readily available. Nevertheless, there are some scenarios where a TEE may be your test of choice, such as in a patient not able to have a CT angiogram because of contrast dye load issues. In addition, in cases where a patient needs to go to the operating room in a more emergent fashion, the anatomy can be delineated intraoperatively with a TEE.

PR: Although the evidence suggests that TEE is accurate, as you point out, it's only as accurate as its availability. I have yet to work in an institution where it's readily available.

DB: We can get a TEE relatively easily, but it requires a cardiologist who specializes in TEE to come in and do the procedure, and this takes time. In addition, the patients often need to be intubated, or at least adequately sedated, to do this comfortably, and this takes even more time. The CTA can be done in just a few minutes in the CT suite in the ED. Therefore, it is unusual, even at our tertiary care center, to reach for a TEE as our first choice for imaging.

PR: These patients' pain is often dramatic in my experience, and undergoing CTA while you are in agonizing pain may be one of the more sadistic things we make patients endure. What is the best method of management while you are trying to obtain a diagnosis?

SG: Assuming the patient is hypertensive, as the majority of these patients are, the initial therapy should be directed toward the hypertension. Treating the hypertension may also lessen the discomfort. I would usually start with a beta-blocker such as esmolol or labetolol. As I start to bring down the blood pressure, I would add some sort of opioid analgesia, such as morphine.

PR: Is there any danger to using blood-pressure-lowering agents with various types of dissection? In other words, if you have an arch dissection, the Type A Stanford, are you in any therapeutic danger if you lower the pressure as opposed to leaving it up? Is there a therapeutic advantage to hypertension with a proximal dissection?

DB: In other words, what happens if the patient has a complication of the dissection that causes immediate cardiogenic shock, such as with acute aortic regurgitation, pericardial tamponade, or a dissection of one of the coronary arteries, which one would only see with a type A dissection and not a type B dissection? Despite

these concerns, the benefits of beta-blockade are undisputed first-line therapy. Their effect is to lower the change in pressure over the change in time (dP/dT), reducing both the blood pressure and even more importantly lowering the heart rate, and in turn reducing the shear stress on the aorta. This then reduces the risk that any of these complications will occur. If you're concerned about these complications, then consider using a short-acting agent such as esmolol.

PR: This patient has a history of COPD; would that be a relative contraindication to using beta-blockade?

SG: I would emphasize that it is a relative contraindication rather than an absolute contraindication. I would start this patient on a short-acting beta-blocker so that if the patient develops some bronchospasm, I would be able to shut it off abruptly. Clearly, beta-blockade is the avenue of choice in beginning pharmacologic therapy in this type of patient.

PR: So we've reduced the shear forces on the aorta, obtained the diagnostic information that hopefully gives us the extent of the dissection, and we've lined up our surgical consultation for correcting the lesion if it's a Type A. When do you need to go the operating room with a Type B dissection, if ever?

DB: Patients with Type B dissections are generally managed medically, unless they develop limb or end-organ ischemia. If a patient develops either a cold extremity or acute impairment of circulation to the mesentery or to one of the kidneys, taking that patient to the operating room to at least fenestrate the aorta and try to restore blood flow to the limb or organ would be appropriate.

PR: Would you, therefore, consult your cardiac surgeon immediately with a Type B, as well as a Type A, dissection?

DB: In our institution, the Type B dissections would be managed by vascular surgery. In a patient with a Type B dissection, we would involve cardiology and vascular surgery. The patients without limb or end-organ ischemia are admitted to the cardiology service for medical management, and those with limb or end-organ ischemia are admitted to the vascular service for operative repair.

PR: Would you consider intubating these patients and taking away the work of respiration so that you could give them higher dosages of analgesia and sedation?

SG: Intubating the patient may also lower your dP/dT (wall stress). If the patient is headed to the operating room anyhow, there is little downside, in my mind, to intubation. Adding a vasodilatator like nitroprusside is also reasonable, as it may offer some additional benefit both from a pain management and a therapeutic management perspective by further reducing the stress on the vessel.

DB: If it's truly pain control that we're after, then I would treat that directly with intravenous narcotics. I would not choose to intubate in the hope that the reduction in need for blood flow to the diaphragm would somehow relieve the patient's pain. I would reserve intubation for those who appear critically ill, or who are otherwise going to need intubation for other problems such as congestive heart failure complicating an aortic dissection.

PR: It is not just pain alone that disturbs these patients, but a tremendous anxiety and sense of impending doom, which often seems very accurate. How often is acute renal failure a problem, and is there anything you can do to avert it while you are trying to deal with the vessel itself?

DB: Acute renal failure is uncommon unless it's an acute complication of contrast in these patients who undergo CTA. More commonly, the flow to the right or left renal artery is impaired by propagation of the dissection down the abdominal aorta, causing ischemia of a single kidney and a lot of pain. Sometimes that pain may be misinterpreted as renal colic. But losing flow to one kidney usually does not cause acute renal failure, at least not during the time in which ED management could effectively change.

PR: What does the emergency physician do who works in remote rural areas or in more remote suburban areas that don't have cardiothoracic surgery or major interventional cardiology?

SG: This is a patient who will require transfer to a center where the surgery can be done, particularly if it's a Type A dissection. If it is a Type B, the patient will often be transferred as well, usually to get a better look at both the patient and at the imaging that was done to make the diagnosis. Your job in the community is to stabilize the patient as best you can, which means again, stabilizing the blood pressure, reducing dP/dT, and to ensure that you are transporting

the patient in an emergent fashion. Often times this means transporting the patient by air, but at a minimum, with critical care and rapid transport.

PR: What packaging requests would you ask your transferring physician to do? What level of blood pressure would you try to reduce the patient to, and how much diagnostic testing do you want the transferring institution to do?

DB: Lowering the heart rate is really more important than lowering the blood pressure, which is why the first drug to be reached for is a beta-blocker or a mixed alpha- and beta-blocker. If the heart rate can be slowed down, then one markedly reduces aortic wall stress. If there is room to lower the blood pressure after the heart rate has been slowed to the low 60s or high 50s, then I would add an agent such as nitroprusside or a very short acting vasodilatator, and be satisfied with whatever blood pressure the patient could tolerate from a mental status standpoint. A young patient may tolerate very low blood pressures, but an older person with fixed atherosclerotic lesions in the cerebrovascular circulation will need a higher blood pressure.

PR: Would you be willing to accept a patient who clinically appears to be having a dissection, but for whom you haven't gotten proof with a CTA or a transthoracic echocardiogram?

DB: If you're in an institution where obtaining a CTA is easy, I think that the scan ought to be done, unless the patient has complications that already make it imperative to transfer the patient, such as an acute stroke, ST elevation myocardial infarction, or acute aortic regurgitation we think secondary to a dissection. However, for patients who simply have chest pain radiating to the back, if we recommend transfer for diagnostic imaging, we are going to be transferring many patients from small hospitals to large ones who don't have an aortic dissection, and in the process use up scarce resources at those larger hospitals.

PR: Should therapy be any different for a younger patient with a vascular connective tissue disorder such as Marfan's or Ehlers-Danlos syndrome, since hypertension is probably not triggering this dissection? Do we manage these patients in any different fashion?

SG: I would manage these patients in very much the same way. Remembering that these are often younger patients should remind one to consider illicit drug use

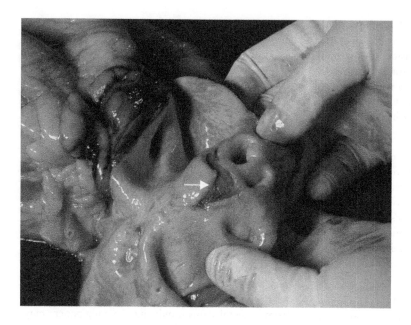

Figure 19.1 Pathologic specimen of the inner aortic surface of a patient who presented with a spontaneous tear in the arch of the aorta (arrow). The takeoff of the arch vessels were uninvolved; however the lesion dissected in a retrograde fashion through the media layer to the pericardial sac, causing pericardial tamponade.

and its association with aortic dissection. Cocaine users might benefit from benzodiazepines as an additional therapy. Beyond that, maximizing control of the heart rate and blood pressure remains appropriate in this patient population as well.

Case resolution

The patient underwent operative repair of a type A aortic dissection and cardiac tamponade. She was initially unstable in the postoperative period, developing mild renal insufficiency and suffered a small non-ST elevation MI. She was discharged to a rehabilitation facility on postoperative day ten.

Section III: Concepts

Epidemiology and pathophysiology

Aortic dissection is defined as a dissection of the wall of the aorta with formation of a false lumen or hematoma within the dissected layer. The aortic wall contains three layers, with dissection generally occurring in the middle (media) layer of the wall, usually emanating from a tear in the intimal layer of the vessel (Figure 19-1). Related variations from the typical mechanism of intimal tear and media dissection include an intramural hematoma with no evidence of intimal tear, dilated thoracic aortic

aneurysm without dissection, and atherosclerotic ulceration that can cause a dissection into the descending aorta. Aortic dissection is defined as acute if the symptoms began within the previous 14 days.

The incidence of the disease is approximately 3 in 100,000 people/year, and thus it is estimated that there are 7,000–10,000 cases per year in the U.S.[2,3] Although relatively rare, the importance of the disease is characterized by its severity. If left untreated, mortality is at least 1% per hour, and 50% within the first 48 hours of symptoms.[3,4] Even with appropriate treatment, overall mortality remains approximately 27%.[5]

The etiology, presentation, treatment, and prognosis of aortic dissection vary depending on whether the dissection involves the ascending, descending, or both areas of the aorta. For this reason, the commonly used Stanford and DeBakey classification schemes are based on the geographic involvement of disease (Figure 19-2). Regardless of the location of the intimal tear, any dissection that involves the ascending aorta is classified as Stanford Type A. Dissection involving only the descending aorta is classified as Stanford Type B. DeBakey Type I dissection involves both the ascending and descending aorta, while Debakey Type II, only the ascending aorta, and Type III, only the descending aorta.

The approximate geographic distribution of dissections is as follows: 65% ascending, 20% descending,

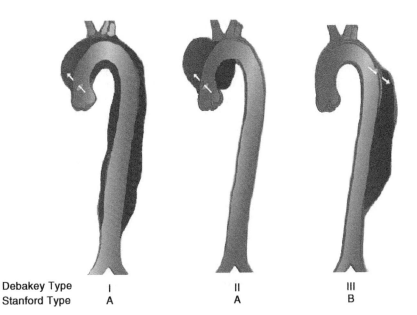

Debakey Type	I	II	III
Stanford Type	A	A	B

Figure 19.2 Schematic diagram of the Debakey and Stanford classification schemes of aortic dissection. Adapted from http://en.wikipedia.org/wiki/Aortic_dissection. Accessed 9/5/09.

10% aortic arch, and 5% confined to the abdominal aorta. It is useful for the emergency physician to appreciate the distinctions between dissections involving the ascending and descending aorta, as only ascending dissections routinely require surgical repair.

Dissection is thought to occur most commonly from a combination of weakening of the aortic wall, increased shear forces, or localized and iatrogenic trauma. Weakening of the aortic wall may be caused by cystic medial necrosis, which is described as disorganization and degeneration of the elastic and collagen components.

Clinical factors most commonly associated with aortic dissection include advanced age (approximately one-third of patients are over the age of 70); a history of hypertension, which is elicited in approximately two-thirds of patients; male gender; and atherosclerosis.[3,5,6] Dissection is also associated with the connective tissue disorders Marfan's Syndrome, Ehlers-Danlos Type IV, osteogenesis imperfecta, the congenital variant bicuspid aortic valve and coarctation of the aorta, prior cardiovascular and particularly aortic or aortic valve surgery, inflammatory or syphilitic aortitis, third trimester or postpartum pregnancy, cocaine abuse, and possibly isometric exercise such as weight lifting.[4,5,7,8] Blunt trauma, such as a motor vehicle accident, may rarely cause aortic dissection or even complete transection, most commonly

in the descending aorta just distal to the left subclavian artery.

A range of complications can result from an acute aortic dissection, and these complications can lead to diverse presentations of illness. Intimal flap formation and distortion of the aortic and associated branch vessel walls can cause critical compromise of arterial flow. This can lead to myocardial infarction, cerebrovascular accident, renal or spinal cord infarction, or ischemic bowel. Involvement of the aortic root can cause acute aortic valvular insufficiency and subsequent left heart failure. Retrograde extension of the dissection into the pericardial space can lead to pericardial effusion and tamponade with syncope, hypotension, and sudden death.[9] Rupture of the aortic wall may cause massive internal hemorrhage and exsanguination.

The differential diagnosis of acute aortic dissection is diverse. Acute coronary syndrome may be the most important differential diagnosis. It can sometimes be distinguished by the crescendo/decrescendo, exertional, and pressure-like nature of pain. Acute myocardial infarction is approximately 100 times more common than aortic dissection, but as noted above, it can actually be a complication of dissection. Pericarditis may also be confused with dissection, although it is associated with a slower pace of symptom onset, positional discomfort, and characteristic EKG abnormalities. Other relevant cardiologic differentials include acute congestive heart failure and aortic valvular disease or failure. Pulmonary conditions including pulmonary embolism and pneumonia, cerebrovascular accident, mediastinal tumor, esophageal disease, and other gastrointestinal causes of upper abdominal pain are also important differentials. Finally, thoracic or abdominal aortic aneurysms may present similarly to a type B dissection.

History

The history of aortic dissection is classically sudden, severe, sharp, stabbing, tearing, or ripping pain in the chest, back, or upper abdomen.[10] The intensity of pain may be maximal at onset. Radiation or migration of the pain to the interscapular region and elsewhere often reflects the anatomy of the disease and progressive propagation of the dissection. Consequently, the pain of ascending dissection tends to present in the anterior chest, while descending dissection may cause pain in the central back or upper abdomen. Many patients do not present with "classic" pain as described above, and 5–10% of patients may have no pain at all.

Approximately 10% of patients have neurologic complaints. This includes a history of acute syncope, which is associated with hemopericardium and cardiac tamponade. Other complaints include the symptoms of an acute cerebrovascular accident, usually due to ascending dissection extension and involvement of the origin of the cerebral vessels, or acute paraplegia from spinal vessel involvement. Dyspnea may occur as a result of acute aortic regurgitation and heart failure. Any recent history of iatrogenic aortic manipulation or trauma such as left heart catheterization is important, as this may be the cause of the dissection. The relation of acute dissection to recent exertion or heavy lifting remains uncertain.[4,11]

Relevant past medical history includes a survey for the contributing causes described above. In particular, a history or phenotype suggestive of Marfan's Syndrome or previous cardiac or aortic surgery should point to a possible dissection, as these are present in approximately 5% and 15% of cases, respectively.[5]

Physical examination

The blood pressure may be elevated, normal, or depressed in the setting of acute aortic dissection.

The majority of patients with type B dissection are hypertensive on presentation. In one series, 35% and 25% of patients with type A dissection present with hypertension and hypotension, respectively.[5] Up to one-third of patients may have a weak pulse in an extremity (pulse deficit), or a greater than 20 mmHg differential systolic blood pressure between arms.[10] Up to one-third of patients may have a diastolic murmur suggestive of aortic regurgitation. These findings are generally associated with Type A dissection.

Transthoracic echocardiography demonstrates an approximate sensitivity and specificity of only 60% and 80%, respectively, for acute aortic dissection.[12] Nevertheless, the technology, skill, and importance of bedside ultrasonography performed by emergency physicians as an extension of the physical examination have grown steadily. Identification of pericardial effusion can be made confidently, and this should suggest an ascending dissection.[13] A definitive diagnosis of aortic dissection with identification of an intimal flap can even sometimes be made, and the resulting time saved to operative repair may be life saving.[14]

EKG

The EKG has limited utility in diagnosing acute aortic dissection. Approximately one-third of dissection patients have evidence of left ventricular hypertrophy on EKG and approximately 5% of dissection patients have an associated acute MI. Ascending dissection most commonly originates along the greater curvature of the right wall of the ascending aorta, and when it dissects in a retrograde fashion, it most commonly involves the origin of the right coronary artery, causing an inferior myocardial infarction. Nevertheless, left main involvement and anterior myocardial infarction can occur too.[15]

Laboratory studies

Traditionally, laboratory studies have had limited utility in diagnosing acute aortic dissection. Anemia could suggest ongoing subacute internal hemorrhage, and hematuria may suggest renal artery involvement, but neither of these findings is sensitive nor specific. Investigators have explored the potential utility of a number of newer markers, including smooth muscle myosin, elastin fragments, and the serum D-dimer.[16–18]

The most promising marker for the identification of acute aortic dissection appears to be the serum D-dimer. D-dimer is a breakdown product of intravascular clot destruction. It seems intuitive that this marker may be elevated in conditions of intravascular clot formation and destruction, such as pulmonary embolism and acute aortic dissection. Advantages of the test are that it is readily available, inexpensive, and can be performed rapidly. Some disadvantages are that there are multiple test methodologies with differing test characteristics; it is known to have poor specificity in patients with malignancy, chronic disease, or advanced age; and it may be elevated in precisely the conditions that must be differentiated from acute dissection, including pulmonary embolism and acute myocardial infarction.[19,20]

Using a threshold cutoff of 500 ng/ml, the sensitivity of the serum D-dimer for acute aortic dissection appears to be approximately 95%, while the specificity is likely in the 40–50% range, depending on the methods used to identify a control group; thus, a negative D-dimer test would lower the odds of disease by a factor of approximately 9.[20,21] Analogous to the use of serum D-dimer for pulmonary embolism, the test may be most useful in patients with a low pretest probability of acute aortic dissection based on the history, physical examination, and chest X-ray study. Patients who then have a serum D-dimer of less than 500 ng/ml would effectively be "ruled out" for the disease. Patients with a positive test would require further urgent imaging studies. The negative likelihood ratio of the test is 1 to 9, insufficiently low to rule out disease in patients with a moderate or high pretest probability of disease, and the test would not be useful in this circumstance.

The goal of using the serum D-dimer would be to identify more accurately the group of patients at risk for acute dissection who require advanced imaging, but this would not necessarily decrease the number of advanced imaging studies performed. A number of questions regarding this use of the serum D-dimer remain, including: the optimal test methodology and threshold value, sensitivity of the test for intramural dissections isolated from the aortic lumen, the test specificity, the time dependence of the test characteristics with respect to symptom onset, and the independence of the test's predictive value from other clinical and radiologic predictors of disease.[22,23]

Imaging studies

Emergency imaging is used to suggest and to diagnose acute aortic dissection. A number of findings on the chest X-ray study may suggest acute dissection, including a widened mediastinum, a widened or abnormal (tortuous, kinking, lump appearance) aortic contour, a blurred aortic knob, displacement of the outer surface of the aortic contour from the intimal aortic calcification, tracheal deviation to the right or distortion of the left main bronchus, and pleural effusion.[10,24] Attempts have been made to quantitate some of these findings. A widened mediastinum may be defined as a ratio of the mediastinum to the chest of greater than 0.25–0.31, or a mediastinal width greater than 8 cm at the level of the aortic knob.[23,24] Displacement of the intimal aortic calcification greater than 6 mm may be considered positive.

Unfortunately, when subjected to rigorous blinded testing, chest X-ray findings have proven neither highly reliable nor discriminatory. Von Kodolitsch and colleagues find the overall sensitivity and specificity of the chest X-ray to be 64% and 86%, respectively.[24] The pooled overall sensitivity from multiple studies appears to be approximately 90%.[10] A widened aortic knob or contour and widened mediastinum may be the most sensitive and reliable findings.[10,24,25] The effect of radiologic technique such as posterior-anterior (PA) or anterior-posterior (AP) view on test characteristics is uncertain. It is critical to appreciate the limited sensitivity of the chest X-ray study for aortic dissection, and the potential delay in diagnosis a false negative may cause.[26] A normal chest X-ray study does not rule out disease.

Advanced imaging studies used to diagnose acute aortic dissection include transthoracic and transesophageal echocardiography (Figure 19-3a and 19-3b), computed tomographic scan (CT scan) (Figure 19-4), magnetic resonance (MR) angiography, and conventional angiography. While the primary goal of these studies is to diagnose aortic dissection if it is present, there are a number of important secondary goals. These include: identifying the location of the dissection (ascending, descending, arch, or combination), its extent and size, the site of the intimal tear, evidence of aortic regurgitation, branch vessel or coronary artery involvement, or pericardial effusion. Methodologic considerations of the imaging test include its diagnostic accuracy, safety, speed, convenience, contraindications, and the ability to identify alternative diagnoses.

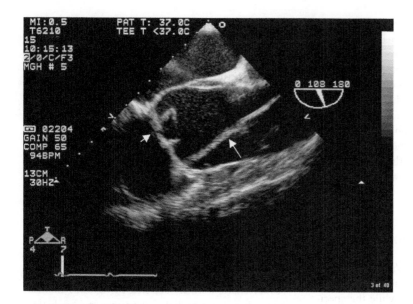

Figure 19.3a Transesophageal echocardiogram longitudinal view of the ascending aortic root: the long arrow identifies an ascending aortic dissection flap that sits diagonally along the length of the aortic root, ending at the aortic valve inferiorly. The short arrow identifies the leaflets of the aortic valve which, in this case, continue to demonstrate good apposition despite mild dilatation of the aortic root.

The technology and test characteristics of the various imaging modalities have steadily improved over the past two decades.[27,28] The sensitivity and specificity of dedicated transesophageal echocardiography, CT scan, and MR angiography are now all at 95% or above at major centers, while transthoracic echocardiography remains distinctly less sensitive (59–85%). Emergency physicians today most commonly use CT scan, followed by transesophageal echocardiography, to diagnose acute dissection.[29] The facilities and time required to perform MR angiography may be the most important hindrances to its widespread use.

Conventional angiography has long been considered the reference standard for aortic imaging. In the setting of ST elevation myocardial infarction and possible causative aortic dissection, it may be desirable to perform aortography in the catheterization laboratory prior to coronary angiography and possible percutaneous intervention. The sensitivity of this procedure for dissection is presumed high, though not precisely

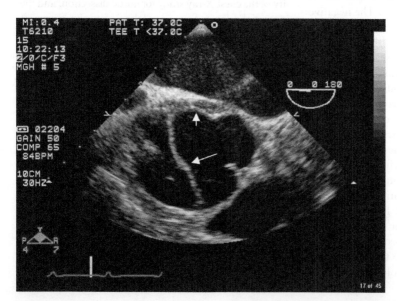

Figure 19.3b Transesophageal echocardiogram transverse view of the ascending aortic root: the long arrow identifies the dissection flap just superior to the level of the tricuspid aortic valve. The short arrow identifies thrombosis underneath the dissection flap along the wall of the aortic root. In this patient, the thrombosed dissection flap involved the origin of the left main coronary artery, causing an associated anteroseptal STEMI.

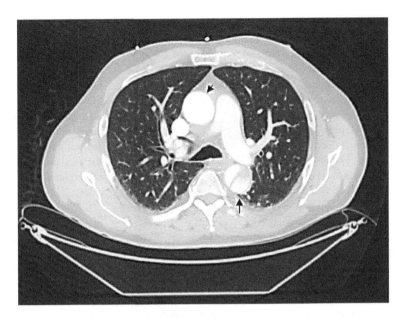

Figure 19.4 Chest CT image including the ascending and descending aorta: the descending aorta demonstrates a dissection flap with heterogeneously decreased contrast consistent with some stasis in the posterior false lumen portion of the vessel (long arrow). The homogeneous appearance of the ascending aorta suggests no dissection involvement (short arrow).

defined. Alternatively, a patient with chest symptoms and elevated serum D-dimer may be referred for pulmonary embolism (PE) CT scan. This involves a contrast bolus timed to highlight the pulmonary arterial, not the systemic arterial circulation. Approximately 0.5% of PE CTs demonstrate aortic dissection, but the sensitivity of this alternate protocol CT angiography for acute dissection is uncertain.[30]

Multidetector CT (MDCT) coronary angiography represents an important technological advance with implications for aortic dissection diagnosis. Timed gating of CT image acquisition to the diastolic phase of the EKG cycle allows for high resolution imaging of the coronary arteries. MDCT coronary angiography can be reliably used to assess for the presence of coronary artery disease and the likelihood of an acute coronary syndrome (ACS).[31]

The simultaneous MDCT assessment for three of the most dangerous and important conditions responsible for chest symptoms (acute aortic dissection, ACS, and PE) is now being explored with "triple rule out" protocols. These protocols extend the coronary angiography technology by using multiple timed contrast boluses and a larger imaging field to include the heart, lungs, and aorta.[32,33] Potential advantages of this technique include a relatively rapid test with high diagnostic accuracy for all three conditions, and the ability to identify a broad spectrum of other possible chest and upper abdominal conditions. For those patients with ascending aortic dissection, EKG gating that effectively freezes cardiac motion allows for evaluation of the aortic perivalvular area and the coronary arteries.[34]

A number of challenges remain in the development of the "triple rule out" protocol. Acquisition time with associated breath hold in the scanner is approximately 20 seconds. Contrast dose (approximately 125 cc) and radiation (approximately 12–30 millisievert) are larger than conventional imaging protocols. Patient limitations include known coronary calcifications or stents, obesity, renal insufficiency, contrast allergy, atrial fibrillation, or the inability to achieve a necessarily slow heart rate to successfully gate image acquisition. Finally, it is rare that emergency physicians seriously entertain the possibility of all three diagnoses in a single patient.[35]

Emergency department diagnosis

Despite the array of advanced technology available to practitioners today, the rapid and correct diagnosis of all acute aortic dissections remains a tremendous challenge. The correct diagnosis is still delayed or determined postmortem in a significant minority of cases.[6,36,37] The most difficult cases seem to be patients who present with isolated epigastric, abdominal, or flank pain.[36] Isolated chest pain without radiation to the back can also be difficult and doubly problematic.

279

Dissection is often misdiagnosed as cardiac ischemia and treated with anticoagulant therapy, which may increase hemorrhage into and expansion of the false lumen. As noted above, some dissections may cause secondary cardiac ischemia such that both conditions exist simultaneously, making appropriate management even more challenging.

To increase the proportion of aortic dissection patients correctly diagnosed in the ED, the first priority is to liberally consider the diagnosis in all patients with pain in the torso, syncope, or focal neurologic complaints. While all dissection patients do not have pain, a combination of pain and neurologic complaints should suggest this diagnosis. A second priority is to consider dissection in all patients with isolated chest pain, and to consider factors that differentiate dissection from ACS. The description of pain, its severity at onset, its radiation, and suggestive physical examination findings may all be helpful. It is also useful to differentiate ascending versus descending dissection. While emergency physician bedside transthoracic ultrasound, EKG, chest X-ray, and serum D-dimer test may all be helpful in assessing the likelihood of disease, none of these studies alone is sufficiently sensitive to rule out disease. When in doubt, a definitive imaging study must be performed.

Emergency treatment

Once the diagnosis of acute aortic dissection is suspected, antiplatelet and anticoagulant therapies that may be routinely administered for ACS or PE should be withheld until the diagnosis is clear.[38] For hypertensive patients, blood pressure control with a goal of 100-120 mmHg systolic pressure is considered essential to minimize further extension of the dissection. Decreasing the force of cardiac contraction (inotropy) and the heart rate may also be protective.[39] For these reasons, medicines with beta-adrenergic receptor blocking activity such as labetalol, propanolol, and esmolol are commonly used first. Other choices include calcium channel blockers such as diltiazem and verapamil, or after heart rate control, a short acting angiotensin-converting enzyme (ACE) inhibitor such as enalaprilat, or nitroprusside. Renal artery compromise with secondary excessive renin excretion may particularly benefit from ACE inhibition. Appropriate analgesia should also be administered.

Hypotension can be treated with intravenous fluid, and an immediate search for underlying causes, including cardiac tamponade, aortic regurgitation, acute myocardial infarction, internal hemorrhage, or another process. The clinician should be wary of pseudo-hypotension due to isolated arterial insufficiency from dissection flap compromise of a subclavian or iliac artery takeoff. All of the complications described above generally require urgent operative intervention. If pressor medicines are required, primary vasoconstrictors with relatively less inotropic effect, such as phenylephrine and norepinephrine, are preferred.

Cardiac tamponade complicates approximately 18% of acute aortic dissections. It is associated with syncope and altered consciousness, and the associated mortality is approximately 50%.[40] Pericardiocentesis may be a useful short-term temporizing measure for pericardial tamponade, but there is some concern that relief of tamponade without definitive repair will promote further hemorrhage.[41]

Surgical treatment

Untreated, the mortality of type A dissection is greater than 50% within 30 days of onset. For this reason, surgical treatment is usually indicated. Uncomplicated type B dissections may be treated with blood pressure control only. The following complications of type B dissection may merit surgical intervention: vital organ or limb ischemia, an expanding hematoma, retrograde extension to the ascending aorta (by definition, this converts to type A), Marfan's syndrome, or uncontrolled hypertension or pain.

Emergent surgical treatment of acute aortic dissection may involve repair of the intimal tear and closure of the false lumen, graft replacement of the involved aortic segment, aortic valve repair or replacement, coronary artery bypass grafting (if the coronary arteries are involved or diseased), or endovascular stent placement in the aorta or involved branches. Transfemoral intraluminal aortic covered stent-graft placement is a relatively new technique. The goals of stent placement are to halt the flow of blood into the false lumen and promote thrombosis, and to keep the true lumen open. This has been used for type B and the distal portion of type A dissections.[42,43] Other advanced endovascular techniques include balloon or scissors treatment to widen the reentry site from the false to the true lumen, and bare metal stenting for static or dynamic obstruction of branch arteries.[7]

Prognosis

The prognosis for patients who receive a timely diagnosis and modern therapy continues to improve. Thirty-day survival postsurgery is approximately 70%. For patients with type B dissection treated medically, 30-day survival is 92%.[5] Five-year survival for all groups discharged from the hospital is 75–82%.

Section IV: Decision making

- Consider aortic dissection in all patients with pain in the torso, syncope, or focal neurologic complaints, and in all patients with both chest and back pain.
- Blood pressure control with a goal of 100–120 mmHg systolic pressure is essential to minimize extension of the dissection. Decreasing the force of cardiac contraction and heart rate are also protective.
- Beta-adrenergic receptor blockers such as labetalol, propanolol, and esmolol should be used initially.
- After heart rate control, enalaprilat or nitroprusside can be used.
- CT scan, MRI, and transesophageal echocardiography all have similar high sensitivities; however, CT scan is generally the test of choice due to time constraints.
- D-dimer is a promising diagnostic tool that can be used to assess further the likelihood of disease in patients at relatively low risk based on the history, physical examination, and chest X-ray.
- Type A and B dissection should both have emergent surgical consultation, although only Type A will routinely require emergent surgery.

References

1 Dihmis WC, Ridley P, Dhasmana JP, Wisheart JD. Acute dissection of the aorta with amphetamine misuse. *BMJ.* 1997;314(7095):1665.
2 Clouse WD, Hallett JW Jr, Schaff HV, et al. Acute aortic dissection: Population-based incidence compared with degenerative aortic aneurysm rupture. *Mayo Clin Proc.* 2004;79(2):176–180.
3 Meszaros I, Morocz J, Szlavi J, et al. Epidemiology and clinicopathology of aortic dissection: A population-based longitudinal study over 27 years. *Chest.* 2000;117(5):1271–1278.
4 Hirst AE Jr, Johns VJ Jr, Kime SW Jr. Dissecting aneurysm of the aorta: A review of 505 cases. *Medicine.* 1958;37(3):217–279.
5 Hagan PG, Neinaber CA, Isselbacher EM, et al. The International Registry of Acute Aortic Dissection (IRAD): New insights into an old disease. *JAMA.* 2000;283(7):897–903.
6 Spittell PC, Spittell JA Jr, Joyce JW, et al. Clinical features and differential diagnosis of aortic dissection: Experience with 236 cases (1980 through 1990). *Mayo Clin Proc.* 1993;68(7):642–651.
7 Golledge J, Eagel KA. Acute aortic dissection. *Lancet.* 2008;372(9632):55–66.
8 Slater EE, DeSanctis RW. The clinical recognition of dissecting aortic aneurysm. *Am J Med.* 1976;60(5):625–633.
9 Gilon D, Mehta RH, Oh JK, et al. Characteristics and in-hospital outcomes of patients with cardiac tamponade complicating type A acute aortic dissection. *Am J Cardiol.* 2009;103(7):1029–1031.
10 Klompas M. Does this patient have an acute thoracic aortic dissection? *JAMA.* 2002;287(17):2262–2272.
11 Hatzaras I, Tranquilli M, Coady M, et al. Weight lifting and aortic dissection: More evidence for a connection. *Cardiology.* 2007;107(2):103–106.
12 Nienaber CA, von Kodolitsch Y, Nicolas V, et al. The diagnosis of thoracic aortic dissection by noninvasive imaging procedures. *N Engl J Med.* 1993;328(1):1–9.
13 Mandavia DP, Hoffner RJ, Mahaney K, Henderson SO. Bedside echocardiography by emergency physicians. *Ann Emerg Med.* 2001;38(4):377–382.
14 Perkins AM, Liteplo A, Noble VE. Ultrasound diagnosis of type A aortic dissection. *J Emerg Med.*2008 Nov 25 [Epub ahead of print].
15 Pinney SP, Wasserman HS. Anterior myocardial infarction, acute aortic dissection, and anomalous coronary artery. *J Interv Cardiol.* 2002;15(4):293–296.
16 Shinohara T, Suzuki K, Okada M, et al. Soluble elastin fragments in serum are elevated in acute aortic dissection. *Arterioscler Thromb Vasc Biol.* 2003;23(10):1839–1844.
17 Suzuki T, Katoh H, Tsuchio Y, et al. Diagnostic implications of elevated levels of smooth-muscle myosin heavy-chain protein in acute aortic dissection. The smooth muscle myosin heavy chain study. *Ann Intern Med.* 2000;133(7):537–541.
18 Weber T, Hogler S, Auer J, et al. D-dimer in acute aortic dissection. *Chest.* 2003;123(5):1375–1378.
19 Bayes-Genis A, Mateo J, Santalo M, et al. D-Dimer is an early diagnostic marker of coronary ischemia in patients with chest pain. *Am Heart J.* 2000;140(3):379–384.

20 Suzuki T, Distante A, Zizza A, et al. Diagnosis of acute aortic dissection by D-dimer: The International Registry of Acute Aortic Dissection Substudy on Biomarkers (IRAD-Bio) experience. *Circulation.* 2009;119(20):2702–2707.

21 Marill KA. Serum D-dimer is a sensitive test for the detection of acute aortic dissection: A pooled meta-analysis. *J Emerg Med.*2008;34(4):367–376.

22 Ohlmann P, Faure A, Morel O, et al. Lower circulating Sta-Liatest D-Di levels I patients with aortic intramural hematoma compared with classical aortic dissection. *Crit Care Med.* 2009;37(3):899–901.

23 Hazui H, Fukumoto H, Negoro N, et al. Simple and useful tests for discriminating between acute aortic dissection of the ascending aorta and acute myocardial infarction in the emergency setting. *Circ J.* 2005;69(6):677–682.

24 Von Kodolitsch Y, Nienaber CA, Dieckmann C, et al. Chest radiography for the diagnosis of acute aortic syndrome. *Am J Med.* 2004;116(2):73–77.

25 Jagannath AS, Sos TA, Lockhart SH, Saddekni S, Sniderman KW. Aortic dissection: A statistical analysis of the usefulness of plain chest radiographic findings. *Am J Roentgenol.* 1986;147(6):1123–1126.

26 Luker GD, Glazer HS, Eagar G, Gutierrez FR, Sagel SS. Aortic dissection: Effect of prospective chest radiographic diagnosis on delay to definitive diagnosis. *Radiology.* 1994;193(3):813–819.

27 Nienaber CA, von Kodolitsch Y, Nicolas V, et al. The diagnosis of thoracic aortic dissection by noninvasive imaging procedures. *N Engl J Med.* 1993;328(1):1–9.

28 Shiga T, Wajima Z, Apfel CC, Inoue T, Ohe Y. Diagnostic accuracy of transesophageal echocardiography, helical computed tomography, and magnetic resonance imaging for suspected thoracic aortic dissection: systematic review and meta-analysis. *Arch Intern Med.* 2006;166(13):-1350–1356.

29 Moore AG, Eagle KA, Bruckman D, et al. Choice of computed tomography, transesophageal echocardiography, magnetic resonance imaging, and aortography in acute aortic dissection: International Registry of Acute Aortic Dissection (IRAD). *Am J Cardiol.* 2002;89(10):1235–1238.

30 Richman PB, Courtney DM, Friese J, et al. Prevalence and significance of nonthromboembolic findings on chest computed tomography angiography performed to rule out pulmonary embolism: A multicenter study of 1,025 emergency department patients. *Acad Emerg Med.* 2004;11(6):642–647.

31 Hoffmann U, Bamberg F, Chae CU, et al. Coronary computed tomography angiography for early triage of patients with acute chest pain: The ROMICAT (Rule Out Myocardial Infarction using Computer Assisted Tomography) trial. *J Am Coll Cardiol.* 2009;53(18):1642–1650.

32 Johnson TRC, Nikolaou K, Wintersperger BJ, et al. ECG-gated 64-MDCT angiography in the differential diagnosis of acute chest pain. *Am J Roentgenol.* 2007;188(1):76–82.

33 Gallagher MJ, Raff GL. Use of multislice CT for the evaluation of emergency room patients with chest pain: The so-called "triple rule-out." *Catheter Cardiovasc Interv.* 2008;71(1):92–99.

34 Frauenfelder T, Appenzeller P, Karlo C, et al. Triple rule-out CT in the emergency department: Protocols and spectrum of imaging findings. *Eur Radiol.* 2009;19(4):789–799.

35 Rogg JG, Neve JW, Huang C, et al. The triple work-up for emergency department patients with acute chest pain: How often does it occur? *J Emerg Med.* 2008 Sep 12 [Epub ahead of print].

36 Sullivan PR, Wolfson AB, Leckey RD, Burke JL. Diagnosis of acute thoracic aortic dissection in the emergency department. *Am J Emerg Med.*2000;18(1):46–50.

37 Rapezzi C, Longhi S, Graziosi M, et al. Risk factors for diagnostic delay in acute aortic dissection. *Am J Cardiol.* 2008;102(10);1399–1406.

38 Davis DP, Grossman K, Kiggins DC, Vilke GM, Chan TC. The inadvertent administration of anticoagulants to ED patients ultimately diagnosed with thoracic aortic dissection. *Am J Emerg Med.*2005;23(4):439–442.

39 Kodama K, Nishigami K, Sakamoto T, et al. Tight heart rate control reduces secondary adverse events in patients with type B acute aortic dissection. *Circulation.* 2008;118(14 Suppl):S167–S170.

40 Gilon D, Mehta RH, Oh JK, et al. Characteristics and in-hospital outcomes of patients with cardiac tamponade complicating type A acute aortic dissection. *Am J Cardiol.* 2009;103(7):1029–1031.

41 Isselbacher EM, Cigarroa JE, Eagle KA. Cardiac tamponade complicating proximal aortic dissection: Is pericardiocentesis harmful? *Circulation.* 1994;90(5):-2375–2378.

42 Verhoye JP, Miller DC, Sze D, Dake MD, Mitchell RS. Complicated acute type B aortic dissection: Midterm results of emergency endovascular stent-grafting. *J Thorac Cardiovasc Surg.* 2008;136(2):424–430.

43 Parker JD, Golledge J. Outcome of endovascular treatment of acute type B aortic dissection. *Ann Thorac Surg.* 2008;86(5):1707–1712.

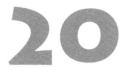

20 Abdominal aortic aneurysm

David A. Peak[1] & David F. M. Brown[2]

[1] *Assistant Professor, Division of Emergency Medicine, Harvard Medical School, Attending Physician and Assistant Residency Director, Department of Emergency Medicine, Massachusetts General Hospital, Boston, Massachusetts, USA*
[2] *Vice Chair, Department of Emergency Medicine, Massachusetts General Hospital, Associate Professor, Harvard Medical School, Boston, Massachusetts, USA*

Section I: Case presentation

A 68-year-old man with a history of hypertension and tobacco use presented to the emergency department (ED) after a syncopal event. He was at home when he abruptly developed right back, flank, and groin pain that was severe in onset. Within about 30 seconds, he developed nausea and passed out. EMS was called. On arrival of the EMS unit, he was awake and alert in a supine position complaining of ongoing right flank and groin pain. Vital signs were: heart rate 90 beats/min, blood pressure 110/60 mmHg, respiratory rate 18 breaths/min. A large bore IV was inserted, and the patient was placed on a monitor that showed a sinus rhythm. He was transported to the local ED.

On ED arrival, he still described the pain as above. The past medical history was notable for hypertension and prostatic hypertrophy. He smoked a pack per day for 50 years. Alcohol use was minimal. Medications were lisinopril and proscar. On physical examination the vital signs were unchanged. The head and neck examinations were normal, the chest was clear to auscultation, the heart sounds were a regular S1 S2 with an S4, and no murmurs. The abdomen was soft but tender in the epigastrium to palpation with a pulsatile mass. Carotid, radial and femoral pulses were 2+. The extremities had no edema. The back had no spinal or costovertebral angle tenderness. The neurological examination was normal. The EKG showed sinus rhythm with voltage

criteria for left ventricular hypertrophy. A bedside ultrasound performed by the emergency physician (EP) showed an abdominal aortic aneurysm.

Section II: Case discussion

Dr Peter Rosen: This is an interesting history that is easy, in retrospect, to diagnose accurately, but prospectively, I think it is much harder to focus upon a vascular event in this patient, especially if the patient focuses on his varied complaints. I've seen a number of these patients who say "I felt a little bit dizzy, but it's really from the pain in my back and the back pain is really killing me," "I've never felt pain this severe," or just "get rid of my back pain." I've also had patients in whom the pain did not start abruptly but who had back pain for months to years, had been treated for spinal stenosis or spinal arthritis, and again, minimize the vascular components of their pain. I think that the issue that helps us the most in this case is the history of syncope. But I believe that many patients are either not aware of it, or dismiss it as a dizzy spell, and don't help us by telling us about the event. Are than any clues that you like to use that put you in the direction of vascular disease when you see a patient like this?

Dr Shamai Grossman: A patient who has a chief complaint of abdominal and flank pain accompanied by syncope: together these are classic symptoms that go with vascular disease. If the patient had a history of hypertension, this would further point you in this direction. If you obtain a history of coronary or peripheral arterial disease, or when examining the patient you note other signs common in vascular disease, such as bruits or signs of peripheral vascular disease, and certainly if you have a pulsatile mass, you should be very concerned that this patient may have a significant vascular problem, such as an abdominal aortic aneurysm that at this point may be ruptured.

PR: In this case the patient was not only cooperative in terms of historical findings, but also physical findings. I think it is probably rare to have a palpable pulsatile mass with an aortic aneurysm. If you have ever palpated one of these during surgery, what you find is a large tube filled with soft toothpaste-like material. The flow through that aneurysm may be slow enough so that you don't get any pulsation or any sensation of a mass when you palpate through the abdomen. In fact, fewer than 25% of these patients have a palpable mass. We were further helped here because this patient didn't come in with normal vital signs, and patients who have renal colic almost never present with lowered blood pressures; they come in with elevated blood pressures. Is the presence of a bruit over the patient's abdomen a helpful physical finding?

Dr David Brown: I find the presence of bruits helpful, but again I find the absence of bruits does not help me eliminate a vascular diagnosis. Although feeling a palpable enlarged aorta is unusual, and certainly can't be considered the norm, the absence of this finding on physical examination should also not reassure the physician that this is not a symptomatic or enlarging abdominal aortic aneurysm (AAA). In addition, a person with a history of hypertension who presents with a blood pressure in the normal range for someone without hypertension should be a red flag, particularly if you are considering the other major disease on the differential list, nephrolithiasis, as this usually presents with hypertension. Furthermore, this patient is old for a first presentation of renal colic, and doesn't give a history of prior renal colic, so that makes this diagnosis unlikely. He also doesn't give a history of spinal disease, making this unlikely as well.

PR: Bruits over the aorta are uncommon. Occasionally we hear bruits over the downstream circulation because they have atherosclerotic narrowing as well,

and I think it's well worth listening for a bruit over the carotid arteries, as these patients often have diffuse vascular disease and have potential for stroke and coronary artery disease. However, I have never made the diagnosis of an abdominal aneurysm from an abdominal bruit. Bruits in the abdomen are mostly seen in women with renal artery stenosis, as they tend to be younger and thinner. Gastrointestinal bleeding is another important diagnosis that must be considered; this too may often be given to you historically, but sometimes syncope can be an initial presentation. I can remember a patient who presented exactly with this history except that he came in somewhat confused; had we not done a rectal on this patient we wouldn't have picked up that he was having both a gastrointestinal (GI) bleed and an aortic aneurysm. One of the things about aneurysms that helps muddy the presentation of the disease is that abdominal aneurysms can have anatomical proximity to the third portion of the duodenum. Therefore, some of these patients present with an upper GI bleed as a sign of their aortic aneurysm erosion. Although GI bleeding doesn't rule out an aneurysm, this presentation may also be consistent with a different disease entity, like peptic ulcer disease, rather than aneurysmal disease.

PR: What is the utility of bedside ultrasound? In this case it seems to have been useful, because it found an aortic aneurysm, but in obese people who have an ileus from an eroding aneurysm it may be very difficult to see aortic enlargement.

DB: I think it is worth doing a bedside ultrasound as part of the secondary survey in patients like this, and if one sees an enlarged aorta, that's extremely helpful. However, unless you can see a normal aorta from the transition through the diaphragm all the way through the bifurcation, one cannot reliably exclude aortic aneurysm with a bedside ultrasound. It is a common pitfall to exclude the diagnosis simply because you didn't see the aorta well on ultrasound. Not seeing the aorta well on ultrasound is a common finding, and not because there is no aneurysm, but because there is gas in the gastrointestinal tract or a lot of fat, which makes the examination of the patient with ultrasound difficult.

SG: I would make the argument that if you have a positive ultrasound it is so helpful that at that point, I would call the surgeon and say that you have a patient who needs to go directly to the operating room (OR).

PR: I couldn't agree more, but I think we have to be somewhat realistic here. When we first started doing vascular surgery, we were in a surgical climate where there was much less reluctance to go the OR without precise diagnoses. Over the past 20 years, we've seen increasing reluctance to take patients to the OR without imaging information. We can ask our surgical colleagues to go directly to the OR, and there seems to be a literature to suggest that outcomes, especially for leaking aneurysms, can be improved by not delaying for further imaging studies, but I would say that it would be rare to find a vascular surgeon who would take this patient based on an ultrasound image alone. I think it is unfortunate, because I think this is precisely the kind of patient who needs to be in an operating room instead of a CT scanner. My guess is that he is going to get a CT scan before he goes to the OR.

One of the reasons so many of these aneurysms are amenable to endovascular repair is because the vast majority are not thoraco-abdominal, as 95% of them originate in the abdomen distal to the renal arteries. It is very rare for them to involve the renal arteries, and it is very rare for them to be two separate aneurysms. For the most part, thoracic aortic aneurysms are visible on a chest X-ray study, if not on an ultrasound, by sliding your probe up into the chest, rather than just looking into the abdomen. So I think that is kind of a weak argument for a CT scan. However, I don't think it matters whether we think the patient should go directly to the operating room or not; we are not the ones doing the surgery, and I think it is important for the person who has that responsibility to feel comfortable about what the patient requires for surgery.

SG: I've seen quite a number of these patients deteriorate rapidly. To better define the anatomy expeditiously, one can bring them to the operating room where they can perform transesophageal echocardiography in the OR; while we have the patient draped, you can better define the anatomy in a setting where if you need to open up the abdomen immediately, you can.

PR: For the thoracic aneurysm that is probably sensible. I don't think you need it for the abdominal aneurysm, but again, I think we are dependent on the person who has the skill set and responsibility for the surgical procedure; it's been 20 years since I've worked with a surgeon who was willing to take a patient like this directly to the operating room. Frankly, it's not easy to repair a leaking aneurysm surgically, and if it can be done endovascularly, there is a tremendous advantage to the patient in terms of morbidity and mortality. With this in mind, it may make sense to get more imaging information before you go to the operating room.

We have a patient who's been a long-term smoker. We know that there is an association between peripheral vascular disease and smoking, and a lesser association between smoking and aortic aneurysmal development. It has been my experience that patients who have Buerger's disease have distal vascular problems usually without aneurysms. In contrast, with aneurysmal disease, while there may be downstream atherosclerotic plaques, for the most part have the disease is primarily confined to the aorta. This is one of the reasons that bypass works so successfully for them. Can you tell the difference in the ED?

DB: Buerger's disease, or thomboangitis obliterans as it's also known, generally presents with limb ischemia. It is a peripheral vascular disease problem with thrombosis and distal embolization. It is strongly associated with smoking, and the only treatment I know of, short of bypass and amputation, which are often not very successful, is smoking cessation. In contrast to abdominal aortic aneurysm, Buerger's disease tends not to rupture. We don't encounter these patients presenting with hemorrhagic shock, but rather with ischemia of a distal limb. Buerger's disease may overlap with popliteal artery aneurysms, which tend to thrombose and embolize, and may present with distal extremity ischemia. There also may be some overlap with Buerger's disease, smoking, and other atherosclerotic aneurysms of the aorta or popliteal arteries.

PR: Many patients who have emergent repair of abdominal aneurysms will sustain non-ST-segment elevated myocardial infarctions (NSTEMIs) during surgery. Is there any point in obtaining a set of enzymes on this patient before he goes to the OR?

SG: Are you considering enzymes before he goes to the OR because you are hoping to ascertain whether he is having a concomitant infarct preoperatively rather than peri- or postoperatively?

PR: Although you would still need to go to the OR even if the patient was in the process of evolving an infarct, would you be able to define a change in troponin level more rapidly if you had a baseline?

SG: Unfortunately, cardiac enzymes tend not to elevate until 6–8 hours after the event. Were you to send preoperative cardiac enzymes, they would very likely be normal and fail to indicate ischemia. How important is it to actually recognize ischemia as preoperative vs. perioperative? I don't believe it makes much difference when the patient became ischemic, as ultimately he will need to be cared for in much the same way, whether it was from a preoperative or perioperative event. In addition, enzymes may elevate anyhow from some myocardial leak connected with the surgery.

PR: The proposed mechanism of the myocardial infarction during surgery is the hypoxia produced by the low blood pressure from the leak, which he already has. Additionally, during surgery when you take the clamps off to start reperfusing the graft, there is often a drop in blood pressure. While there are great efforts made to prevent this using blood transfusion or pressors right before you unclamp, there frequently is a drop in blood pressure. Unfortunately, this can cause diminished flow in a coronary artery that is already stenosed, or even in the carotid arteries. This reminds us that as much as we would hope that it is, vascular disease is not a localized problem.

Often one has access to vascular surgeons fairly ubiquitously, but there are institutions that are reluctant to take care of critical postoperative patients, and that often might be a reason for transfer. What would you do with this patient if you had to transfer him before you could arrange a surgery for him?

DB: I would call the local helicopter and tertiary care center immediately after the results of my bedside ultrasound, even if I decided to proceed with a CT scan. I wouldn't feel compelled to keep the patient in a community hospital ED if I had a reliably positive finding on ultrasound, and a CT scan would delay moving the patient to a center where definitive care could be given. In reality, usually one can get a CT scan in a community hospital before the tertiary center has agreed to accept the patient and transport has been arranged, so most of the time I think the CT scan is done at the referring hospital.

PR: How high would you want his blood pressure during transfer?

DB: This is a somewhat controversial area. Most of the data about fluid resuscitation and hemorrhagic shock are from the trauma model, using pigs, so we don't know as much about this as we would like to. I would keep blood pressures as low as the patient can tolerate, meaning I would not over-resuscitate with crystalloid and blood if the patient had a normal mental status, was making urine, and not complaining of chest pain or stroke symptoms. Even if the systolic blood pressure is 100 mmHg or a little less, there is a theoretical concern that by giving fluid or blood, we could increase the perfusion pressure and the bleeding that has been tamponaded in the retroperitoneum will restart and cause fatal hemorrhage. We also may dilute out clotting factors and disrupt the body's ability to create thrombus in the area of rupture that in the same way could cause a fatal hemorrhage.

PR: We used to use medical antishock trouser (MAST) suits in the field and perhaps in the ED before bringing patients we thought might have a leaking aneurysm to the operating room. Would you consider that as a therapy in a patient who had to be transferred?

SG: Today MAST suits aren't readily available, and we aren't accustomed to using them. I think we would waste too much precious time trying to locate one and getting it on the patient, and lose a fair amount of the benefit of arranging for the patient to be transferred.

PR: The data on whether or not it helped was also pretty muddy. I remember seeing a few patients in whom I thought the MAST suit actually increased hemorrhage when it was inflated. When one uses a MAST suit, you have to take it down compartment by compartment, starting with the abdomen, and you have to make sure you are giving fluid resuscitation simultaneously, otherwise you will have an acute precipitous drop in blood pressure leading to the development of an acute lethal dysrhythmia. There isn't much you can do to make this patient safe during transfer; it is worth transferring the patient if you don't have critical care or vascular surgery capacity, but it is much better if you can go from the ED directly to the OR rather than to another ED.

PR: Many of these patients are misdiagnosed as spinal arthritis, as the symptoms of spinal stenosis and vascular disease overlap; both have claudication. It may require imaging studies to differentiate the two, or even an MRI of the spine. Our patient, who presents with syncope, moves us away from spinal disease; however, in a patient with known spinal disease, it makes it harder to jump to a vascular diagnosis. Does this patient need any additional workup besides the ultrasound and a type and cross before going to the OR?

DB: I don't think so; if you only have one vial of blood to send to the laboratory it ought to be a type and cross. I don't think it matters what the initial hematocrit is, but it is very likely that the patient will need blood.

SG: It would be useful to know the patient's baseline renal function, especially if this turns out to have some involvement of the renal artery.

PR: I would also forgo preoperative imaging studies such as carotid duplex studies in a patient who might have a bruit, as this is a patient who needs to go to the OR, and needs to go there very quickly.

DB: I would argue to do a noncontrast CT. You can get enough information from a noncontrast CT scan to know whether there an aneurysm, and if it is rupturing. Some emergency physicians may prefer a contrast-enhanced CT for better delineation of pathology, but I think the time that it takes to wait for the creatinine to come back, convince the radiologist to push the contrast, and then give the contrast is time poorly spent.

PR: Some institutions have a protocol that mandates oral and rectal contrast as well; a bowel full of contrast is the last thing you need in a surgical patient.

SG: The only test I would do on this patient in addition would be a 12-lead EKG, particularly with concern for concomitant cardiac dysrhythmia after this patient's syncopal event.

PR: Our biggest responsibility in emergency medicine is the recognition of the aneurysm, and the expeditious involvement of the service that can give definitive care. I think where we fall into error is going down the pathway of renal colic or spinal disease, and overlooking the time constraints of a vascular repair. When would you pursue a pulmonary embolism (PE) as the cause of the syncopal episode?

SG: If the physical examination was less compelling for an aortic aneurysm, and the ultrasound and CT were negative, then you'd have to ask yourself if this

flank pain is really pleuritic chest pain and rethink the differential, but with this patient's presentation, I would not consider a PE.

What if the patient presented without syncope, but with flank pain and dizziness, and a CT scan showed an unruptured 5–6 cm AAA. What should one do then?

DB: This is a symptomatic AAA until proven otherwise, and needs to be treated in much the same way as a ruptured AAA, with urgent vascular surgery referral. Telling patients that less than 5 cm aneurysms tend not to rupture and putting off an evaluation to the outpatient setting, I think, is a mistake.

PR: If the aneurysm is <5 cm, I would have a hard time believing that it is the cause of his symptoms, but that doesn't mean he isn't having a vascular catastrophe. He could have a mesenteric artery occlusion obstructing his renal blood flow, causing pain in the groin and kidney region. Thus, I would still consider this a vascular emergency and regardless of whether it requires immediate operative repair, it requires immediate consultation.

To conclude, I would emphasize the confusion we create by treating aortic dissection and aortic thoracic aneurysm as the same diseases. A dissection is a disease of the lining of the aorta, probably caused by hypertension, and it is not an aneurysm; it's a totally different pathology than atherosclerosis of the thoracic aorta that can behave like an abdominal aneurysm. Atherosclerosis of the thoracic aorta is less common, can also rupture, and needs to be evaluated and treated as if it were an abdominal aneurysm. The treatment is totally different and the course is totally different than a dissection of the aorta. The distinction can be made by imaging studies, as a thoracic aortic atherosclerotic aneurysm will be demonstrated as enlargement of the aorta. It has the same kind of deformity of the entire wall of the vessel as does the abdominal aneurysm, and it requires either stenting endovascularly, or resection and replacement with an artificial graft. We need to stop talking about dissecting aneurysms, refer to them as dissecting aortas, and confine the term aneurysm to atherosclerotic disease.

Case resolution

A stat vascular surgery consult was called, and a second large bore IV was placed. Uncrossmatched blood was sent for from the blood bank, while a blood sample was sent for type and cross matching. The patient was brought to the CT scanner and underwent a noncontrast scan that showed a ruptured AAA with a right retroperitoneal hemorrhage. He was taken directly to the OR from the CT scanner for repair. He underwent an open procedure with aortic graft placement. Postoperatively he developed transient renal failure that resolved over several weeks. He was discharged on hospital day seven and was doing well at 6 month follow-up.

Section III: Concepts

Introduction

The definition of an aneurysm is a focal dilatation of the blood vessel compared to the normal state or adjacent blood vessel. The definition of an abdominal aortic aneurysm (AAA) is an aortic diameter at least 1.5 times the diameter measured at the level of the renal arteries. The normal value at this level is approximately 2.0 cm with a range of 1.4 to 3.0 cm.[1,2] A diameter greater than 3.0 cm is usually considered aneurysmal. Abdominal aortic aneurysms involve all the layers of the aorta and do not create intimal flaps or false lumens. Most (75%) AAAs are infrarenal.

An abdominal aortic aneurysm is the most common site of an arterial aneurysm. The aorta, like most arterial vessels, is made up of the intima, the media, and the adventia. The intima is a single layer of endothelial cells resting on a subendothelial tissue composed of collagen, elastin, fibroblasts, and mucoid ground substance. The media provides strength and elasticity, and is composed of smooth muscle cells within a matrix of elastin, collagen, and ground substance arranged in complex lamellar units. Degenerative changes within the media are thought to be the etiology of abdominal aortic aneurysms. The abdominal aortic media is composed of 28 lamellar units, compared to 45–56 in the thoracic aorta. The human abdominal aortic media lacks a vasa vasorum and has relatively fewer lamellar units for its diameter than abdominal (or thoracic) aortas of other species, resulting in a relatively elevated estimated mean tension per lamellar unit.[3] Finally, the adventia is a loose connective tissue around the outer diameter and contains the nerve supply.

Approximately 15,000 deaths per year in the United States are attributed to abdominal aortic aneurysm rupture, making it a leading cause of death.[4] Only 10–15% of patients will survive a rupture of an AAA;

most die before presenting for care, and only half will survive emergency surgery.[5] The prevalence of AAA is negligible in persons under age 60, and then rises dramatically with advancing age. By age 65, approximately 1.7% of women and 5% of men will have an abdominal aortic diameter ≥3 cm.[6] Clinically important aneurysms (over 4 cm diameter) occur in about 1% of men between the ages of 55 and 64, and the incidence increases approximately 2–6% per decade thereafter.[7-9] There is a male predominance of at least three-fold, with white men being the most highly represented group. Studies that use a definition of maximum external diameter (e.g., ≥3cm) may underestimate the prevalence of AAA in women.

While age and male gender are obviously epidemiologic risk factors, there are many others. Smoking is the strongest risk factor for the presence of AAA, and is a major risk for growth and rupture of an existing AAA.[8-10] More than 90% of patients with AAA have been smokers.[11] Current American College of Cardiology/American Heart Association (ACC/AHA) guidelines recommend smoking cessation for all patients with an AAA or a family history of an AAA.[1] Other, lesser identified risks include a family history of an AAA, hypertension, claudication, hypercholesterolemia, cerebral vascular disease, and increased height.[1,9-13] Decreased risk factors include female gender, diabetes mellitus, and black race.

The true pathogenesis of an AAA is currently unknown, it is probably multifactorial and systemic, and is being actively studied. A genome scan of families with an AAA identifies a possible gene locus on chromosome 19q13.[14] Multiple studies have focused on vascular structural proteins, especially elastin and collagen, degradation by various proteases, including metalloproteinases derived from endovascular and smooth muscle cells, and inflammatory cells that infiltrate the media and adventitia. These studies hold promise for better understanding the pathogenesis of an AAA, and potentially earlier therapeutic possibilities in the future.

Over the final few decades of the 20th century, much has been learned about the natural history of an AAA that, when coupled with advances in surgical modalities, has changed management for an unruptured AAA. Although some aneurysms may become symptomatic with back or abdominal discomfort, many remain asymptomatic until rupture.[5] Given the high incidence of death from a ruptured AAA, and the fact that most patients (>75%) are unaware they have an aneurysm prior to complications, there has been a major push for screening.[15] In 2005, the United States Preventive Services Task Force published a recommendation for one-time screening with an ultrasound imaging study for men aged 65–75 who have ever smoked at least 100 cigarettes in their lifetime.[16] In 2007, Medicare started offering a one-time screening AAA ultrasound study to men ages 65–75 who have smoked or have a family history of an AAA as part of their covered initial preventive physical examination.[17] Ultrasound screening approaches a sensitivity and specificity of 100% and 95%, respectively, for the detection of an infrarenal AAA.[18]

An asymptomatic, unruptured AAA is not an emergency, but should invoke a thoughtful discussion with a qualified physician, preferably a vascular surgeon. Individualized decision-making for an AAA is complex, and requires careful assessment of factors that affect the risk of rupture, as well as perioperative mortality, life expectancy, and patient preference.[19] The goals of management are to prevent rupture and to prolong life. Current guidelines suggest surveillance of an AAA up to 5.5 cm is acceptable in men unless symptoms or tenderness develop or rapid expansion (>1 cm/year) occurs.[1,8,19] Selective repair should be effective when the risk of rupture exceeds the risks of perioperative mortality. Optimal surveillance interval recommendations have varied, but the 2005 American College of Cardiology/American Heart Association published guidelines recommend surveillance with ultrasound or computed tomography for 3–4 cm diameter AAAs every 2–3 years, and every 6 months to 1 year for an AAA with diameters of 4–5.4 cm.[1] In the largest surveillance studies to date, 60–65% of patients randomized to surveillance require surgery at 5 years and 70–75% at 8 years.[20–22] Ultimately, patient preference is a major determinant in the decision to proceed with early elective surgery versus surveillance.

Rupture risk

The great variability in estimates for risk of rupture for a particular size of AAA reflect that other factors besides absolute size should be considered for each individual case.[23–25] Many surgeons consider the ratio of the aneurysm diameter compared to the native vessel, or some other adjustment to account for body size to be important, but the improvement in predicting

rupture using these techniques has been minimal.[26] Asymmetrical bulges compared to more uniform cylindrical aneurysms seem to increase local wall stress, and likely increase the risk of rupture.[27,28] Computer generated calculated wall stress may become a valuable predictor of an individual AAA rupture risk as these techniques become more widely adopted.

The best predictor of an AAA rupture is size. The risk of rupture up to a diameter of 5.5 cm in men is low, but substantially increases above this threshold.[29] In men, the estimated annual rupture risk is almost zero for aneurysms less than 4 cm and increases from 0.5% to 5% percent per year between a diameter of 4 and 5 cm. With a diameter of 5–6 cm, the risk increases to 3–15%/year. The annual risk of rupture becomes 10–20% per year for aneurysms 6–7 cm diameter, 20–40% per year for aneurysms 7–8 cm diameter, and 30–50% per year for aneurysms greater than 8 cm diameter.[5,19,29–33] Women are more likely to rupture at any given AAA diameter.[5,34] Continued smoking, chronic obstructive pulmonary disease (COPD), bronchiectasis, hypertension, a family history of an AAA, and a larger initial diameter of an AAA, all seem to increase the relative risk of an AAA rupture.[5,34–38] Localized blisters/blebs where the medial elastin is diminished likely increase the risk of rupture, whereas intraluminal thrombus does not appear to affect rupture rates.[39–41] Intraluminal thrombus does, however, seem to be associated with a rapid expansion rate of an AAA, as does continued smoking, poorly controlled hypertension, advanced cardiac disease, stroke, advanced age, and a large initial AAA diameter.[37,42–47]

Perioperative risk

Perioperative risk is an important consideration when discussing an individual management plan, and depends on patient factors, surgical training, and experience as well as the anatomy of the AAA itself. A review of multiple studies reveals an average operative mortality for open elective AAA repair of approximately 5.5%, with a range from less than 1% to over 50%.[47–59] Cardiac complications are the primary cause of perioperative death, and thus existing cardiac disease is thought to be a major risk factor. Individual risk factors for a poor outcome include electrocardiographic evidence of ischemia, COPD, an elevated creatinine, low FEV$_1$ (forced expiratory volume in 1 second), congestive heart failure, advanced age, and female gender.[48,50,60–65] Predictive models based on patient factors have been developed to stratify patients into low- and high-risk categories. Perioperative mortality is markedly higher with emergency surgery as compared to elective surgery.[66]

Operator training and experience also play a role in risk assessment, with subspecialty training in vascular surgery along with high volume surgeons and centers portending a better prognosis.[49,53–55,60,61,67] Adjusted inhospital and 30-day mortality for elective open AAA repair has been found to be inversely proportional to volume.[68] Finally, less quantitative pathologic factors of the aneurysm itself, such as extensive atheromatous disease, thrombus formation, calcifications at the anastomosis or clamp sites, extension to the juxtarenal level, and adhesion of the AAA to surrounding structures, make surgery more technically challenging, and would be expected to increase morbidity/mortality.[69–74] Previous abdominal surgeries may make also make AAA repair technically more difficult.

Lastly, endovascular aneurysm repair (EVAR) has changed the landscape of both elective and emergency repair of AAA. EVAR has demonstrated equal or better early safety and efficacy, as well as reduced intensive-care and hospital length of stays, fewer major complications, more rapid recovery, and less blood loss during the procedure compared with traditional open techniques.[75–81] Because of the lower perioperative complication rate and faster recovery, EVAR may be particularly well suited for older, high-risk patients compared to open repair.[82–84] Anatomic eligibility for EVAR varies from 14–54%.[85,86] Factors that influence eligibility include the axial length of the aortic neck, the diameter and condition of the iliac and femoral arteries, and the degree of calcification, tortuosity, angulation, as well as the degree of thrombosis that exists, all of which can influence the seal of the endoluminal device. EVAR requires preoperative CT angiography with three-dimensional reconstruction, which is repeated immediately postprocedure, at 1 month postoperatively, 6 months, and then yearly thereafter. The cost of an endoluminal device is also significant. The durability of EVAR has also been questioned. Secondary procedures are required in 10–27% of patients at 2 years as reported in 2 large series.[87,88] More long-term studies of newer endoluminal devices are needed to make conclusions about the durability of EVAR. For now, EVAR is an option for elective surgery when anatomically feasible, and may provide an alternative for patients at a very high risk for an open repair.

Presentation

The majority of AAAs are asymptomatic. Symptoms related to mass effect or compression of spatially related structures may manifest as discomfort, or vague gastrointestinal symptoms. An AAA may present with complications from intraluminal thrombus or distal embolization, and with erosion into adjacent structures. A large AAA may also present with disseminated intravascular coagulation causing bleeding or thrombosis.[89,90] New or progressive symptoms are worrisome for rapid expansion and impending rupture. Asymptomatic patients may be inappropriately referred to acute settings after a serendipitous diagnosis during studies for other conditions, a screening radiographic study, or physical examination. Available data suggest that approximately 50% of 4.0–4.9 cm AAA and 76% of ≥5 cm AAA may be palpated with careful physical examination close to the umbilicus.[91] Patients with a known AAA with back, abdominal, flank, or groin pain or new onset of tenderness over the AAA should be evaluated urgently.

After rupture, only one-quarter of the patients will reach a hospital alive, and only 10% will reach the operating room alive, with an additional 40% emergent operative mortality rate.[92,93] Presenting patients will usually complain of acute onset of back or abdominal pain, may have a palpable abdominal mass, and often have palpable tenderness on examination.[94,95] Almost half the patients will present with hypotension. Less common presentations include syncope and vomiting. In the rare case of a partially contained rupture, patients may complain of vague discomfort for days, even weeks, prior to presentation, making the diagnosis challenging. A vascular catastrophe such as an AAA rupture should be considered in the differential diagnosis of every patient who presents with shock, syncope, and abdominal or flank pain. The most common misdiagnoses in patients with a proven AAA rupture, according to one study, are renal colic, diverticulitis, and gastrointestinal bleeding.[96]

Diagnosis

Effectively making the diagnosis of a ruptured AAA, given the grim prognostic data, is of critical importance. A delay in diagnosis or operative intervention is expected to increase the morbidity and mortality of this lethal condition. Rapid diagnosis in order to organize

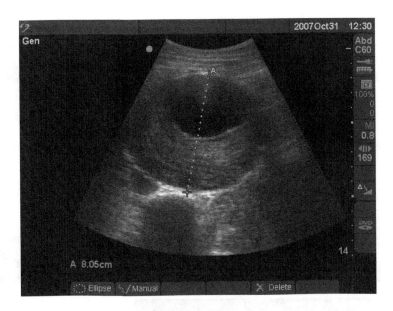

Figure 20.1 Ultrasound, transverse view, of the abdomen shows an abdominal aortic aneurysm measuring 8 cm in anteroposterior diameter. Note the laminated thrombus along the posterior wall.

prompt surgical repair is the patient's only chance for success. In the last few decades, bedside ultrasound imaging study has proven useful in this regard. In one study, the time to an AAA rupture diagnosis is reduced from 83 minutes to 5 minutes, and time from presentation to reaching the operating room is reduced from 90 minutes to 12 minutes.[97] Even emergency providers with limited ultrasound experience are able to visualize large ($\geq$4 cm) AAAs more than 85% of the time.[98] The goal in a symptomatic patient is simply to visualize an AAA by measuring the anteroposterior, longitudinal, and transverse dimensions (Figure 20-1). Intramural thrombus and calcifications may also be appreciated. Most of the AAA ruptures are retroperitoneal, and will not result in intraperitoneal abdominal free fluid. Visualizing an AAA in a symptomatic patient should prompt immediate vascular surgery consultation along with other emergent management. Signs of an AAA on a plain abdominal radiograph, including calcification of the aortic wall, paravertebral mass, and loss of psoas or renal outlines, can be seen in approximately 75% of patients, and may prompt vascular surgical consultation and emergent management in a symptomatic patient.[94] Both ultrasound and plain X-ray studies can be done rapidly and portably with minimal interruption in assessment and treatment of these gravely ill patients.

Computed tomography (CT) scan offers advantages including the detection of real or impending rupture, and providing anatomic detail useful in preoperative planning (Figures 20-2, 20-3A–C). Disadvantages include time, availability, and the need for an interruption in assessment and management of the patient, and often a transfer to a site outside of the ED. Contrast is not required to make the diagnosis, but may be preferred by some (Figure 20-4). Angiography and MRI are generally not used in the acute setting.

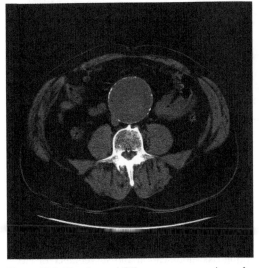

Figure 20.2 Unenhanced CT scan, transverse view, of the abdomen shows a large unruptured abdominal aortic aneurysm. Note the calcified aortic wall.

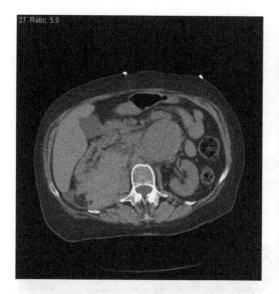
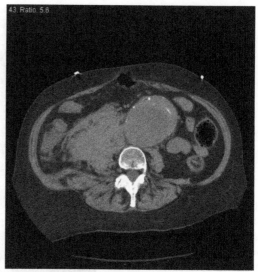
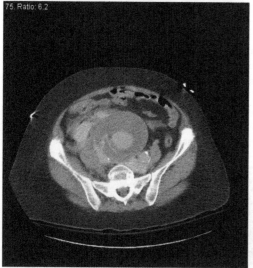
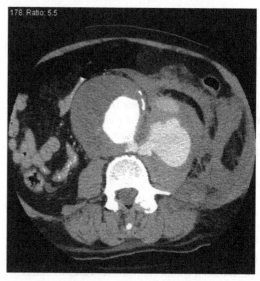

Figure 20.3 Unenhanced CT scan, transverse view, of the abdomen shows a ruptured abdominal aortic aneurysm with extensive blood in the right retroperitoneum.

Figure 20.4 Contrast-enhanced abdominal CT scan, transverse view, shows a ruptured abdominal aortic aneurysm with active extravasation into the left retroperitoneum.

Treatment

For asymptomatic, unruptured AAA patients, diagnosis prompting risk modification and surveillance or elective surgery is essential. Timely diagnosis can prompt surgical consultation to discuss surgical options and facilitate counseling regarding smoking cessation, as well as appropriate hypertension and hypercholesterolemia control as per current ACC/AHA guidelines.[1] Current guidelines also recommend beta-blocker therapy for patients being followed nonoperatively. Elective or urgent repair should be considered at an

AAA diameter of 5.5 cm, or with rapid expansion (>0.5cm in 6 months) of the AAA.[1]

For ruptured AAA patients, the goal is rapid transfer to the operating room. Any factors that may delay going to the operating room should be omitted. In settings without surgical capability, time should not be wasted to confirm the diagnosis when the clinical presentation is that of a leaking or ruptured AAA. Once the diagnosis is entertained, prompt consultation (or referral to a site with surgical capabilities) is essential in concert with stabilization. Large-bore intravenous access should be obtained, and preoperative laboratory studies sent stat.

Symptomatic but unruptured AAA patients should be treated like those with contained rupture: immediate surgical consultation is mandated along with rapid standard preoperative testing. The use of blood pressure agents (beta-blockers) for blood pressure control prior to surgery should be decided in conjunction with vascular surgery on a case-by-case basis, and administered in a well-monitored setting.

Section IV: Decision making

- Most AAAs are asymptomatic.
- Screening protocols may assist in identifying an AAA, allowing discussion about the risks or benefits of elective repair.
- In symptomatic patients, flank pain and back pain may suggest less dangerous diagnoses.
- Avoid narrowing the differential diagnosis too early, and discounting the possibility of an AAA.
- With a ruptured AAA, the goal is prompt control of the bleeding vessel in the operating room as soon as possible.
- In an unruptured symptomatic AAA, immediate surgical consultation is also mandatory—here, the emergency physician can make the biggest difference.

References

1 Hirsch AT, Haskal ZJ, Hertzer NR, et al. ACC/AHA 2005 practice guidelines for the management of patients with peripheral arterial disease (lower extremity, renal, mesenteric, and abdominal aortic): A collaborative report from the American Association for Vascular Surgery/Society for Vascular Surgery, Society for Cardiovascular Angiography and Interventions, Society for Vascular Medicine and Biology, Society of Interventional Radiology, and the ACC/AHA Task Force on Practice Guidelines (Writing Committee to Develop Guidelines for the Management of Patients With Peripheral Arterial Disease); endorsed by the American Association of Cardiovascular and Pulmonary Rehabilitation; National Heart, Lung, and Blood Institute; Society for Vascular Nursing; TransAtlantic Inter-Society Consensus; and Vascular Disease Foundation. *Circulation.* 2006;113:e463.

2 Ouriel, K, Green, RM, Donayre, C, et al. An evaluation of new methods of expressing aortic aneurysm size: relationship to rupture. *J Vasc Surg.* 1992;15:12.

3 Wolinsky H, Glagov S. Comparison of abdominal and thoracic aortic medial structure in mammals: deviation of man from usual pattern. *Circ Res.* 1969;25:677–686.

4 Creager, MA, Halperin, JL, Whittemore AD. Aneurysmal disease of the aorta and its branches. In: Loscalzo, J, Creager, MA, Dzau, VJ, eds. *Vascular Medicine.* New York: Little, Brown; 1996:901.

5 Brown LC, Powell JT. Risk factors for aneurysm rupture in patients kept under ultrasound surveillance. *Ann Surg.* 1999:230:289.

6 Scott RA, Ashton HA, Kay DN. Abdominal aortic aneurysm in 4237 screened patients: prevalence, development and management over 6 years. *Br J Surg.* 1991;78:1122.

7 Singh K, Bonaa KH, Jacobsen BK, et al. Prevalence of and risk factors for abdominal aortic aneurysms in a population-based study: The Tromso Study. *Am J Epidemiol.* 2001;154:236.

8 Powell JT, Greenhalgh RM. Small abdominal aortic aneurysms. *N Engl J Med.* 2003;348:1895.

9 Lederle FA, Johnson GR, Wilson SE, et al. Prevalence and association of abdominal aortic aneurysm detected through screening. *Ann Intern Med.* 1997;126:441.

10 Lederle FA, Johnson GR, Wilson SE, et al. The aneurysm detection and management study screening program: validation cohort and final results. Aneurysm Detection and Management Veterans Affairs Cooperative Study Investigators. *Arch Intern Med.* 2000;160:1425.

11 Greenhalgh RM, Powell JT. Endovascular repair of abdominal aortic aneurysm. *N Engl J Med.* 2008;358:494.

12 Salo JA, Soisalon-Soininen S, Bondestam S, et al. Familial occurrence of abdominal aortic aneurysm. *Ann Intern Med.* 1999;130:637.

13 Fleming C. Whitlock EP, Beil T, Lederle F. *Primary care screening for abdominal aortic aneurysm.* Evidence Synthesis No. 35. Rockville, MD: Agency for Healthcare Research and Quality; February 2005.

14 Shibamura H, Olson JM, van Vlijmen-Van Keulen C, et al. Genome scan for familial abdominal aortic aneurysm using sex and family history as covariates suggests genetic

heterogeneity and identifies linkage to chromosome 19q13. *Circulation.* 2004;109:2103.

15 Rose WM 3rd, Ernst CB. Abdominal aortic aneurysm. *Compr Ther.* 1995;21:339.

16 Fleming C, Whitlock EP, Beil T, Lederle F. Screening for abdominal aortic aneurysm: a best-evidence systematic review for the U.S. Preventive Services Task Force. *Ann Intern Med.* 2005;142:203–211.

17 http://www.wpsic.com/medicare/part_b/policy/cv041.pdf

18 Kent KC, Zwolak RM, Jaff MR, et al. Screening for abdominal aortic aneurysm. *J Vasc Surg.* 2004;39:267.

19 Brewster DC, Cronenwett JL, Hallett JW, et al. Guidelines for the treatment of abdominal aortic aneurysms. Report of a subcommittee of the Joint Council of the American Association for Vascular Surgery and Society for Vascular Surgery. *J Vasc Surg.* 2003;37:1106.

20 Lederle FA, Wilson SE, Johnson GR, et al. Mortality results for randomized controlled trial of early elective surgery or ultrasonographic surveillance for small abdominal aortic aneurysms. The UK Small Aneurysm Trial Participants. *Lancet.* 1998;353:1649.

21 Brady AR, Brown LC, Fowkes FGR, et al. Long-term outcomes of immediate repair compared to surveillance of small abdominal aortic aneurysms. The UK Small Aneurysm Trial Participants. *N Engl J Med.* 2002;346:1445.

22 Lederle FA, Wilson SE, Johnson GR, et al. Immediate repair compared with surveillance of small abdominal aortic aneurysms. *N Engl J Med.* 2002;346:1437.

23 Cronewett JL, Murphy TF, Zelenock GB, et al. Actuarial analysis of variables associated with rupture of small aortic aneurysms. *Surgery.* 1985;98:472.

24 Limet R, Sakalihassan N, Albert A. Detertmination of the expansion rate and incidence of rupture of abdominal aortic aneurysms. *J Vasc Surg.* 1991;14:540.

25 Guirguis EM, Barber GG. The natural history of abdominal aortic aneurysms. *Am J Surg.* 1991;162:481.

26 Ouriel K, Green RM, Donayre C, et al. An evaluation of new methods of expressing aortic aneurysm size: relationship to rupture. *J Vasc Surg.* 1992;15:12.

27 Vorp DA, Raghavan ML, Webster MW. Mechanical wall stress in abdominal aortic aneurysm: influence of diameter and asymmetry. *J Vasc Surg.* 1998;27:632.

28 Fillinger MF, Raghaven ML, Marra SP, et al. In vivo analysis of mechanical wall stress and abdominal aortic aneurysm rupture risk. *J Vasc Surg.* 2002;36:589.

29 Lederle FA, Johnson GR, Wilson SE, et al. Rupture rate of large abdominal aortic aneurysm refusing or unfit for elective repair. *JAMA.* 2002;287:2968.

30 Nevitt MP, Ballard DJ, Hallett JW Jr. Prognosis of abdominal aortic aneurysms. A population-based study. *N Engl J Med.* 1989;321:1009.

31 Reed WW, Hallett JW Jr, Damiano MA, Ballard DJ. Learning from the last ultrasound: a population-based

study of patients with abdominal aortic aneurysm. *Arch Intern Med.* 1997;157:2064.

32 Scott RA, Tisi PV, Ashton HA, Allen DR. Abdominal aortic aneurysm rupture rates: a 7-year follow-up of the entire abdominal aortic aneurysm population detected by screening. *J Vasc Surg.* 1998;28:124.

33 Jones A, Cahill D, Gardham R. Outcome in patients with a large abdominal aortic aneurysm considered unfit for surgery. *Br J Surg.* 1998;85:1382.

34 Heikkinen M, Salenius J-P, Auvinen O. Ruptured abdominal aortic aneurysm in a well-defined geographical area. *J Vasc Surg.* 2002;36:291.

35 Sterpetti AV, Cavallaro A, Cavallari N, et al. Factors influencing the rupture of abdominal aortic aneurysms. *Surg Gynecol Obstet.* 1991;173:175.

36 Strachan DP. Predictors of death from aortic aneurysm among middle-aged men: the Whitehall study. *Br J Surg.* 1991;78:401.

37 Cronenwett JL, Sargent SK, Wall MH, et al. Variables that affect the expansion rate and outcome of small abdominal aortic aneurysms. *J Vasc Surg.* 1990;11:260.

38 Darling RC III, Brewster DC, Darling RC, et al. Are familial abdominal aortic aneurysms different? *J Vasc Surg.* 1989;10:39.

39 Hunter GC, Smyth SH, Aguirre ML, et al. Incidence and histologic characteristics of blebs in patients with abdominal aortic aneurysms. *J Vasc Surg.* 1996;24:93.

40 Faggioli GL, Stella A, Gargiulo M, et al. Morphology of small aneurysms: definition and impact on risk of rupture. *Am J Surg.* 1994;168:131.

41 Schurink GW, van Baalen JM, Visser MJ, van Bockel JH. Thrombus within an aortic aneurysm does not reduce pressure on the aneurismal wall. *J Vasc Surg.* 2000;31:501.

42 Chang JB, Stein TA, Liu JP, Dunn ME. Risk factors associated with rapid growth of small abdominal aortic aneurysms. *Surgery.* 1997;121:117.

43 MacSweeney ST, Ellis M, Worrell PC, et al. Smoking and growth rate of small abdominal aortic aneurysms. *Lancet.* 1994;344:651.

44 Wolf YG, Thomas WS, Brennan FJ, et al. Computed tomography scanning findings associated with rapid expansion of abdominal aortic aneurysms. *J Vasc Surg.* 1994;20:529.

45 Krupski WC, Bass A, Thurston DW, Dilley RB. Utility of computed tomography for surveillance of small abdominal aortic aneurysms. *Arch Surg.* 1990;125:1345.

46 Hallin A, Bergqvist D, Holmberg L. Literature review of surgical management of abdominal aortic aneurysm. *Eur J Vasc Endovasc Surg.* 2001;22:197.

47 Schewe CK, Schweikart HP, Hammel G, et al. Influence of selective management on the prognosis and the risk of rupture of abdominal aortic aneurysms. *Clin Investig.* 1994;72:585.

48 Heller JA, Weinberg A, Arons R, et al. Two decades of abdominal aortic aneurysm repair: have we made any progress? *J Vasc Surg.* 2000;32:1091.

49 Cronenwett JL, Birkmeyer JD, eds. *The Dartmouth Atlas of Vascular Healthcare.* Chicago: AHA Press; 2000.

50 Akkersdijk GJM, van der Graaf Y, van Bockel JH, et al. Mortality rates associated with operative treatment of infrarenal abdominal aortic aneurysms in the Netherlands. *Br J Surg.* 1994;81:706.

51 Hertzer NR, Avellone JC, Farrell CJ, et al. The risk of vascular surgery in a metropolitan community. With observations on surgeon experience and hospital size. *J Vasc Surg.* 1984;1:13.

52 Katz DJ, Stanley JC, Zelenock GB. Operative mortality rates for intact and ruptured abdominal aortic aneurysms in Michigan: an eleven-year statewide experience. *J Vasc Surg.* 1994;19:807.

53 Hannan EL, Kilburn H Jr, O'Donnell JF, et al. A longitudinal analysis of the relationship between in-hospital mortality in New York State and the volume of abdominal aortic aneurysm surgeries performed. *Health Serv Res.* 1992;27:517.

54 Manheim LM, Sohn MW, Feinglass J, et al. Hospital vascular surgery volume and procedure mortality rates in California, 1982-1994. *J Vasc Surg.* 1998;28:34.

55 Tu JV, Austin PC, Johnston KW. The influence of surgical specialty training on the outcomes of elective abdominal aortic aneurysm surgery. *J Vasc Surg.* 2001;33:447.

56 Amundsen S, Trippestad A, Viste A, Soreide O. Abdominal aortic aneurysm—a national multicentre study. *Eur J Vasc Surg.* 1987;1:239.

57 Ernst CB. Abdominal aortic aneurysm. *N Engl J Med.* 1998;328:1167.

58 Zarins CK, Harris EJ Jr. Operative repair for aortic aneurysms: the gold standard. *J Endovasc Surg.* 1997;4:232.

59 Hertzer NR, Mascha EJ, Karafa MT, et al. Open infrarenal abdominal aortic aneurysm repair: the Cleveland Clinic experience from 1989 to 1998. *J Vasc Surg.* 2002;35:1145.

60 Huber TS, Wang JG, Derow AE, et al. Experience in the United States with intact abdominal aortic aneurysm repair. *J Vasc Surg.* 2001;33:304.

61 Dardik A, Lin JW, Gordan TA, et al. Results of elective abdominal aortic aneurysm repair in the 1990s: a population-based analysis of 2335 cases. *J Vasc Surg.* 1999;30:985.

62 Johnston KW. Multicenter prospective study of nonruptured abdominal aortic aneurysm. Part II. Variables predicting morbidity and mortality. *J Vasc Surg.* 1989; 9:437.

63 Brady AR, Fowkes FG, Greenhalgh RM, et al. Risk factors for postoperative death following elective surgical repair of abdominal aortic aneurysm: results from the UK Small Aneurysm Trial. On Behalf of the UK Small Aneurysm Trial Participants. *Br J Surg.* 2000;87:742.

64 Steyerberg EW, Kievit J, De Mol Van Otterloo JCA, et al. Perioperative mortality of elective abdominal aortic aneurysm surgery: a clinical prediction rule based on literature and individual patient data. *Arch Intern Med.* 1995;155:1998.

65 Katz DJ, Stanley JC, Zelenock GB. Gender differences in abdominal aortic aneurysm prevalence, treatment, and outcome. *J Vasc Surg.* 1997;25:561.

66 Ashton HA, Buxton MJ, Day NE, et al. The Multicentre Aneurysm Screening Study (MASS) into the effect of abdominal aortic aneurysm screening on mortality in men: a randomized controlled trial. *Lancet.* 2002;360:1531.

67 Pearce WH, Parker MA, Feinglass J, Ujiki M, Manheim LM. The importance of surgeon volume and training in outcomes for vascular surgical procedures. *J Vasc Surg.* 1999;29:768.

68 Birkmeyer JD, Siewers AE, Finlayson EV, et al. Hospital volume and surgical mortality in the United States. *N Engl J Med.* 2002;346:1128.

69 Crawford ES, Becket WC, Greer MS. Juxtarenal infrarenal abdominal aortic aneurysms: special diagnostic and therapeutic considerations. *Ann Surg.* 1986;203:661.

70 Green RM, Ricotta JJ, Ouriel K, DeWeese JA. Results of supraceliac aortic clamping in the difficult resection of infrarenal abdominal aortic aneurysm. *J Vasc Surg.* 1989;9:125.

71 Nypaver TJ, Shepard AD, Reddy DJ, et al. Supraceliac aortic crossclamping determinants of outcome in elective abdominal aortic reconstruction. *J Vasc Surg.* 1993;17:868.

72 Sarac TP, Clair DG, Hertzer NR, et al. Contemporary results of juxtarenal aneurysm repair. *J Vasc Surg.* 2002;36:1104.

73 Pennell RC, Hollier LH, Lie JT, et al. Inflammatory abdominal aortic aneurysms: a thirty-year review. *J Vasc Surg.* 1985;2:859.

74 Nitecki SS, Hllett JW Jr, Stanson AW, et al. Inflammatory abdominal aortic aneurysm: a case-control study. *J Vasc Surg.* 1996;23:860.

75 Brewster DC, Geller SC, Kaufman JA, et al. Initial experience with endovascular aneurysm repair: comparison of early results with outcome of conventional open repair. *J Vasc Surg.* 1998;27:992.

76 May J, White GH, Yu W, et al. Concurrent comparison of endoluminal versus open repair in treatment of abdominal aortic aneurysms: analysis of 303 patients by life-table method. *J Vasc Surg.* 1998;27:213.

77 Zarins CK, White RA, Schwarten D, et al. AneuRx stent graft versus open surgical repair of abdominal aortic aneurysms: multicenter prospective clinical trial. *J Vasc Surg.* 1999;29:292.

78 Moore WS, Brewster DC, Bernhard WM, for the EVT/ Guidant Investigators. Aorto-uni-iliac endograft for

complex aortoiliac aneurysms compared with tube/bifurcation endografts: results of the EVT/Guidant trials. *J Vasc Surg.* 2001;33:S11.

79 Matsumura JS, Brewster DC, Makaroun MS, Naftel DC, for the Excluder Bifurcated Endoprosthesis Investigators. A multicenter controlled clinical trial of open versus endovascular treatment of abdominal aortic aneurysms. *J Vasc Surg.* 2003;37:262.

80 Moore WS, Kashyap VS, Vescera CL, Quinones-Baldrich W. Abdominal aortic aneurysm: a 6-year comparison of endovascular versus transabdominal repair. *Ann Surg.* 1999;230:298.

81 Zarins CK, White RA, Moll FL, et al. The AneuRx stent graft: four-year results and worldwide experience 2000. *J Vasc Surg.* 2001;33:S135.

82 Sicard GA, Rubin BG, Sanchez LA, et al. Endoluminal graft repair for abdominal aortic aneurysms in high risk patients and octogenarians: is it better than open repair? *Ann Surg.* 2001;234:427.

83 Chuter TA, Reilly LM, Faruqi RM, et al. Endovascular aneurysm repair in high-risk patients. *J Vasc Surg.* 2000;31:122.

84 Buth J, van Marrewijk CJ, Harris PL, et al. for the EUROSTAR Collaborators. Outcome of endovascular abdominal aortic aneurysm repair in patients with conditions considered unfit for an open procedure. A report on the EUROSTAR experience. *J Vasc Surg.* 2002;35:211.

85 Cotroneo AR, Iezzi R, Gicancristofaro D, et al. Endovascular abdominal aortic aneurysm repair: how many patients are eligible for endovascular repair? *Radiol Med.* (Torino) 2006;111:597.

86 Elkouri S, Martelli E, Gloviczki P, et al. Most patients with abdominal aortic aneurysm are not suitable for endovascular repair using currently approved bifurcated stent-grafts. *Vasc Endovascular Surg.* 2004;38:401.

87 Brewster DC, Jones JE, Chung TK, et al. Long-term outcomes after endovascular abdominal aortic aneurysm repair: the first decade. *Ann Surg.* 2006;244:426.

88 Becquemin JP, Kelley L, Zubilewicz T, et al. Outcomes of secondary interventions after abdominal aortic aneurysm endovascular repair. *J Vasc Surg.* 2004;39:298.

89 Aboulafia DM, Aboulafia ED. Aortic aneurysm-induced disseminated intravascular coagulation. *Ann Vasc Surg.* 1996;10:396.

90 Fisher DF Jr, Yawn DH, Crawford ES. Preoperative disseminated intravascular coagulation associated with aortic aneurysms. A prospective study of 76 cases. *Arch Surg.* 1983;118:1252.

91 Lederle FA, Simel DL. The rational clinical examination. Does this patient have abdominal aortic aneurysm? *JAMA.* 1999;281:77.

92 Brown MJ, Sutton AJ, Bell PR, Sayers RD. A meta-analysis of 50 years of ruptured abdominal aortic aneurysm repair. *Br J Surg.* 2002;89:714.

93 Brown PM, Pattenden R, Vernooy C, et al. Selective management of abdominal aortic aneurysm in a prospective measurement program. *J Vasc Surg.* 1996;23:213.

94 Donaldson RC, Rosenberg JM, Bucknam CA. Factors affecting survival after ruptured abdominal aortic aneurysm. *J Vasc Surg.* 1985;2(4):564–570.

95 Wakefield TW, Whitehouse WM Jr, Wu SC, et al. Abdominal aortic aneurysm rupture. *Surgery.* 1982;91:586–596.

96 Marston WA, Ahlquist R, Johnson G Jr. Misdiagnosis of ruptured abdominal aortic aneurysm. *J Vasc Surg.* 1992;16:17.

97 Plummer D, Brunette D, Asinger R, et al. Emergency department ultrasound improves time to diagnosis and survival in ruptured abdominal aortic aneurysm. *Acad Emerg Med.* 1998;5:417.

98 Brown DFM, Rosen CL, Rhee R, et al. Bedside abdominal ultrasound scanning to detect critically enlarged abdominal aortic aneurysms in elderly emergency department patients: a preliminary report. *Ann Emerg Med.* 1998;32:S28.

21

Hypertensive emergencies

Russell Berger[1] & Edward Ullman[2]

[1] *Children's Hospital Boston, Junior Toxicology Fellow, Harvard Medical Toxicology Fellowship, Children's Hospital Boston, Massachusetts, USA*
[2] *Assistant Professor of Medicine, Harvard Medical School, Director of Medical Student Education, Division of Emergency Medicine, Beth Israel Deaconess Medical Center, Boston, Massachusetts, USA*

Section I: Case presentation

A 56-year-old woman was brought to the emergency department (ED) in respiratory distress. She awoke at 4 a.m. gasping for breath. Her husband called 911. The EMS team found the patient seated upright, diaphoretic, and laboring to breathe. The patient denied chest pain, abdominal pain, fever, or chills. Initial vital signs were: blood pressure 240/134 mmHg, heart rate 102 beats/min, respiratory rate 28 breaths/min, oxygen saturation 89% on room air. The patient was placed on a non-rebreather mask at 15 L/min, an IV line was established, and the patient received 325 mg of aspirin and 40 mg of IV furosemide. Upon arrival at the ED, the patient continued to be short of breath; vital signs were: blood pressure 220/128 mmHg, heart rate 104 beats/min, respiratory rate 25 breaths/min, temperature 98.6°F, oxygen saturation 96% on a non-rebreather mask. Medical records showed a past history of uncontrolled hypertension, chronic kidney disease, and diabetes mellitus type 2. Current medications included hydrochlorothiazide, labetalol, and insulin.

On physical examination, the patient was agitated with an elevated jugular venous distension (JVD); bilateral rales to the apex on chest examination; tachycardia without murmurs, rubs, or gallops on cardiac auscultation; and minimal pedal edema. An EKG was performed.

A nitroglycerin drip was started, and the patient was placed on positive pressure ventilation, with improvement in symptoms. The patient continued to be hypertensive with systolic pressure 190 mmHg, and esmolol was added for improved blood pressure control. A chest X-ray study showed evidence of acute heart failure. Pertinent laboratory tests were elevated nl-BNP 1300 pg/mL, Troponin T 0.25 ng/ml. The patient was admitted to the coronary care unit, where she continued on positive pressure ventilation and a nitroglycerin drip. An echocardiogram showed evidence of decreased anterior wall motion. The following morning the patient underwent a cardiac catheterization that showed an 80% occlusion of the left anterior descending (LAD) artery, which was dilatated and successfully stented.

Section II: Case discussion

Dr Peter Rosen: I normally don't ask what race the patient is, but in a case like this, does it help you to think of the underlying disease if the patient is African American, since the incidence of hypertension is so high in this race?

Dr William Brady: We have the luxury of being color-blind in emergency medicine. In the acute management phase, the race is not going to impact how I approach this patient.

Cardiovascular Problems in Emergency Medicine: A discussion-based review, First Edition.
Edited by Shamai A. Grossman and Peter Rosen.
© 2011 John Wiley & Sons, Ltd. Published 2011 by John Wiley & Sons, Ltd.

PR: I wouldn't think of hypertension as my initial concern in this patient. This case sounds more like a patient who is presenting with acute pulmonary edema. When you're dealing with a hypertensive emergency, we usually think of the brain or the kidney as the end-organ target, but do you find that many of the patients who have problems with their hypertension present with acute pulmonary edema?

Dr David Brown: It is difficult to know what is driving what in a case like this. Congestive heart failure from underlying heart disease, whether it be coronary artery disease, valvular disease or some other kind of structural heart disease, which leads to an elevation in blood pressure is more common than uncontrolled hypertension leading to a hypertensive emergency that presents with pulmonary edema. Yet, the initial approach is much the same, unless you suspect an acute coronary syndrome, which is also possible here. Otherwise, the approach is always the same: oxygenating the patient, controlling the blood pressure, and providing some diuretics. Together, these three treatments will probably improve the situation while you sort out what is driving what.

PR: What is the drug that you reach for first in trying to stabilize a patient such as this, after you put them on some oxygen?

Dr Amal Mattu: As this patient sounds like she is in acute cardiogenic pulmonary edema, and it seems it was relatively abrupt in onset, I'm less worried about worsening fluid overload. The best way to treat this patient is with aggressive preload and afterload reduction. If you are going to reach for one drug, I would go with nitroglycerin, and use it aggressively, perhaps starting with sublingual nitroglycerin and then moving to a nitroglycerin drip, titrating up fairly rapidly. If you can lower the preload and afterload, then you can turn these patents around very quickly in many cases.

PR: What should be used in the prehospital setting?

WB: I would probably start with sublingual nitroglycerin, follow with some topical nitrate, and if possible, move on to the IV nitroglycerin, if this can be done easily. Next, I would move to positive pressure ventilation. I think this is an excellent therapeutic approach, and we should really think about using it both out-of-hospital and in the ED. It is very powerful, and can be very beneficial to the patient if applied early in their management, as it was in this case.

PR: Once the patient arrives in the ED, what other medications might you use?

WB: After nitroglycerin I would use an ACE inhibitor and either oral or sublingual captopril or intravenous enalapril or enalaprilat. ACE inhibitors, if used early in the patient's course, can make a significant difference in her response, and ultimately her hospital course.

PR: There seems to be a significant number of patients who can't tolerate ACE inhibitors because of their association with cough, angioedema, and renal failure. Are these problems that occur over time in multiple doses of the drug, or a problem that may be seen in a single administration of the drug in the ED?

WB: The allergic issues here should be no different than with other agents. You're probably not going to know enough about the angioedema or cough to have it enter into your medical decision making. Hemodynamically, I would like to see the patient very hypertensive, as she is in this case. That gives you a range for maneuvering and a cushion so you don't have to worry too much about perfusion issues. The state of Maryland has now moved to ACE inhibitor therapy for out-of hospital treatment of pulmonary edema, and in central Virginia at several EMS agencies we've done the same thing. Our numbers are small, but we've not had any untoward events in patients with respect to renal function, whether they've had any preexisting renal insufficiency or the development of new renal insufficiency. In the out-of-hospital setting and early in the ED with a critical patient, you're not going to have the ability to determine what the renal function is, but nevertheless, I would feel comfortable with starting an ACE inhibitor without being aware of the renal.

PR: Given that this patient may have an acute ischemic coronary syndrome, is there anything that you would do differently in terms of the initial management of the patient with a high blood pressure, other than to try to lower the blood pressure somewhat?

Dr Shamai Grossman: There are a couple of things that I might think about. If I were going to use an ACE inhibitor, one of the options you have is to try a test dose of captopril. The way that I would do that is to give 6.25 mg, breaking the pill down to about a quarter, administering it sublingually, which has rapid onset, and then you can get an idea of how effective it is at lowering the patient's blood pressure and the extent of the hemodynamic response that you can expect from that drug. If there is a profound drop, then you don't want to give a whole lot more. The traditional antihypertensive agent I would avoid in this patient is nitroprusside. Although it is an excellent medication to use to lower blood pressure, if we're worried that this is a patient with concomitant ischemia, then this is a dangerous drug to use, because nitroprusside is notorious for causing coronary steal syndrome, and can exacerbate ischemia. Nitroglycerin is useful regardless of whether or not this patient is ischemic, particularly in the intravenous form, because you can turn it off quickly if you have a precipitous drop in blood pressure without the patient having absorbed too much. For this reason, I would not use nitropaste, and I might be a little more reluctant to use sublingual nitroglycerin, again, because you may overshoot your desired blood pressure.

PR: The patient is described as being agitated, and we don't have any real evidence that it is from hypoxia. We used to give these patients morphine, and tried to justify it on the basis of it being an unloading drug. Do you think that it helps a patient's agitation, and perhaps some of the potential chest pain that can be induced by ischemia?

DB: She is likely agitated because she feels so short of breath, and I do not think morphine is a good choice here. The prevailing opinion of our specialty is moving away from morphine as a treatment for agitation, ischemic chest pain, or for any other type of chest pain. Although there may be a small effect on preload by morphine, with increased venous capacitance, and dropped preload, which in some ways may be efficacious, the sedation can be deleterious to the patient, and I would not choose morphine here.

WB: In this case, I too read agitation to mean that this patient had air hunger and was fighting for breath, and that's an appropriate and understandable situation here. But there is also agitation where the patient is combative and fighting, and that's intimating a much more pronounced hypoxia. If we feel the extreme agitation is resulting from respiratory failure, then you have a very short window of opportunity to reverse them before you need to proceed to endotracheal intubation. We

don't intubate the vast majority of patients who come in with cardiogenic pulmonary edema because we have such effective tools now to correct that quickly, but in the patient who is truly agitated and combative, you have to move quickly to avoid intubation.

PR: Rotating tourniquets used to be a major effort of our therapy. They even had some technologically elaborate means for having four limb tourniquets that serially inflated and deflated. Is there ever any benefit from this?

AM: Essentially, rotating tourniquets enable you to reduce preload, and there is benefit from rotating tourniquets if you don't have other means of preload reduction. If you are on an airplane or in the wilderness, and you don't have medications or noninvasive ventilation, then rotating tourniquets or even phlebotomy may be reasonable methods to decrease preload.

PR: I would argue against phlebotomy. I lived through the years when we did this, and it's hard to withdraw enough blood to get an effect, it's extraordinarily messy, and in modern medicine we're probably best off with minimal exposure to blood. Rotating tourniquets did seem to work, although the biggest problem was remembering to deflate them periodically.

DB: Another way to effectively use non-pharmacologic approaches is to use gravity: sit the patient up and let the legs hang over the side of the stretcher. Patients are often brought into the ED, and we immediately put them on their backs. Yet, a patient like this would be much more comfortable sitting up, and if you let her legs hang over the side of the stretcher, you get a little pooling in the legs as well. Again, in the ED with medications we don't need to do this, but airplanes are common places to find a patient like this, and by the time the doctor gets there, the flight attendants often have laid the patient down in the aisle.

PR: You indicated that we don't intubate these patients very much anymore, and I want to clarify that. I think that's true for the patient who has high-resistance failure, but are you implying that we also wouldn't rapidly intubate a patient who was in pump failure?

WB: In a pump failure case, your ability to maneuver with cardioactive medications is markedly constrained, and these patients probably will need some form of positive pressure ventilation, likely intubation, in addition to vasopressor and inotropic support.

They're a very ill group and often don't do well, and I would advocate intubation of these patients early on, but in the hypertensive presentation, I believe that if we can appropriately treat the patient early in the course, we very frequently can avoid intubating these patients.

PR: I noticed that the patient is on both hydrochlorothiazide and labetalol, although the chances are that she's technically not on either. Do you find that when patients are on the thiazide diuretics that they often present with hypokalemia?

DB: Hypokalemia is common when the patient is using a non-potassium-sparing diuretic; it is not usually of much consequence, and when it is noted, it can be corrected with supplemental potassium.

PR: This is an interesting change in our practice, because I can remember 30 years ago we saw a stunning number of patients who would present in digitalis toxicity because of hypokalemia induced by non-potassium-sparing diuresis, and that always complicated the management of their pulmonary edema.

AM: Very few patients are being put on digoxin anymore, which at least for us I think is a good thing.

SG: If you knew this patient had normal left ventricle (LV) function, but presented now with profound hypertension and pulmonary edema, would you do anything differently, assuming the patient had diastolic dysfunction?

DB: I considered giving the patient labetalol when I first read the case. The patient was already taking it, so you know she tolerated it. If there has been no known coronary artery disease, and the patient is profoundly hypertensive with presumably hypertension-induced diastolic dysfunction, then this would not be a bad choice.

PR: What is the risk of the beta-blockade-induced failure in a patient who is already in failure?

DB: In a patient without preexisting depressed LV function, beta-blockers are a reasonable choice. The problem in the ED is that we often don't know. If the patient has no known coronary artery disease, normal R wave progression and prominent R waves throughout the EKG, then a mixed alpha- and beta-blocker like labetalol is a reasonable choice, and probably safe

in someone who presents with what you're describing as resistance-induced pulmonary edema rather than pump failure.

AM: Adding further to that question: A lot of this is the old chicken versus the egg query. Did the heart failure put the patient into a cascade of events resulting in increasing catecholamines because of myocardial ischemia, which produced severe hypertension? If that's the case, then you've got to focus on treating the heart failure, and that will bring the blood pressure down. On the other hand, if the patient's primary problem is the hypertension and a stiffening ventricle, and that led to the heart failure, then that patient might benefit from bringing the blood pressure down with a medication like labetalol. The teaching that we all go by is: let's use a medication that has the least possible harm to the ejection fraction (EF), and will definitely benefit the heart failure. That's why we usually go with nitroglycerin and captopril.

WB: I think that beta-blockers are underused. We've all seen situations where patients receive an intravenous beta-blocker, and have had decompensation, but if you're in a situation where you think beta-blockers might be of benefit, then esmolol is an excellent choice, given it is short-acting with a short half-life. If the patient isn't tolerating it, you can turn the drip off and it will clear rather rapidly.

PR: Would you do anything differently if the initial EKG showed you an ST-segment elevation myocardial infarction (STEMI)?

SG: If the EKG showed an ST elevation MI, and the patient presented within 6 hours of the onset of symptoms, then that patient deserves an emergent primary percutaneous intervention; if that's not feasible, then the patient deserves thrombolytics, and so this EKG would make a big difference.

DB: The other point to make about STEMIs is that that may make noninvasive ventilation contraindicated if the patient were acutely ischemic, and I would move very quickly to intubation.

SG: That's a controversial point; there's conflicting data about bi-level positive airway pressure (BiPAP) and very limited data about continuous positive airway pressure (CPAP) and ischemia. It's hard to call it contraindicated, but you at least need to think about possible associated worsening ischemia before you use it.

WB: Nevertheless, I would move to intubation quickly. If nothing else, it helps to take the work of breathing out of the equation as additional strain on the patient's heart.

PR: We tend to overlook the cost of the work of breathing. Perhaps we think a little bit more about it when the patient is hypotensive, but it is well worth considering if the patient does not respond rapidly to CPAP.

A BNP was ordered. Why do you need a BNP in this case to prove what the clinical appearance of the patient proves?

AM: I don't think that you need a BNP in this case. In all likelihood, this was sent off as part of a comprehensive laboratory panel.

SG: I would make the argument, although I don't particularly agree with it, that a BNP would help you get a baseline, and that you could follow that BNP as an indicator for both prognostic information and to evaluate the patient's progress. I don't think there is adequate literature to support either, but those are two of its uses currently being touted.

PR: I have observed that the incidence of myocardial infarction (MI)-inducing failure is uncommon; is that truly the case?

WB: The cases where acute coronary syndrome (ACS) presents with pulmonary edema tend to be with pump failure caused by very large infarctions. These are the patients presenting with cardiogenic shock, or situations bordering cardiogenic shock. A pure, acute coronary syndrome with thrombosis, rupture, or vasospasm is less likely to present with such extreme blood pressure elevations. Patients do come in with STEMIs, anxious and hypertensive, but with a little calm bedside approach and a little pharmacologic manipulation, the blood pressure often comes down very quickly and rapidly. I think that blood pressure here is largely anxiety-mediated. You could see troponin elevation without true ACS, but it may not demonstrate the typical rise and fall of an acute myocardial infarction, and is just an indication of the myocardial injury from the hypertensive state. This will not be sorted out in the ED, but over time during the hospitalization, when the typical rise and fall of the serum marker is not observed.

PR: If this patient had a dialysis catheter in place and presented like this, would you be in a great rush to get her dialyzed?

AM: The dialysis would help the pulmonary edema, and probably the blood pressure as well, so this would be one of those times where I get the nephrologist out of bed and get them moving towards the ED. In the meantime, I would still do everything else that we've talked about.

I can't help wondering whether the 80% LAD lesion is essentially an incidental finding here. It's not clear to me that although she has some anterior wall hypokinesis, that it is an acute process. While I don't disagree with placing a stent in an 80% LAD lesion, I'm not prepared at this point, based on the information provided, to call this a hypertensive emergency caused by an acute coronary syndrome.

PR: Perhaps we uncovered an incidental finding, which may or may not have warranted stenting. At any rate, I think this is a case that combines a number of different diseases that we have to think about. I'm particularly concerned with the patients, like this one, who have renal failure who then develop end-organ failure in the brain or in the heart. Is there any point in looking at her retinas to see if she has any signs of papilledema?

WB: A well-rounded, thorough physical examination would include the eyes. For the initial ED approach, we already have enough information to identify this as a hypertensive urgent or emergent state, with the pulmonary edema and the very high blood pressure measurements accompanying the chest findings. If we did look in the eyes and they demonstrated papilledema, it would just be one other manifestation of the hypertensive emergency. We're already approaching the patient rather aggressively and effectively lowering the pressure, so it would not alter my therapy. Arterial findings of long-term hypertension would also only support my belief that this is an acute exacerbation of a chronic problem in this patient.

SG: What would you do with this blood pressure without pulmonary edema?

WB: With this level of blood pressure and no pulmonary edema, no respiratory distress, normal mental status, and the absence of focal neurologic findings, if I found papilledema, I would still consider that a hypertensive emergency, and I would approach the patient rather aggressively. Labetalol might be a good choice here.

PR: If the patient had no pulmonary edema and had no papilledema, I wouldn't even treat her blood pressure in the ED. I would presume that she came because she had stopped taking her medications, and got worried about it or because she had a headache. We are hyperaggressive in emergency medicine about treating the blood pressure cuff, and I think that we need to treat the patient's symptoms. This is a blood pressure that she may walk around with, and while it's not good for her, it doesn't need to be treated acutely. I don't worry about a diastolic pressure until it is in the 140 range, unless we have a patient with concomitant end-organ failure.

DB: In the asymptomatic patient without end-organ damage, I would ask if she had remembered to take her medication in the morning, and if she hadn't, I would probably administer to her the usual medications. It would be hard to do nothing at all as a diastolic blood pressure of 134 is very high. I might administer an additional dose of the oral labetalol, even if she had taken it that morning, and I would be happy if her blood pressure came down over an hour of sitting in a quiet room in the ED. Then I would let her go home and follow up with her primary care doctor.

SG: What would be your target blood pressure?

DB: I would like the diastolic blood pressure to come down to 100 or less.

PR: We used to have blind limits on these patients where a diastolic above 120 meant that the patient had to be admitted, and we would reach for a sublingual calcium channel blocker or an IV beta-blocker and treat the blood pressure cuff, but we ended up harming more patients than we helped. Different blood pressures tend to set at different thermostatic points, and we don't always help when we move it back down in an acute fashion to what we think is normal. It may take time for the blood pressure to reset back to lower values, so moving slowly is reasonable, unless you have end-organ failure where you are obligated to act quickly to bring the diastolic pressure down. That's one of the indications today for hospital admission for these patients.

SG: One still must be cautious, even if the patient has end-organ damage, to avoid precipitously lowering the blood pressure, because even if you do have an ongoing end-organ process, you can still induce a stroke by lowering the blood pressure too fast. The number used in the literature is lowering the mean arterial pressure by about 10–25% in the first hour, assuming the patient has end-organ damage. Without end-organ damage, there isn't a number to quote, because as mentioned, we shouldn't be lowering her blood pressure. On the other hand, you don't want to send someone out with a diastolic of 130 when you know the patient is not compliant with medications, but even here, you have to be very cautious about giving an extra dose of her medications. Someone who is not used to taking her medications, and is suddenly given a little more, may ultimately experience more harm than good.

Case resolution

Following the percutaneous intervention, the patient recovered well and was discharged on hospital day six after a lengthy education session about hypertension and heart disease, and with prescriptions for hydrochlorothiazide and labetalol.

Section III: Concepts

Background/epidemiology

Hypertension (HTN) affects 50 million people in the United States, and one billion people worldwide[1]. Over half of people aged 60–69 and 75% of those older than 70 have hypertension.[1] Thirty percent of patients with elevated blood pressure are unaware that they are hypertensive, while 37% percent of coronary artery disease (CAD) in men and 27% of CAD in women is attributable to HTN.[2,3]

African Americans are 3–5 times more likely to suffer HTN morbidity and mortality than Caucasians, and twice as likely to experience a hypertensive crisis.[4,5] Poverty, combined with poor access to health care, predisposes to hypertensive crisis.[4] Of all individuals with HTN, 1–2% will develop hypertensive emergencies; while this appears low, given the prevalence of the disease, this accounts for approximately 500,000 patients per year.[1,4]

Table 21-1. Examples of Hypertensive Emergencies by Organ System

Brain	Hypertensive encephalopathy, CVA
Cardiac	Aortic dissection, Myocardial infarction, ACS
Lung	Pulmonary edema
Renal	Acute renal failure
Blood	Microangiopathic hemolytic anemia
Gravid Uterus	Eclampsia

Hypertensive emergency is defined as a sudden increase in systolic or diastolic blood pressure associated with end-organ damage to the central nervous system, the heart, or the kidneys.[5] Acute heart failure and associated pulmonary vascular overload are the presenting findings in 11% of patients with hypertensive emergency. Ischemic heart disease manifests as either angina or MI, representing 4.1% and 3.7%, respectively, of patient presentations. Elevations in serum creatinine to greater than 2.3mg/dl occur in 31% of people at presentation (Table 21-1).[4]

No specific blood pressure criteria define a hypertensive emergency; in general, absolute blood pressure is not as important as the rate of increase of that pressure. However, organ dysfunction is uncommon with diastolic blood pressures less than 130 mmHg.[6] Despite the alarming numbers of individuals with hypertension, long term prognosis for individuals with hypertensive crisis has improved from a 5-year survival rate of 1% to a 5-year survival rate of greater than 75%, due to the rapid, effective lowering of blood pressure.[1,7]

Unique etiologies

Hypertensive emergencies may result from progressive degradation of the renal parenchyma. In this setting, autoimmune diseases like scleroderma and lupus are known culprits. Pre-renal pathology, such as polyarteritis nodosa or fibromuscular dysplasia, may also be associated with the development of a hypertensive emergency.[1]

The ingestion of illicit or prescribed medications such as sympathomimetics, cyclosporine, or erythropoietin can lead to the emergency. Conversely, drug withdrawal may result in the development of rebound hypertension, which can turn into a hypertensive emergency; clonidine and propranolol are particularly linked to this phenomenon.[8]

Hypertensive emergencies may also stem from endocrine processes, including pheochromocytoma, Conn's syndrome, or Cushing's syndrome.[1]

Pathophysiology

Specific precipitants of hypertensive emergency are poorly understood and multifactorial. The final common pathway, however, is fibrinoid necrosis of small arterioles and a cycle of worsening endothelial damage, ultimately producing tissue ischemia.

The vascular beds of the heart, the kidneys, and the brain rely on autoregulation to ensure constant perfusion pressure. With extreme pressures, high or low, autoregulation is impaired. Higher systemic pressures found in hypertensive emergency lead to capillary bed vasodilatation, and these pressures ultimately damage the vascular base of the endothelium, increasing its porosity. In this milieu, fibrin is able to deposit within the affected vessels' walls. The presence of fibrin in the vessel wall activates the coagulation cascade, and stimulates cell proliferation. The combination of endothelial damage, fibrin deposition, coagulation cascade activation, and myointimal proliferation leads to progressive arteriolar narrowing, inhibiting oxygen delivery and producing tissue ischemia.[4,9,10]

Initial workup history and physical

The goal is to expeditiously identify those patients who exhibit evidence of end-organ damage. The workup must start with accurate blood pressure measurement; cuff selection and standardized measurement of pressure are important considerations. The blood pressure bladder should be 80% of the patient's arm circumference, as cuffs that are too small will artificially exaggerate blood pressure measurement.[8,10] The blood pressure should be obtained in both arms in a seated position with the patient's arm at the level of the heart.[10] The automated measurement of blood pressure is inaccurate in patients with concomitant atrial fibrillation, and therefore, in this case, a manual blood pressure should be obtained.[10]

Once an accurate blood pressure is obtained, the history should focus on the degree of previous blood pressure control, medication compliance, previous hypertensive emergencies, drug use, chest pain, back pain, shortness of breath, and neurologic symptoms.

In women of childbearing age, special attention should be directed to the date of last menstrual period, as preeclampsia may be present.[1,6]

The physical examination should be directed toward identifying target organ dysfunction. Significant blood pressure asymmetry suggests aortic dissection.[8]

The eyes should be examined for the presence of papilledema, and the patient's level of consciousness should be assessed; visual fields and focal neurologic deficits should be ascertained and documented. New retinal hemorrhages, exudates, or papilledema suggest hypertensive emergency, regardless of changes in vision.[5,8]

The neck veins should be scrutinized for evidence of jugular venous distention (JVD). The cardiac examination should focus on the detection of either an S3 or S4, heart sound evidence of cardiomegaly, or a displaced point of maximal impulse. The pulmonary examination should focus on the presence or absence of crackles. In younger patients, special attention should be directed toward identifying abdominal bruits, as these may point to hypertension from renal artery stenosis, and can be amenable to surgical therapy.[1]

Laboratory evaluation should include a blood smear, electrolytes, complete blood count (CBC), urinalysis, pregnancy test (where applicable), EKG, chest X-ray study, and, when there is concern for a neurologic event, a noncontrast head CT scan. A blood smear and CBC can help characterize the presence of microangiopathic anemia, while renal pathology may be detected by an elevated serum creatinine and a urinalysis demonstrating a nephritic pattern. The chest X-ray study can identify evidence of pulmonary edema or a widened mediastinum, which is indicative of a potential acute aortic dissection.[1,4,5,8]

Treatment

Precipitous decreases in the level of the blood pressure in chronic hypertensive patients, as well as in the elderly patient, may cause ischemic complications. As such, the goal of therapy for the treatment of a hypertensive emergency is a maximum rapid reduction in mean arterial pressure, by 20–25% in the first 1–2 hours, to prevent further ischemic damage.

All patients with a hypertensive emergency require large bore IV access for fluid resuscitation and dedicated access for antihypertensive drug administration.

Intraarterial blood pressure measurement should be established in patients with labile pressures. The ideal antihypertensive drug acts rapidly and predictably with minimal agent toxicity and a short half-life. While the optimal medication therapy for hypertensive emergencies is vast, preferred agents include labetalol, esmolol, nicardipine, and fenoldopan.[2,5,8] Clevidipine, a new agent, may be useful as well.

Labatolol is both an alpha- and beta-blocker, with a large beta predominance. It acts quickly, but its effects may persist for up to 5 hours.[8,9] This agent preserves cerebral, coronary, and renal perfusion and is safe for pregnancy, but boluses of 1–2 mg/kg are not recommended, and have been linked to hypotension.[8] In addition, labetalol is contraindicated in patients with bradycardia, heart block, bronchospasm, cocaine ingestion, and heart failure.[4]

Esmolol, a cardioselective beta-blocker, is another reasonable choice for hypertensive emergency management, as esmolol achieves beta-blockade in 5 minutes, and a decrease in beta-antagonism can be appreciated in 2 minutes when the drip is turned off. A huge benefit of esmolol is its metabolism by serum esterases. Therefore, it is useful in patients with renal disease and hepatic dysfunction. Like other beta-blockers, this agent is not recommended for treating patients with hypertensive emergency from cocaine ingestion secondary to theoretical concern for unopposed alpha activity.[8,9]

Nicardipine is a dihydropyridine calcium channel blocker, which is helpful in preserving cardiac and cerebral perfusion, and does not significantly interrupt myocardial oxygen balance.[8] However, it acts relatively slowly, and its effects last approximately 40 minutes. This agent should be avoided in patients with aortic stenosis because these patients are preload dependent, and the agent leads to smooth muscle relaxation and venous pooling.

Fenoldopan acts at peripheral D1 receptors, and is rapidly metabolized by the liver. It acts in approximately 4 minutes, and the agent remains in the system for 8–10 minutes. Fenoldopan has a desirable renal profile as it increases creatinine clearance and sodium excretion. The agent may cause an increase in intraocular pressure, and therefore should be avoided in glaucoma patients, and it should also be avoided in patients who have been given acetaminophen, as these levels may increase up to 70%.[1] Side effects are mild and include headache and facial flushing in up to 25% of patients.[5,6,8,9]

Nitroprusside once was routine therapy in hypertensive emergencies; however, the agent has fallen into disfavor recently. It is advantageous because it acts rapidly, within 1–2 minutes, and has a half-life of 4 minutes. Despite this favorable profile, nitroprusside decreases cerebral blood flow while increasing intracerebral pressure. Nitoprusside is also contraindicated in the setting of cardiac ischemia as it can cause a coronary steal phenomenon exacerbating the ischemia. Nitroprusside can only be used for a maximum of 48 hours secondary to production of thiocyanate as a byproduct of its metabolism. Logistically it also poses both storage and handling issues, as it is light sensitive and rapidly degrades. Since the agent crosses the placenta, it should not be used in patients who are pregnant.[1,5,6,8,9]

Clevidipine is a new dihydropyridine calcium channel blocker that may be useful in the treatment of hypertensive emergency. The drug has an onset of action of 2–4 minutes and a half life of 5–15 minutes. Like esmolol, clevidipine is rapidly hydrolyzed by plasma esterases, and therefore may be particularly helpful in patients with renal and hepatic dysfunction. As with other calcium channel blockers, it is not indicated in patients who suffer from severe aortic stenosis or for patients in congestive heart failure (CHF). It may have a niche in treating hypertensive emergencies in patients who cannot tolerate beta-blockade.[8]

Hydralazine is a popular drug for rapid blood pressure lowering, but with the exception of pregnancy, is probably best avoided in the management of hypertensive crises. Hydralazine works within 10 minutes, but its blood pressure effects may persist for greater than 12 hours.[5] This prolonged activity relates to the rate of acetylation of hydralazine; 50% of the population acetylates slowly.[9] In addition, hydralazine should never be used in aortic dissection, as it increases vascular shear forces.

Special cases

Aortic dissection

In the specific case of aortic dissection, goals for blood pressure reduction differ from other hypertensive emergencies. Rather than a 20–25% reduction in blood pressure over the first 2 hours, the goal is emergent lowering of blood pressure and heart rate to limit vascular shear forces and dissection progression. Goal blood pressure should be a systolic blood pressure of 100–120, or lower if tolerated. First line antihypertensives in this setting are either propranolol or labetalol. In patients who cannot tolerate beta-blockade, verapamil or diltiazem may be employed. In patients with an intact mental status and no signs of renal dysfunction, sodium nitroprusside may be employed to achieve further blood pressure decrease.[10]

Congestive heart failure

Congestive heart failure can result primarily from an acute cardiac insult, but it can also result from a rapid increase in afterload from a cholinergic surge. In this setting of acute onset of CHF, therapy should be directed toward acute afterload and preload reduction. This is best accomplished with nitroglycerin or ACE inhibitors, and ultimately with furosemide. By decreasing preload and afterload, there will be a decrease in cardiac wall stress and oxygen consumption, and allow for systemic perfusion.

Disposition

All patients with a hypertensive emergency should be admitted to the hospital, with the majority sent to the intensive care unit for careful hemodynamic monitoring and titration of antihypertensive therapy. An arterial line may be useful for second-to-second pressure management, particularly in patients with labile blood pressures.

Section IV: Decision making

- Look for evidence of hypertensive emergency target organ damage.
- Do not lower blood pressure in the ED simply because the blood pressure is elevated.
- If end-organ damage is found, blood pressure should be lowered within the first 1–2 hours by 20–30%.
- Choice of blood pressure-lowering agent should be directed toward the specific clinical needs of the patient (Table 21-2).

Table 21-2. Pharmacological Management for Hypertensive Emergencies

Drug	Dosage Reference	Avoid in
Labetalol	20 mg IV push over 2 minutes followed by 40–80 mg at 10-minute intervals for max of 300 mg	Cocaine ingestion, bradycardia, bronchospasm, heart failure
Esmolol	Initial bolus: 80 mg (~1 mg/kg) over 30 seconds, followed by a 150 mcg/kg/minute infusion	See Labetalol (can be used in renal/liver patients)
Fenoldopan	Initial: 0.1–0.3 mcg/kg/minute. May be increased in increments of 0.05–0.1 mcg/kg/minute every 15 minutes	Elevated intraocular pressure
Nitroprusside	Initial: 0.3–0.5 mcg/kg/minute; increase in increments of 0.5 mcg/kg/minute. Usual dose: 3 mcg/kg/minute	Elevated ICP, pregnancy
Nicardipine	Initial: 5 mg/hour increased by 2.5 mg/hour every 15 minutes to a maximum of 15 mg/hour	Aortic stenosis
Clevidipine	Initial: 1–2 mg/hour	CHF, severe AS, impaired lipid metabolism

References

1 Mcgowan C. Hypertensive emergencies. In: Hemphill RR, ed. *Emedicine*, Boston: Emedicine; 2007:1–5.

2 Varon J. Diagnosis and management of labile blood pressure during acute cerebrovascular accidents and other hypertensive crises. *Am J Emerg Med.* 2007;25:949–959.

3 Fleming J, Meredith C, Henry J. Detection of hypertension in the emergency department. *Emerg Med J.* 2005;22: 636–640.

4 Kitiyakara C, Guzman NJ. Malignant hypertension and hypertensive emergencies. *J Am Soc Nephrol.* 1998;9: 133–142.

5 Varon J, Marik PE. Clinical review: The management of hypertensive crises. *Crit Care.* 2003;7(5):374–84.

6 Varon J and Marik PE. The diagnosis and management of hypertensive crises[see comment]. *Chest.* 2000;118(1): 214–227.

7 Edmunds E, Landray MJ, Li-Saw-Hee FL, et al. Dyslipidaemia in patients with malignant-phase hypertension. *QJM.* 2001;94(6): 327–332.

8 Marik PE, Varon J. Hypertensive crises: Challenges and management. *Chest.* 2007;131:1949–1962.

9 Tintanelli J, Gabor K, Stapczynski S. *Emergency Medicine: A Comprehensive Study Guide.* New York: McGraw Hill Book Company; 2003.

10 Kaplan NM, Rose BD. Hypertensive emergencies: Malignant hypertension and hypertensive encephalopathy. In: Bakris GL, ed. *UpToDate.* Waltham, MA: UpToDate; 2008. Available at: www.UpToDate.com. Accessed June 8, 2010.

11 Wolfson AB, Linden CH, Rosen CL, Shaider J. In: Harwood Nuss, ed. *Clinical Practice of Emergency Medicine.* Philadelphia: Lippincott Williams and Wilkins; 2005.

Cardiac Testing

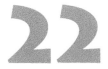

22

The electrocardiogram in acute coronary syndromes

Laura Oh[1] & William J. Brady[2]

[1] Department of Emergency Medicine, University of Virginia School of Medicine, Charlottesville, VA, USA
[2] Vice Chair, Department of Emergency Medicine, Professor of Emergency Medicine and Medicine, University of Virginia Health System, Charlottesville, VA, USA

Section I: Case presentation

A 43-year-old man presented to the emergency department (ED) with chest pain. He had noted progressive chest discomfort over the prior several days with exertion. Now, the chest pain had come at rest approximately 30 minutes prior to presentation, and resolved soon after presentation. He also complained of dyspnea and mild nausea. The past medical history was significant for hypertension, tobacco use, and a parental history of coronary disease. The physical examination was unremarkable. The patient received an aspirin. The initial 12-lead EKG was minimally abnormal with nonspecific ST-segment–T-wave changes. The first troponin level was normal.

The patient was admitted to an ED-based chest pain center for serial biomarkers and further observation. The patient remained pain free during the initial 4 hours of observation; the second troponin level was still normal. However, he then developed recurrent chest pain accompanied by diaphoresis. The electrocardiogram (EKG) (Figure 22-1) demonstrated an inverted T wave in lead aVl. Despite nitrates and morphine, the chest discomfort continued. With the recurrent chest pain accompanied by a new, although minimal, alteration of the EKG, the management strategy changed to hospital admission.

While awaiting an inpatient bed, the patient's pain worsened. ST-segment trend monitoring revealed progressive change in the ST-segments of the inferior leads. Ultimately, significant ST-segment elevation was noted in the leads II, III, and aVf, consistent with an inferior ST-segment elevation myocardial infarction (STEMI) (Figure 22-2).

The patient received thrombolytics, with resolution of the chest pain and normalization of the ST-segments. Repeat biomarker testing was positive, indicating acute myocardial infarction (MI).

Section II: Case discussion

Dr Peter Rosen: We see a lot of patients who come in with a similar history to the opening of this case: chest pain that sounds like an acute coronary syndrome, maybe a couple of risk factors, perhaps a past history of ischemic cardiac disease, an EKG that is nondiagnostic, and a set of cardiac biomarkers that is normal. What is a safe protocol for these kinds of patients?

Dr Richard Harrigan: At our institution, we do not have a chest pain center, so we have to make the decision of whether to admit these patients, or send them home. We do have a prolonged ED rule-out protocol that involves two sets of cardiac biomarkers and two EKGs. The problem of potentially putting this patient into that protocol would be that his pretest probability for cardiac disease seems rather high. He is not that old, but he has risk factors, a story consistent

Cardiovascular Problems in Emergency Medicine: A discussion-based review, First Edition.
Edited by Shamai A. Grossman and Peter Rosen.
© 2011 John Wiley & Sons, Ltd. Published 2011 by John Wiley & Sons, Ltd.

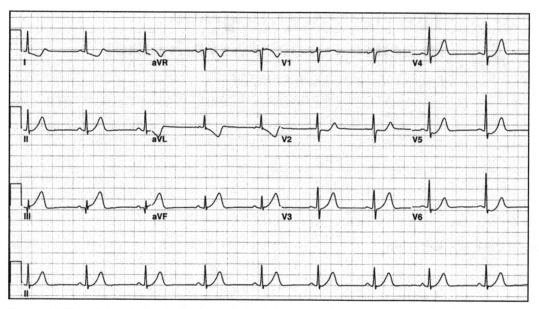

Figure 22.1 Normal sinus rhythm (NSR) with "reciprocal" ST-segment depression with T wave inversion in leads I and AVL—a potential early warning sign of inferior wall ST-segment elevation myocardial infarction.

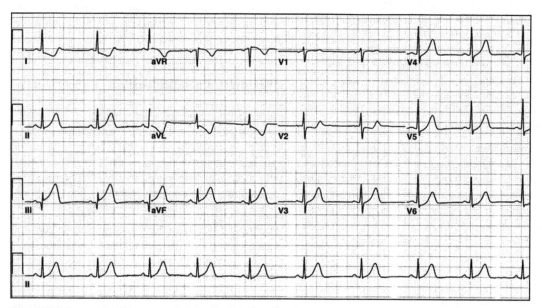

Figure 22.2 Progressive ST-segment elevation in the inferior leads consistent with inferior wall ST-segment elevation myocardial infarction.

with possible myocardial ischemia, and it seems likely that he has presented in-between episodes of ischemia. I favor the application of the two sampling rule-out over 6 hours after presentation more in a patient with an atypical presentation than in the patient with

typical anginal symptoms; these latter patients should be considered for admission.

Dr Shamai Grossman: I think the problem here is that we often don't differentiate between what is classically called a "rule-out myocardial infarction," and what was traditionally called "unstable angina." Unstable angina suggests you are not done with your workup when you've decided the patient is not having a myocardial infarction. You clearly need to do more investigations. Having ruled out myocardial infarction is not going to be useful if the patient has unstable angina. In that sense, observation units do not always fill the appropriate role for all chest pain that is possibly cardiac ischemia. If you want to know if a specific event was a myocardial infarction, then, obtaining serial biomarkers 6 hours apart is reasonable. If you want to know whether the recurrent events the patient is having every day were actually ischemic in nature, then a chest pain unit may not be the best idea for the patient, and hospital admission may still be the most appropriate strategy.

PR: The difficult problem that can lead to missed diagnosis of myocardial infarction in the emergency department is not the STEMI presentation, but rather patients like this one in our case today—they are having unstable angina, yet an objective test is not always positive or diagnostic in this presentation.

Dr William Brady: When a patient presents to the ED with chest pain or with an anginal equivalent; who looks ill, diaphoretic, or pale; and has obvious ST-segment elevation on the electrocardiogram; I do not think that anyone questions the diagnosis, nor fails to understand the time sensitivity of the treatment. On the other side of the spectrum is the group of patients who have non-ST elevation acute coronary syndrome presentations. In this situation, you must ask yourself which diagnostic strategy are you following: ruling out an MI, ruling out acute coronary syndrome, or ruling out asymptomatic coronary obstructive lesion? For some patients, you may need all three strategies. Early on, in the first minutes of presentation to the ED, you are ruling out STEMI, then you progress into ruling out acute coronary syndrome, at least one that is marker-positive with an evolving EKG. After that, with continued stability of the patient, you are evolving into "Is this an ischemic coronary syndrome with obstructive coronary lesions?"

I believe that in patients with atypical presentations who have an EKG that is normal, minimally abnormal, or unchanged; negative serial biomarkers; and a stable ED course; you have safely completed the ED evaluation. These patients have a very low 30-day

event rate, and can be safely discharged from the ED with appropriate follow-up. A patient who has a higher pretest probability can still be put into an ED chest pain or observation unit if a risk-stratification study can be done at the end of marker sampling, regardless of the ED rule-out protocol. Higher risk patients likely should be admitted to the hospital or, at least, be referred to a cardiologist for evaluation that day.

PR: How do you define "unstable angina"? What is it about the history that allows us to say that this patient is no longer having stable angina, or has developed an unstable event?

SG: Traditionally, unstable angina had two meanings: the first, new onset angina that was considered unstable because it was new in onset, and the second is "crescendo angina," or angina that is progressing over a number of days, ultimately ending in infarction. Where that terminology becomes problematic is the scenario where a patient presents with a single episode of chest pain, and we decide to call it "chest pain, rule out myocardial infarction"; we obtain serial biomarkers, and then decide that perhaps the process is complete and negative. The problem with that is, if it is truly unstable angina, then you are putting a patient who has an unstable lesion on a treadmill, and you may end up with an infarction during the testing study, or a progression of the disease. The historical management of the patient with unstable angina was that patient needs admission to the hospital, needs to be "cooled down" with heparin, ultimately with a plan to have more diagnostic testing when the patient is no longer symptomatic. Here, more diagnostic testing would be either a risk stratification study, such as a stress test with nuclear scan, to define if significant coronary obstructive lesions are present, or going to the catheterization laboratory to define and treat the coronary artery pathologies and related obstruction.

PR: We are constantly told that a common error that we make in emergency medicine is missing myocardial infarction, and I do not believe it. I do not think we are missing STEMIs, perhaps what we are missing are some of the MIs that are very hard to define, the non-ST-segment elevation myocardial infarctions (NSTEMIs), the right ventricular infarction, the posterior MI, and the MI in the face of bundle branch block. When would you do special additional lead testing on a patient who comes in with a history like our man today with nonspecific changes on the EKG?

RH: I would not have been tempted to do special lead testing on this patient as he presented. He does lie in a group that we have termed "prone to classic angina": not elderly, not female, not diabetic, and so he should present with classic symptoms, and indeed, he does. Whereas his EKG does not show ischemia initially, at that time he was not having ongoing symptoms, so that is not surprising. There is no proven benefit to additional lead EKGs in any certain subpopulation in terms of decreasing mortality. However, I would be tempted to add leads when I have ongoing ischemic symptoms without any findings on the 12-lead EKG. If I have ongoing symptoms of ischemia, but the presentation is not one of STEMI, but rather in the right precordial leads, and I see some degree of ST-segment depression, maybe a taller-than-expected R wave, signaling that this may be a posterior myocardial infarction, then, in this instance, the addition of leads V8 and V9 would allow you to visualize the ST-segment elevations you are looking for to diagnose a posterior wall infarction. Lastly, in patients who present with ongoing ischemic symptoms who have difficult to interpret inferior changes (i.e., borderline ST-segment elevation or ST-segment elevations that are subtle with more atypical characteristics), right-sided V leads may demonstrate ST-segment elevation suggesting a right ventricular infarction.

WB: A review looked at ST-segment depression in the right precordial leads. The current standard approach for patients who present with ST-segment depression syndromes, either with or without a positive marker, is not to provide a fibrinolytic agent, but perhaps take them to the catheterization laboratory within 24 hours. While this approach is appropriate in patients with NSTEMI, patients with acute posterior wall infarction should not be managed with this strategy of delayed coronary angiography. We need to get out of the idea of looking exclusively for anatomic segment infarctions, meaning anterior wall, inferior wall, or lateral wall. Instead, we need to get into the mindset of looking for an occluded artery syndrome. This review considered patients who presented with right precordial ST-segment depression, and notes that more than a quarter of these patients have an

occluded epicardial artery responsible for their syndrome. Interestingly and unfortunately, none of these patients had percutaneous coronary interventions (PCIs) or urgent reperfusion therapy within 6 hours. These patients had higher cardiovascular complications and mortality rates compared to patients without obstruction of an epicardial artery.

PR: Carrying on with our case, the patient has a normal set of biomarkers, but then becomes symptomatic again. What is the next most appropriate diagnostic step?

RH: Recurrent chest discomfort: here you almost have to restart the evaluation, which is a challenge to the culture in the ED where we seem to think that, if we've done the work, we've done the EKG, and we've done the initial set of cardiac markers, that we're done; we find it hard to reset the clock and begin again with new EKGs and reevaluation. I do not know exactly where that mindset comes from. In this case, ST-segment trend monitoring was revealing in this patient; if you do not have that technology available, the poor man's ST-segment trend monitoring is the serial EKG. When you have a patient with either recurrent or ongoing chest pain, such a scenario should trigger a response similar to that of a new patient reevaluation, including a repeat EKG. The most important thing you can do is to get another EKG at that time.

SG: This situation is exactly why we do serial EKGs. I find repeating an EKG is far more valuable than extra EKG leads, particularly when your data do not quite provide an answer. If the patient has a classic story for unstable angina, and the initial EKG is not revealing, then repeat it. Now, when you obtain a cardiology consultation, you can demonstrate serial changes: normal to nonspecific to worrisome ST-segments. With this information, you have now proven that the patient not only should be admitted to the hospital, but directly to the catheterization laboratory to address an unstable plaque.

RH: It's easy data; it's free, noninvasive, and easy to obtain. One additional closing thought: from an electrocardiographic point of view, I find it interesting that in our case the first EKG abnormality this patient showed us was the change in lead aVL. This finding can be an early warning of impending inferior wall STEMI.

Section III: Concepts

Historical background of the electrocardiogram

The electrocardiogram (EKG) is one of the most widely applied and cost-effective tests in emergency medicine. Dutch scientist Willem Einthoven (1860–1927) is credited with the discovery of the EKG, as well as its ability to graphically record the electrical activity of the heart.[1] In 1895, Einthoven himself questioned whether efforts to fully interpret the EKG should be abandoned, given the uncertainty of the recording; yet, by 1908, Einthoven had successfully interpreted the EKG in the clinical setting, for which he eventually won the 1924 Nobel Prize.[2] In the presentation speech of Einthoven's Nobel Prize, it was noted that Einthoven had developed a tool of "the greatest clinical significance: that different forms of heart disease reveal themselves characteristically in the electrocardiogram."[2] Today, 100 years after Einthoven's initial EKG interpretations, the EKG continues to play a pivotal role in the management of the patient with suspected cardiovascular disease, guiding not only diagnosis, but also the treatment and disposition.

Definition of acute coronary syndrome

In the ED, the most frequent reason for obtaining an EKG is chest pain. According to a 2007 Centers for Disease Control report, 120 million patients are seen annually in the ED, with 5.4% of these patients presenting with chest pain.[3] Approximately 1 million of these patients will develop an acute myocardial infarction (AMI). Although only a minority of patients will have pain of cardiac origin, the priority for a patient presenting with chest pain suspected of acute coronary syndrome (ACS) is identification of ST-segment elevation myocardial infarction. The term acute coronary syndrome is used to describe a spectrum of myocardial injury syndromes inclusive of unstable angina (UA), non-ST elevation myocardial infarction, and ST elevation myocardial infarction. In UA, the EKG is consistent with reversible ischemia and the biomarkers are normal. In NSTEMI, the EKG may initially be indistinguishable from UA, but biomarkers will be elevated in a "typical rise and fall pattern." In STEMI, the EKG will show ST elevation and biomarker elevation. AMI and UA (along with aortic dissection, pulmonary embolism, tension pneumothorax, and esophageal rupture) represent two of the six priority diagnoses,

or catastrophic causes, of acute chest pain that are both life-threatening in outcome and time-sensitive in management.[4]

In 2007, the Joint Task Force of the European Society of Cardiology, American College of Cardiology Foundation, the American Heart Association, and the World Health Federation (ESC/ACC/AHA/WHF) redefined myocardial infarction as evidence of myocardial necrosis in a clinical setting consistent with myocardial ischemia. In addition to serum biomarkers and pathologic evidence on autopsy, EKG changes (e.g., new ST-segment–T-wave changes, new left bundle branch block, and pathological Q waves) are recognized as central criteria in the diagnosis of MI.[5]

The initially normal or minimally abnormal EKG

The single EKG is more powerful diagnostically at ruling in than ruling out myocardial infarction. The EKG is a highly specific test (at least 94%, thus its power in the rule-in approach), but it is also highly insensitive (25–50%, hence its inability to conclusively rule-out).[6] Fifty percent of patients who are ultimately diagnosed with MI will have a nondiagnostic initial EKG. A frequent pitfall of EKG interpretation and application is to assume that the initially normal EKG is equivalent to a nonspecific EKG; further, neither of these entities can be used to exclude the diagnosis of MI by themselves (i.e., to the exclusion of other clinical data). In the adult ED population, 1–4% of patients with an absolutely normal EKG have a final diagnosis of AMI; patients with nonspecific EKG findings (e.g., T-wave flattening or subtle ST-segment deviations [<0.5 mm]) experience AMI in 4–8% of cases.[7] Thus, the EKG cannot be used by itself to rule out MI, yet the EKG, when used in the context of other clinical data, can be useful as negative evidence to answer the question: is the patient having an MI?

In a 2001 study by Welch et al. examining prognostic value of a normal or nonspecific initial EKG in AMI, patients with an initially normal EKG have a 41% lower risk of in-hospital death. The 30-day mortality rate, however, is still substantial; the patients with AMI and normal or nonspecifically abnormal initial EKGs experience a composite rate of mortality and life-threatening adverse event of 19.2% and 27.5% respectively, compared with the 34.9% rate experienced by patients with AMI and initially diagnostic EKG.[8]

Roughly 2% of patients who present to the ED with AMI are incorrectly discharged, and these patients do less well than their admitted counterparts. A study by Pope et al. examined the incidence and clinical outcome of failure to hospitalize patients with acute cardiac ischemia. Nonhospitalized patients with MI have a 30-day risk of death that is 1.9 times that of hospitalized MI patients, and nonhospitalized patients with UA have a 30-day risk of death that is 1.7 times that of hospitalized UA patients.[9] The missed MI also accounts for a significant portion of malpractice dollars in the United States.[4]

The EKG and risk stratification

The EKG is best used with Bayesian principles in mind: the interpretation of the EKG is a biologic test, and the result depends on the patient's pretest probability of disease.[10] In a patient with a 90% pretest probability of infarction, a negative EKG would only decrease posttest probability of infarction to 80%.[4] A patient with a 10% pretest probability and the same negative EKG would have a different management plan. This Bayesian approach is best summed in the following statement: interpret the EKG within the context of the clinical presentation.

Pretest probability is either derived by the clinician's individual judgment or by clinical decision rules. Assigning a patient's pretest probability of disease based on experience is no easy task. In a 2004 study by Miller et al., ED physicians were asked to predict based on history, physical, and EKG whether chest pain in 17,737 patients was cardiac or noncardiac in nature; 2.8% of patients whom physicians believed to have noncardiac chest pain experience an adverse event.[11] Up to one-third of patients with ACS do not experience chest pain, and atypical features often used by clinicians to exclude the diagnosis of ACS (reproducible chest wall pain, pleuritic pain) carry odds ratios (0.6 for each) that cannot exclude the diagnosis reliably.[8] According to Pope et al., preconceptions about heart disease in women and nonwhite populations and atypical presentation likely contribute to misdiagnosis of ACS. Women less than 55 years old have an odds ratio of 6.7 for inappropriate discharge, while nonwhite persons have an odds ratio of 4.5. Patients with an initial normal or nondiagnostic EKG have an odds ratio of 7.7.[9]

Several ACS risk stratification algorithms have been developed to aid the clinician, such as the Thrombolysis in Myocardial Infarction (TIMI) risk score, Global Registry of Acute Events (GRACE) score, Goldman Criteria, Sanchis score, and the Vancouver Chest Pain Rule.[12–17] One of the clinical questions that the ED physician seeks to answer in evaluating patients with suspected ACS is determining which patients can be safely discharged from the ED. Unfortunately, the first four algorithms above were not designed for this purpose; they are primarily used for risk stratification in admitted patients, and cannot be applied to determine if discharge of an ED patient is appropriate. The Vancouver Rule is unique in that it identifies with 98.8% sensitivity very low-risk patients who are able to be discharged early from the ED; these include patients under 40 who have a normal EKG and no prior history of ischemic chest pain, those over 40 and low-risk pain characteristics (no radiation of pain, no increase with deep breath or palpation) with an initial CK-MB under three, and those over 40 and low-risk pain characteristics with a CK-MB over three but no change in EKG or CK-MB 2 hours after arrival.[16] The Vancouver rule, however, has yet to be prospectively validated.

New algorithms, serial biomarker rule-out protocols, and chest pain units all hold promise as means to decrease the 2% diagnostic error rate in AMI. Twenty-five percent of the patients who are mistakenly discharged, however, are sent home likely because of a more fundamental error—an error in the interpretation of the EKG itself.[14]

EKG changes reflecting non-ST-segment elevation syndromes: T-wave inversion, ST-segment depression, and the U wave

T-wave inversion
Repolarization is more sensitive to ischemia than depolarization; therefore, ST-segments and T waves are the portions of the EKG primarily affected when there is an increased myocardial demand for oxygen.[18,19] The myocardium normally depolarizes from endocardium to epicardium, and repolarizes in the opposite direction. When there is extensive ischemia, it causes a delay in the repolarization so that the direction of repolarization reverses, resulting in a T-wave inversion.[20] In a normal EKG, the T wave is upright in most leads and inverted in lead aVR. Normal T-wave inversions may

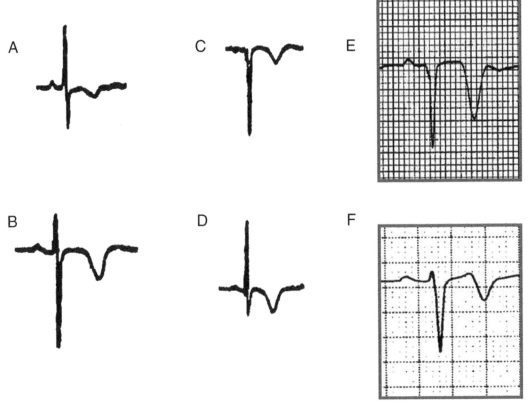

Figure 22.3 T-wave inversion in acute coronary syndrome. A–D. Typical ischemic T-wave inversions with symmetric downsloping and upsloping configurations. E–F. Wellens' syndrome T-wave inversions. (E. with the deeply inverted T-wave pattern and F. with the biphasic T-wave pattern).

be seen in leads III and aVF. T-wave inversions may also be seen in leads V1 and V2 and, more rarely, in leads V3 and V4, particularly in younger populations.[21]

In the healthy population, T-wave abnormalities may be seen in the setting of glucose ingestion, body positioning, deep inspiration, tachycardia, or obesity.[22] In the ill ED population, T-wave change that is new, dynamic, >1 mm, or present in >1 lead in a coronary distribution may represent myocardial ischemia in the patient who presents with chest pain.[21] In a 2008 study by Lin et al., the presence or absence of T-wave flattening or inversion was examined in 5,582 patients who presented to the ED with a potential ACS. The study concludes that there is a higher 30-day rate of cardiovascular event (death, AMI, invasive procedure, or positive stress test) in those patients with T-wave abnormalities. Risk increases with the degree of T-wave change; T-wave flattening carries a relative risk of 1.41

(95% CI 1.07 to 1.85), while T-wave inversion of 1–5 mm carries a relative risk of 2.37 (95% CI 1.78 to 3.14), and T-wave inversion >5 mm carries a relative risk of 3.36 (95% CI 1.67 to 6.14).[23] Refer to Figure 22-3A–D for examples of inverted T-waves associated with ACS.

When T-wave inversion is seen in the undifferentiated ACS patient, it increases the patient's mortality risk because of its association with ACS. However, in the STEMI patient, minimally inverted (>1 mm) static T-wave inversion does not predict a worse outcome.[23]

One pattern of T-wave inversion deserves special attention. In Wellens' syndrome, a patient with a history of anginal chest pain presents with marked T-wave inversion in leads V2 and V3 (occasionally in leads V1 and V4 to V6), or less commonly a biphasic T-wave in leads V2-V3. These findings suggest a critical stenosis in the left anterior descending (LAD)

artery. The EKG will not show Q waves or significant ST-segment elevation, biomarkers will be normal or only slight elevated, and the patient will be
chest pain-free at the time of the EKG. However, this
patient will be at high risk for acute anterior MI and
death, and requires admission.[24] Refer to Figure 22-3
E–F for examples of inverted T-waves associated with
Wellens' syndrome.

ST-segment depression

When T-wave inversion is combined with ST depression, it predicts a worse outcome. In a study by Larsen
et al., ST depression with T-wave inversion carries a
relative risk of 1.98 (1.21–3.26) for cardiovascular
disease mortality during a 7-year follow-up period,
while negative T-wave alone has a relative risk of
1.82 (1.35–2.45).[25] Risk of MI also increases with a
greater number of leads involved and greater degree
of ST-segment depression. Savonitto et al. conclude
that in patients with an NSTEMI, the greater the sum
of ST-segment depression in all leads, the greater the
risk of 30-day mortality.[26]

ST-segment depression with T-wave inversion
accompanied by ST elevation in lead aVR signifies left
main coronary artery involvement, and is a potential
indication for an emergent coronary angiography.[27–30]
In the Savonitto et al. study, the extent of ST depression shows a highly significant correlation with the
degree of three-vessel or left main coronary disease.[26]

Although left main occlusion is a rare entity, because
this vessel provides the blood supply to a large portion
of the heart, it is associated with a high mortality rate.
Patients generally present catastrophically with pulmonary edema, cardiogenic shock, or sudden death
due to ventricular dysrhythmias.[31] Medical management of acute left main occlusion is largely ineffective.
In this situation, the presence of intercoronary collat-
erals, a dominant right coronary artery, or incomplete
occlusion increase chance of survival, but the key to
survival is the time to reperfusion by invasive methods (PCI and coronary artery bypass graft surgery).

Not all ST-segment depression is due to subendocardial ischemia. The ST-segment depression of reversible
ischemia is usually flat or downsloping, similar to the
ST-segment depression associated with hypokalemia
(typically with serum potassium level <3.0 mmol/L)
or digitalis effect. Both hypokalemia and digitalis may
cause positive U waves in contrast to the new negative
U waves that can be seen in ischemia.[21] In addition,

digitalis effect can be associated with a "scooped"
appearance of the ST depression and can be associated with QT shortening (in contrast to the QT prolongation that may be present in ACS).[21]

U waves

U waves are small deflections that follow T-waves.
In general, they demonstrate the same polarity as
T waves; U-wave inversion in leads other than leads
aVR, III, and aVF can signal myocardial ischemia.
U waves may also been seen in cases of uncontrolled
hypertension, left ventricular enlargement, and valvular heart disease.

Serial electrocardiogram and continuous ST-segment trend monitoring

A 12-lead EKG records only 10 seconds of electrical
activity; therefore, a single EKG may fail to capture
dynamic changes of early ACS. Comparison of the
new EKG to an old EKG in the medical record or a
prehospital EKG, or performing serial EKGs in the
ED, may help identify ACS earlier, which can lead to
a more rapid delivery of therapy. Fesmire et al., in a
study of 1000 patients admitted for chest pain, demonstrate that serial EKGs are more sensitive (68.1%
versus 55.45%) and more specific (99.4% versus
97.1%) compared to a single EKG for detection
of AMI. Serial EKGs detect injury in an additional
16.2% of AMI patients. High-risk patients benefit the
most from additional EKGS; they are 15 times more
likely to have their therapy changed when compared
to low-risk patients.[32] In a high-risk patient, the intervals between EKGs may be taken 5–10 minutes apart,
versus 30 minutes to 2 hours in a lower-risk patient.[33]
Serial EKG monitoring does not require extra equipment, but does require additional staffing.

Another option for monitoring change of the
ST-segment is continuous ST-segment monitoring.
Continuous ST-segment monitoring requires specialized equipment that monitors ST-segment trends
every few seconds to minutes; alarm thresholds
typically include a change of 200 μV in one lead
or 100 μV in two contiguous leads.[34] Continuous
ST-segment monitoring is of value in distinguishing dynamic change of the ST-segment in AMI from
other causes of static ST-segment elevation. A 1999
study by Moons et al. also suggests that the area
under the curve of the ST-segment has prognostic

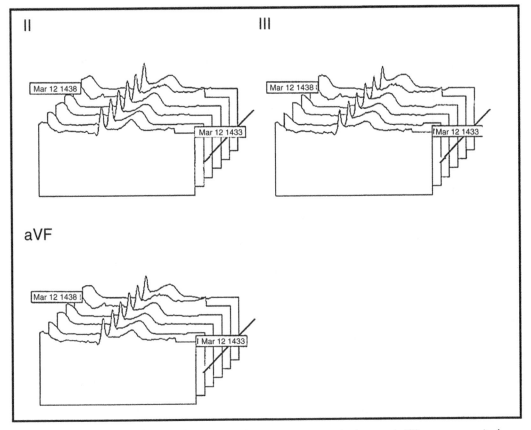

Figure 22.4 ST-segment trend monitoring—progressive ST-segment changes in a patient with inferior wall ST-segment elevation myocardial infarction. Note the progressive increase in ST-segment magnitude over a 5 minute period of observation.

significance; in the study, a greater area under the ST trend curve is associated with larger infarct size and lower resultant left ventricular ejection fraction.[35] Refer to Figure 22-4 for an example of a patient with evolving inferior wall STEMI.

Evolution of the EKG in STEMI: hyperacute T waves, dynamic change of the ST-segment, and Q waves

The EKG in STEMI evolves in a classic progression over a time course of minutes to months. During the first few minutes of a STEMI, the QT interval may prolong, followed by an increasing prominence in the T wave that is out of proportion to the preceding QRS complex. This prominent, or "hyperacute," T wave appears within 5 to 30 minutes of AMI, but may persist for several hours. Next, the ST-segment elevates, typically in the first several hours. A Q wave can develop within the first hour after coronary artery occlusion; it will be fully developed within 8 to 12 hours postocclusion. Over the following 2–5 days, the ST-segment elevation resolves, but with persistent T-wave inversion that may recover over weeks to months, or last indefinitely. Q waves persist for months to years postinfarction. In a subset of STEMI patients, the ST-segment elevation persists, most often resulting from left ventricular aneurysm.

Hyperacute T waves

Although the hyperacute T wave is an early indicator of STEMI, other clinical syndromes, such as hyperkalemia and benign early repolarization (BER), can cause hyperacute T waves; these prominent T waves are non-ischemic in origin. The hyperacute T wave in

CHAPTER 22

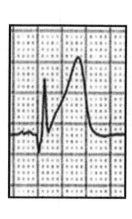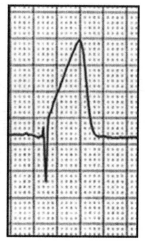

Figure 22.5 Hyperacute T waves of early ST-segment elevation myocardial infarction: tall, broad-based, blunt apex, and asymmetric.

AMI is asymmetric, broad based, rounded at the apex, and dynamic in nature. It may be accompanied by reciprocal ST-segment depression in the inferior leads. The hyperkalemic T wave, in contrast, is symmetric, narrow, peaked, and static (static in terms of alterations of the serum potassium level). T waves in BER are asymmetric, and have a "notching" or concavity of the J point. The J point is the transition point at the end of the QRS complex and the beginning of the ST-segment. The amplitude of the T wave may change, yet the T wave should not become biphasic or inverted. In addition, the T wave of BER may be associated with a shorter QT interval and ST-segment elevation <2 mm in leads V2-V5 and <0.5 mm in the limb leads, but is unaccompanied by reciprocal ST-segment depression in other anatomic regions. BER has a high prevalence in young, African-American, athletic men. Hyperacute T waves in the elderly with ACS symptoms are unlikely to be attributed to BER, particularly when the ST-segment elevation is limited to the limb leads.[36] Refer to Figure 22-5 for examples of prominent T waves ("hyperacute") associated with early STEMI.

ST-segment elevation
The hyperacute T wave in AMI may precede or develop concurrently with ST-segment elevation. The ST-segment elevation seen in STEMI is called a "current of injury" because the damage done to the heart alters the electrical charge on the myocardial cell membranes, causing the ST-segment deviation from its normal, isoelectric position. The Joint Task Force of the ESC/ACC/AHA/WHF defines ST-segment elevation according to the following criteria: new ST elevation at the J point in two contiguous leads with cut off points >0.2 mV (2 mm) in men or >0.15 mV in women in leads V2-V3, or <0.1 mV in men and women in other leads.[5] They define lead contiguity as follows: Anterior: V1-V6; Inferior: II, III, and aVF; Lateral: I and aVL; and Frontal: aVL, I, aVR, II, III, and aVF. As ST-segment elevation progresses, it may become indistinct from the T wave, resembling a monophasic action potential: the so-called monophasic R wave.

Only 15–25% of patients with ST-elevation have AMI. The differential diagnosis for causes of ST elevation other than infarction is broad, including acute myopericarditis, Prinzmetal's angina, left ventricular hypertrophy, left ventricular aneurysm, bundle branch block, ventricular paced rhythm, benign early repolarization, hyperkalemia, Wolff-Parkinson-White syndrome, and Brugada's syndrome, among many others. The ability to distinguish these noninfarction causes of ST-segment elevation from AMI is important, since the under-diagnosis of STEMI prevents timely life-saving therapy while overdiagnosis of infarction can lead to unnecessary, expensive, and dangerous interventions.

In a study by Brady et al., the authors describe a technique of morphologic analysis of the ST-segment that acts as a diagnostic aid in the patient with ST-segment elevation suspected of STEMI.[37] By drawing a line between the J point and the apex of the ST-segment–T-wave complex, the clinician can determine if the ST-segment morphology is concave (EKG waveform below the line) or nonconcave (EKG waveform above or on the line). The presence of a nonconcave ST-segment has a poor sensitivity (77%) but a high specificity (97%) for ruling in acute MI. This technique is best used as an adjunct to the EKG diagnosis of STEMI; with its high specificity, the clinician can rule in STEMI. Refer to Figure 22-6 for examples of ST-segment elevation syndromes (both STEMI and noninfarction causes of ST-segment elevation).

In addition to ST-segment elevation, reciprocal ST-segment depression (Figures 22-7 and 22-8), also known as reciprocal change, may be present in STEMI; this is a mirroring phenomenon observed on the ventricular wall opposite injury.[38] Yet, its cause remains unknown, with distant ischemia and

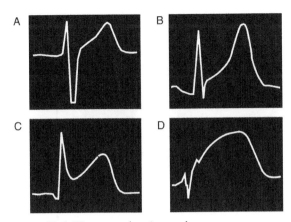

Figure 22.6 ST-segment elevation syndromes.
A. Benign early repolarization with concave morphology.
B. Acute myopericarditis with concave morphology.
C. Obliquely straight morphology of STEMI. D. Convex morphology of STEMI.

electrophysiologic effect as likely possibilities. If ST-segment elevation is accompanied by reciprocal change, the presence of the reciprocal change improves specificity for the EKG diagnosis of STEMI.

Anterior STEMI will have reciprocal change in the inferior leads 40–70% of the time; in inferior STEMI, ST-segment depression is seen in leads I and aVL in approximately 30% of such patients.[38]

Q waves

A normal, or nonpathologic, Q wave represents the depolarization of the septal wall between two ventricles; an abnormal Q wave usually signifies myocardial necrosis, and is both wider and deeper.[19,39] The 2007 Joint Task Force of the ESC/ACC/AHA/WHF defines an abnormal Q wave as any Q wave in leads V2-V3 >20 msec, a QS complex in leads V2-V3, any Q wave >30 msec and >0.1 mV deep, or QS complex in leads I, II, aVL, aVF, or V4-V6. These changes must be present in any two contiguous leads.[5] A Q wave in lead V1 is considered normal.[5]

While Q waves usually develop within 12 hours of infarction, they can also develop early in the course of the infarction, at a time in which urgent reperfusion therapy is still of benefit; thus, the mere appearance of pathologic Q waves does not preclude the consideration for emergent reperfusion therapy. Further, early

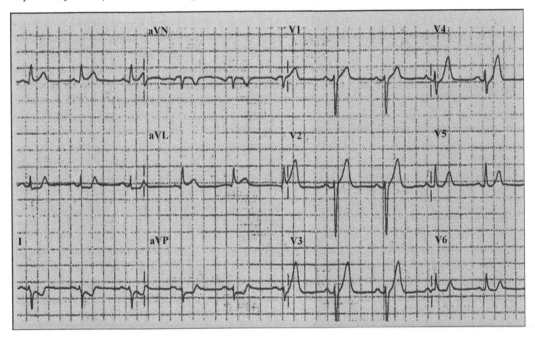

Figure 22.7 Subtle ST-segment elevation myocardial infarction of the lateral wall with ST-segment elevation in leads I and AVL. ST-segment depression, termed reciprocal ST-segment depression or reciprocal change, is seen in the inferior leads. The presence of the reciprocal change strongly supports ST-segment elevation myocardial infarction in this patient with subtle ST-segment elevation in the lateral leads.

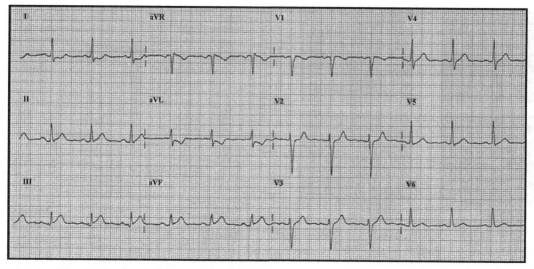

Figure 22.8 Subtle inferior wall ST-segment elevation myocardial infarction with minimal ST-segment elevation and reciprocal ST-segment depression in leads I and AVL.

appearance of abnormal Q waves within 6 hours of symptom onset in acute anterior infarction is associated with larger infarct size and increased hospital mortality.[40] The subset of STEMI patients who never develop Q waves has a better prognosis in terms of left ventricular function and survival.

Role of additional EKG leads

Due to the insensitivity of the EKG, an infarct in certain anatomic segments can be missed electrocardiographically; there are certain regions of the heart that are electrographically silent (i.e., under reflected): the inferior wall, the lateral wall, the posterior wall, and the right ventricle. "Electrographically silent" refers to the 12-lead EKG's limited ability to portray these anatomic segments of the heart.

The inferior and lateral walls of the left ventricle are reflected, yet these regions are less than optimally scrutinized by the standard 12-lead EKG; they are electrocardiographically "near silent." STEMI in these two anatomic distributions can be subtle electrocardiographically. Refer to Figures 22-7 and 22-8 for STEMI of the lateral and inferior walls, respectively, with subtle ST-segment elevation.

Electrocardiographically "silent" regions of the heart include the posterior wall of the left ventricle and the right ventricle. The posterior wall is supplied by the circumflex artery and its obtuse marginal branches or the right coronary artery and its posterior descending branch. Approximately 3–9% of all MIs diagnosed by biomarkers are posterior infarctions that present without ST-segment elevation on the 12-lead EKG.[41] Posterior MI may present as persistent ST-segment depression in leads V1-V4; ST depression >2 mm in leads V1-V3 is 90% specific for posterior STEMI.[41] In the presence of inferior AMI, anterior ST-segment depression almost always signifies posterior STEMI.[42,43] Posterior STEMI also frequently accompanies lateral wall AMI. A posterior infarction pattern may be more easily discernable by using the reverse transillumination technique or the mirror test; both techniques require inversion of the EKG and either back-illumination by a strong light source or viewing the EKG in a mirror. Another aid to diagnosing posterior wall infarction is the application of additional EKG leads V7-V9, which should be placed on the left back of the patient in the same horizontal plane as leads V4-V6. Lead V7 is placed at the posterior axillary line, lead V8 inferior to the scapular tip, and lead V9 at the paravertebral border. Figure 22-9 demonstrates the classic 12-lead EKG findings of posterior wall STEMI; it also demonstrates ST-segment elevation in the additional posterior leads V8 and V9.

In the majority of right ventricle (RV) infarction presentations, the right coronary artery or one of

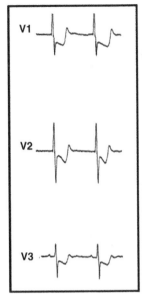

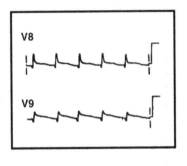

Figure 22.9 Posterior wall ST-segment elevation myocardial infarction. Leads V1, V2, and V3 demonstrate horizontal ST-segment depression with prominent R wave and upright T wave. Additional EKG leads V8 and V9, the posterior leads, demonstrate ST-segment elevation, consistent with ST segment elevation myocardial infarction of the posterior wall.

its branches is occluded. Isolated RV infarction only accounts for 3% of MI cases, but should be suspected when there is ST-segment elevation in lead V1 or when there is evidence of inferior STEMI, since 50% of those patients will have associated RV MI.[43] Right-sided leads V1R-V6R are placed on the anterior chest wall in a mirror image to the standard chest leads. Lead V4R is the key lead in diagnosing RV infarction; ST-segment elevation >1 mm is both sensitive (90–100%) and specific (68–95%). In the setting of concurrent posterior MI, this sensitivity and specificity decreases.[43] Identification of RV infarct patients is important because they can be more susceptible to nitrate and diuretic-related hypotension resulting from the preload dependence.[44]

Notable challenges to EKG interpretation in presumed ACS presentations: the confounding patterns

In addition to the presence of electrographically silent areas of the heart, EKG interpretation can also be obscured by patterns of new ST-segment and T-wave abnormality seen in several common clinical scenarios: left bundle branch block, ventricular paced rhythms, and left ventricular hypertrophy.[45]

Left bundle branch block

Left bundle branch block (LBBB) represents approximately 7% of myocardial infarctions. Patients with LBBB in ACS have significantly higher mortality, as not only do patients with LBBB tend to be older with more comorbid conditions, but the EKG itself is more difficult to interpret correctly, leading to delays in diagnosis and therapy.

In normal conduction of a cardiac electrical impulse, the right ventricle and left ventricle are simultaneously depolarized via the right and left bundle of His. In LBBB, normal conduction through the left bundle of His is blocked; the left ventricle is depolarized in a delayed fashion from impulses traveling through the right ventricle to the interventricular septum and then to the left ventricle. This progression is represented on the EKG by negative QS waves in leads V1, V2, or V3 with a large monophasic R wave (large, prolonged QRS complex) in leads I, aVl, and V6. The sequence of repolarization is also altered, causing ST-segment and T-wave changes that can mimic ACS.

The patient with LBBB has a "new normal EKG." The ST-segment and T-wave configurations will be in the opposite direction (discordant) with the major, terminal portion of the QRS complex. For

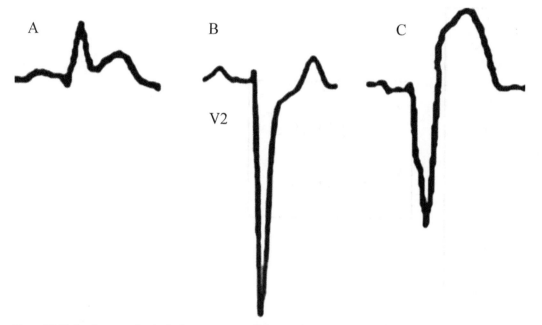

Figure 22.10 Sgarbossa et al. criteria for acute myocardial infarction in left branch bundle block. A. Concordant ST-segment elevation. B. Concordant ST-segment depression limited to the right precordial leads. C. Excessive, discordant ST-segment elevation.

instance, in the anterior leads (leads V1-V3) that have negative QRS complexes, we expect to see ST-segment elevation and an upright T wave. In the lateral leads (leads I, aVl, V5, and V6) with positive QRS complexes, we expect to see ST-segment depression and T-wave inversion. This relationship is known as the "rule of appropriate discordance."[46] Loss of this relationship may indicate ACS in the appropriate patient.

Whether or not it is possible to diagnose AMI in the patient presenting with ACS symptoms and LBBB has been a subject of great research and clinical interest. In a 1996 study, Sgarbossa et al. attempted to establish a set of criteria for diagnosing acute infarction in the setting of LBBB.[47] The EKGs of patients enrolled in the GUSTO-1 (Global Utilization of Streptokinase and Tissue Plasminogen Activator for Occluded Coronary Arteries) trial had LBBB and AMI confirmed by biomarkers compared to EKGs of control patients with known, stable coronary heart disease and LBBB taken from an outpatient database. Sgarbossa et al. report three EKG criteria of potential independent value in diagnosis of AMI as well as a scoring system (0–5 points):

1 ST-segment elevation of 1 mm or more concordant with QRS complex (Five points; Figure 22-10a)
2 ST-segment depression of 1 mm or more in lead V1, V2, or V3 (Three points; Figure 22-10b)
3 ST-segment elevation of 5 mm or more discordant with QRS complex. (Two points; Figure 22-10c)

A Sgarbossa et al. EKG algorithm score of three or greater (i.e., either of the first two criteria) is highly specific in diagnosing AMI in patients with LBBB. A score of two, representing the last Sgarbossa et al. criterion, is not helpful in diagnosis. However, a score of zero cannot exclude AMI. The criteria were applied to the American College of Emergency Physicians clinical policy in modified form as a decision rule for when to initiate emergent reperfusion therapy.[48]

Subsequent studies that have tested the Sgarbossa et al. criteria have mixed conclusions about their utility, with some studies saying that they are no better than clinical judgment. In 2008, Tabas et al. published a meta-analysis that reevaluated data from 11 studies (2100 patients) since 1996; they conclude that when one of the first two Sgarbossa et al. criteria are present, the specificity for AMI is 98% with a positive likelihood ratio of 7.9, but that the presence of the third criteria in isolation is not sensitive or specific enough to diagnose acute MI. Although the research of Tabas et al. lends support to the criteria, it also reaffirms that the lack of Sgarbossa et al. criteria does not rule out infarction. As is true with most EKG characteristics and AMI, the Sgarbossa et al. criteria are specific and thus helpful with ruling in infarction; the criteria are not sensitive and therefore are of little value in ruling out MI.

Right ventricular paced rhythm

In a right ventricular paced rhythm (VPR), similar to LBBB, the depolarization of the left ventricle is delayed in comparison to the right ventricle. The impulse propagates from the right ventricle to the interventricular septum to the left ventricle, resulting in a greater time of total depolarization and a wide QRS complex. The EKG of the right ventricular paced rhythm differs from LBBB in leads V5 and V6; in such paced rhythms, a QS complex replaces the monophasic R wave seen in LBBB.

The rule of appropriate discordance, however, still applies. In right ventricular paced rhythms, the QRS complex is positive in leads I and aVl; the ST-segment is depressed with T-wave inversion in those leads. Similarly, in leads with a negative QRS complex (leads II, III, aVf, and V1-V6), the ST-segment is elevated and the T wave is upright. Similarly to LBBB, a lack of discordance could signify ACS, although the lack of these findings does not rule out ACS.

Sgarbossa et al.'s criteria can also be applied in the right ventricular paced rhythm presentation. Returning to the GUSTO-1 data, there were 17 patients with pacemakers and AMI in the study; of the three criteria previously discussed above, the most useful in diagnosis of AMI and RV paced rhythm is the third: ST-segment elevation ≥5 mm discordant to the QRS complex.[49] This finding has a specificity of 88% and a positive likelihood of diagnosis of AMI of 4.41.[50] It is speculated that the reason that the excessive discordance (the third Sgarbossa et al. criterion) is helpful in the EKG interpretation of right ventricular paced rhythms, in contrast to the LBBB presentation, is that it results from the fact that most such rhythms have predominantly negative QRS complexes, so that there is more "opportunity" to witness a discordant change in the ST-segment.[51] As with LBBB, the Sgarbossa et al. criteria can help rule in infarct in right ventricular paced rhythms, yet not rule out AMI.

Left ventricular hypertrophy

The Sokolow-Lyon Index (the S-wave amplitude in V1 plus the R wave amplitude in lead V5 or V6 >35 mm) is one of many methods of diagnosing the left ventricular hypertrophy (LVH) pattern by EKG. LVH can produce the following EKG changes: increased QRS voltage, widened QRS complex, poor R-wave progression, and repolarization abnormalities of the ST-segment and T wave. Importantly, ST-segment and T-wave abnormalities are seen in approximately 75% of LVH cases. The repolarization abnormalities, which mimic AMI, can be divided into two categories: those associated with ST elevation and hyperacute T waves, and those associated with ST-segment depression and T-wave inversion.[46] Morphologic analysis of the ST-segment can help distinguish STEMI from LVH. The ST-segment of LVH is typically concave (rather than the "tombstone" convexity of AMI).[46]

In a 2004 study by Pope et al., having LVH does not alter the true-positive rate for ACS, but it does increase the false-positive rate by almost 50%.[52] A feature of LVH that may help distinguish it from AMI is the static nature of its ST-segment and T-wave abnormalities, unlikely to change during the course of ED evaluation. Serial EKG monitoring or ST-segment trend analysis may assist the clinician with diagnosis.[40]

Section IV: Decision making

- A normal or nonspecifically (i.e., minimally) abnormal EKG does not rule out AMI.
- The EKG must be interpreted within the context of the clinical presentation.
- With regards to AMI, the EKG is most useful in ruling in acute myocardial infarction, but is not particularly sensitive and should not be used alone to rule out AMI.
- Additional EKG leads, such as leads V4R, V8, and V9, can add diagnostic information in ACS, particularly with a moderate to high suspicion for AMI and a nondiagnostic EKG.
- ST-segment elevation in chest pain patients does not always result from STEMI; sound EKG interpretation, ST-waveform analysis, reciprocal change, and serial monitoring, can assist in this EKG differentiation.
- Confounding EKG patterns such as bundle branch block, LVH, and ventricular paced rhythms reduce

the impact of, but do not invalidate, using the EKG in chest pain evaluation.

References

1 O'Connor RE. Foreword. In: Mattu A and Brady W, eds. *ECGs for the Emergency Physician 2*. Malden, MA: Blackwell Publishing; 2008:1–2.

2 *Nobel Lectures, Physiology or Medicine 1922-1941*. Amsterdam: Elsevier Publishing Company; 1965.

3 Pitts SR, Niska RW, Xu J, Burt CW. *National Hospital Ambulatory Medical Care Survey: 2006 emergency department summary*. National Health Statistics Reports; no. 7. Hyattsville, MD: National Center for Health Statistics. Available at: http://www.cdc.gov/nchs/data/nhsr/nhsr007.pdf. Accessed June 16, 2010.

4 Hamilton GC, Malone S, Janz TG. Chest pain. In: Hamilton, GC, Sanders, AB, Strange, GR, Trott AT, eds. *Emergency Medicine: An Approach to Clinical Problem Solving*. 2nd ed. Philadelphia: Saunders: An Imprint of Elsevier; 2003:131–152.

5 Thygesen K, Alpert JS, White HD. Universal definition of myocardial infarction. *J Am Coll Cardiol*. 2007; 50(22):2173–2178.

6 Body R. Emergent diagnosis of acute coronary syndromes: Today's challenges and tomorrow's possibilities. *Resuscitation*. 2008;8:13–20.

7 Brady WJ, Roberts D, Morris F. The nondiagnostic ECG in the chest pain patient: Normal and nonspecific initial ECG presentations. *Am J Emerg Med*. 1999;17(4):394–397.

8 Welch RD, Zalenski RJ, Frederick PD, et al. Prognostic value of a normal or nonspecific initial electrocardiogram in acute myocardial infarction. *JAMA*. 2001;286(16): 1977–1984.

9 Pope JH, Aufderheide TP, Ruthazer R, et al. Missed diagnoses of acute cardiac ischemia in the emergency department. *N Engl J Med*. 2000;342(16):1163–1170.

10 Grunkemeier GL and Payne N. Bayesian analysis: A new statistical paradigm for new technology. *Ann Thorac Surg*. 2002;74:1901–1908.

11 Miller CD, Lindsell CJ, Khandelwal S, et al: Is the initial diagnostic impression of "noncardiac chest pain" adequate to exclude cardiac disease? *Ann Emerg Med*. 2004;44(6): 565–574.

12 Morrow DA, Antman EM, Charlesworth A. TIMI Risk Score for ST-elevation myocardial infarction: A convenient, bedside, clinical score for risk assessment at presentation. *Circulation*. 2000;102:2031–2037.

13 Fox KA, Dabbous OH, Goldberg RJ, et al. Prediction of risk of death and myocardial infarction in the six months after presentation with acute coronary syndrome: Prospective multinational observational study (GRACE). *BMJ*. 2006;333:1079–1080.

14 Manini, AF, Dannemann N, Brown DF. Limitations of risk score models in patients with acute chest pain. *Am J Emerg Med*. 2009;27:43–48.

15 Sanchis J, Bodi V, Nunez J, et al. New risk score for patients with acute chest pain, non-ST-segment deviation, and normal troponin concentrations. *J Am Coll Cardiol*. 2005;46:443–449.

16 Christenson J, Innes G, McKnight D, et al. A clinical prediction rule for early discharge of patients with chest pain. *Ann Emerg Med*. 2006;1:1–10.

17 Goldman L, Kirtane A. Triage of patients with acute chest pain and possible cardiac ischemia: The elusive search for diagnostic perfection. *Ann Intern Med*. 2003;139:987–995.

18 Dubin D. *Rapid Interpretation of EKGs*, 6th ed. Tampa, FL: Cover Publishing Company; 2000;1–30.

19 Wagner GS, ed. *Marriott's Practical Electrocardiography*. 9th ed. Baltimore: Williams & Wilkins; 1994:116–170.

20 Ehrling BF, Perron AD. Waveform genesis in acute coronary syndromes. In: Chan TC, Brady WJ, Harrigan RA, Ornato JP, Rosen P, eds. *ECG in Emergency Medicine and Acute Care*. Philadelphia: Elsevier; 2005: 151–169.

21 Bertog SC, Smith SW. What ECG changes might myocardial ischemia cause other than ST-segment elevation or Q waves, and what are the differential diagnoses of these changes? In: Brady WJ, Truwit JD, eds. *Critical Decisions in Emergency & Acute Care Electrocardiography*. West Sussex, UK: Wiley-Blackwell; 2009:103–114.

22 Lin KB, Shofer FS, McCusker C, et al. Predictive value of T-wave abnormalities at the time of emergency department presentation in patients with potential acute coronary syndromes. *Acad Emerg Med*. 2008;15:537–543.

23 Whitman W, Taha N, Bachour, K. Can the ECG be used to predict cardiovascular risk and acute complications in ACS? In: Brady WJ, Truwit JD, eds. *Critical Decisions in Emergency & Acute Care Electrocardiography*. West Sussex, UK: Wiley-Blackwell; 2009:216–224.

24 Rhinehardt J, Brady WJ, Perron AD, et al. Electrocardiographic manifestations of Wellens' Syndrome. *Am J Emerg Med*. 2002;20:638–643.

25 Larsen CT, Dahlin J, Blackburn H, et al. Prevalence and prognosis of electrocardiographic left ventricular hypertrophy, ST-segment depression and negative T-wave. *Eur Heart J*. 2002;23:315–324.

26 Savonitto S, Cohen MG, Politi A, et al. Extent of ST-segment depression and cardiac events in non-ST-segment elevation acute coronary syndromes. *Eur Heart J*. 2005;26:2106–2113.

27 Szymanski FM, Grabowski M, Filipiak KJ. Admission ST-segment elevation in lead aVR as the factor improving

complex risk stratification in acute coronary syndromes. *Am J Emerg Med.* 2008;26:408–412.

28 Williamson K, Mattu A, Plautz CU, et al. Electrocardiographic applications of lead aVR. *Am J Emerg Med.* 2006;24:864–874.

29 Yamaji H, Iwasaki K, Kusachi S, et al. Prediction of acute left main coronary artery obstruction by 12-lead electrocardiography. *J Am Coll Cardiol.* 2001;38(5):1348–1354.

30 Yan AT, Yan RT, Kennelly BM, et al. Relationship of ST elevation in lead aVR with angiographic findings and outcome in non-ST elevation acute coronary syndromes. *Am Heart J.* 2007;154(1):71–78.

31 Yip H, Wu C, Chen M, et al. Effect of primary angioplasty on total or subtotal left main occlusion. *Chest.* 2001;120:1212–1217.

32 Fesmire FM. Which chest pain patients potentially benefit from continuous 12-lead ST-segment monitoring with automated serial ECG? *Am J Emerg Med.* 2002;18(7):773–778.

33 Velez J, Brady WJ, Perron AD, Garvey L. Serial electrocardiography. *Am J Emerg Med.* 2002;20(1):43–49.

34 O'Laughlin D. Is serial electrocardiography (serial ECGs and ST-segment monitoring) of value in the ECG diagnosis of ACS? In: Brady WJ, Truwit JD, eds. *Critical Decisions in Emergency & Acute Care Electrocardiography.* West Sussex, UK: Wiley-Blackwell; 2009:148–154.

35 Moons K, Klootwijk P, Meij SH, et al. Continuous ST-segment monitoring associated with infarct size and left ventricular function in the GUSTO-1 trial. *Am Heart J.* 1999;138 (3):525–532.

36 Herbert M, ed. *EMRAP TV* "Episode 34: Big T-waves." Available at: www.emraptv.com. Accessed May 14, 2010.

37 Brady WJ, Syverud SA, Beagle C, et al. Electrocardiographic ST-segment elevation: The diagnosis of acute myocardial infarction by morphologic analysis of the ST-segment. *Acad Emerg Med.* 2001;8:961–967.

38 Whitwam W, Taha N. Can the ECG be used to predict cardiovascular risk and acute complications in ACS? In: Brady WJ, Truwit JD, eds. *Critical Decisions in Emergency & Acute Care Electrocardiography.* West Sussex, UK: Wiley-Blackwell; 2009:216–229.

39 Smith SW, Whitman W. Acute coronary syndromes: Acute myocardial infarct and ischemia. In: Chan TC, Brady WJ, Harrigan RA, Ornato JP, Rosen P, eds. *ECG in Emergency Medicine and Acute Care.* Philadelphia: Elsevier; 2005:151–169.

40 Birnbaum Y, Chetrit A, Sclarovsky S, et al. Abnormal Q waves on the admission electrocardiogram of patients with first acute myocardial infarction: Prognostic implications. *Clin Cardiol.* 1997;20:477–481.

41 Stellpflug SJ, Holger JS, Smith SW. What are the electrographically silent areas of the heart? In: Brady WJ, Truwit

JD, eds. *Critical Decisions in Emergency & Acute Care Electrocardiography.* West Sussex, UK: Wiley-Blackwell; 2009:167–175.

42 Whitwam W, Smith SW. Does localization of the anatomic segment/identification of the infarct-related artery affect early care? In: Brady WJ, Truwit JD, eds. *Critical Decisions in Emergency & Acute Care Electrocardiography.* West Sussex, UK: Wiley-Blackwell; 2009:204–215.

43 O'Laughlin DT, Bachour K, Whitwam W. What are the ECG indications for additional electrocardiographic leads (including electrocardiographic body-surface mapping in Chest Pain Patients?) In: Brady WJ, Truwit JD, eds. *Critical Decisions in Emergency & Acute Care Electrocardiography.* West Sussex, UK: Wiley-Blackwell; 2009:128–137.

44 Moye S, Carney MF, Holstege C, et al. The electrocardiogram in right ventricular myocardial infarction. *Am J Emerg Med.* 2005;23:793–799.

45 Brady WJ, Perron AD, Ullman EA, et al. Electrocardiographic ST-segment elevation: A comparison of AMI and non-AMI ECG syndromes. *Am J Emerg Med.* 2002;20(7):609–612.

46 Brady WJ, Lentz B, Barlotta K, et al. ECG patterns confounding the ECG diagnosis of acute coronary syndrome: Left bundle branch block, right ventricular paced rhythms, and left ventricular hypertrophy. *Emerg Med Clin N Am.* 2005;23:999–1025.

47 Sgarbossa EB, Pinski, SL, Barbagelata A, et al. Electrocardiographic diagnosis of evolving acute myocardial infarction in the presence of left bundle-branch block. *N Engl J Med.* 1996;334(8):481–487.

48 Tabas JA, Rodriguez RM, Seligman HK, et al. Electrocardiographic criteria for detecting acute myocardial infarction in patients with left bundle branch block: A meta-analysis. *Ann Emerg Med.* 2008;52:329–336.

49 Klimczak A, Wranicz JK, Cygankiewicz I, et al. Electrocardiographic diagnosis of acute coronary syndromes in patients with left bundle branch block or paced rhythm. *Cardiol J.* 2007;4:207–13.

50 Sgarbossa EB, Pinski SL, Gates KB, et al. Early electrocardiographic diagnosis of acute myocardial infarction in the presence of ventricular paced rhythm. *Am J Cardiol.* 1996;77:423–424.

51 Harrigan RA, DeAngelis MA. Evaluation and management of patients with chest syndromes. In: Mattu A, Goyal D, eds. *Emergency Medicine: Avoiding the Pitfalls and Improving the Outcomes.* Malden, MA: Blackwell Publishing; 2007:1–14.

52 Pope JH, Ruthazer R, Kontos MC. The impact of electrocardiographic left ventricular hypertrophy and bundle branch block on the triage and outcome of ED patients with a suspected acute coronary syndrome: A multicenter study. *Am J Emerg Med.* 2004;22:156–163.

23 Cardiac markers

J. Stephen Bohan

Executive Vice Chair, Department of Emergency Medicine, Brigham and Women's Hospital, Assistant Professor of Medicine, Harvard Medical School, Boston, Massachusetts, USA

Section I: Case presentation

A 45-year-old woman who complained of substernal chest pain radiating to the left arm, neck, and back presented to the emergency department (ED). The pain began about 12 hours before presentation. She had a history of "microvascular angina," and had been seen and evaluated multiple times for similar symptoms by the cardiology service at this hospital. There was a recent cardiology note in the electronic record stating that they have attempted to control her symptoms with nitroglycerin on a prn basis. The patient had taken 15 nitroglycerin tables on the day of presentation, and noted that she did have some relief, but it did not completely resolve the pain, so she came in for further evaluation. She also stated that she had right upper quadrant pain that is chronic for her. She specifically denied any diaphoresis, headache, or visual change. She denied nausea, dizziness, syncope or near syncope, weakness, dyspnea, ankle swelling, orthopnea, or paroxysmal nocturnal dyspnea. She did not have a cough.

The past medical history was significant for long-standing chest pain with a negative cardiac catheterization 18 months ago, along with no hypertension, diabetes, oral contraceptive use, or hyperlipidemia. She had two pregnancies, and has two living children. She had regular periods that ended two years prior. There was no history of venous thrombosis or cancer. Her only medication was a daily aspirin. The family history was noteworthy for a father who died at age 66 of a heart attack; he had been a life-long smoker. The patient was a nonsmoker. She drank 2–4 glasses of wine per month.

On physical examination she was comfortable while recumbent on a gurney. The vital signs were: pulse 74 beats/min and regular; blood pressure 180/103 mmHg; respirations 15 breaths/min; temperature 98.6°F; O_2 saturation 98%. There was no jugular venous distention at 30 degrees; the point of maximum impulse was normal, and there was no thrill. The peripheral pulses were normal. There was a normal S1S2 without murmur, rub, or gallop. The chest cardiac sound was without crackles or wheezes. The abdomen had no scars, and was soft and nontender, despite the complaints of chronic pain mentioned above. Laboratory evaluation showed a normal complete blood count, metabolic panel, and cardiac enzymes. The chest X-ray study was normal with no infiltrates and a normal hilum. The EKG was normal in all respects.

The patient was given one dose of IV metoprolol, and the blood pressure fell to 158/93 mmHg. The patient's cardiologist was inclined to discharge the patient, but he and the emergency physician concluded that it would be more prudent to ensure that the patient's blood pressure was better controlled before discharge. The plan was as follows: "We have decided to admit to the Observation Unit for both blood pressure control with her oral antihypertensives,

---

Cardiovascular Problems in Emergency Medicine: A discussion-based review, First Edition.
Edited by Shamai A. Grossman and Peter Rosen.
© 2011 John Wiley & Sons, Ltd. Published 2011 by John Wiley & Sons, Ltd.

in addition to the one dose of IV metoprolol that we gave her, and also pain control so that we hope to get her pain free. Once this is accomplished, and after she has two sets of negative markers, we will discharge her home. The pain has been going on for approximately 13 hours, and given this, I feel that two sets of markers are appropriate. Disposition: Admit to Observation Unit for pain control . . ."

Subsequently an addendum was dictated: "This is an addendum to the note I dictated earlier on this patient. The patient initially had a set of negative cardiac markers, and had remained chest pain free throughout her entire stay in the observation unit; however, her B set of cardiac markers shows a troponin of 64 and a repeat to ascertain whether or not this was a true value showed a troponin level of 114. EKGs throughout this interval have not shown any ST-segment changes, and the patient remains pain free. We discussed this with her cardiologist, and she will be admitted."

Section II: Case discussion

Dr David Brown: How much stock do you place in the initial set of cardiac biomarkers being normal, particularly in the context of her symptoms persisting for 12 hours?

Dr Shamai Grossman: The issue of a single set of cardiac markers is a controversial one, and unfortunately there is little data that look specifically at a single set of cardiac markers as a reliable test to demonstrate a patient has not had an acute myocardial infarction. There is one study, by a group of us at Massachusetts General Hospital, in which we find that a single set of cardiac markers drawn about 8 hours from the onset of symptoms is very sensitive, in a range of about 95%, a number quite similar to serial cardiac markers.[1] This data makes sense logically given that the sensitivity of serial troponins drawn 3 and 9 hours from the onset of symptoms is about 95%. The problem with a single set of cardiac markers is that the average patient arrives about 3 hours from the onset of symptoms, and at 3 hours a single set of markers has a very low sensitivity. In this particular case, the patient came approximately 12 hours after the onset of symptoms, which places her outside the norm, and because she was no longer the average patient,

a single set of enzymes may be useful, as we showed in our study.

Dr Peter Rosen: The problem is often timing the onset of the symptoms that relate to the present problem. It is possible that this patient's symptoms were stuttering, and that the true ischemia did not start 12 hours prior, but rather just before she came to the ED.

DB: Does a normal cardiac catheterization 18 months previous help you in your confidence that she does not have an acute coronary syndrome at this point?

Dr Stephen Bohan: It would boost my confidence, but not to 100%. About 90% of people who have a normal cardiac catheterization will, when repeated, even up to 7 or 8 years later, still have normal coronary arteries. However, there is a recent phenomenon of women who have a "chest pain syndrome," and cardiac catheterization shows normal or minimally-diseased coronary arteries. The outcome in this patient population 5 years later turns out to be worse than women who are asymptomatic, so there's probably something different about women, particularly in the subset of women who have a recurrent chest pain syndrome.

PR: About 30 years ago, there was a description of women who had chest pain but no EKG changes, and who on coronary angiography had right coronary artery spasm. This was prior to troponin measurements, so it is not possible to know if the lack of flow during spasm was producing necrosis, although some of the patients did evolve an inferior wall myocardial infarction.

DB: Does the combination of the normal coronary artery angiogram 18 months ago, coupled with the normal initial set of cardiac markers, make you feel comfortable sending this patient home without further treatment or evaluation?

SB: This is an interesting phenomenon. Here, we're unable to tell when ischemia ended and infarction began. Almost all people short of an unequivocal ST-segment elevation myocardial infarction (STEMI) and a complete occlusion have some degree of ischemia before the heart shows evidence of an infarct. We don't know when that transition occurs. In addition, there's a fundamental question we must ask when practicing emergency medicine, which is why did she come now, why did she not come at hour four, hour seven, or hour nine? Why did she wait 12 hours? What happened at 12 hours to make her come?

SG: What you're really saying is that you cannot trust the patient who tells you that it's been the same for 12 hours. Maybe it's not really the same.

SB: In addition, a joint statement from the American College of Cardiology and the European Society of Cardiology recommends a set of biomarkers on presentation and another 6 hours later. It does admit that the symptoms may exist a while before that.

SG: Is there a way in your mind to identify which of those women are more likely to actually have microvascular disease, and which are less likely to have this process?

SB: I don't know that there's any way to really detect them, other than that they're symptomatic. Although the overall event rate is low, it is still substantially higher than the rate in a group of asymptomatic women who were the control group.

DB: Does that leave us in the position of having to admit and rule out that cadre of patients—young women with normal EKGs and atypical stories?

SB: I think that sometimes it is a gut feeling or a clinical judgment. Remember, the prevalence of coronary heart disease in pre-menopausal women is extremely low, but at the same time we know that symptomatic women, even with normal coronary arteries, do have a higher rate of incidence than asymptomatic women.

SG: If you look at the various studies that have studied the patients inadvertently discharged home from the ED with an unrecognized myocardial infarction, one of the more common misses is the young woman. Clearly, we do need to be more discerning and pay closer attention to these patients.

DB: Why don't we go ahead and discuss the emergency department course?

SB: Her cardiologist was consulted on the basis of the initial biomarkers and EKG. The cardiologist felt that she could probably be safely discharged, given the negative catheterization, but the emergency physician concluded that the blood pressure was substantially high on presentation, and was still abnormal after treatment. He suggested that they put her in the observation unit for both blood pressure control, and to see if they could control her pain, and rule out a very unlikely myocardial infarction (MI). The physician

thought that once this was accomplished, and after a second set of negative markers, they would be able to discharge her home.

SG: Can you identify patients who you think are the appropriate population for an ED observation unit? Are there certain patients who you think belong there?

SB: In our ED, if you have a normal initial set of markers and a normal EKG, you're suitable for the observation unit, and if we think that it's important to control mildly elevated blood pressure, the observation unit would also be suitable.

SG: What would it take to make that patient ineligible for the observation unit? Who would you not put in there?

SB: Our exclusion criteria are an abnormal set of biomarkers, particularly troponin, because that's a myocardial infarction by definition, and new EKG changes or an abnormal EKG, not known to be old.

DB: As many patients come in with a story that is atypical and abnormal EKGs with no access to their old tracings, we tend to be a little less restrictive in our observation unit, and place patients there whom we believe to be low likelihood to have positive testing, and have a high likelihood of going home in 18–24 hours.

SG: I would tend to concur with you, as did the Faroukh et al. study a number of years ago. This study demonstrates the safety of an intermediate-risk patient population in an observation unit.[2] The idea is that if you're not sending the patient home, then you have most of the same monitoring capacities in the observation unit that you have anywhere else in the hospital, and if the patient evolves evidence of an infarction or more evidence of an acute coronary syndrome, then you can always transfer the patient to a higher acuity bed.

SB: It's just that we happen to be quicker and cheaper in the observation unit than upstairs.

PR: I wonder whether approaching this patient as having cardiac ischemia is the right approach at all. This is a patient who is described as having ongoing abdominal discomfort as well as chest discomfort, and we need to be concerned that perhaps this is not cardiac ischemia at all, and maybe what is being missed here is gall bladder disease. We do know there is overlap of symptoms between cardiac and gall bladder diseases, and sometimes we become so focused upon the cardiac diagnosis that we forget the possibility of alternative concomitant diseases.

DB: The way that this case is described, the pain is unchanged from her baseline right upper quadrant pain. I think that it becomes more of an issue if the pain in the right upper quadrant is different or if the examination is concerning.

SB: I agree. Her principal complaint is unequivocally chest pain. She notes the abdominal pain as being chronic, but what brought her to the ED was persistent chest pain. Someone once said that a lot of people have had coronary bypasses for gall bladder disease, and a lot of people have had their gall bladder out for coronary heart disease.

DB: You're right that gallbladder disease can present with chest pain, back pain, or flank pain in addition to, or instead of, right upper quadrant pain, but in my experience, the discomfort can be elicited on physical examination, either in the right upper quadrant or in the flank when the gallbladder is inflamed. In addition, in this particular case, the woman is able to make a distinction between her chest pain, which is different and new in onset, from her abdominal pain, which is chronic and unchanged. Couple that with a physical examination that elicits no right upper quadrant or flank tenderness, gallbladder disease has considerably lower probability, and should not require any further evaluation in the ED in the absence of vomiting, fever, or other concerning findings on examination.

PR: Nevertheless, given the increasing capacity of the emergency physician to utilize bedside ultrasound imaging, it wouldn't take much time to examine the gall bladder with an ultrasound in the ED, and order a formal study only if something abnormal is discovered.

DB: This patient was admitted to the observation unit, was given an intravenous beta-blocker, and I presume started on an oral antihypertensive agent, since previously she had not been on one. She was then observed for a period of several hours, and had a second set of cardiac markers. The second set of cardiac markers showed a troponin of 64 µg/L, and when repeated to ascertain whether or not this was a true value, the

troponin was 114 µg/L. The EKGs throughout this interval did not show ST-segment changes and the patient remained painfree. At this point she is admitted to cardiology. I'm very troubled by this case. At times, I have decided that a single set of cardiac markers in a low-risk patient with continuous chest pain, particularly when they have had prior testing, is adequate to exclude the presence of a myocardial infarction, and been satisfied that the chest pain was noncardiac. In this case, a cardiac catheterization, the most definitive of tests, was done within the last 18 months, which I think is a reasonable time interval. Now, despite the negative coronary angiogram and what sounds like multiple evaluations, she's ruling in for some myocardial necrosis or a non-ST-segment elevation MI, without any significant clues other than a prolonged episode of chest pain.

SB: No matter what we think about, there's always one person, out of the entire population we see, who is going to upset our theories. Judd Hollander has tried to look for a group of people who he felt could safely be discharged from the ED after presenting with chest pain; the criteria were no risk factors, age less than 40 years, a normal EKG, and one set of normal enzymes. He found no bad outcomes at 30 days.[3] This patient doesn't fulfill these criteria exactly because she's over 40. Secondly, it comes back to what I mentioned earlier, which is that there's something about this patient that brought her to the ED this time.

SG: Perhaps we don't understand what microvascular angina is on a pathophysiologic basis. She does carry this strange diagnosis, and perhaps that actually should have raised some red flags, and that's the key to this case. There's reassuring data using a protocol consisting of a single set of enzymes and rapid stress testing in the ED. Looking at this patient, do you think this might have been an appropriate approach?

DB: I would not have chosen that protocol in this particular patient because my pretest probability that she has epicardial coronary artery disease with a negative catheterization 18 months ago is so low that I feel it wouldn't be necessary. Frankly, if she weren't hypertensive, I would have sent her home based on a single negative marker, the history of the normal coronary angiogram, the normal EKG, and the normal set of markers. The hypertension seemed to help in this case, in a way, because it got her admitted. I might still have sent her home if her blood pressure fell on its own, without much treatment, and I would have ascribed the hypertension to anxiety or pain or fear.

I have occasionally used a single set of markers and a stress test. For example, if the duration of pain was sufficiently long enough ago in onset that the first set of markers should have been accurate, and if she was pain free after 12 hours of symptoms in the ED and had a negative set of markers, she could have gotten a stress test in our institution. If she were still having pain, or if her pain were only within 2–3 hours of symptom onset, then she would not have gotten a stress test. A low-risk patient like this, with no known coronary disease, a normal EKG, and symptoms that are somewhat atypical, is a good candidate for a coronary CT scan. If the test is completely normal, you can feel comfortable with the patient not having coronary artery disease.

SB: In this case I would argue as Goldman and Kirtane did in 2003, in the Annals of Internal Medicine, "If you think enough to do the first set, then you are obliged to do the second set."[4]

DB: Is that 6 hours after the first set or 6 hours after the resolution of pain?

SB: People used to talk about the resolution of pain, but the ACC guidelines for myocardial infarction in 2007 talk about after the first set.

DB: What then would you recommend to the practicing emergency physician who walks into a patient's room, hears the story, feels that it is atypical, with an EKG that is normal, but as part of the standard chest pain protocol, the first set of markers has already been sent off?

SB: I think that the emergency physician needs to ask himself four questions sequentially for any patient who could be having cardiac ischemia or infarction, and the first question is, "Is this patient having an ST-segment elevation MI, and do I need to do anything about it right now?" If the answer to that is no, then the next question is, "Could this patient be having a myocardial infarction of the type that I don't need to deal with right now, but a myocardial infarction nonetheless?" That question, in my mind, is only answerable by enzymes, and the current literature supports two sets taken 6 hours apart. Then there is a third question: "If those are negative, does this patient have ischemia as

the cause of a disease that did not cause infarction?" The answer to that has to be a separate question, with a separate testing mode, and that is where CT angiography and provocative testing may come in. Although the CT scan is a very attractive test, there's only one ED study, containing 568 patients, that says that if you have a TIMI score of one or less, with one set of enzymes and a CT angiography that is normal (by definition less than a 40% obstruction), then those patients can go home and will have no adverse events within 30 days.[5]

SG: I might look at this case a little differently. People often mistakenly call normal coronary angiography a catheterization where there was no significant disease, and it's likely this patient really did have coronary disease, but it was insignificant. The patient may have had 30 or 50% stenoses 18 months ago, and, therefore, it was a relevant study 18 months ago, but not as relevant today.

SB: When we say normal, obviously every study has a different definition of normal. There's "perfectly normal," meaning no disease at all, then there is some disease. In 2009, in an article termed "Adverse cardiac outcomes in women with non-obstructive coronary artery disease," Gulati and Cooper-DeHoff divided the patients into those who had 1–50% obstruction and those who had zero obstruction, followed them for 5 years, and compared them to asymptomatic women.[6] Of the women who did have some disease, they had a higher incidence of adverse events compared to those who had no demonstrable anatomic disease. Nevertheless, patients who had no demonstrable anatomic disease still had a higher event rate than the asymptomatic patients. This case does emphasize the utility of two sets of enzymes, as somewhere in those 12 hours, this patient infarcted, and we otherwise couldn't tell that.

SG: I might make the argument that perhaps that we are all at fault for being unable to get enough history from this patient about what happened in the course of those 12 hours. Clearly, if she's bumping her enzymes now, there was something that did change over the course of those 12 hours. Unless she's truly, truly an outlier, the inciting event was probably somewhere around hour six or so.

SB: In our department we can exercise people based on their history, without evidence of enzyme elevations, when we think that the history that they are giving us is very much like what you would get in an office visit. "Oh yes, doctor, when I go up to get my mail in the morning up the hill, I get pain, but it doesn't happen in the summer, but in the winter it comes, and my wife sent me here . . ." and that's an office visit. In that kind of situation, you're not wondering if this patient has an infarction; you just want to know if this patient has obstructive coronary heart disease, and we can send patients for exercise testing on this basis.

SG: I would argue that despite Goldman and Kirtane's concerns, simply because someone sent a test in error doesn't mean that you need to make a second error. We don't always have control over every test in the ED, but that shouldn't change what our thinking was in the first place. We don't need to say that we base all of our thinking and all of our clinical judgment on testing; rather, our thinking is based on our clinical judgment.

SB: Are we, as a group or as an industry, trying to push for one enzyme because we are being forced by overcrowding rather than the literature supporting this decision making, or do we feel deprived in our judgment? A doctor's clinical judgment in assigning a diagnosis of noncardiac chest pain is clearly fallible. About 3% of people who have been determined, by physicians from six academic centers, to have noncardiac chest pain experience cardiac events within 30 days.

SG: I think the argument is a logical one. We know the pharmacokinetics of troponin, and we know that troponin peaks 6–8 hours from the onset of symptoms. If we can clearly define when the symptoms were, then we should know when the enzymes should be elevated, and have an idea that when enzymes are negative, they are negative. I think that this is the argument that people have used, and although it's true that logic doesn't always work in medicine, it's always the way we try and practice.

SB: Two newer, more-sensitive troponin assays have recently been described. These assays allow earlier detection of MI; however, whether they improve patient outcomes remains to be seen. With the new assays, as with current assays, sensitivity for unstable angina is inadequate, and discharging a patient after a single troponin test may still be imprudent.[7-9]

PR: Since we don't know if the patient has been having coronary artery spasm, and since we don't know what

spasm does to enzyme elevation, perhaps the clue to this case is a woman with persistent, but increasing, pain. Rather than trying to decide with a single set of enzymes, serial enzymes would then make a lot of sense. Moreover, while most patients may have a slower rate of progression than 18 months, that surely can't fit all patients. I would have been much happier about the normal angiogram if it were 3–6 months ago. Finally, as was already mentioned, we don't know what negative meant in that study.

Case resolution

During admission, the patient was sent for a cardiac catheterization that showed a totally occluded obtuse marginal branch of the left circumflex artery. This was successfully opened, and a stent was placed. On review of the prior catheterization, a 40–50% occlusion of that artery was evident. The patient had an uneventful recovery, and was symptom free at 30 days.

Section III: Concepts

"The sobering bottom line is that two decades of research has taught us that without compelling evidence of a noncardiac cause, there is no absolutely fail-safe way to exclude myocardial ischemia or infarction at the time of a patient's initial presentation." The emergency physician, when faced with a patient whose symptoms suggest cardiac ischemia or infarction, needs to answer four questions:

1 Is this patient having a myocardial infarction?
2 If not, does this patient have unstable angina?
3 If not, does this patient have cardiac ischemia as the cause for his/her symptoms?
4 Is it safe to send this patient home?

Answering these questions sequentially enables risk stratification, as the three entities that form the basis of these questions have sequentially less risk of adverse outcomes. We can never achieve a zero risk because of the vagaries of human diseases, our abilities to interpret the histories, and the reality that we can never practice perfect medicine, but at some level of risk it is safe to send a patient home.

In 1979 the World Health Organization defined acute myocardial infarction with three parts: characteristic chest pain of greater than 10 minutes duration, evolutionary EKG changes (ST-segment elevation with subsequent normalization and the development of Q waves), and a rise in the total creatine kinase (CK), with greater than 5% identified as the MB band.[2,3,7-10] Subsequently, it became apparent that there were individuals who incurred myocardial cell death who did not manifest the defined EKG changes, (and in some cases had no EKG changes). This group of non-ST-segment MIs had heterogeneous EKG changes, and were initially termed non-Q wave MIs; these patients were found to have a worse prognosis than the archtypical ST elevation MI. These heterogeneous variants came to be grouped together as non-STEMIs, or NSTEMI.

Twenty-one years later, and about 10 years after the introduction of troponin testing (which had proven to be both more sensitive and more specific than CK-MB and had a much greater prognostic accuracy), the American College of Cardiology and the European Society of Cardiology developed a new definition based almost exclusively on troponins.[11] This definition requires a rise and fall in the troponin level in a patient who has presenting features that could be consistent with myocardial ischemia. This definition was revised in 2007 to reflect the growing awareness of the phenomenon of small rises in the troponin level resulting from procedures, as well to include those patients who die before any testing can be done.[12] EKG changes are no longer a necessary element of the diagnosis of acute myocardial infarction (Table 23-1).

By this definition, all patients with symptoms compatible with ischemia who are troponin positive at any level of abnormality (higher than the 99th percentile of a healthy cohort) have had a myocardial infarction. A further classification was done to organize clinical events according to pathophysiology (Table 23-2).

The chemical diagnosis of myocardial infarction

There are three markers used in contemporary testing: myoglobin, creatine kinase, and troponin. Myoglobin is present at about 2.5 hours after cardiac injury, and while highly sensitive, it is notably nonspecific. It does, however, have a high negative predictive value (99%) when the degree of rise is considered in the decision.[13]

Creatine kinase and its subunits have been the workhorse markers of the past 40 years; however, they have been replaced by troponin testing as the preferred marker, as noted in the 2007 definition document.[12]

There are two cardiac troponins: troponin T and troponin I; they are proteins that control the interaction between actin and myosin during muscle contraction. A form of troponin T exists in skeletal muscle as well (though is not detected by the latest generation troponin T testing), while the troponin I is not found outside the heart.

The methodology for troponin T testing is a patented process, and therefore the same irrespective of the location of testing. As a result, the range of normal values is also the same. Conversely, there are multiple patented methods for testing for troponin I, and each has its own range of normal values, which are not comparable to other methods or institutions. The ESC/ACC consensus document recommends that each institution establish its own 99th percentile of the normal population.[12] The ESC/ACC also states that there is a binary classification for troponin I levels: normal and abnormal, with no intermediate levels in between. There is evidence to support this convention (Figure 23-1), as even the lowest levels of abnormality are associated with worse cardiac outcomes in patients with acute coronary syndromes than those

Table 23-1. Criteria for acute myocardial infarction.

The term myocardial infarction should be used when there is evidence of myocardial necrosis in a clinical setting consistent with myocardial ischemia. Under these conditions any one of the following criteria meets the diagnosis for myocardial infarction: Detection of rise and fall of cardiac biomarkers (preferably troponin) with at least one value about the 99th percentile of the upper reference limit (URL) together with evidence of myocardial ischemia with at least one of the following:
- Symptoms of ischemia
- EKG changes indicative of new ischemia (new ST-T or new left bundle branch block [LBBB])
- Development of pathological Q waves in the ECG
- Imaging evidence of new loss of viable myocardium or new regional wall motion abnormality

Source: *Eur Heart J.* 2007;28:2525–2538.

Table 23-2. Clinical classification of different types of myocardial infarction.

Type 1
Spontaneous myocardial infarction related to ischemia due to a primary coronary event such as plaque erosion or rupture, fissuring, or dissection.

Type 2
Myocardial infarction secondary to ischemia due to either increased oxygen demand or decreased supply, e.g., coronary artery spasm, coronary embolism, anemia, dysrhythmias, hypertension, or hypotension.

Type 3
Sudden unexpected cardiac death, including cardiac arrest, often with symptoms suggestive of myocardial ischemia, accompanied by presumably new ST elevation, or new LBBB, or evidence of fresh thrombus in a coronary artery by angiography or at autopsy, but death occurring before blood samples could be obtained, or at a time before the appearance of cardiac biomarkers in the blood.

Source: *Eur Heart J.* 2007;28:2525–253.

with normal levels; this phenomenon continues across all levels of abnormality (the higher the abnormality, the worse the prognosis). Moreover, there is some evidence that the presence of any detectable troponin (by current methods) is abnormal, and is associated with a worse natural history. Studies have shown that individuals who have detectable but normal troponin levels often have heart failure, diabetes, or left ventricular hypertrophy.[14,15] The full clinical implications of this phenomenon are as yet unknown, and should not enter into the decision making in the ED.

The release of small amounts of intracellular troponin from the injured cell is not immediately detectable by assays in current use. Nevertheless, these assays can detect larger amounts resulting from degradation of structural troponin within 3 hours of release in 80% of patients. This interval is not much different than that achieved by the inclusion of myoglobin in the testing scheme, and troponin also provides a much higher specificity.[16] Serial testing of troponin levels, beginning at 6 hours, captures the remainder of cases, and testing for peak troponin

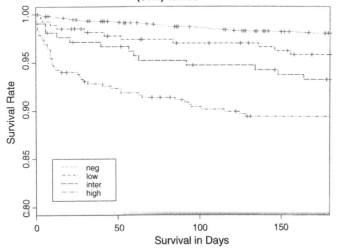

Kaplan-Meier curves of six-month cardiac mortality for the different cardiac troponin I (cTnI) values

Kontos, M. C. et al. J Am Coll Cardiol 2004;43:958-965

Figure 23.1 Kaplan-Meier curves of six-month cardiac mortality for the different cardiac troponin I (cTnI) values. The trend toward increased mortality and increased cTnI is highly significant (p < 0.001). In addition, mortality is significantly different (p < 0.01) between the negative (neg) cTnI and low, intermediate (inter), and high cTnI groups.

aids in prognostication and choice of therapy, as troponin-positive NSTEMI patients experience distinct, well-proven benefit from anticoagulants and invasive therapy.[17]

Because troponin stays in the serum for as long as 14 days, it can be difficult to detect a later reinfarction, this long half-life is the only reason in contemporary practice for ordering a CK, as CK is cleared rapidly within 36–48 hours, and thus, allows for detection of reinfarction if used after this time period. CK does not provide earlier detection of MI than current troponin assays, and has shown to be normal when the troponin is positive. The prognosis of patients with discordant markers is related solely to troponin positivity, as troponin positive and CK negative patients have a worse prognosis than those patients who are troponin negative and CK positive.[18] The latter group has a relative risk very close to baseline (Figure 23-2). It is because of these test characteristics that troponin is now the preferred maker in current guidelines, and has come to form the definition of myocardial infarction.[12]

The degree of troponin elevation is of interest, in that it appears to reflect two separate pathophysiologic processes. Coronary artery plaque rupture, either on a macro level resulting in a STEMI, or on a micro level resulting in a shower of microemboli, yields troponin elevations at high multiples of normal, and patients with the highest troponin levels usually have visible thrombosis and depressed left ventricular function. Conversely, in patients whose symptoms are not predominately of cardiac ischemia, but who are seriously ill with other syndromes (e.g., sepsis, pulmonary edema), troponin levels may only be 3–4 times normal levels, known colloquially as a "troponin leak." These microinfarctions are thought to result more from demand/supply mismatch (type 2 infarction) (Table 23-2) than active vessel wall disease.[11] However, because of the inherent seriousness of the active pathophysiology, the prognosis of these patients is as poor as or worse than those with higher troponin levels resulting from active vessel wall disease.[3,19]

Patients with renal failure often have particularly high baseline troponin levels, more often when troponin T is measured than with troponin I. Usually these patients also have substantial vascular disease, and thus are prone to acute coronary syndrome, resulting in a confounding situation for the clinician. Nevertheless, in a group of more than 7,000 selected patients, "troponin T elevation is an independent predictor of death or myocardial infarction within 30 days across the entire spectrum of renal function."[20] Additionally, in a study of more than 800 patients (including some on dialysis) troponin I levels are independent of renal function, and no false positive elevations of troponin I occur.[21] In contrast, CK-MB and myoglobin elevations in this study are related to renal function.

Low but abnormal levels of troponin are also detectable in patients with trauma, and in marathon runners, but this does not appear to mark a deleterious effect.[22] The current hypothesis is that in otherwise healthy individuals, repair takes place. Because these patients do not have symptoms of ischemia, or evidence of supply/demand mismatch, they do not fit the operative definition of myocardial infarction. Additionally, the elevated troponin in these otherwise well, nonacute coronary syndrome cases is cleared within 24 hours, in marked distinction to those with an acute coronary syndrome.[23]

Patients who are troponin negative after serial testing have not had a myocardial infarction, and question one of the four questions above has been answered. However, this does not mean that they do not have ischemia as the cause of their symptoms, and except for a small segment of the patient population who are less than 40 years old and have certain other

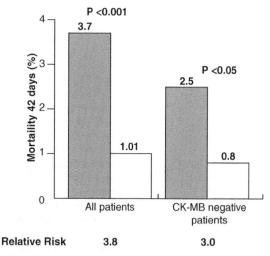

Figure 23.2 Relative risk of death at 42 days in troponin positive vs. troponinnegative patients related to CK MB status

characteristics, they should undergo further testing before discharge in order to answer the remaining questions.[24]

Summary

In the current practice environment, missing an MI or ischemia is not an option. Fortunately, a structured approach, using the currently available technology, provides a safety net for the patient and the physician, as long as entry into the structured diagnostic scheme is kept wide with respect to symptoms. This wide entry and use of a protocol approach overcomes the demonstrably fallible judgment of physicians.[1]

Clearly, risk factors were not useful in assessing the patient discussed in the case above. The physicians caring for her did think enough of her symptoms, despite a "negative" catheterization only 18 months prior, to order an EKG and a marker. Ordering a marker is a manifestation of attempting to answer the question "Does this patient have an MI?", and that question can only be answered by serial troponins. If the answer to that question is no, then the remaining questions (Does this pain represent unstable angina? Does this symptom represent coronary ischemia? Can I safely send this patient home?) must still be answered.

The diagnosis of unstable angina is purely clinical, combining patient's history, serial EKGs, and the patient's course in the ED. The search for ischemic disease with stress testing or a CT scan should be done promptly (general agreement is within 72 hours), and can be done as an outpatient if the patient is given a scheduled test time before leaving, and is thought to be reliable with respect to keeping the appointment. Otherwise, the patient should be kept for further testing to detect ischemia or structural vascular disease.

Section IV: Decision making

- Ordering a marker may only answer the question "Does this patient have an MI?"
- The only cardiac markers that can rule out MI are serial troponins.
- Other criteria, such as clinical presentation, past medical history, stress testing, or cardiac

catheterization, must be employed to decide whether these symptoms represent unstable angina or coronary ischemia and whether a patient can safely be discharged home.

References

1 Goldman L, Kirtane AJ. Triage of patients with acute chest pain and possible cardiac ischemia: The elusive search for diagnostic perfection. *Ann Intern Med.* 2003;139:987–995.

2 Giillum RF, Fortmann SP, Prineas RJ, Kottke TE. International diagnostic criteria for acute myocardial infarction and acute stroke. *Am Heart J.* 1984;108: 150–158.

3 Marsan RJ, Shaver KJ, Sease KL, et al. Evaluation of a clinical decision rule for young adult patients with chest pain. *Acad Emerg Med.* 2005:12(1):26–31.

4 The Joint European Society of Cardiology/American College of Cardiology Committee. Myocardial infarction redefined: A consensus document of the Joint European Society of Cardiology/American College of Cardiology Committee for the redefinition of myocardial infarction. *Eur Heart J.* 2000;21:1502–1513.

5 Hollander JE, Chang AM, Shofer FS, et al. Coronary Computed Tomographic Angiography for Rapid Discharge of Low-Risk Patients with Potential Acute Coronary Syndromes. *Ann Emerge Med.* 2009;53:295–304.

6 Gulati M, Cooper-DeHoff RM, McClure C, et al. Adverse cardiovascular outcomes in women with nonobstructive coronary artery disease. *Arch Intern Med.* 2009;169: 843–850.

7 Thygesen, Alpert J, White HD, et al. Universal definition of myocardial infarction. *Eur Heart J.* 2007;28: 2525–2538.

8 Brogan GX, Friedman S, McCuskey C, et al. Evaluation of a new rapid quantitative immunoassay for serum myoglobin versus CK-MB for ruling out acute myocardial infarction in the emergency department. *Ann Emerg Med.* 1994;24:665–671.

9 Schulz O, Kirpal K, Stein J, et al. Importance of low concentrations of cardiac troponins. *Clin Chem.* 2006;52: 1614–1615.

10 Jaffe AS. Chasing troponin: How low can you go if you can see the rise? *J Am Coll Cardiol.* 2001;48:1763–1764.

11 Newby KL, Storrow AB, Gibler BW, et al. Bedside multimarker testing for risk stratification in chest pain units: The Chest Pain Evaluation by Creatinine Kinase-MB, Myoglobin and Troponin I (Checkmate) Study. *Circulation.* 2001;103(14):1832–1837.

12 Anderson JL, Adams CD, Antman EM, et al. ACC/AHA 2007 guidelines for the management of patients with

unstable angina/non ST-elevation myocardial infarction: A report of the ACC/AHA Task Force on practice guidelines. *Circulation.* 2007;116(7):e148–e304.

13 Storrow AB, Lindsell CJ, Han JH, et al. Discordant cardiac biomarkers: Frequency and outcomes in emergency department patients with chest pain. *Ann Emerg Med.* 2006;48: 660–665.

14 Lim W, Qushmaq I, Devereaus PJ, et al. Elevated cardiac troponin measurements in critically ill patients. *Arch Intern Med.* 2006;166:2446–2454.

15 Alcalai R, Planer D, Afsin C, et al. Acute coronary syndrome versus nonspecific troponin elevation: Clinical predictors and survival analysis. *Arch Intern Med.* 2007; 167(3):276–281.

16 Aviles RJ, Askari AT, Lindah B, et al. Troponin T levels in patients with acute coronary syndromes, with or without renal dysfunction. *N Engl J Med.* 2002;346: 2047–2052.

17 Kontos MD, Garg R, Anderson FP, et al. Outcomes in patients admitted for chest pain with renal failure and troponin I elevations. *Am Heart J.* 2005;150(4): 674–680.

18 Siegel AJ, Sholar M, Yang J, et al. Elevated serum cardiac markers in asymptomatic marathon runners after competition: Is the myocardium stunned? *Cardiology.* 1997; 88:487–491.

19 Hermann M, Scharhag J, Miclea M, et al. Post-race kinetics of cardiac troponin T and I and N-terminal pro brain natriuretic peptide in marathon runners. *Clin Chem.* 2003;49(5):831–832.

20 Nagurney J, Brown D, Chae C, et al. The sensitivity of cardiac markers stratified by symptom duration. *J Emerg Med.* 2005;29:409–415.

21 Farkouh ME, Smars PA, Reeder GS, et al. A clinical trial of a chest-pain observation unit for patients with unstable angina. *N Engl J Med.* 1998:339:1882–1888.

22 Reichlin T, Hochholzer W, Bassetti S, et al. Early diagnosis of myocardial infarction with sensitive cardiac troponin assays. *N Engl J Med.* 2009;361(9):858–867.

23 Keller T, Zeller T, Peetz D, et al. Sensitive troponin I assay in early diagnosis of acute myocardial infarction. *N Engl J Med.* 2009;361(9):868–877.

24 Morrow DA. Clinical application of sensitive troponin assays. *N Engl J Med.* 2009;361(9):913–915.

24 Stress testing

Jefferson Williams[1] & Shamai Grossman[2]

[1] EMS Fellow and Clinical Instructor, University of North Carolina Department of Emergency Medicine, Chapel Hill, North Carolina, USA
[2] Director, Cardiac Emergency Center and Clinical Decision Unit, Beth Israel Deaconess Medical Center, Assistant Professor of Medicine Harvard Medical School, Boston, Massachusetts, USA

Section I: Case presentation

A 49-year-old woman presented to the emergency department (ED) on a Friday evening asking to be evaluated for her recent chest discomfort. She stated that over the past few months, she had been under greater stress at work as a business executive, and had been rushing out the door to catch the early commuter train. Over the prior several weeks, she had occasionally felt a burning sensation in her chest while she was walking quickly, or jogging to catch the train. She had also been skipping breakfast and drinking more coffee, and initially attributed the chest burning to worsening of her known gastroesophageal reflux disease. She reported having to run to catch the train 2 days in a row, and on both days, she had severe chest burning that was associated with shortness of breath, which only resolved after 10–15 minutes of rest while sitting on the train. She was concerned about her heart, as her father died of a myocardial infarction at age 69.

In the ED, the patient was not currently complaining of any discomfort. She described the episodes of chest discomfort as epigastric and substernal burning, occasionally radiating as a sharp pain to her throat when severe, exacerbated by exercise and lasting 20–30 minutes, then relieved by rest. She had a past medical history of esophageal reflux, and has been told that she has a "minor valve problem" in her heart. The cholesterol level was "borderline" at her last primary care visit 1 year ago. She occasionally drank wine with dinner. She took no medications other than omeprazole. She neither smoked nor used illicit drugs. She was otherwise healthy.

The physical examination was notable for a BMI of 29. The vital signs were: resting heart rate 93 beats per minute, blood pressure 141/92 mmHg, respiratory rate 16 breaths per minute, and oxygen saturation 95%. There was a faintly audible mid-systolic click on cardiac auscultation. The remainder of the physical examination was unremarkable. A resting EKG demonstrated ST depression of 1 mm in lead III, T-wave flattening in leads III and aVF, and flipped T-waves in V1 and V2, with no prior tracing available for comparison. The ED physician was appropriately concerned regarding possible angina, and observed the patient for two sets of cardiac enzymes, which were normal, and serial EKGs, which were unchanged.

A standard exercise treadmill EKG stress was ordered, as that was the only stress test available on the weekend. During the stress test, the patient exercised for 6.5 minutes under a standard Bruce protocol, at which time she stopped due to fatigue and leg cramping. The maximal heart rate during the test was 140 beats per minute, just under 85% of predicted. She did not complain of any chest burning or abnormal shortness of breath, and the EKG showed ST depressions of

Cardiovascular Problems in Emergency Medicine: A discussion-based review, First Edition.
Edited by Shamai A. Grossman and Peter Rosen.
© 2011 John Wiley & Sons, Ltd. Published 2011 by John Wiley & Sons, Ltd.

1.5 mm in lead III and avF and flipped T waves in V1–V3. The patient had symptoms concerning for angina, and a borderline or indeterminate exercise tolerance test without imaging. It was Saturday morning, and the patient wanted to go home.

Section II: Case discussion

Dr Peter Rosen: Does this patient's BMI suggest that she's in the obese range?

Dr Shamai Grossman: Yes, it does.

PR: This is a very common history, a very common kind of patient to see in the ED, where we have to start by trying to distinguish between gastrointestinal and cardiac disease. Here we have a patient who could easily have both. And what are our obligations? Do you have any clues for separating out these two histories: the pain that she has now on exertion when going to the train, and the pain that she has had in the past thought to be esophageal reflux?

Dr Amal Mattu: It's interesting you pointed out that she actually may have both. There's a study that was done a few years ago that suggests that patients with underlying cardiac disease have a higher prevalence of underlying reflux disease as well.[1] Acute coronary syndrome (ACS) and reflux may then tend to coexist more often than they exist individually. The cardiology literature going back to the 1950s and 1960s has indicated that there is a "gastro-cardiac reflex" in which acute episodes of reflux can induce some cardiac ischemia on an EKG and cardiographic monitoring.[2] This makes distinguishing between the ACS and reflux very difficult. One must also keep in mind that reflux is the most common misdiagnosis in malpractice cases for a missed myocardial infarction (MI), hence physicians have to be extremely careful when discharging a patient with a diagnosis of reflux without fully considering the possibility that maybe they're missing an ACS. Unfortunately, I don't think there are reliable ways to tell the difference, and that's why we make the mistake so often in assuming the benign diagnosis. Therefore, in emergency medicine we must always first consider the worst case scenario, and assume it's ACS initially to be prudent. If we can acquire some negative evidence that it is not ACS, then we can conclude the problem is reflux. That negative evidence may require a stress test, or even a cardiac catheterization, as I don't think there are any good descriptions that patients can use that tell you that they have reflux and not ACS. Often patients will say they have "indigestion," yet rule in for ACS.

PR: A generic error in emergency medicine is to assume a patient has a diagnosis that can't be proved or disproved in the ED, and reflux is one of them. Many of our colleagues use the diagnosis of "reflux" because it requires much less workup, and enables a rapid discharge of the patient. However, I too, do not believe this diagnosis can be made based on history alone. Do you think that there's any utility in ordering a plain chest X-ray study to look for a hiatal hernia as evidence that the patient has reflux disease?

Dr William Brady: In the common undefined ED chest pain patient, a chest X-ray study can be helpful in providing alternative diagnoses, including the occasional hiatal hernia or other esophageal pathology, but there still may be coexisting ischemic heart disease. This is similar to obtaining a plain abdominal film to demonstrate constipation as the cause of abdominal pain. I would be very wary of this practice.

PR: President Eisenhower, when he had his first heart attack in office, was treated for 3 days for indigestion! Our patient has a history not only of reflux disease, but also has a history of a minor valve problem, and a click on examination. We know that floppy mitral valves can be associated not only with pain that sounds like angina, but can also evolve into other cardiac problems. How helpful is it that you hear the click, and that she has had this diagnosis in the past, or is this another confounder?

Dr David Brown: I believe the possible diagnosis of mitral valve prolapse to be another confounder here. Although patients with mitral valve prolapse may have chest pain syndromes not related to other cardiovascular disease, I would not rely on that as the diagnosis, particularly in a patient for whom you don't have definitive prior evaluation data to confirm that diagnosis. Given that there is so much overlap between ACS and all these other conditions, I believe these patients must have a period of evaluation in an ED or an ED-based observation area, and have some kind of provocative testing before it's safe to send them home.

PR: Along with an investigation of a potential ischemic coronary syndrome, would you send blood cultures and order an echocardiogram to be sure this isn't new-onset endocarditis?

WB: If there was some point in the history that would make me think of endocarditis, such as IV drug abuse, bacteremia, or ongoing subacute symptomatology like weakness, malaise, fever, a generic feeling of being unwell, or stigmata of embolization, I might explore it. Reading this story, I would not suspect endocarditis, so I would not pursue this diagnosis in this particular patient.

PR: Isn't endocarditis associated with mitral valve prolapse?

WB: Only if there is associated valvular dysfunction. Without other symptoms in the information we are given, I wouldn't explore it.

PR: Our European colleagues often do echocardiography on patients as part of their ischemic evaluation, as well as for other reasons. Is that a test that you think might have some utility in separating the gastrointestinal from the cardiac pathology?

SG: Sabia studied the utility of echocardiography to discern ischemic chest discomfort from nonischemic chest discomfort, and finds echocardiography to be a highly sensitive tool.[3] If a patient were to have a regional wall motion abnormality that disappears when the symptoms go away, that would be a very useful test to help discern whether this is ischemic symptomatology or nonischemic symptomatology. The problem with using echocardiography routinely in the ED is that it's operator dependent. In order to adequately identify a regional wall motion abnormality, one needs to be technically very adept at performing echocardiography and at reading echocardiography.

Echocardiography could potentially be very useful if we were all expert sonographers with vast expertise in identifying a regional wall motion abnormality. For valvular heart disease, one would also need expertise to utilize echocardiography.

WB. What about contrast echocardiography? My understanding is that although detecting wall motion abnormality is a difficult call to make for anyone, and clearly expertise is needed to make that call, with contrast echocardiography it's much easier to identify the endocardium, thus, wall motion abnormalities are easier to detect.

SG: I believe that although contrast may make identifying regional wall motion abnormalities easier, I am not convinced that it would adequately enable emergency physicians to become as facile as they are in using bedside ultrasound for abnormalities such as trauma and central line placement. I hope I am proven wrong.

PR: In this case we have an abnormal EKG with nothing to compare it to. How much trouble should you go to in trying to find another tracing? Do you need to call other hospitals, or doctors' offices? Are you comfortable enough in your decision making that in the absence of enzyme changes, it doesn't really matter what the prior EKG looked like?

DB: I would not go through a lot of trouble in this case tracking down old EKGs if they were not readily available in my own healthcare system. These findings aren't so worrisome to trigger a trip to the cardiac catheterization laboratory or something along those lines. And even if old EKGs were identical, it wouldn't reassure me enough to allow immediate discharge from the ED.

PR: This is the patient who is the curse of emergency medicine. We all agree that this patient needs investigation for an ischemic cardiac syndrome, but I doubt that any of us agree about what that investigation should be. Moreover, if we ask 100 cardiologists, we'd get 100 different answers depending on the time of the day, and whether or not they were responsible for doing the work. I doubt any cardiologist would take this patient to the catheterization laboratory. I think some cardiologists might admit the patient in order to obtain the next study, but there are many cardiologists who wouldn't even do that. Do you have any advice from your own institutions and your own cardiologists as to what the emergency physician can hope for next in the evaluation of this patient?

AM: That's a tough question. I think at our institution this patient would at the very least get a stress test, if not go directly to the catheterization laboratory, given that she has an abnormal EKG at rest, and a concerning story for what could be called true unstable angina with exertional chest pressure, even if it also sounds like reflux. I think most cardiologists would agree that this history is consistent with unstable angina, and she has a baseline abnormal EKG. Alternatively, the next best options would be to arrange very close follow up or even transfer to another institution where the cardiologists are more aggressive about their workups. I wouldn't feel comfortable discharging this patient home even after an observation period unless I knew that this patient was going be seen again in the next day or two. Even that would not be ideal.

DB: Before a stress test, would this patient go for a cardiac catheterization at your institution?

AM: At our institution, at the very least, she would get a stress test, and there are some cardiologists who would take her directly for catheterization given the abnormal EKG, cardiac risk factors, and history of worsening exertional symptoms over the past couple of weeks.

PR: Would they do the procedure at night? Or would they admit her, and perform it the next day?

AM: If she's asymptomatic and hemodynamically stable, I don't think any of them would perform the procedure that night nor in the next few hours, even if it was daytime. Nevertheless, I think that they would be fairly aggressive with this patient (even though there is no indication that she should be treated like a ST-segment elevation myocardial infarction, and go to the catheterization laboratory immediately).

WB: In someone who presents and remains symptom free, doesn't evolve the electrocardiogram, and has two markers that are negative in sequential fashion, I think you've clearly ruled out the presence of a ST-segment elevation myocardial infarction, non-ST-segment elevation myocardial infarction, and likely a more severe form of unstable angina, but you still haven't answered the question: "Are there symptomatic obstructive coronary lesions present?" I would admit her to an observation unit, and arrange an exercise test. But an exercise stress test in this population, particularly in a younger woman, may not be revealing. Many hospitals will not have this resource available on a Friday evening, and might not do anything with these patients until Monday. This hospital actually has the capability of stressing her, so that's what I would do. But, if you have a nondiagnostic result, then I think you need to take the next couple of steps, which would either be catheterization or a nuclear study or exercise echocardiography. I would be very uncomfortable discharging her. If you look at this patient, she is a very busy woman, and she's

already put this off for a probably excessively long period of time. She's going to have in her mind that she feels better, and the doctors let her go home, and therefore she doesn't need to follow up. I think we've all seen people who were discharged with the hope of near immediate follow up who end up back in the ED sick, or worse yet, arrest outside the hospital.

PR: I would have a hard time getting this patient admitted to a cardiologist in Jackson Hole, probably in Tucson, and also probably in Boston. I think that they might be willing to hold the patient in the ED to do a stress test, but I don't think they would be willing to put the patient in the hospital to obtain an exercise test or an imaging study.

SG: There are data that suggest that if a patient can go 6 minutes worth of exercise utilizing a standard Bruce protocol, then regardless of the results of that stress test the patient has an excellent prognosis, and should able to go home. Some of our cardiologists would say, "Well, the patient was able to do 6 and half minutes worth of exercise, so it doesn't matter what the stress test shows. She is going to do fine, and you can send her home. We'll follow her up on Monday."

DB: I think that it depends on how you're using the stress test, and how you present it to the patient. If we're using it to diagnose coronary artery disease, then we are using the test improperly. A nonimaging stress test is not a good diagnostic test for coronary artery disease. If we are using it to determine whether the patient is safe to go home once she has ruled out for an MI, and continue her activities of daily living while undergoing a reasonably prompt outpatient evaluation for a chest pain syndrome, then I think it is appropriate to do what you just described. In my institution, you would have three options with this patient. She would never get admitted to the hospital, and cardiology would never hear about her, unless you decide to choose option three. In my mind, she gets admitted to an observation unit, she gets ruled out for an MI, she gets a stress test (which would have the described equivocal results), and then you either keep her to do a stress test with imaging (option one), or (option two) you do a CT scan of her coronary arteries to determine whether she has coronary artery stenosis or not. She may be a great candidate for that considering she is young, and doesn't have any previous diagnosis of coronary artery disease. If her coronary arteries are clean, then she can be discharged quite safely. The third option is to send her home with a scheduled stress test or arrange with her cardiologist or internist to make sure they schedule her a stress test with imaging on the next business day. The ACC/AHA guidelines for patients like this recommend provocative testing within 72 hours if the patient is pain free. In my institution, the cardiologists would not admit her from the observation unit after this nondiagnostic treadmill test.

WB: I agree that it would be hard to get a cardiologist involved until she infarcted, and then we're all incorrect for having sent her home in the first place. Nevertheless, you really haven't answered the ultimate question as to whether this patient had cardiac ischemia. You've demonstrated that she is stable with a normal to near-normal electrocardiogram and two negative markers. There are some data to suggest that this person has a low negative 30-day event rate. Should you really obtain an advanced imaging study, like a stress test with a radionuclide, MIBI, or a stress ECHO before she goes home, or can we be comfortable doing these tests within 72 hours?

DB: I would be comfortable waiting 72 hours because I know I can personally schedule these tests for Monday morning. I think if she has good follow up with an internist or a cardiologist who can make sure this happens, that would be perfectly reasonable. In many institutions, if a patient had a nondiagnostic stress test, that patient would automatically be rolled over to a MIBI to get a better answer. But I think it's within the standard of care to allow her go home with the understanding that we haven't excluded coronary artery disease, but we have given her the opportunity to continue with her activities of daily living without much risk while she completes this workup as an outpatient.

PR: I am somewhat concerned about using a stress test on an obese patient whose only exercise is catching a train. I would predict that we would not be able to get a diagnostic treadmill test. In my mind, the real problem here is not whether she is having an MI; I think that we have successfully answered this question. I also would say that we have successfully answered that she's not having truly unstable angina. She almost falls into my definition of stable angina, in that she has to do something unusual in order to

get the discomfort. But we have not answered the question of, "Do we need to worry about this patient to the point of pushing her toward coronary catheterization?" I believe short of that, we are never going to get a good answer for this patient. However, I think the reality in most EDs in this country is that this woman is not admissible. So what it really boils down to in my mind is: if you can do an imaging study or a CT scan and get more evidence for plaque-coronary artery disease, you may have acquired enough evidence to get her an elective coronary angiography. If you can't get either of those, then the best that you can hope for is a cardiologist who will get her in early in the next week.

AM: I wonder if the reason we tend to be more aggressive is because our patients cannot get good follow up. In some ways this may be a blessing in disguise, because we tend to go ahead and try to get the workup sooner rather than discharging them for a 72-hour follow up despite the ACC/AHA guidelines. I wonder whether if in Boston there is a higher percentage of insured patients, and ironically, they end up waiting longer for a definitive workup than our uninsured patients.

DB: I would take the opposite approach. Let's say you catheterize this patient, and she has 60 or 70% lesion in her right coronary artery. We have no idea whether that is causing her symptoms or not, and in an aggressive institution she's going to get a stent placed, she is going to be on clopidogrel for a year, and then she's going to be at risk for in-stent stenosis in 2 years, and when and if that occurs, she will really need a procedure. In a less aggressive institution she's going to get a functional study, either a stress ECHO or a stress MIBI, in some reasonable time frame, either the next day, or in 72 hours, or even in the next week, and then if she has ischemia that's documented in that region, then proceeding with cardiac catheterization and placing a stent makes sense to me. But the alternative of catheterization based on a non-specific finding on a nonimaging stress test, I think, puts large groups of patients at risk for procedures they don't need.

SG: The literature bears this out somewhat. When they looked at the number of cardiac procedures in New England versus the rest of the United States, they find that the physicians in New England were far more conservative in performing invasive cardiac procedures, yet the outcomes in New England and the rest of the United States were the same. So we tend to do less, but our patients seem to do just as well, or perhaps just as poorly. The literature also suggests that with regards to stress testing, if a patient gets a stress test as an outpatient, or if a patient is scheduled for a stress test from the ED as an outpatient, they tend to have poorer outcomes when compared with patients who had their stress tests done in the ED. This makes sense in a patient population where most of those patients would not be compliant with a previously outpatient scheduled stress test that is easily scheduled. In Boston, our patients are well connected with their insurers and primary care physicians so that they will likely get their stress test regardless of whether it is as an inpatient, or in the ED, or shortly afterward as an outpatient. I think this too might influence the outcome in which the less aggressive physicians in Boston do not have worse outcomes than anyone else anywhere else in the country.

Yet there is another problem with taking many of the patients directly for catheterization. The literature also suggests that patients with angina have the same mortality rates when maximized on medical therapy when compared to invasive therapy.

PR: I have some problem with that data; mortality may not be the most appropriate endpoint, as I don't think medical therapy will permit the same magnitude of physical activities. To my mind it is a life quality question, not just a mortality question.

PR: If you were talking to a rural Virginia physician about this patient, would you accept her in-transfer on a Friday or Saturday, or would you just make an arrangement for her to come up on Monday?

WB: I wouldn't accept her in-transfer to the ED. If the transferring physician had concerns, and wanted the patient admitted to the hospital, I would refer that to the cardiologist. The initial ED evaluation process has been taken care of, and all I could offer is a parking spot waiting for her to be evaluated in some further fashion.

PR: Unfortunately, many of our emergency medicine colleagues are faced with this transfer decision because they can't get cardiologists to accept patients like this, and more unfortunately, sometimes they just arrive at your door.

WB: I think you have to put yourself in the position of a small five-bed ED where you don't even have a cardiologist, and they do stress tests Monday through Friday during bankers' hours; it is a very difficult situation for an emergency physician to be in.

DB: In a way that situation is almost easier. As an emergency physician in that situation, you have to admit the patient to the hospital. You can't get the stress test, you can't keep her in the ED for 12 hours to rule her out, and the patient can't go home without some sort of stress test. I think it's harder if you have some of the resources, but not all of the resources. It's harder if you get to the point where this case ends, but you can't obtain either a stress imaging test or schedule one for the first business day after she goes home.

WB: That's assuming that you can get a family practitioner or internist to admit these patients to the hospital. We have a number of small feeder hospitals in the area that don't want to take anything even close to unstable angina, no matter how stable it might be, so then you're almost back in that same position.

DB: This case is a perfect example of a case where I believe the standard of care for our specialty is going to change over the next few years. I think that she is a great candidate for a coronary CT scan. There is a large group of patients with no known coronary artery disease, a story that is both typical and atypical, and an EKG that is nondiagnostic, who will have a negative coronary CT angiography. The CT scan can be done 24/7 and the images sent anywhere in the world to be read by a competent radiologist. I personally think that we are going to see a change in practice over this next 3–5-year interval for patients just like this.

PR: One last question based on the facts of this case as presented. We have a patient who is going to move on to another kind of imaging study, and we have a weekend facing us. If you are working at an institution where the best you could arrange for this patient is home with a 72-hour follow-up, is there any special therapy that you would place the patient on while she is awaiting the stress test: plavix, low-molecular weight heparin, aspirin, or nothing?

DB: My vote would be for aspirin.

AM: My vote would be for aspirin, and a prescription for nitroglycerin with the instructions to return if she needs to take a couple.

AM: In conclusion, the standard of care is not determined by the four or five of us at major centers, but rather by what resources people have where they are. Patients need to understand that we're not going to be right every time. The standard of care means to be reasonable and prudent, but not necessarily ideal. The standard in hospitals with five-bed ERs may be very different, and perhaps discharging this patient is their standard. Patients need to be reasonable and understand that in this scenario, their doctor maybe doing the best this weekend that he can.

PR: What we're trying to do here is not define a legal standard of care, which after all is what a prudent physician in the same circumstances would do. What we're trying to do is medically define what is safe for the patient in most cases. Obviously, there are going to be outliers, and we'll have been wrong. But, for the most part, with the workup that we've described, it is safe to discharge this patient even if it is suboptimal compared to what we can achieve at a more aggressive tertiary care center. Nevertheless, I don't believe that what we are advising people to do here is unsafe for the patient.

Case resolution

The patient was admitted to the hospital and had myocardial perfusion testing before and after exercise, which was normal. At 6-month follow up, the patient had been taking a proton pump inhibitor daily and was symptom free.

Section III: Concepts

Background

Chest pain and related symptoms constitute the second most common reason (behind abdominal pain) for ED visits in the United States, with approximately 6 million visits annually, or 5% of all ED visits.[4] Nevertheless, over half of these patients do not have a cardiac cause for their symptoms.[5-7] Yet, heart disease remains the leading cause of death in the United States.[8]

Determining which ED patients presenting with symptoms concerning for possible myocardial ischemia

actually have coronary heart disease or an acute coronary syndrome represents a serious challenge to the emergency physician. Although the rates of missed diagnoses of acute cardiac ischemia in the ED are low and are improving, a missed diagnosis may be associated with increased morbidity and mortality.[7] On the other hand, the evaluation of patients for possible myocardial ischemia represents a significant financial burden to the healthcare system.[5,9] The development of rapid, cost-effective, and accurate strategies for risk stratification and diagnosis of patients presenting with chest pain and associated symptoms remains an important goal.

What is the role of cardiac stress testing in these patients? The key questions for the emergency physician are to determine who requires cardiac testing, which testing modality should be used, and what should be done with the results of the test.

Initial workup

Once an emergency physician determines that a patient is hemodynamically stable, and does not require immediate intervention or resuscitation, a detailed history begins the evaluation for possible coronary artery disease. The patient in this case illustrates a common scenario: the patient presents symptom-free and hemodynamically stable with an unremarkable physical examination, has a normal or nonspecific EKG, and has a normal initial laboratory profile. In these patients, suspicion for an acute ischemic coronary syndrome (ACS) may be based solely on the history. The patients whose history is concerning for possible myocardial ischemia, but whose initial evaluation is otherwise normal, represent a diagnostic challenge, and are the patients who should undergo extended observation and timely cardiac stress testing.[10,11]

Etiology and differential diagnosis

The differential diagnosis for chest pain is broad. Many potential non-ACS cardiovascular etiologies must be considered, as well as musculoskeletal, gastrointestinal, and respiratory disorders.[12] Features of the initial evaluation and the clinical history of a patient lead the ED physician to establish the likelihood, or pretest probability, of each disease process in the differential diagnosis. The concept of pretest probability is an initial estimate of the likelihood that a patient has a given disease.

After further evaluation and subsequent testing is performed, the resulting likelihood of disease is the posttest probability, which the physician uses to make decisions regarding therapy and disposition. Pretest probability is combined with test characteristics such as sensitivity and specificity, and the results of a given test, to determine the posttest probability that a patient has a given disease. For example, a patient who describes chest pain of sudden onset that is sharp, pleuritic, and associated with shortness of breath may have an intermediate pretest probability of pneumothorax. If a subsequent CT scan, which is highly sensitive and specific for pneumothorax, shows findings concerning for pneumothorax, then the patient's posttest probability for the disease has increased substantially, and should lead the physician to treat the patient for pneumothorax.

In cases of suspected coronary heart disease such as the present one, patient-specific features of the clinical history create the pretest probability of coronary heart disease or ACS. This pretest probability guides the physician in choosing the next step in evaluation, with the understanding that no test is perfectly sensitive and specific. For example, a patient with a very high pretest probability of ACS should undergo extensive and perhaps invasive evaluation for ACS, while a patient with very low pretest probability for ACS may not require any further testing.

The medical literature has extensively reviewed the concept of estimating the pretest probability of coronary heart disease.[13-16] Historical factors ("cardiac risk factors") that can assist in determining pretest probability include age, gender, smoking, diabetes, hypertension, and hypercholesterolemia. One of the most important historical factors is the character of the patient's symptoms.[12,16] Classic cardiac chest pain may be defined as substernal in location with the three following characteristics: of a typical quality and duration, incited by physical or emotional stress, and relieved by rest or nitroglycerin. Atypical angina may have two of the three characteristics, and noncardiac chest pain may have one or none. The difficulty is that the description of the pain is not constant between patients, and is often hard for the patient to describe. Often, the closest generalization is the pain makes the patient restless. While the patient often cannot exactly describe the pain, it can be severe, is usually something the patient wants to be rid of, and not something they stoically tolerate.

Once a patient's pretest probability is estimated, the physician must decide upon the next step in evaluation. For example, a 25-year-old nonsmoking female patient with intermittent sharp chest pain lasting seconds, whose pretest probability for significant coronary artery disease is likely less than 5%, would not warrant further evaluation with cardiac stress testing.[13,16] A positive finding on a cardiac stress test in this patient is likely to be a false positive given the low probability for coronary ischemic disease as well as the imperfect sensitivity and specificity of diagnostic testing.[13,16,17] Similarly, a 65-year-old male smoker with substernal aching radiating to the left arm lasting for 30 minutes after exercise (typical angina, with pretest probability likely greater than 90%) should also not undergo stress testing for the purpose of diagnosing suspected coronary artery disease.[13,16] A negative finding on this patient's exercise stress test is likely to be a false negative, and would not lower the posttest probability to a degree that would reassure the physician that coronary artery disease is absent. Cardiac stress testing is most useful for the patients who, based on clinical history and pretest probability, are at intermediate risk for coronary artery disease (e.g., a middle-aged person with atypical angina).[11,17,18]

Testing

Once a cardiac stress test is indicated, the physician must decide which test to choose. If the patient cannot or does not adequately complete the appropriate protocol, the results of the test may not be interpretable. In general, three options are available: standard exercise radionuclide exercise EKG testing, exercise echocardiography, and myocardial perfusion testing. Pharmacologic stress may also be available for patients unable to physically exercise. Each testing modality has advantages and disadvantages, as well as differences in sensitivity, specificity, and cost effectiveness.

Exercise EKG testing, typically on a treadmill, has been extensively studied, and is generally reported to have a sensitivity of around 70% and specificity of around 80%, with broad variability across studies.[6,18-20] It is the least expensive, and possibly the most cost-effective method, of cardiac stress testing, and is widely available.[6] However, this modality has a lower sensitivity than stress imaging tests (see below). Another disadvantage, given that test results rely on EKG changes, is that nonspecific abnormalities on the resting EKG (i.e., ST depression at baseline or left bundle branch block) may render the test uninterpretable.[19,20]

Exercise echocardiography has both a sensitivity and specificity of 80–90%.[6,18,21] It has a lower associated cost than nuclear imaging, and can assess location and extent of heart disease, even with EKG abnormalities at baseline. However, disadvantages of this modality are that it is highly operator- and interpreter-dependent. Results may be difficult to interpret due to poor image quality in certain patients, such as those who are obese, or who have underlying heart or lung disease at baseline.

Myocardial perfusion testing before and after exercise is generally reported to have a sensitivity of 80–90% and a specificity of 70–80%.[18,21] Depending on the isotope and methodology used, this modality may be the most sensitive cardiac stress test.[18,22] Results are generally reproducible and provide detailed information regarding location of disease and overall cardiac function. However, disadvantages of this modality are that it the most expensive cardiac stress test, and may not be widely available.

In addition to differences in modality, physicians must choose whether a patient should exercise (i.e., walk on a treadmill or ride a stationary bicycle) or undergo pharmacologic stress. In general, patients who are able to do so should exercise. In the case of a positive test, an exercise test can document the functional capacity at which symptoms occur, and there are no concerns about possible side effects of stress-inducing medications. However, in patients who cannot exercise due to musculoskeletal disease or other limitations, pharmacologic stress may be indicated. While pharmacologic stress testing may aid in the diagnosis of coronary artery disease in patients unable to exercise, care should be taken to screen patients who should not receive cardiac agonist medications. For example, dobutamine may cause dysrythmias, and dipyridamole should not be given to patients with severe reactive airway disease.

Disposition

As discussed, patients with a very low or very high pretest probability of coronary artery disease should not undergo cardiac stress testing for the diagnosis of coronary artery disease. Patients with chest pain and very low pretest probability should undergo evaluation for noncardiac causes of chest pain, and their disposition depends on the appropriate management of their noncardiac diagnosis. Patients with very high pretest probability of a new diagnosis of coronary artery disease should be admitted to the hospital for close monitoring and further observation and examination. These patients may undergo evaluation and treatment with an invasive strategy that may include coronary angiography, or a conservative strategy with standard medical therapy.[11]

Patients who have been appropriately selected for cardiac stress testing (those with intermediate pretest probability, nondiagnostic serial EKGs, and normal serial cardiac biomarkers) should undergo an appropriate cardiac stress test in the ED, in an observation unit, or as an outpatient within 2–3 days. Those with a negative stress test, probably have a low posttest probability of coronary artery disease, and may be discharged home with short-term primary care follow up for further evaluation of their symptoms. Those with a positive stress test, probably have a high posttest probability of coronary artery disease, and should be admitted to the hospital for further evaluation and treatment.[11]

Patients who present to the ED with chest pain concerning for ACS, who have had a prior normal stress test, present a disposition challenge for the emergency physician. Assuming that the patient's initial evaluation is normal, and that the patient would otherwise be referred for cardiac stress testing, the physician may consider whether or not stress testing has a "warranty period." For example, is another stress test indicated if the patient had a normal stress test 1 year ago? In other words, how long after a negative stress test does the patient remain at low risk of an adverse cardiac event such as myocardial infarction or even death?

Unfortunately for the emergency physician, the medical literature has not been able to establish a broad-based consensus warranty period for a normal stress test.[23–26] In general, studies use an adverse event rate of less than 1% per year to define an acceptable risk or benign prognosis.[23,24,26] Nevertheless, comparison across studies of the duration of a benign prognosis is difficult because of differing study populations, testing protocols, and follow-up periods with regard to the normal index test. One review and meta-analysis indicates that adverse event rates after normal exercise myocardial perfusion imaging and normal exercise echocardiography are fewer than 1% throughout an approximately 3-year follow-up period.[26] This suggests that the warranty period of normal stress echo and stress myocardial perfusion may be 2–3 years. However, another study suggests that the warranty period for stress echo may only be 18 months.[23]

Furthermore, patient history likely alters the warranty period of a normal test. In other words, the duration of a benign prognosis may differ between individual patients. For example, one study regarding the warranty period of a normal myocardial perfusion scan suggests that clinical factors (such as diabetes and increasing age) may change the risk of adverse events over time.[24]

Little prospective data exists regarding the warranty period of exercise EKG testing; nonetheless, at least one study demonstrates the superior prognostic ability of stress echocardiography when compared to stress EKG.[25] In addition, given the decreased sensitivity of

stress EKG compared with imaging stress, it is intuitive that the warranty period should be shorter.

Summary

The patient discussed at the beginning of this chapter, a 49-year-old woman with a history suggestive of typical angina, likely has a pretest probability for coronary artery disease between 50 and 60%.[13,16] The most appropriate initial test in this patient would be cardiac stress imaging, either with echocardiography or myocardial perfusion, depending on local availability and expertise. Additionally, the emergency physician should make a frank determination regarding whether the patient can adequately exercise for the test. A more accurate imaging test would also

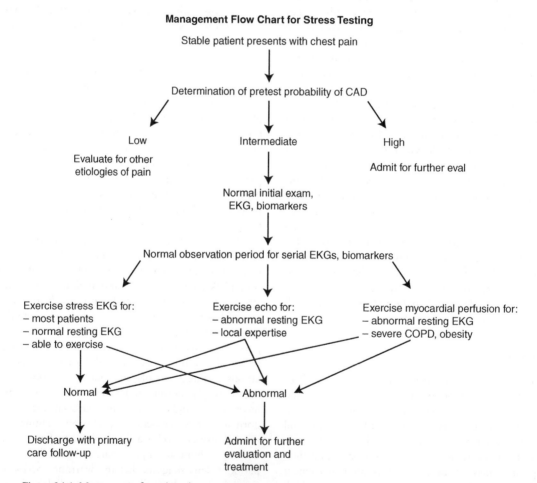

Figure 24.1 Management flow chart for stress testing.

be useful in diagnosing coronary artery disease in the setting of an abnormal baseline EKG.

At this point in the case, after a concerning but indeterminate exercise EKG, the physician had not definitively changed the patient's posttest risk for coronary artery disease. The patient still warranted further testing, and as well, a cardiology consultation based on the abnormal EKG findings on the indeterminate stress test. In consultation with the cardiologist, one reasonable approach would be to admit the patient for further evaluation of her cardiac risk and close monitoring while awaiting stress imaging. Furthermore, based on the ST depressions on her stress EKG, the cardiologist may have admitted the patient for angiography and an early invasive treatment strategy.[11] Another reasonable approach, in consultation with a cardiologist who will follow the patient closely, would be to discharge the patient with instructions for rest and return on Monday (less than 72 hours) for a stress-imaging test. Thorough and direct communication with the patient and cardiologist is paramount in ensuring that the patient will present for and receive close follow up and further evaluation for her possible coronary artery disease.

Section IV: Decision making

See Figure 24-1.

References

1 Dobrzycki S, Baniukiewicz A, Korecki J, et al. Does gastro-esophageal reflux provoke the myocardial ischemia in patients with CAD? *Int J Cardiol.* 2005;104:67–72.

2 Smith KS, Papp C. Episodic, postural and blinked angina. *BMJ.* 1962;II:1425–1430.

3 Sabia P, Afrookteh A, Touchstone DA, et al. Value of regional wall motion abnormality in the emergency room diagnosis of acute myocardial infarction: A prospective study using two-dimensional *echocardiography. Circulation.* 1991;84:I85–I92.

4 Nawar EW, Niska RW, Xu J. *National Hospital Ambulatory Medical Care Survey: 2005 Emergency Department Summary.* Vol No. 386. Hyattsville, MD: National Center for Health Statistics; 2007.

5 Hollander JE, Chang AM, Shofer FS, et al. Coronary computed tomographic angiography for rapid discharge of low-risk patients with potential acute coronary syndromes. *Ann Emerg Med.* 2009;53: 295–304.

6 Lau J, Ioannidis JPA, Balk EM, et al. Diagnosing acute cardiac ischemia in the emergency department: a systematic review of the accuracy and clinical effect of current technologies. *Ann Emerg Med.* 2001;37: 453–460.

7 Pope JH, Aufderheide TP, Ruthazer R, et al. Missed diagnosis of acute cardiac ischemia in the emergency department. *N Engl J Med.* 2000;342:1163–1170.

8 Heron M. Deaths: leading causes for 2004. *Natl Vital Stat Rep.* Nov 20 2007;56(5):1–95.

9 Bayley MB, Schwartz JS, Shofer FS, et al. The financial burden of emergency department congestion and hospital crowding for chest pain patients awaiting admission. *Ann Emerg Med.* 2005;45:110–117.

10 Antman EM, Anbe DT, Armstrong PW, et al. ACC/AHA guidelines for the management of patients with ST-elevation myocardial infarction: a report of the American College of Cardiology/American Heart Association task force on practice guidelines (committee to revise the 1999 guidelines for the management of patients with acute myocardial infarction). *J Am Coll Cardiol.* 2004;44:e1–211.

11 Anderson JL, Adams CD, Antman EM, et al. ACC/AHA 2007 guidelines for the management of patients with unstable angina/non-ST-elevation myocardial infarction: a report of the American College of Cardiology/American Heart Association task force on practice guidelines (writing committee to revise the 2002 guidelines for the management of patients with unstable angina/non-ST-elevation myocardial infarction). *J Am Coll Cardiol.* 2007;50:e1–157.

12 Wolfson AB, et al. *Harwood-Nuss' Clinical Practice of Emergency Medicine.* 4th ed. Philadelphia: Lippincott Williams & Wilkins; 2005:58–61.

13 Diamond GA, Forrester JS. Analysis of probability as an aid in the clinical diagnosis of coronary-artery disease. *N Engl J Med.* 1979;300:1350–1358.

14 Pryor DB, Harrell FE, Lee KL, et al. Estimating the likelihood of significant coronary artery disease. *Am J Med.* 1983;75(5):771–780.

15 Pryor DB, Shaw L, McCants CB, et al. Value of the history and physical in identifying patients at increased risk for coronary artery disease. *Ann Intern Med.* 1993;118:81.

16 Weiner DA, Ryan TJ, McCabe CH, et al. Exercise stress testing: Correlations among history of angina, ST-segment response, and prevalence of coronary-artery disease in the Coronary Artery Surgery Study (CASS). *N Engl J Med.* 1979;301(5):230–235.

17 Patterson RE, Horowitz SF. Importance of epidemiology and biostatistics in deciding clinical strategies

for using diagnostic tests: a simplified approach using examples from coronary artery disease. *J Am Coll Cardiol.* 1989;13(7):1653–1665.

18 Garber AM, Solomon NA. Cost-effectivenes of alternative test strategies for the diagnosis of coronary artery disease. *Ann Intern Med.* 1999;130:719–728.

19 Gianrossi R, Detrano R, Mulvihill D, et al. Exercise-induced ST depression in the diagnosis of coronary artery disease: a meta-analysis. *Circulation.* 1989;80:87–98.

20 San Roman JA, Vilacosta I, Castillo JA, et al. Selection of the optimal stress test for the diagnosis of coronary artery disease. *Heart.* 1998;80:370–376.

21 Fleischmann KE, Hunink MGM, Kuntz KM, et al. Exercise echocardiography or exercise SPECT imaging? A meta-analysis of diagnostic test performance. *JAMA.* 1998;280:913–920.

22 Ioannidis JPA, Salem D, Chew PW, et al. Accuracy of imaging techniques in the diagnosis of acute cardiac ischemia in the emergency department: a meta-analysis. *Ann Emerg Med.* 2001;37(5):471–477.

23 Bangalore S, Yao S, Puthumana J, et al. Incremental prognostic value of stress echocardiography over clinical and stress electrocardiographic variables in patients with prior myocardial infarction: "warranty time" of a normal stress echocardiogram. *Echocardiography.* 2006;23(6):455–464.

24 Hachamovitch R, Hayes S, Friedman J, et al. Determinants of risk and its temporal variation in patients with normal stress myocardial perfusion scans: what is the warranty period of a normal scan? *J Am Coll Cardiol.* 2003;41:1329–1340.

25 Mahenthiran J, Bangalore S, Yao S, et al. Comparison of prognostic value of stress echocardiography versus stress electrocardiography in patients with suspected coronary artery disease. *Am J Cardiol.* 2005;96:628–634.

26 Metz LD, Beattie M, Hom R, et al. The prognostic value of normal exercise myocardial perfusion imaging and exercise echocardiography: a meta analysis. *J Am Coll Cardiol.* 2007;49:227–237.

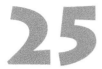

Coronary computed tomography

J. Tobias Nagurney[1] & David F.M. Brown[2]

[1] *Assistant Professor of Surgery, Division of Emergency Medicine, Harvard Medical School, Attending Physician and Director of Research, Department of Emergency Medicine, Massachusetts General Hospital, Boston, Massachusetts, USA*
[2] *Vice Chair, Department of Emergency Medicine, Massachusetts General Hospital, Associate Professor, Harvard Medical School, Boston, Massachusetts, USA*

Section I: Case presentation

A 38-year-old man presented to the Emergency Department (ED) with left-sided chest pain. The pain began the prior morning during some exertion, lasted about 15 minutes, and recurred intermittently during the afternoon and evening. On the day of admission, he awakened with a similar pain that lasted about an hour prior to coming to the ED. The pain was dull, nonpleuritic, and nonradiating. There was no associated shortness of breath, nausea, or palpitations. There was some diaphoresis. The patient had no prior history of similar chest pain, and no known coronary artery disease. His past medical history was notable for migraine headaches that were relieved with Fioricet. He had smoked about one pack of cigarettes per day for 20 years, did not use drugs, and worked as a fork lift operator. He had a positive family history for coronary artery disease—his father had suffered from a myocardial infarction (MI) at age 50.

On ED arrival, he was pain free. The vital signs were: blood pressure 140/85 mmHg, heart rate 80 beats/min, respiratory rate 12 breaths/min, temperature 98.6°F, and oxygen saturation 99% on room air. There was neither jugular venous distention nor bruits. The breath sounds were clear. The chest wall was nontender. The cardiac auscultation revealed a normal S1 and S2 without murmurs, gallops or rubs. The abdomen was soft and nontender without masses. The

extremities had no edema. The pulses were 2+ and symmetric. The EKG demonstrated a normal sinus rhythm with normal intervals and axis. There were no ST or T-wave changes suggestive of ischemia.

The patient was placed on oxygen and a cardiac monitor, given 325 mg of aspirin by mouth, and intravenous access was obtained. Laboratory tests showed normal electrolytes, a normal blood urea nitrogen and creatinine, and a normal complete blood count. The cardiac enzymes and troponin levels were normal. A chest radiograph was normal.

The patient was admitted to observation status for cardiac monitoring and further testing.

Section II: Case discussion

Dr Peter Rosen: I would submit that unless they are lucky enough to work in an ED that has a chest pain unit, providers in most institutions would not admit this patient. There is a divergence of opinion in many EDs about whether they would hold this patient for a second set of biomarkers, or whether they would say that he's been pain free and the time interval is long enough, and this first set of cardiac tests is adequate information. Assuming the history was clear enough for this emergency physician to decide that this patient needed to be ruled out for an ischemic

Cardiovascular Problems in Emergency Medicine: A discussion-based review, First Edition.
Edited by Shamai A. Grossman and Peter Rosen.
© 2011 John Wiley & Sons, Ltd. Published 2011 by John Wiley & Sons, Ltd.

coronary syndrome, is there an optimal way to manage this patient?

Dr Shamai Grossman: This presentation is typical of many patients we see in the ED. They present with chest discomfort. While there are some components that are suggestive of cardiac ischemia, there are other components that are not; coupled with a nondiagnostic EKG, we are left with trying to decide: Does the patient need further ED evaluation, or are we comfortable enough that this is not cardiac ischemia that we are willing to discharge the patient home? The problem with discharging the patient home is that we know the literature: the number one source of malpractice in emergency medicine is missing acute MIs. If we send home all of these patients, we will certainly miss some acute MIs. The cautious practitioner of emergency medicine will recognize these realities, and act conservatively. Acting conservatively leaves you with a number of options, one of which might be admitting the patient to the hospital, one of which might be admitting the patient to an observation unit, and another might be doing further evaluation in the ED with tests such as a coronary CTA.

PR: I would submit that, if your question is, "Is this patient having a heart attack," the answer is no. This patient does not meet criteria for either an ST elevation or non-ST elevation MI (STEMI or NSTEMI), and perhaps that is the wrong question. You still have the possibility that this is an ischemic coronary syndrome, and that this patient could go home and fare badly. However, this is not a reason to conclude that this patient needs to be admitted to the hospital. I don't think that there are all that many hospitals that have beds for a patient like this, nor will many cardiology services be willing to admit a patient with a story like this.

DB: I don't agree that at this point you can conclude from this workup that this person is not having an acute MI. The symptoms today lasted an hour, and then the patient came to the ED. It's not clear what the interval is between that hour of symptoms and the arrival in the ED, but unless it's 6 or more hours, the first troponin can be discounted because it takes at least 4 and probably 6 or 8 hours for a troponin to become positive after myocardial cell death. Altogether I don't think we have excluded an MI sufficiently in this patient, yet I don't think that is the

right question. I think that the right question is, "Is this an acute coronary syndrome?," which here should include a NSTEMI or unstable angina. I disagree with you as well on the disposition of this patient. I think that most of our colleagues feel compelled to keep this patient at least for 6 hours to get a second set of markers, and then either perform some sort of provocative or anatomic test, or arrange to have one performed within 72 hours. This is consistent with the recommendations of the ACC/AHA guidelines for patients who present to the ED with chest pain.

Dr J. Tobias Nagurney: There are a number of important issues here that may influence our decision making. The first is the age of the patient. If this were a female patient, we need to know her pre-, peri-, or postmenopausal status. Here the age is 38, which is young but would place a man into the cardiac risk age group. Secondly, the clinical story raises a couple of red flags. We know from the chest pain literature that two of the more important characteristics that suggest that chest pain is from an acute coronary syndrome (ACS) are exertional chest pain and chest pain that is accompanied with diaphoresis, both of which were present in this case. Thirdly, even if this patient has angina pectoris, new-onset angina has a poor prognosis and a high major adverse cardiac event rate. There are some other clues that this patient has an unstable cardiac chest pain: it began the day prior for 15 minutes, which is semiprolonged; it occurred intermittently throughout the day, so there is a crescendo quality to it; on the morning of presentation, while the patient was at rest, he developed pain upon awakening; and there was not only an episode at rest, but a prolonged episode. Therefore if this is ischemic pain, it's very unstable angina or an infarction that has not been picked up because the biomarkers were sent too early. We also know that having a normal initial EKG in the ED does not completely eliminate the possibility that the patient is having an acute MI. I don't think we have enough data in this patient to conclude that it's clearly not ACS.

PR: To be more prudent, you could argue that the real meaningful pain was on the admission morning, and that the prior day's symptoms were a teaser, and therefore we do need a second set of biomarkers. I wouldn't argue strongly with anyone who wanted to hold the patient for a second set of enzymes, but I still feel that there are very few EDs who would admit this patient unless they had no way to set up a stress test or obtain close follow up within the next 24 hours. Many departments would hold this patient to get a second set of biomarkers and a stress test, and if there were no further symptoms or EKG changes, they would feel comfortable about dismissing the patient. Nevertheless, I think there are too many patients who present like this for us to take the easy path out for the emergency physician and say, "Just admit the patient and let cardiology sort it out on the inpatient service". In reality, we don't have enough inpatient beds, and we don't have that kind of support from most cardiologists.

PR: Let's assume we get a second set of normal biomarkers, the EKG is unchanged, and he does not have further symptoms; what would you do next?

JTN: A second negative troponin at the 8-hour mark has over 95% sensitivity for ruling out an MI. Coupled with a normal repeat EKG, I would agree with you that the patient has not had a NSTEMI. However, he still could have unstable angina. This too needs to be ruled out, because that can have a poor prognosis, even short term. I would evaluate this patient with some sort of risk stratification scheme: an observation unit may be ideal here to avoid keeping this patient in the ED for 4–6 more hours while someone is arranging an exercise tolerance test. If this cannot be done, I am left with a very difficult decision: do I send this person home and hope he will return for their risk stratification test in 72 hours or do I admit him to a regular floor?

PR: Is a coronary CT scan appropriate in this patient? Is it a replacement for the stress test?

SG: We have all alluded to the fact that we are not truly comfortable saying that this patient's discomfort is noncardiac based on the initial presentation, as well as based on what we know in the literature of these patients. So we decided that we need to risk stratify this patient a bit more. One of the options that we just mentioned is simply to do a second set of cardiac biomarkers to reinforce that this patient is not having an acute MI. Even if we do this, we still haven't answered the question of whether this patient is having an acute coronary syndrome or not. We now can utilize a CT scan, and look directly at the coronary arteries. The advantage of doing a CT scan is that it is an imaging modality that is available in just about every ED in the United States, and can potentially be done 24 hours a day, 7 days a week. The disadvantages of the CT scan, and there are a number of them, begin with the literature. Is CT an adequate tool to rule out coronary artery disease? The studies are ongoing, and we don't have a conclusive answer as yet. Some literature suggests that if a patient has less than 50% stenosis by coronary CT, then that patient is very unlikely to have acute coronary disease. The idea would seem to be that if the patient has the CT scan performed while in the ED, and it doesn't demonstrate coronary disease, the patient should not need a stress test, and we can be reassured that the patient is not having an acute coronary syndrome. We should be further reassured that if we send that patient home, then we are not sending a patient home who is going to have an adverse outcome shortly after we discharge the patient.

PR: I recently saw a paper from Italy which suggested that CT is actually more accurate than angiography. Yet, we also know from prior experience that angiography can sometimes fool us, and find lesions that are perhaps not the cause of the patient's symptoms thereby forcing our hand into treating them because we don't really know what the source of the patient's symptoms is. How do you feel about the accuracy of finding a cardiac lesion on CT scan?

DB: Although CT scanning is universally available, the technology to do a high-resolution coronary CT scan may not be readily available in many EDs or hospitals at this point. Even if a coronary CT is available, having someone who is competent to read the CT is not necessarily a given. In our group, a select group of cardiologists and cardiac radiologists read these scans. This is not to say that it can't be learned by a broader group of general CT radiologists just as, for example, appendicitis has. You might recall that initially, appendiceal CTs were read by gastrointestinal radiology in our institutions, but are now read by emergency and general radiologists everywhere. Having said that, coronary CT scan is more rapidly available in many institutions then stress testing.

We are also starting to see data that suggest that coronary CT images do approach the resolution of conventional coronary angiography, which is the gold standard for determining whether or not a patient has coronary artery disease. I sense they will be much more accurate than conventional stress testing, and perhaps even more accurate than stress testing with imaging.

However, when you use the test on the moderate- to high-risk groups of patients and find plaques with stenosis, it may not be clear whether that stenosis is causing the patient's pain, and so you will have to add other testing such as sestamibi testing. For the moment, with low-risk patients primarily being selected for this test, this would be an unusual result, but if we broaden the testing population too quickly, we'll be left with a lot of patients who will need additional testing, and we won't have a more efficient system.

JTN: The reason that cardiac CT scan is on the table as a discussion point is because the existing tests haven't really filled our needs in the ED. Whether an institution uses a plain exercise tolerance test, a sestamibi imaging (nuclear imaging), or a rest and stress echo, they all have limitations of sensitivity and specificity. Moreover, they are not generally available 24/7. CT results have also been shown to add to the differential information beyond that provided by the risk factors and chest pain story in an ED. In particular, whether there is any plaque at all, and if so, how many coronary artery segments are involved, have both been shown to have predictive value in diagnosing ACS. The newest literature demonstrates that if the CT shows only plaque but not significant stenosis (less than 50–70% luminal occlusion, and there are different points of view on that), these patients are quite safe to go home and do well for the short (2 weeks) and longer term (6 months). Nevertheless, there are a lot of exclusion criteria for utilizing CT scans: for example, atrial fibrillation, renal insufficiency or elevated creatinines, and patients who are at moderate or high risk of having an ACS event. Evaluating this group with a CT scan is not totally contraindicated, but the data suggest they are not a good group to study. Related to this are patients with known coronary disease. When there is a coronary artery calcification, reading the scan is technically difficult.

Another limitation is that across the literature about 10% of these scans have results that are indeterminate. And when you get an indeterminate scan, the patient ends up getting a second study, a second dose of radiation, and a second charge (remember these are not inexpensive tests). These false positives can lead all the way to cardiac catheterization and generate the spending of more healthcare dollars.

PR: Almost nowhere in medicine do we have evidence for a negative test that stands out, and yet this would sound like this is such an instance. We have been searching for many years as to how can we safely prove these patients negative for ischemia so that we aren't going to send them out to drop dead of an ischemic coronary syndrome. But how do you define low probability? Is it several sets of negative biomarkers, a lack of EKG changes, or is there something else that identifies a low-probability patient who will benefit from having this negative evidence?

DB: A number of instruments can be used to assist the physician's clinical prediction, although I suspect that most of the time, that assessment is purely based on the history that is obtained, the EKG, and the physician's clinical judgment. But, one could use TIMI risk scores, which was the approach used in one paper that limited coronary CT testing to patients with a TIMI risk scoring of zero or one. One finds, when risk-stratified by a negative coronary CT scan, none of them had adverse outcomes at 6 months. The ACI TIPI score, a computer-based algorithm based on the EKG and some clinical questions, also can help the clinician. Like TIMI scores, it is not in widespread use. One is left with the physician's gestalt, based on risk factors, the history, and the findings on the EKG. I think we can assume that cardiac markers are always negative when this discussion is being had, since any patient with positive cardiac markers is no longer low risk.

PR: I see CT scanning being used as a screening tool. I have been told that this has become part of the "executive workup," and that once a year if you are over the age of 50, you ought to have a coronary artery CT scan. I am not pleased with using it that way because if you find calcifications, I don't know whether or not this translates into significant stenosis if the patient is asymptomatic.

JTN: I agree in general, but that doesn't mean that patients shouldn't get CT scans in the ED. My concern is that this is a very powerful tool, but is very expensive, and incurs a lot of radiation exposure for the patient, though the newer CT scanners have decreased that radiation dose. If we aren't prudent about who gets it, as we have seen with other tests that have been applied to ED populations, it will be used more and more broadly until just about everyone is getting one. While today's discussion is about how can we apply CT scanning to our own undifferentiated ED patients, the CT scan is being used by cardiologists to follow patients with known coronary artery disease. They are beginning to study not only the anatomy of the coronary arteries, but actual perfusion imaging with the CT scan. Cardiologists may actually use this data in ambulatory patients to track their ejection fraction and their perfusion. The CT scan has dozens of potential legitimate uses. The concierge aspect that you mentioned is just one of the abuses.

SG: What do you do with the argument that patients who receive a CT scan in the ED could have just as easily had a stress test? The stress test would have exposed them to no radiation. What do you tell your patient, and how do you tell your practitioner of emergency medicine that you should be doing a CT rather than a stress test?

JTN: I ask them a question, and I tell them two things. The question I ask the ED practitioner is, "How sensitive do you think an exercise tolerance test is in an undifferentiated ED population?" Depending on who I ask, I get different results. There are some data that exercise stress tests are actually quite insensitive for coronary artery disease. There is a contrary literature that shows that a negative stress test in the ED is associated with an enormous positive or good prognostic potential for a lack of cardiac events for six months or even longer. It really depends on what you believe is the value or the sensitivity in predicting untoward outcomes of the exercise tolerance test. I would tell the patient, "You can have a stress test tomorrow morning when it is available. Stay with us overnight and have that test, which will cost your health insurance company less money and deliver no radiation to you, or you can have a test now and possibly go home in 3 hours. This test may be superior to the one we would do in the morning, but does expose you to radiation and costs a great deal more. What would you prefer?" Only a handful of papers have begun to address how cardiac CT compares to alternative testing like an exercise tolerance test, a nuclear imaging test, or a resting and stress echocardiogram.

SG: Would you be more inclined to image patients with CT scan who are at less risk of adverse effects toward radiation, such as limiting your patient population to patients who are not women of childbearing age?

JTN: Yes, but I think that question is easy because women of childbearing age rarely develop acute coronary syndrome. I wouldn't use a CT scan to look for coronary disease in a woman of childbearing age. The good news about all of the literature addressing radiation exposure is that the people who are at higher risk for radiation exposure are young and female, but the people who get coronary disease tend to be old and male. Thus, radiation exposure is not a major concern to me in implementing this test.

PR: If I understood you correctly, you were using the CT coronary angiogram as a substitute for an exercise stress test. Do you think it would be more prudent to use it only on those patients for whom the stress test either was not sufficient, because they couldn't reach maximum exercise tolerance or the patients' obesity, or some reason that kept them from performing the stress test? We know that the stress test, when negative, is not necessarily useful, certainly not as useful as when it's positive. I'm not sure that I would trust a stress test for 6 months, although that may be a safe timeframe. I don't think we truly know at what rate coronary artery disease progresses, and although 6 months sounds reasonable, it may in fact be a shorter time frame than that.

SG: Given the current literature, I don't think I would use a coronary CT scan as my follow-up study for an indeterminate stress test. That may change as the literature evolves, but at this point, I think we are talking about coronary CT scan in the same situations that we have used a stress test, and perhaps in patient populations where we can't do a stress test. So, for instance, in a patient who returns to an ED who has had an indeterminate or even a negative stress test and who presents with the same symptoms, I am still concerned that the symptoms may be cardiac in etiology. Then, perhaps doing a different test, such as a coronary CT scan, will be more useful rather than, as some times we are forced to do, referring that patient for a coronary angiogram. The other patient population where it might be useful is in the patient with cocaine-related chest pain where, perhaps, doing a stress test in an emergent fashion may not be useful but a coronary CT might be. The true utility of coronary CT scan is dependent on literature that is yet to come.

PR: Can coronary CT be used to assist in diagnosing the patient who might have been suffering from coronary artery spasm, or do we really need angiography for that?

DB: The answer to your question is not really known, but I believe that coronary CT scan is not going to be particularly useful in excluding underlying coronary vasospasm as the cause for someone's angina or chest pain. The CT scan may show you nonobstructive coronary artery disease. You could surmise, I suppose, that those patients might have coronary vasospasm that would make non-obstructive disease obstructive during the period of spasm. I don't think there's any way to know that. With coronary angiography the opportunity to do some sort of chemical stimulation test to test for vasospasm is an option, but with CT scan, I don't think it is.

Case resolution

The patient received a CT scan of the coronary arteries. All 17 coronary artery segments were clearly visualized. Three segments had a small amount of calcified plaque, but no lumen was obstructed by more than a 25% cross section. There was no wall motion abnormality. The patient was discharged home to receive a tailored medical regimen for mild coronary artery disease and was doing well at 6-month follow-up.

Section III: Concepts

Scope of the problem

A large percentage of patients presenting to EDs complain of chest pain.[1] Distinguishing those with an acute myocardial infarction and acute coronary syndrome from those with noncardiac chest pain is difficult.[2,3] A history of risk factors for coronary disease may not be helpful.[4]

Certain parts of the chest pain story may contribute to establishing a diagnosis, but are neither sensitive nor specific enough to allow providers to discharge patients directly home from the ED.[5] The EKG changes that are diagnostic of an acute MI are both insensitive and nonspecific.[6-8] Biomarkers are time dependent, and the patient may arrive in the ED too early for them to be helpful.[9] Clinical factors and laboratory results have been combined in attempts to predict which patients have ACS, but with varying success.[10,11]

Because all of the diagnostic tools available to the ED clinician are imperfect, less than 40% of patients admitted to the inpatient service to ruleout ACS turn out to have this disease.[1] Conversely, approximately 2–8% of patients with either acute myocardial infarction or unstable angina are erroneously discharged home from the ED.[12] Missed myocardial infarctions represent a major source of medical malpractice dollars.[13] In an effort to diagnose ACS accurately and to minimize admissions and inappropriate discharges, many technologies had been evaluated in ED populations. Among them are exercise tolerance tests, nuclear scans, and echocardiograms.[14-20] However, most of these tests are not available all hours of the week. A routinely-available test that would accurately distinguish ED patients with ACS from those without it would represent an important diagnostic tool.

Characteristics of an ideal diagnostic test

An ideal diagnostic test would have excellent test characteristics: sensitivity, specificity, positive predictive value, negative predictive value, overall accuracy, and positive and negative test-likelihood ratios. It would be safe to perform and require a minimal amount of time outside the monitored ED environment. It would be available nights and weekends, with results reported soon after completion. It would demonstrate good interrater reliability and be inexpensive. At this time, there is no such test, and we therefore have to accept a degree of imprecision in any strategy that we pursue. Despite the claims of the plaintiff bar and those who think we can eliminate all error from medicine, it is impossible to eliminate all error in the decisionmaking about possible ischemic coronary disease.

Cardiac computed tomography (CCT) angiography: overview

Advances in temporal and spatial resolution of new multidetector CT scanners allow accurate visualization of the coronary arteries in the motion-free state. Its primary value is to determine whether the coronary arteries contain atherosclerotic plaque, and if so, whether significant stenosis is present or not. In particular, the degree of luminal obstruction by plaque in any of the four major coronary arteries (left main, left anterior descending, circumflex, and right) can be estimated. Plaque can be identified as calcified (hard), noncalcified (soft), or mixed. Both the intra- and extracardiac contents of the entire thoracic cavity are visualized and additional noncardiac or "incidental" findings outside the coronary vascular tree may be discovered.[21]

Image acquisition and interpretation

The CT image is constructed from an X-ray source that rotates around the patient to be imaged, and a detector array that is positioned on the opposite side. In a multidetector CT scanner, a detector array may contain many rows of detectors or sensors. As a patient is passed through the X-ray source and these sensors, multiple cross sectional images (slices) are obtained. They are then reorganized by computers to create three-dimensional reconstructions of the anatomic area of interest. Based on the generation of the scanner, these source images typically contain 16, 64, or 128 parallel cross sections. Modern CT scanners provide isotropic or near-isotropic spatial resolution of 0.4–0.5 mm, with a temporal resolution of 83–250 milliseconds. This allows visualization of the complete coronary tree in a single breath hold over several heart beats.[22]

To visualize the coronary arterial tree, an initial test bolus of approximately 10–20 ml of intravenous imaging contrast is given to determine timing, followed by a full bolus of 80–100 ml (depending on the scan range). While most imaging protocols inject contrast, some acquisition protocols obtain a non-contrast CT first to calculate a calcium (Agatston) score. A calcium score is measured in Hounsfield units, and if high, suggests the presence of advanced coronary artery disease. Due to the blooming artifact from calcification, a high calcium score can suggest that the scan will be more difficult to interpret.[23] Sublingual nitrates are usually administered to maximally dilatate the coronary vessels.[24] EKG gating allows the CT angiography to be timed to the cardiac cycle to provide motion-free images. Due to the limited temporal resolution of certain CT scanners, slower heart rates are needed to achieve the desired motion-free images. Thus, for 64-slice CT scanners or older generation scanners, oral or intravenous beta-blockers are often administered to patients with heart rates above 65 beats per minute (bpm), with a goal heart rate below 60 bpm for optimal image

quality. As the temporal resolution of the newer generation CT scanners improve, strict heart rate control has become less critical. Patients in atrial fibrillation (which makes gating more difficult) are usually excluded, but this restriction is less stringent with the newer, faster CT scanners. If functional data is desired, a cine data set can be obtained with certain acquisition protocols that permit the assessment of global and regional left ventricular function in the hope that this information may add diagnostic and prognostic value to information on the coronary arterial tree.

The patient is typically out of the ED for 30 minutes, of which approximately 20 minutes is for patient preparation and image acquisition. The remaining time is for transportation. Besides cardiac dysrhythmias, other important exclusion criteria include elevation in serum creatinine or other concerns for contrast-induced nephropathy, allergy to iodinated contrast, pregnancy, and unwillingness to withhold use of metformin for 48 hours after the contrast administration. The radiation dose delivered by CT angiography has been estimated to be approximately 10–20 mSieverts per examination, but this is decreasing with newer generation scanners and employment of dose-saving techniques (such as lower tube voltage for thinner patients, minimizing the scan range, and EKG-tube current modulation).[25,26] This compares to approximately 12 mSieverts of radiation exposure with nuclear isotope (i.e. sestamibi) utilization.

The cross-sectional or transaxial images obtained (called source images) are reviewed by CT readers, typically general or cardiac radiologists or cardiologists. These source images are reconstructed into multi-planar reformations (MPR) that are oriented into three standard planes (coronal, sagittal, and axial), and can be manipulated and viewed by the user into any obliquity. A maximum intensity projection (MIP) image can be reconstructed using larger slice thickness to produce better contrast differentiation between the contrast and noncontrast enhanced structures. Three-dimensional volume-rendered techniques (VRT) can provide visually pleasing images that graphically demonstrate the location of lesions. The reader typically comments first on whether the study is interpretable, meaning that all 17 segments of the coronary arterial system, as described by the AHA, are clearly visualized. Due to the blooming

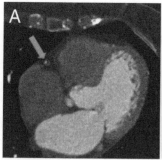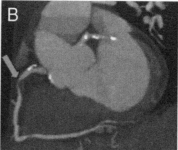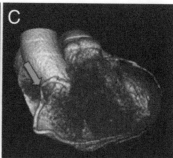

Figure 25.1 Images of CCT CAS: Source Images, multiplanar reformat; 3D image all with pathology. CT images of the right coronary artery (RCA) show high-grade stenosis of a noncalcified plaque in its mid segment (arrow). A. Multi-planar reformation (MPR) image in the axial view. B. Maximum intensity projection (MIP) image with also calcification in the right coronary cusp, as well as mild calcified plaques in the proximal RCA, left main and proximal left anterior descending artery but no significant stenosis. C. 3D-volume rendering technique (VRT) image. Courtesy of Quynh Truong, MD, Massachusetts General Hospital, Boston, MA.

and beam-hardening artifacts, a high burden of coronary artery calcification makes the degree of luminal obstruction difficult to interpret, as do prior open or percutaneous (i.e., coronary stent) revascularization procedures. For this reason, patients with a history of coronary artery bypass graft surgery or percutaneous coronary interventions with stenting are often excluded. Other causes of uninterpretable coronary artery segments involve technical issues, such as respiratory or motion artifacts.[27]

A typical report will comment on which if any of the four main coronary arteries (CA) contain plaque, and how much of their lumen is obstructed. Luminal obstruction may be reported quantitatively or qualitatively. Qualitative description of luminal obstruction is typically preferred, but may vary significantly depending on the CT reader and local institutional protocol for interpretation. Depending on CCT interpreter or author, a plaque burden considered "mild" may be reported as causing luminal narrowing of between 1% and 25%, or sometimes up to 40%. The term "moderate" severity may be used either for lesions obstructing from 26–50% or from 41–70% of the CA lumen. The term "severe" has been applied by some interpreters for any luminal narrowing greater than 50%, but is usually reserved for lesions causing greater than 70% obstruction. This high grade or "severe" obstruction is also referred to as "significant stenosis." Complete or total occlusion is reported when no contrast appears to traverse a lesion.[28–35] A final report may describe wall motion abnormality and incidental intra-and extracardiac findings as well (see Figure 25-1 for examples).[21]

Scientific basis for the use of CCT in ED populations

The utility of the CCT to rule out ACS rests on evidence that ACS usually occurs in the context of coronary artery disease.[36,37] Hence, a test that demonstrates that a patient has no or minimal coronary artery disease decreases the likelihood that this patient is suffering from ACS. The original research on CCT compared its ability to identify lesions in the coronary arteries to coronary arteriography, and compared its sensitivity and specificity to this criterion (gold) standard. The ability of the CCT to detect both plaque and stenosis was measured. Test characteristics such as sensitivity or specificity were reported either by the number of coronary artery segments or by the number of patients evaluated correctly. For the finding of CA stenosis by evaluable segment, both individual studies and meta-analyses suggest sensitivities of 80–95% and even higher, with specificities around 90–95%.[10,28–35,38,39] However, the percentage of CA segments that can be evaluated vary from 80–100% depending on the generation of the scanner.[40–43] For the finding of CA stenosis on a per patient analysis, ranges for sensitivities are 95–100%, with specificities of 84–100%.[35,41,44,45] The sensitivity of CCT for finding both CA plaque and stenosis varies by whether plaque is calcified or not, the size of the CA being examined, and the generation of scanner used.[34,41] Newer generation scanners provide higher sensitivity.[41,46] Since a scan that accurately characterizes 16 of the 17 CA segments but misses a stenosis in the 17th would affect patient care, per patient data may be more relevant to clinicians, particularly since studies vary on how they include unevaluable segments in a per patient analysis. Since stenosis has not been ruled out in a patient with even only one unevaluable segment, patients with these indeterminate scans often receive another risk stratification test such as a cardiac nuclear-imaging test.

Once it was established that CCT measured CA plaque and stenosis reliably compared to coronary arteriography, a number of studies examined the clinical usefulness of this information. These studies demonstrate the ability of the CCT to diagnose ACS in undifferentiated ED population with sensitivities from 0.83–1.00 and specificities from 0.74–1.00.[28–30,33,35,47–49] Summary estimates from pooled data suggest sensitivities of 0.95 and specificities of 0.90.[27,41] Furthermore, the extent of plaque adds to the diagnosis of ACS and contributes diagnostic information beyond that of traditional risk factors or clinical estimates of the probability of ACS.[29,30]

The most recent published studies have examined how well CCT results predict short and long-term safety in patients discharged from an ED. Patients studied were typically at low or moderate risk for ACS; in fact, it has been demonstrated that the CCT is most helpful in patients with low or medium pretest probabilities of ACS, and has less value in those with high pretest probabilities.[50,51] While the definition of low or moderate risk varies, patients in these studies are typically those with nondiagnostic ED evaluations, including normal initial troponin measurements and nonischemic EKGs.[52] Risk-stratification scores, such as the TIMI risk score indicating low risk for subsequent adverse events, have been used for patient selection as well. Depending on the availability of the scan and interpreters, the CCT is obtained from the ED or from an observation unit or medical floor. Patients with no or non-obstructing plaque, typically occluding less than 50% of any CA lumen (i.e., no stenosis), are discharged without any further cardiac testing. Their calcification score is often used for decision making as well.[47,52,53]

Study populations were followed for the development of Major Adverse Cardiac Events (MACE),

typically death, acute MI, or a coronary artery revascularization procedure. Patients with no or nonobstructing plaque are shown to be free of MACE events for at least 2 weeks and up to 12 months.[47,52] The change in ED length of stay varies by study, but there is some suggestion that time in the ED decreased.[52,54] This literature suggests that patients with a negative biomarker 8 hours after onset of symptoms, a non-diagnostic initial EKG, a low TIMI score, and no or mild coronary artery disease on CCT can be safely discharged from the ED. Patients with severe or total obstruction should receive additional cardiac risk-stratification testing per institutional guidelines. The best approach for patients with CCTs displaying moderate stenosis remains unclear.[47,52,53]

Unresolved issues regarding CCT in ED populations

It appears that CCT offers a unique and accurate ability to provide information on the status of an ED patient's CAs in real time. It has a good to excellent sensitivity and predictive negative value both to diagnose ACS and to predict major adverse cardiac events. Why, then, is it not the perfect test? Unresolved issues revolve around the degree to which it changes providers' decisions, and how it compares to traditional cardiac risk stratification tests used in the past. In particular, its cost effectiveness has been called into question.[55,56]

The few articles that exist suggest that CCT has the ability to change clinicians' decisions, and to avoid admissions in patients who do not have ACS.[57,58] In studies that have compared the ability of the CCT to cardiac nuclear imaging to reach the correct clinical diagnosis, the sensitivities of these tests are comparable.[47,59] Limited data also suggest that the CCT can change clinical diagnoses from ACS to other diagnoses and possibly lead to discharge from the ED in 20–40% of patients.[57,58] The cost effectiveness of CCT may vary by gender and by its cost.[50,60] In several studies, it appears to be as or more cost effective than alternative diagnostic strategies.[29,47,54] However, these studies were conducted at single sites, and most involved modest study population sizes. Conclusions also vary a great deal depending on the value chosen for input variables.[50,60] While they suggest that CCT may indeed be comparable to or better than alternative imaging strategies and be cost effective, large multicenter trials are needed.[55,56]

With respect to the test's accuracy, while false negative tests do occur, they are relatively few, and the negative predictive value of CCT is high. Sensitivity and specificity depend on which plaque or stenosis criterion is used to define a "positive" or abnormal CCT. The major concerns that have been raised are around the issue of false positives. These are patients who have significant stenosis on CT, but do not turn out to have an ACS event. In these cases, the visualized stenosis did not represent a thrombosis related to a culprit lesion or vulnerable atherosclerotic plaque. For example, in one study, a higher number of coronary arteriograms is associated with use of the CCT.[47] A second area of concern revolves around radiation doses. Modeling studies suggest that the lifetime risk of cancer from CCT is significant, particularly in women and the young.[61] Newer data suggest a decreasing dose of radiation with newer generation scanners.[25] Finally, reactions to IV contrast and contrast-related renal failure have been raised as potential issues.[62]

Section IV: Decision making

- The advantages of CCT are that it can be performed and interpreted relatively quickly, and a result demonstrating absent or only minimal CA plaque has been associated with lack of ACS and a good prognosis.
- To date, there is minimal published data to show how much it changes provider decisions, and how it compares to other available testing.
- Issues of risk, especially with regard to radiation, need to be considered.
- The specific population in which it will be used needs to be clearly defined.

The authors would like to acknowledge Quynh Truong, MD, for her advice on technical issues involving CCT.

References

1 McCaig LF, Nawar EW. National hospital ambulatory medical care survey: 2004 emergency department summary. Adv Data. 2006;372:1–29.
2 Goldman L, Kirtane AJ. Triage of patients with acute chest pain and possible cardiac ischemia: The elusive search for diagnostic perfection. Ann Intern Med. 2003;139(12):987–995.
3 Hollander JE. The continuing search to identify the very-low-risk chest pain patient. Acad Emerg Med. 1999;6(10):979–981.
4 Jayes RL,Jr, Beshansky JR, D'Agostino RB, Selker HP. Do patients' coronary risk factor reports predict acute cardiac ischemia in the emergency department? A multicenter study. J Clin Epidemiol. 1992;45(6): 621–626.
5 Swap CJ, Nagurney JT. Value and limitations of chest pain history in the evaluation of patients with suspected acute coronary syndromes. JAMA. 2005;294(20):2623–2639.
6 Speake D, Terry P. Towards evidence based emergency medicine: Best BETs from the Manchester Royal Infirmary. First ECG in chest pain. Emerg Med J. 2001;18(1):61–62.
7 Goodacre S, Locker T, Morris F, Campbell S. How useful are clinical features in the diagnosis of acute, undifferentiated chest pain? Acad Emerg Med. 2002;9(3):203–208.
8 Fesmire FM, Percy RF, Wears RL, MacMath TL. Initial ECG in Q wave and non-Q wave myocardial infarction. Ann Emerg Med. 1989;18(7):741–746.
9 Nagurney JT, Brown DF, Chae C, et al. The sensitivity of cardiac markers stratified by symptom duration. J Emerg Med. 2005;29(4):409–415.
10 Limkakeng AT, Halpern E, Takakuwa KM. Sixty-four-slice multidetector computed tomography: The future of ED cardiac care. Am J Emerg Med. 2007;25(4): 450–458.
11 Smith SW, Tibbles CD, Apple FS, Zimmerman M. Outcome of low-risk patients discharged home after a normal cardiac troponin I. J Emerg Med. 2004;26(4):401–406.
12 Pope JH, Aufderheide TP, Ruthazer R, et al. Missed diagnoses of acute cardiac ischemia in the emergency department. N Engl J Med. 2000;342(16):1163–1170.
13 Karcz A, Korn R, Burke MC, et al. Malpractice claims against emergency physicians in Massachusetts: 1975–1993. Am J Emerg Med. 1996;14(4):341–345.
14 Hill J, Timmis A. Exercise tolerance testing. BMJ. 2002;324(7345):1084–1087.
15 Kirk JD, Turnipseed S, Lewis WR, Amsterdam EA. Evaluation of chest pain in low-risk patients presenting to the emergency department: The role of immediate exercise testing. Ann Emerg Med. 1998;32(1):1–7.
16 Amsterdam EA, Kirk JD, Diercks DB, Lewis WR, Turnipseed SD. Immediate exercise testing to evaluate low-risk patients presenting to the emergency department with chest pain. J Am Coll Cardiol. 2002;40(2):251–256.
17 Klocke FJ, Baird MG, Lorell BH, et al. ACC/AHA/ASNC guidelines for the clinical use of cardiac radionuclide imaging--Executive Summary: A report of the American College of Cardiology/American Heart Association task

force on practice guidelines (ACC/AHA/ASNC committee to revise the 1995 guidelines for the clinical use
of cardiac radionuclide imaging). *J Am Coll Cardiol.*
2003;42(7):1318–1333.

18 Sabia P, Abbott RD, Afrookteh A, et al. Importance of
two-dimensional echocardiographic assessment of left
ventricular systolic function in patients presenting to
the emergency room with cardiac-related symptoms.
Circulation. 1991;84(4):1615–1624.

19 Varetto T, Cantalupi D, Altieri A, Orlandi C. Emergency
room technetium-99m sestamibi imaging to rule out
acute myocardial ischemic events in patients with nondiagnostic electrocardiograms. *J Am Coll Cardiol.*
1993;22(7):1804–1808.

20 Ingkanisorn WP, Kwong RY, Bohme NS, et al. Prognosis
of negative adenosine stress magnetic resonance in
patients presenting to an emergency department with
chest pain. *J Am Coll Cardiol.* 2006;47(7):1427–1432.

21 Onuma Y, Tanabe K, Nakazawa G, et al. Noncardiac
findings in cardiac imaging with multidetector computed
tomography. *J Am Coll Cardiol.* 2006;48(2):402–406.

22 Ferencik M, Nomura CH, Maurovich-Horvat P, et al.
Quantitative parameters of image quality in 64-slice
computed tomography angiography of the coronary
arteries. *Eur J Radiol.* 2006;57(3):373–379.

23 Scheffel H, Alkadhi H, Plass A, et al. Accuracy of dual-
source CT coronary angiography: First experience in a
high pre-test probability population without heart rate
control. *Eur Radiol.* 2006;16(12):2739–2747.

24 Chun EJ, Lee W, Choi YH, et al. Effects of nitroglycerin on the diagnostic accuracy of electrocardiogram-
gated coronary computed tomography angiography.
J Comput Assist Tomogr. 2008;32(1):86–92.

25 Raff GL, Chinnaiyan KM, Share DA, et al. Radiation
dose from cardiac computed tomography before and
after implementation of radiation dose-reduction techniques. *JAMA.* 2009;301(22):2340–2348.

26 Hausleiter J, Meyer T, Hermann F, et al. Estimated
radiation dose associated with cardiac CT angiography.
JAMA. 2009;301(5):500–507.

27 Vanhoenacker PK, Decramer I, Bladt O, et al. Detection
of non-ST-elevation myocardial infarction and unstable
angina in the acute setting: Meta-analysis of diagnostic
performance of multi-detector computed tomographic
angiography. *BMC Cardiovasc Disord.* 2007;7:39.

28 Sato Y, Matsumoto N, Ichikawa M, et al. Efficacy of
multislice computed tomography for the detection of
acute coronary syndrome in the emergency department.
Circ J. 2005;69(9):1047–1051.

29 Hoffmann U, Bamberg F, Chae CU, et al. Coronary
computed tomography angiography for early triage of patients with acute chest pain: The ROMICAT
(Rule Out Myocardial Infarction using Computer

Assisted Tomography) trial. *J Am Coll Cardiol.*
2009;53(18):1642–1650.

30 Hoffmann U, Moselewski F, Cury RC, et al. Predictive
value of 16-slice multidetector spiral computed tomography to detect significant obstructive coronary artery
disease in patients at high risk for coronary artery disease: Patient-versus segment-based analysis. *Circulation.*
2004;110(17):2638–2643.

31 Hollander JE, Chang AM, Shofer FS, et al. Coronary
computed tomographic angiography for rapid discharge
of low-risk patients with potential acute coronary syndromes. *Ann Emerg Med.* 2009;53(3):295–304.

32 Jeudy J, White CS. Evaluation of acute chest pain in
the emergency department: Utility of multidetector
computed tomography. *Semin Ultrasound CT MR.*
2007;28(2):109–114.

33 White CS, Kuo D, Kelemen M, et al. Chest pain evaluation in the emergency department: Can MDCT provide a comprehensive evaluation? *Am J Roentgenol.*
2005;185(2):533–540.

34 Achenbach S, Moselewski F, Ropers D, et al. Detection
of calcified and noncalcified coronary atherosclerotic
plaque by contrast-enhanced, submillimeter multidetector spiral computed tomography: A segment-based
comparison with intravascular ultrasound. *Circulation.*
2004;109(1):14–17.

35 Miller JM, Rochitte CE, Dewey M, et al. Diagnostic
performance of coronary angiography by 64-row CT.
N Engl J Med. 2008;359(22):2324–2336.

36 Roe MT, Harrington RA, Prosper DM, et al. Clinical
and therapeutic profile of patients presenting with acute
coronary syndromes who do not have significant coronary artery disease.the platelet glycoprotein IIb/IIIa in
unstable angina: Receptor suppression using integrilin therapy (PURSUIT) trial investigators. *Circulation.*
2000;102(10):1101–1106.

37 Patel MR, Chen AY, Peterson ED, et al. Prevalence, pre-
dictors, and outcomes of patients with non-ST-segment
elevation myocardial infarction and insignificant coro-
nary artery disease: Results from the Can Rapid Risk
Stratification of Unstable Angina Patients Suppress
ADverse Outcomes with Early Implementation of the
ACC/AHA guidelines (CRUSADE) initiative. *Am Heart
J.* 2006;152(4):641–647.

38 Runza G, La Grutta L, Alaimo V, et al. Comprehensive
cardiovascular ECG-gated MDCT as a standard diagnostic tool in patients with acute chest pain. *Eur J Radiol.*
2007;64(1):41–47.

39 Schuijf JD, Beck T, Burgstahler C, et al. Differences in
plaque composition and distribution in stable coronary
artery disease versus acute coronary syndromes; noninvasive evaluation with multi-slice computed tomography. *Acute Card Care.* 2007;9(1):48–53.

40 Pugliese F, Mollet NR, Runza G, et al. Diagnostic accuracy of non-invasive 64-slice CT coronary angiography in patients with stable angina pectoris. *Eur Radiol.* 2006;16(3):575–582.

41 Stein PD, Yaekoub AY, Matta F, Sostman HD. 64-slice CT for diagnosis of coronary artery disease: A systematic review. *Am J Med.* 2008;121(8):715–725.

42 Hamon M, Biondi-Zoccai GG, Malagutti P, et al. Diagnostic performance of multislice spiral computed tomography of coronary arteries as compared with conventional invasive coronary angiography: A meta-analysis. *J Am Coll Cardiol.* 2006;48(9):1896–1910.

43 Raff GL, Gallagher MJ, O'Neill WW, Goldstein JA. Diagnostic accuracy of noninvasive coronary angiography using 64-slice spiral computed tomography. *J Am Coll Cardiol.* 2005;46(3):552–557.

44 Budoff MJ, Dowe D, Jollis JG, et al. Diagnostic performance of 64-multidetector row coronary computed tomographic angiography for evaluation of coronary artery stenosis in individuals without known coronary artery disease: Results from the prospective multicenter ACCURACY (Assessment by Coronary Computed Tomographic Angiography of Individuals Undergoing Invasive Coronary Angiography) trial. *J Am Coll Cardiol.* 2008;52(21):1724–1732.

45 Bayrak F, Guneysu T, Gemici G, et al. Diagnostic performance of 64-slice computed tomography coronary angiography to detect significant coronary artery stenosis. *Acta Cardiol.* 2008;63(1):11–17.

46 Pugliese F, Mollet NR, Hunink MG, et al. Diagnostic performance of coronary CT angiography by using different generations of multisection scanners: Single-center experience. *Radiology.* 2008;246(2):384–393.

47 Goldstein JA, Gallagher MJ, O'Neill WW, et al. A randomized controlled trial of multi-slice coronary computed tomography for evaluation of acute chest pain. *J Am Coll Cardiol.* 2007;49(8):863–871.

48 Raff GL, Gallagher MJ, O'Neill WW, Goldstein JA. Diagnostic accuracy of noninvasive coronary angiography using 64-slice spiral computed tomography. *J Am Coll Cardiol.* 2005;46(3):552–557.

49 Rubinshtein R, Halon DA, Gaspar T, et al. Usefulness of 64-slice cardiac computed tomographic angiography for diagnosing acute coronary syndromes and predicting clinical outcome in emergency department patients with chest pain of uncertain origin. *Circulation.* 2007;115(13):1762–1768.

50 Khare RK, Courtney DM, Powell ES, Venkatesh AK, Lee TA. Sixty-four-slice computed tomography of the coronary arteries: Cost-effectiveness analysis of patients presenting to the emergency department with low-risk chest pain. *Acad Emerg Med.* 2008;15(7):623–632.

51 Meijboom WB, van Mieghem CA, Mollet NR, et al. 64-slice computed tomography coronary angiography in patients with high, intermediate, or low pretest probability of significant coronary artery disease. *J Am Coll Cardiol.* 2007;50(15):1469–1475.

52 Hollander JE, Chang AM, Shofer FS, et al. Coronary computed tomographic angiography for rapid discharge of low-risk patients with potential acute coronary syndromes. *Ann Emerg Med.* 2009;53(3):295–304.

53 Gallagher MJ, Ross MA, Raff GL, et al. The diagnostic accuracy of 64-slice computed tomography coronary angiography compared with stress nuclear imaging in emergency department low-risk chest pain patients. *Ann Emerg Med.* 2007;49(2):125–136.

54 Chang AM, Shofer FS, Weiner MG, et al. Actual financial comparison of four strategies to evaluate patients with potential acute coronary syndromes. *Acad Emerg Med.* 2008;15(7):649–655.

55 Redberg RF, Walsh J. Pay now, benefits may follow—the case of cardiac computed tomographic angiography. *N Engl J Med.* 2008;359(22):2309–2311.

56 Newman DH. Computed tomographic angiography for low risk chest pain: Seeking passage. *Ann Emerg Med.* 2009;53(3):305–308.

57 Rubinshtein R, Halon DA, Gaspar T, et al. Impact of 64-slice cardiac computed tomographic angiography on clinical decision-making in emergency department patients with chest pain of possible myocardial ischemic origin. *Am J Cardiol.* 2007;100(10):1522–1526.

58 Nagurney JT, Bamberg F, Nichols JH, et al. The disposition decision on emergency department patients with chest pain is affected by the results of multi-detector computed axial tomography scan of the coronary arteries. *J Emerg Med.* 2009 [e-pub ahead of print].

59 Gallagher MJ, Ross MA, Raff GL, et al. The diagnostic accuracy of 64-slice computed tomography coronary angiography compared with stress nuclear imaging in emergency department low-risk chest pain patients. *Ann Emerg Med.* 2007;49(2):125–136.

60 Ladapo JA, Hoffmann U, Bamberg F, et al. Cost-effectiveness of coronary MDCT in the triage of patients with acute chest pain. *Am J Roentgenol.* 2008;191(2):455–463.

61 Einstein AJ, Henzlova MJ, Rajagopalan S. Estimating risk of cancer associated with radiation exposure from 64-slice computed tomography coronary angiography. *JAMA.* 2007;298(3):317–323.

62 Valls C, Andia E, Sanchez A, Moreno V. Selective use of low-osmolality contrast media in computed tomography. *Eur Radiol.* 2003;13(8):2000–2005.

Cardiac Surgery Complications

26 Postcardiac Surgery Emergencies

Jonathan Anderson[1] & Shamai Grossman[2]

[1] *Instructor of Medicine, Harvard Medical School, Beth Israel Deaconess Medical Center, Boston, Massachusetts, USA*
[2] *Director, Cardiac Emergency Center and Clinical Decision Unit, Beth Israel Deaconess Medical Center, Assistant Professor of Medicine, Harvard Medical School, Boston, Massachusetts, USA*

Section I: Case presentation

A 57-year-old man was brought to the emergency department (ED) by EMS. The paramedics reported that they found the man sitting on a sidewalk a couple of blocks from his apartment. He was diaphoretic, and felt too weak to walk home. A passerby had noticed him, and called 911. On scene, the patient had a blood pressure of 85mmHg/palpation, and a finger-stick glucose of 227 mg/dl. They noted him to be tachycardic with an irregular rhythm at a rate of about 150 beats/min. He denied chest pain or dyspnea, and was transported to the ED immediately; they did not have time to perform an EKG en route, but did establish IV access in one arm, and started a normal saline drip.

The patient appeared flushed and diaphoretic. The initial vital signs were: temperature 37.8°C (100.1°F) orally, heart rate 156 beats/min (irregular), blood pressure 83/52 mmHg, respiratory rate of 18 breaths/min, and oxygen saturation 98% on room air. On physical examination there was a fresh surgical scar, a median sternotomy. The patient stated, "I was just released from the hospital yesterday. I had heart surgery last week, but I felt great this morning so I went for a walk to the donut store." He further complained about palpitations, weakness, and lightheadedness that started suddenly about 30 minutes prior. He stated he was discharged on "a bunch of pills" that he

has been taking faithfully. He again denied chest pain and dyspnea. The review of systems revealed low-grade fevers, which the patient noted he had since surgery. He stated that aside from the heart condition, high blood pressure, and high blood sugars he had no other medical problems, no allergies, and had only had the one surgery in his life.

The patient was an obese male who appeared to be his stated age. He was in mild distress, but was lying nearly supine on the gurney. Pertinent findings included an irregularly irregular and tachycardic cardiac rate. There were no murmurs or rubs. The lungs were clear to auscultation. The sternal incision had some mild erythema extending 1 cm from the incision over the inferior one-third of its length. The abdomen was nontender. The remainder of the physical examination was normal.

A second peripheral IV was established, and blood was sent for complete blood count, chemistries, cultures, and cardiac enzymes. A portable chest X-ray study and a urinalysis were ordered. An EKG revealed atrial fibrillation with a rate of 152 beats/min, a normal axis, normal intervals, and no ST changes. After a 500 cc normal saline bolus, the patients' vital signs improved to a heart rate of 145 beats/min (irregular) and blood pressure of 104/65 mmHg. The decision was made to attempt pharmaceutical control of the patient's heart rate. After 5 mg of IV metoprolol, the *patient's vitals were unchanged. An additional 5 mg of IV metoprolol was administered, with reduction of the rate to 95 beats/min, and improvement of the blood pressure to 110/70 mmHg. The patient noted that his subjective malaise and weakness felt improved.*

The patient's laboratory studies showed a white blood cell count of 18,000 cells/mm³ with a slight left-shift, a blood sugar of 230 mg/dl, and a creatinine of 1.3 mg/dl. The chest X-ray study showed sternal wires from the median sternostomy, and some widening of the mediastinum. The urinalysis was normal. An initial diagnosis of mediastinitis was made, the patient was started on broad spectrum antibiotics, and was admitted to the cardiac surgery service.

Section II: Case discussion

Dr Peter Rosen: Was the patient's cardiac surgery performed at your medical center, or is he new to your hospital?

Dr Shamai Grossman: The surgery was at an outside hospital.

PR: Let's discuss this case from both vantage points. Clearly, if the surgery was performed at your hospital, then you are going to have an easier time evaluating this patient because you will have access to his records. You will be able to find out what the surgery was, what the postoperative course was, and you should be able to contact the surgical service that cared for him expeditiously. If he is new to your hospital, then that's a problem; you don't have easy access to any of these materials, and you will have to retrieve them. While he may be able to tell you which hospital he is from, he may not know the details of his surgery. I am amazed at the number of times patients don't get back to the hospital where they were recently admitted, even though it would clearly be preferable for them to be cared for in that institution. I can understand the constraints upon the EMS system, but an extra 10 minutes of transit time could make hours of difference in the evaluation of a patient.

SG: Would you attempt to transfer this patient after stabilization in the emergency department?

PR: Absolutely. I am a firm believer that surgeons should take care of their own postoperative patients.

This is not work aversion; one cannot care for another surgeon's postoperative problems as successfully as when you are taking care of your own complications.

Dr. Amal Mattu: I think most surgeons would be amenable to transfer, especially when it's after a complicated surgery. Assuming this patient had bypass surgery, I can't imagine a cardiothoracic surgeon who would say anything other than, "Yes, definitely transfer him back to us so we can take care of him."

PR: Before talking about transfer, however, we need to discuss what interventions would be important while the patient is in the ED. I am a little surprised to hear that he was given a beta-blocker with a blood pressure as low as that reported.

AM: I am also a bit surprised. Even though metoprolol is beta-one specific, because of the negative inotropic effect, I would be very hesitant to give a beta-blocker to someone who is already hypotensive. If I did use metoprolol, I would start out with even lower doses than were used in this case. Some might argue for using esmolol instead, since it is titratable, but I'd still be hesitant even with esmolol, because if your patient deteriorates and you turn off the esmolol, its effects may linger for about 15 more minutes. I would prefer diltiazem, because in my experience, premedicating with calcium can be very helpful in avoiding hypotension. In addition, if the patient does drop his blood pressure further, you can always give the calcium afterward to reverse the vasodilatatory effect without reversing the chronotropic effect. Other alternatives might be digoxin, if you're not in a rush, or even amiodarone. Although I think amiodarone is often overused, I've had success utilizing it in patients with this scenario of borderline or low blood pressure plus rapid atrial fibrillation. The final option is cardioversion, which is particularly useful in the unstable patient in rapid atrial fibrillation. However, before any interventions, I would want to know what comprised this patient's daily "bunch of pills." This list might direct me toward using a medication that he is already taking, such as a beta-blocker, calcium channel blocker, or amiodarone.

SG: Would you consider not intervening with this patient's rhythm at all, and instead try to treat the underlying etiology of his atrial fibrillation, such as treating what's likely an infectious process?

AM: I would start by giving IV fluid, although I don't think the heart rate is going to slow to normal just with fluid boluses. I also don't think antibiotics are going to help immediately in terms of rate control for rapid atrial fibrillation.

PR: This is where it would be very useful to know the patient's past history. We don't know whether he was in atrial fibrillation prior to surgery, or even at the time of discharge. If we knew that this was new onset atrial fibrillation, it might give us a reason to consider other possible causes of acute atrial fibrillation, such as "holiday heart." We don't know if he went to the donut shop on the way home from the bar. If I knew this was a patient with new onset atrial fibrillation, I would be more inclined to cardiovert him given the low blood pressure. I would also want to know whether this is new onset diabetes. If the patient had a coronary artery bypass, are we looking at diabetes triggered from a postoperative myocardial infarction (MI), or are we looking at a complication of long-standing diabetes? We don't know if he is on insulin, and perhaps his initial episode was in fact a hypoglycemic episode to which he reacted, and then developed hyperglycemia. It would be useful to know more about the patient's underlying metabolic state before we just focus on the cardiac dysrhythmia. Even if he has a wound infection or a tissue infection that was secondary to the cardiac surgery, most surgical infections don't respond to antibiotics alone, if they do at all, but require drainage of the area of infection. If the infection is due to a contaminated foreign body, then it may need to be removed and replaced.

PR: What else might you do to manage this patient before transferring him to the surgical service?

SG: If the patient is hemodynamically unstable, it behooves us to try and stabilize him as best as we can in the ED. In this case, I would start with fluid resuscitation. If you are unable to improve the blood pressure and ventricular rate with fluid resuscitation and antipyretics, it may be necessary to cardiovert the atrial fibrillation. I would concomitantly try to find other sources that might be able to corroborate some of the history, such as family members, EMS, or records from the other hospital. I think utilizing every piece of information you have to better understand the patient's history will allow you to better treat your patient, and to better stabilize him before you send

him to another institution. Until he gets to that other institution, he is still very much your patient, and you still have complete responsibility to care for him.

PR: Let's just consider for a minute what are the sources of fever postoperatively. In the immediate postoperative 48 hours, fever is most likely to be due to lung problems such as atelectasis, and not sepsis. By a week postoperatively, the fever should have resolved unless it has not been successfully treated, and has evolved into pneumonia. An initial chest X-ray study should help define whether he has developed a pneumonitis from partially or unsuccessfully treated atelectasis.

The second source of fever could be from the surgical wound itself. It takes time for a wound to develop infection. However, I've seen it occur as rapidly as 24 hours after surgery, especially when the patient has some immunosuppression or is diabetic. If the wound is infected with gram-negative anaerobes, you may see an early gas-gangrene infection, which may present as a wound infection away from the wound. It can present with a funny appearance to the skin such as blistering or crepitus. The patient looks like someone in the midst of an inflammatory syndrome with septic shock. While there are some elements of this here in this patient, this case is not typical of this type of infection. A more conventional wound infection is most likely to be caused by *staphylococcus*. It's interesting that it takes between 5 and 7 days for this to develop. This type of infection is usually noted in the wound itself, with a reddened and angry appearance. There may or may not be purulence escaping from the edges of the wound, but it looks like an abscess forming. The best management for that wound, like any other abscess, is to open the incision.

The third source of fever is one that begins to complicate the surgery itself. Here it would be useful to know what type of cardiac surgery this patient had sustained. The infectious complications of coronary artery bypass surgery are less concerning than the infectious complications of valvular surgery, particularly if the valve was being replaced because of destruction from endocarditis. The infectious complications of coronary artery bypass surgery are also less concerning than if the surgery is for a tumor of the heart, or for many other reasons for doing heart surgery besides coronary bypass. Yet, that doesn't mean that wounds post coronary bypass can't become infected and have mediastinitis, especially in a diabetic patient.

I would further question whether was he being operated on to treat dysrhythmias. In this case, pacemaker wires may be a source of his infection. We don't know what sort of vascular support he had during the cardiac surgery. Any of those sites may also be the source of his fever and sepsis. Therefore, we would want to look at the areas that may have had vascular access, such as his legs, to see if he is developing abscesses or infection at these sites.

There are a couple of other things that happen during cardiac surgery that can cause fever that's not due to sepsis. Some patients have a propensity for developing massive pleural effusions, particularly diabetic patients. These patients may have a fever without actually having an empyema. The effusion should show up on our portable chest X-ray study, and therefore we might have had an answer to the infectious source at this point in the patient's workup.

SG: Are these pleural effusions infectious in nature?

PR: They are not infectious. They are a serous fluid outpouring seen after all cardiac surgery, similar to what is seen in joints after they have been operated on. It's a kind of inflammatory response that can be seen in the pericardium as well, but different from Dressler's syndrome seen after MI. Sometimes these effusions need to be drained to control the fever and the patient's symptoms.

I think this is a patient who deserves at a minimum a good upright posterior to anterior (PA) and lateral chest X-ray study. Even with a median sternotomy, a postoperative pneumothorax can occur, and that can cause a low grade fever as well as the hypotension that this patient demonstrated. An anterior pneumothorax is hard to define. A portable supine chest X-ray study, which it sounds like is what was obtained in this patient, may be inadequate for this diagnosis. In truth, this patient will probably require a CT scan of the chest.

Lastly, we often forget about pulmonary embolus in cardiac surgery because it's relatively uncommon. Pulmonary embolus can produce low grade fever as well as all of the other changes that this man has. Although I would not put this at the top of my differential list, I think we might want to consider this as a possible cause of the rapid deterioration. Quick echocardiography might help us in the evaluation of this patient. It would also give us answers to what kind of surgery he had, what kind of foreign bodies he may have, and it might give us answers to whether or not we are dealing with a pulmonary embolus.

SG: Would you get those tests in the ED?

PR: I would get them in conjunction with the cardiothoracic service. If they wanted them from the ED, I wouldn't hesitate to do them there. If they wanted to take this patient to the surgical intensive care unit and obtain them there, I wouldn't hesitate to do that either. I think it is institution dependent. In most of the institutions I've worked at, it's probably easier to get scans from the ED, and it's probably easier to do echocardiograms in the intensive care unit. The surgeon also may want to take this patient directly back to the operating room because he is aware of something from the original surgery that may be appropriate to repair at this time, rather than to delay with imaging studies.

AM: How long after the surgery do you need to start worrying about wound infections? Is your worry going to be different if they are 2 days postoperative versus 2 weeks postoperative? Would it make a difference if the skin doesn't look erythematous, but the patient is complaining of increasing pain at the incision site, and there is a low-grade fever?

PR: The appearance of the wound is perhaps the best indicator of a wound infection. I've never seen a wound infection where the wound looked like it was healing perfectly and the only complaint was pain. That may be true of hidden soft tissue infections such as with an ischiorectal abscess, where patients can present with severe rectal pain but you can't find a source for the fever. Surgical wounds demonstrate inflammation quickly even if they don't always show pus quickly. It's rare for wound infections to occur within the first 2 days. Surgical wounds can also be accompanied by low-grade fevers due to failure to deposit collagen and start laying down the healing structure of the wound; here the wound is trying to dehisce. This probably happens more with abdominal wounds than with chest wounds, but it can occur in the chest as well. This is particularly concerning in the immunosuppressed patients and diabetics. This kind of wound doesn't look normal; it may look swollen and it may leak yellow serous fluid. When you see this, you must be concerned that this wound is about to come apart. This requires immediate surgical repair.

In this case, the time from incision to repair is about 3 weeks, but the time to repair from a previously repaired wound after a dehiscence is about a week and a half. This time difference in wound healing is due to the geometric orientation of the fibroblasts laying down the collagen that will heal the wound. This process is already ongoing in the dehisced wound, but the infection interfered with the collagen deposition. This is something to look for on physical examination rather than with an imaging study.

Most of the decisions concerning infection and the source of infection are not going to be resolved in the ED; they are going to be resolved by the surgical service. This reemphasizes that it's absolutely critical, if at all possible, to contact the surgeon who initially managed this patient.

Case resolution

With the atrial fibrillation controlled, the patient was taken to the operating room, where mediastinitis was definitively diagnosed and the wound was washed out and debrided. The wound was left open initially, and then after several days of antibiotics was closed intraoperatively. Blood cultures remained negative throughout the hospital course. The atrial fibrillation did not recur; it was thought to be a result of the recent coronary artery bypass graft surgery (CABG) and the added stress of an infection and fever. He was discharged from the hospital without further complication.

Section III: Concepts

Background and epidemiology

There are three major complications of cardiac surgery that will be addressed in the chapter: coronary artery bypass graft surgery (CABG), the left ventricular assist device (LVAD), and valvular surgery.

Coronary artery bypass graft
Coronary artery bypass graft surgery is a very common surgical procedure, with nearly 430,000 surgeries being performed each year.[1] Like any surgery, complications occur. One study estimates that about one-tenth of the money spent on CABG procedures goes to pay for complications.[2] It is not uncommon for a post-CABG patient to present to an ED with

complications, and there are some unique issues that must be assessed when evaluating these patients.

The common complications that occur in the perioperative period include dysrhythmias, myocardial ischemia, pericardial effusion, infections, renal failure, and neurological deficits. While many of the complications occur early on, while the patient is still hospitalized, in the ED one would be more likely to encounter those complications found relatively later in the postoperative period, after hospital discharge.

Preventative perioperative therapies
There are some common therapies used to minimize postoperative complications. Most post-CABG patients one may encounter in the ED will be taking many, if not all, of these prescribed medications, and all medications are associated with side effects and complications.

Aspirin is probably the most common and best known of these medications. In post-CABG patients, daily aspirin provides a 44% odds reduction in losing graft patency at 1 year postop.[3] The 2004 ACC/AHA task force on ST-segment elevation myocardial infarctions states that post-CABG aspirin should be prescribed as soon as possible.[4] Aspirin does incur some risks, largely related to bleeding and gastrointestinal complications, and patients often take a concomitant antacid medication. Plavix is also a common post-CABG medication, also with some data supporting better graft patency. Like aspirin, it also comes with an increased risk of bleeding.

Antidysrhythmic drugs are the next common category of post-CABG medication, with beta-blockers like sotalol prescribed to reduce the risk of atrial fibrillation after a CABG. A recent meta-analysis calculates that these drugs reduce the risk from around 35% to around 15%.[5] The 2004 ACC/AHA guidelines on CABG suggest beta-blockers as standard therapy in all patients without contraindication, as there are some data to suggest a true reduction in 30-day mortality in those patients given beta-blockers.[6]

Amiodarone is another antidysrhythmic agent sometimes given after a CABG procedure, also with the intent of preventing post-operative atrial fibrillation. Current ACC/AHA guidelines suggest amiodarone be given to patients who are at high risk of developing atrial fibrillation who cannot receive beta-blockers. Metoprolol therapy comes with some risk of congestive heart failure (CHF), hypotension, and bradycardia, along with lesser side effects. Amiodarone has a black box warning due to its pulmonary toxicity, and has also been associated with photosensitivity and movement disorders.[7]

Statins have proven long-term morbidity and mortality benefits in post-CABG patients. In fact, some recent studies demonstrate a short-term perioperative advantage to continuing (or starting) statin therapy.[8] Fortunately, statin therapy is relatively low risk compared to many other pharmaceuticals.

Neurological complications

Perioperative neurologic complications are both common and particularly devastating in CABG patients. They are divided into two large categories: Type 1 Neurologic Injuries include strokes and transient ischemic attacks, injuries that are focal in nature, while Type 2 Neurologic Injuries are diffuse injuries, often relating to neurocognitive decline.

Type 1 injuries occur in 3.1% of CABG patients, and are the second most common cause of perioperative demise.[9] As age increases, the risk of type 1 injury also increases. Commonly, these injuries are blamed on embolic events. They can arise from proximal aortic plaques, which are commonly manipulated during the surgery itself. Post-operative atrial fibrillation is also a cause of embolic stroke, and patients who demonstrate recurrent atrial fibrillation, or remain in atrial fibrillation for greater than 24 hours, should be anticoagulated with coumadin for at least 4 weeks.[1] Other causes of type 1 injuries include carotid plaques and left ventricular thrombi.

Type 2 injuries are diffuse, and can be recognized in roughly half of patients undergoing CABG.[10] While many of these patients will recover as time passes, there is a significant proportion who will have some permanent neurocognitive effects. This can cause not only morbidity and concern for the patient and their family, but can also be a potential complicating factor in other areas of their health and recovery.

Dysrhythmias

Dysrhythmias are the most common post-CABG complication, with biphasic peaks in incidence. The first peak occurs inside the operating room, and the second around post-op days two through five. The dysrhythmias are multifactoral in etiology. Instigating factors include fevers, hypokalemia, hypomagnesemia, hypocalcemia, anemia, ischemia, increased sympathetic tone, hypertension, pericardial inflammation, and medication side effects.

Atrial fibrillation is the most common symptomatic post-CABG dysrhythmia, occurring in 15–40% of cases.[11] The risk of post-CABG atrial fibrillation has been modeled in a multivariable risk index, breaking the risk of atrial fibrillation into low (<17%), medium (17–52%), and high (>52%). This risk analysis shows a strong correlation between increasing age and risk of atrial fibrillation. There is also a positive correlation between history of prior atrial fibrillation, chronic obstructive pulmonary disorder (COPD), and the withdrawal of beta-blocking or ACE-inhibiting medications. Full details of this index are available in Table 26-1.[12] As mentioned above, beta-blocker or amiodarone therapy successfully reduces the risk of atrial fibrillation following CABG. Patients with recurrent or extended episodes of atrial fibrillation should be anticoagulated with warfarin.

The acute treatment of new onset or symptomatic atrial fibrillation in post-CABG patients is identical to other patients, with the exception that long-term antidysrhythmic therapy is usually not needed. In the stable patient who presents with atrial fibrillation with a rapid rate, rate control can usually be obtained pharmacologically. This can be done either with calcium channel blockers (e.g., diltiazem 15–20 mg IV over 2 minutes, repeat in 15 minutes) or beta-blockers (e.g., metoprolol 5 mg IV every 5 minutes up to 3 doses). The choice of drug is largely up to the clinician, and one must consider the individual circumstances of the patient, such as a history of severe COPD or asthma or home medications. In the hemodynamically unstable patient in atrial fibrillation with rapid ventricular response, the proper treatment is prompt electrical cardioversion. Sedation can be obtained with medications such as Versed, morphine, or Valium as tolerated by blood pressure. Cardioversion should proceed with a direct synchronized current beginning at 50 joules.

Less common post-CABG dysrhythmias, which arise from the same set of precipitating factors, include supraventricular and ventricular tachydysrhythmias. They are treated as per typical Advanced Cardiovascular Life Support protocol. Also occasionally seen are sinus bradyarrhythmias and sinus arrest, either as a medication effect or due to trauma to the sinus node during the operation.[13]

Table 26-1. Causes of Fever in Postop Cardiac Patients

Cause of Fever	Features	Diagnostic Test
Atelectasis	Common in the first 2 days postop	Can be visible on chest X-ray study, CT chest scan
Pneumonia	Cough, change in mucus, fever	Chest X-ray study, CT chest scan
Urinary Tract Infection	Common after catheter use, often symptomatic	Urinalysis, urine culture
Wound Infection	Mediastinitis more common in diabetics; can also involve vein harvest sites	Physical examination, ultrasound if abscess is sought; surgical exploration can be necessary
Endocarditis	In postvalvular surgery patients; fever, superficial lesions, new murmurs	Multiple blood cultures, echocardiography, ESR/CRP
Pulmonary Embolism	Not common after cardiac surgery, low-grade fevers possible. Dyspnea, chest pain	CTA of chest, V/Q scan
Pleural Effusion	Can cause fever without infection	Chest X-ray study, ultrasound, CT chest scan

Myocardial infarction

In CABG patients, there is a roughly 10% chance of a perioperative myocardial infarction. There are a multitude of causes for this ischemia, including distal or diffuse coronary artery disease, spasm, embolism, thrombosis of the graft, technical problems of the anastomosis, or any of the typical causes of ischemia. Initial diagnosis and therapy should proceed as per a nonsurgical patient, but the emergency physician needs to quickly engage the patient's cardiologist and cardiac surgeon, as re-operation or prompt cardiac catheterization may be indicated.[1]

Pericardial effusion

Almost all patients will have some form of a pericardial effusion following a CABG procedure. In the first postoperative month, it is not uncommon to develop a Dressler's-like pericarditis, with the typical features of positional chest pain, elevated inflammatory markers, and a small pericardial effusion. Occasionally these effusions can develop into a cardiac tamponade. This should be near the top of the differential diagnosis list when a postop patient arrives with tachycardia, hypotension, muffled heart sounds, or jugular venous distention. Rapid diagnosis is possible with bedside ultrasound or more formal echocardiography. Treatment does not differ from any other cause of cardiac tamponade; brief stabilization is possible with a fluid bolus, but in a hemodynamically unstable patient immediate pericardiocentesis is mandatory.[1]

Infections

It is common to have a fever for up to 6 days after undergoing a CABG procedure, caused by the operation itself. Aside from infection, other common reasons to have fevers in the first 2 weeks after a CABG procedure include atelectasis, phlebitis, drug reactions, and pulmonary emboli. A typical infectious workup should involve peripheral blood cultures, urinalysis, chest radiograph, and blood cell counts. The post-CABG chest radiograph will be abnormal for some time after the operation, frequently demonstrating small pleural effusions. When searching for a source of fever, it is important to check the leg harvest sites, as wound infections can occur in these locations. Mediastinitis occurs in roughly 2% of patients in the post-CABG period. This disease is marked by fever, leukocytosis, bacteremia, and purulent discharge from the sternal wound. It should be suspected in any post-CABG patient who is febrile without clear source; definitive diagnosis requires exploration of the wound. Mediastinitis is a debilitating complication, with a roughly threefold increased mortality rate over the first 4 years postoperatively as compared to noninfected patients.[14] Diabetes mellitus, which is common in patients undergoing CABG, is an independent risk factor for developing postoperative mediastinitis.[15]

Left ventricular assist devices

Left ventricular assist devices are implantable pumps that offer patients with severe heart failure either a bridge to transplant or a potential terminal therapy for increasing life span. They are used in post-CABG patients, as well in patients with other causes of heart failure. They are proven to extend life as compared to medical therapy alone.[16] There are multiple types of LVADs currently on the market, and they all share certain common traits. They are assist pumps that are implanted into the abdomen that increase the forward flow into the aorta. Generally, the devices take blood from the left ventricle and bypass this blood through the pump and into the aorta. They are battery powered, but can also connect to AC power to either recharge or as their primary power source. These batteries generally provide 4–6 hours of energy per charge. Some versions have emergency hand pumps that can provide forward flow in the case of battery failure. Due to the constant flow of blood through the LVAD, there is frequently no palpable pulse in these patients. There is a high risk of thromboembolic events, so patients are typically triple anticoagulated with warfarin, aspirin, and persantine.[17] These devices typically have an external system controller pack, along with a battery, which is worn in a harness. Sometimes they have a separate AC controller/charger unit, or an extended use emergency battery pack.

Both the patient and the immediate family go through a rigorous training course when preparing to use an LVAD. They should be able to identify a variety of alarms, and provide basic trouble shooting. There is also a 24-hour on-call center for each LVAD that can give a healthcare provider important information on emergency therapy. However, there are some basic techniques all emergency providers should be aware of in case there is a need to care for an LVAD patient.[17,18]

As mentioned, these patients are often pulseless during normal operation of the device. Other signs of circulation, such as warm, pink extremities, must be sought. In the ED, one can use occlusion with a blood pressure cuff and a Doppler distally to listen for flow. This technique allows for good approximation of the systolic blood pressure, which should be from 80–100 mmHg. One should also auscultate the LVAD to ensure it is pumping.

Dysrhythmias, both atrial and ventricular, can severely impede forward flow in these devices, and require aggressive and prompt treatment. They may be treated in typical fashion, via pharmaceuticals or electrical cardioversion. If these patients do need electrical cardioversion or defibrillation, the external control device may need to be disconnected, depending on the type of device; for example, the HeartMate II does not need to be disconnected. Chest compressions are dangerous in patients with LVADs, in that one can dislodge the device from the heart. If an external hand pump is available, one should use it instead.[19,20]

Valvular surgery

After prosthetic valve placement, patients commonly have postoperative fevers, dysrhythmias, wound infections, and the other above complications, which are managed identically to patients after a CABG procedure. However, surgical placement of a prosthetic valve can trigger specific complications aside from those commonly seen in post-CABG patients. Late complications that may present to an ED include CHF secondary to new functional strains on the heart, thromboembolic events such as strokes, endocarditis, and valve failure.[21]

Prosthetic valve endocarditis is often secondary to nosocomial bacteremia. It is a complication in some 2–4% of valve replacements in the United States. Roughly one-half of cases are early, defined as less than 60 days postoperative, and half are late. In early cases, a variety of staphylococcal bacteria are the cause over half of the time. Other common infectious agents include gram-negative bacteria, diptheroids, and fungi. Just like native endocarditis, prosthetic valve endocarditis can be a difficult diagnosis to make.[22] Salient features are fevers, rigors, septic physiology, and characteristic lesions such as Roth spots, which are oval white spots seen on the retina in SBE. Draw multiple (at least three) blood cultures for maximum yield, since identification of the causative organism is extremely important for therapy. Emperic antibiotics should be given after these blood drawings, and should include vancomycin, gentamycin, and either carbapenem or cefepime.[23] Clinical features that indicate a more serious course include new heart failure, a fungal organism, a drug-resistant organism, or need for removal of hardware.[22]

Valvular failure can be an immediately life-threatening occurrence. It is suspected when the patient complains of sudden dyspnea or weakness, and generally presents with muffled heart sounds, a mechanical valve without a click, or with a new murmur. Exact symptoms vary based on the degree of stenosis and regurgitation in the valve's stuck position, and more importantly, depend on which valve is affected. Treatment includes aspirin, a heparin drip, and often a thrombolytic drip. Management should include emergent echocardiography and cardiac surgery consultation.[22]

References

1 Eagle KA, Guyton RA, Davidoff R, et al. ACC/AHA 2004 guideline update for coronary artery bypass graft surgery: A report of the American College of Cardiology/American Heart Association Task Force on Practice Guidelines. *Circulation.* 2004;110:340–437.

2 Mangano DT. Cardiovascular morbidity and CABG surgery—a perspective: Epidemiology, costs, and potential therapeutic solutions. *J Card Surg.* 1995;10: 366–368.

3 Antiplatelelet Trialists' Collaboration. Collaborative overview of randomized trials of antiplatelet therapy—II: Maintenance of vascular graft or arterial patency by antiplatelet therapy. *BMJ.* 1994;308:159–168.

4 Antman EM, Anbe DT, Armstrong PW, et al. ACC/AHA guidelines for the management of patients with ST-elevation myocardial infarction. *J Am Coll Cardiol.* 2004;44:671–719.

5 Crystal E, Connolly SJ, Sleik K, et al. Interventions on prevention of postoperative atrial dibrillation in patients undergoing heart surgery: a meta-analysis. *Circulation.* 2002;106:75–80.

6 Ferguson TB, Coombs LP, Peterson ED. Preoperative beta-blocker use and mortality and morbidity following CABG surgery in North America. *JAMA.* 2002;287:2221–2227.

7 *Micromedex® Healthcare Series.* [Internet database]. Greenwood village, Colo: Thomson Healthcare. Updated periodiacally. 24 Jan. 2006. Available at: http://www.thomsonhc.com. Accessed May 14, 2010.

8 Collard CD, Body SC, Shernan SK, Wang S, Mangano DT. Preoperative statin therapy is associated with reduced cardiac mortality after coronary artery bypass graft surgery. *J Thorac Cardiovasc Surg.* 2006;132(2):392–400.

9 Gardner TJ, Horneffer PJ, Manolio TA, et al. Stroke following coronary artery bypass grafting: a ten-year study. *Ann Thorac Surg.* 1985;40:574–581.

10 Newman MF, Kirchner JL, Phillips-Bute B, et al, for the Neurological Outcome Research Group and the Cardiothoracic Anesthesiology Research Endeavors Investigators. Longitudinal assessment of neurocognitive function after coronary-artery bypass surgery. *N Engl J Med.* 2001;344:395–402.

11 Maisel WH, Rawn JD, Stevenson WG. Atrial fibrillation after cardiac surgery. *Ann Intern Med.* 2001;135:1061–1073.

12 Mathew JP, Fontes ML, Tudor IC, et al. A multicenter risk index for atrial fibrillation after cardiac surgery. *JAMA.* 2004;291:1720–1729.

13 ECC Committee, Subcommittees and Task Forces of the American Heart Association. 2005 American Heart Association guidelines for cardiopulmonary resuscitation and emergency cardiovascular care. *Circulation.* 2005;112(24 Suppl):IV1–203.

14 Braxton JH, Marrin CA, McGrath PD, et al. Mediastinitis and long-term survival after coronary artery bypass graft surgery. *Ann Thorac Surg.* 2000;70:2004–2007.

15 Slaughter MS, Olson MM, Lee JT, Ward HB. A fifteen-year wound surveillance study after coronary artery bypass. *Ann Thorac Surg.* 1993;56:1063–1068.

16 Rose EA, Gelijns AC, Moskowitz AJ, et al. Long-term mechanical left ventricular assistance for end-stage heart failure. *N Engl J Med.* 2001;345:1435–1443.

17 Seemuth SC, Richenbacher WE. Education of the ventricular assist device patient's community services. *ASAIO J.* 2001;47:596–601.

18 Stahl MA, Richards NM. Ventricular assist devices: developing and maintaining a training and competency program. *J Cardiovasc Nurs.* 2002;16:34–43.

19 Bond AE, Nelson K, Germany CL, Smart AN. The left ventricular assist device. *Am J Nurs.* 2003; 103(1):32–40.

20 Riddle WA. The high-tech heart: LVAD emergencies in the pre-transplant patients. *JEMS.* 2007;32(8): 58–63.

21 Schwartz, et al. *Principles of Surgery.* 7th ed. New York, McGraw-Hill; 1999.

22 Libby P, Bonow RO, Mann DL, Zipes DP. *Braunwald's Heart Disease: A Textbook of Cardiovascular Disease.* 7th ed. Philadelphia, Elsevier Sanders; 2005.

23 Baddour LM, Wilson WR, Bayer AS, et al. Infective endocarditis: diagnosis, antimicrobial therapy, and management of complications: a statement for healthcare professionals from the Committee on Rheumatic Fever, Endocarditis, and Kawasaki Disease, Council on Cardiovascular Disease in the Young and the Councils on Clinical Cardiology, Stroke and Cardiovascular Surgery and Anesthesia, American Heart Association. *Circulation.* 2005;111:e394–434.

27 Pediatric cardiac emergencies

Shannon Straszewski[1] & Carrie Tibbles[2]
[Chapter Consultant: Kenneth J. Bramwell]

[1] Chief Resident, Harvard Affiliated Residency in Emergency Medicine, Beth Israel Deaconess Medical Center, Boston, Massachusetts, USA
[2] Associate Director, Graduate Medical Education, Beth Israel Deaconess Medical Center, Associate Residency Director Harvard Affiliated Emergency Medicine Residency, Assistant Professor of Medicine, Harvard Medical School

Section I: Case presentation

A 3-day-old boy was brought to the emergency department (ED) by his mother. She reported that the child had been feeding poorly the prior day, had become less active, and was having trouble breathing. Prior to this, the mother was nursing him without difficulty. She stated the patient had not had any noticeable changes in the number of wet diapers, and had not been febrile. The baby had no sick contacts, and all the siblings were healthy. The child was the product of a normal, spontaneous, vaginal delivery at 40 weeks gestational age. The patient weighed 7 lbs 8 oz (3.12 kg) at birth. He took no medications, and had no allergies. There was no family history of cardiopulmonary disease in childhood. The baby lived with his mother, father and 3-year-old brother in a smoke-free household.

The vital signs were: temperature 37.2°C (99°F), pulse 190 beats/min, blood pressure 50/30 mmHG, respiratory rate 56 breaths/min, and oxygen saturation 85% on room air.

On physical examination, the patient appeared listless in his mother's arms, making no spontaneous movements. He appeared pale with some central cyanosis. The head was unremarkable, with normal fontanelles. The heart rate was tachycardic, with no appreciable murmurs. The lungs were clear to auscultation, but the breathing was tachypneic and labored. The abdomen was soft, *nontender, and nondistended with normal bowel sounds. The extremities were cyanotic, but no rash was present; the pulses were thready, and more prominent in the upper extremities compared to the lower.*

The patient was placed on a non-rebreather oxygen mask with no improvement of oxygen saturation. An initial fingerstick glucose was normal. The serum bicarbonate level was low, while electrolytes and complete blood count were otherwise normal. A urinalysis was normal. An EKG showed a sinus tachycardia with a right heart strain. The chest X-ray study did not show any abnormalities in the lungs or cardiac silhouette.

Section II: Case discussion

Dr Peter Rosen: It is rare to get a blood pressure on an infant, and because of that, most of us are probably not going to know what to make of this blood pressure. Do you have any rules for what a blood pressure ought to be in a 3-day-old, and when would you recommend taking one?

Dr Kenneth Bramwell: There are a number of rules that have been offered. The one that is used most commonly is to double the age in years and add 70 ([age in years × 2] + 70); some will use the age in years times 2 plus 80 ([age in years × 2] + 80) as well, so you'll capture even more patients who have abnormal blood

Cardiovascular Problems in Emergency Medicine: A discussion-based review, First Edition.
Edited by Shamai A. Grossman and Peter Rosen.
© 2011 John Wiley & Sons, Ltd. Published 2011 by John Wiley & Sons, Ltd.

pressures. In practice, very few people obtain blood pressures unless the infant is unresponsive. Most of the time we will not attempt a blood pressure in a patient less than 5 years old, although there are no set rules.

PR: Given our inexperience with pediatric blood pressure, I am more concerned about the pulse rate. Here we have a little more experience with children, and even though they generally have tachycardias by adult standards, it shouldn't be up to 190. Since we have a normal fingerstick glucose even though the child looks like he's not perfusing well, given the age of the child and that the child is limp, my first thoughts would be about sepsis. How do we move away from sepsis in children, which is probably the most common cause of a critically-ill child, to any other etiology of disease in a child?

Dr Carrie Tibbles: Sepsis is very high on the differential diagnosis. It is very common for a child who later ends up diagnosed with a congenital heart lesion to be initially misclassified as sepsis. The one study that looked at sepsis versus congenital heart disease finds that babies with congenital heart disease can have elevated white blood cell counts and fevers similar to those who are septic.

KB: We always think of sepsis first. For every infant who we see with a congenital heart lesion, we probably see somewhere in the neighborhood of 10–100 times as many children who are septic, or at least have beginning signs of sepsis.

CT: However, the oxygen saturation of 85%, with a normal chest X-ray study, may begin to move you toward another diagnosis. The other finding that helps you is that the cyanosis seems worse in the lower extremities than in the upper; if you check the pulses and they are a little bit different in the upper extremities, that can help you as well. The rapidity of change is also noteworthy. He was feeding well, then suddenly he became tachypneic and blue; however, he is not really coughing, and doesn't have respiratory distress. This begins to make you suspect that maybe this is congenital heart disease.

PR: I always thought that the most probable presentation of congenital heart disease in an infant is heart failure, yet this child does not appear to be in failure, although he does appear to be failing, if you can accept the distinction. Are there other clues to the presence of congenital heart disease in infants that we should be more alert to?

KB: I don't think that heart failure is the most common presentation of these newborns with congenital heart disease. It would seem that it should be, but the problem is generated by ductal-dependent lesions; on days 2–5 the ductus arteriosus closes, and all of a sudden, a child who has been doing reasonably well becomes acutely ill. Some of the lesions that these children can have will ultimately end up causing heart failure symptoms, but many of them do not. Many of these lesions, particularly the ductal-dependent types, cause listlessness, differential pulses, and somewhat surprising or severe cyanosis, without the development of heart failure.

PR: I've seen a number of infants who have presented with a supraventricular tachycardia (SVT) from which they were failing. Is there any way to predict who should be looked at for that purpose, just in terms of the pulse rate, before you acquire an EKG?

Dr Shamai Grossman: This is a patient with a fast heart rate; who therefore deserves an EKG to evaluate the rhythm. One way or another you're going to need an EKG, and that will make your diagnosis if there is an SVT. I would be very surprised to see an adult with this oxygen saturation with an SVT as the sole etiology of the hypoxia. Is this true of children as well?

PR: In Denver, we were somewhat blasé about oxygen saturations because of the altitude. Patients could present with an oxygen saturation of around 90% without us being particularly concerned about it. Do infants follow the adult pattern in terms of changes of their oxygen saturation?

KB: When I was in Salt Lake City, we were similarly unimpressed with low oxygen saturations in the 90–91%, or even in the 89%, range, particularly during respiratory syncytial virus (RSV) season, where we were somewhat sad that we had even obtained those numbers in a well-appearing child. Having said that, I think that a lot of people base their concern about oxygen saturation on where they did their residency, and not so much as where they are presently practicing. A saturation of 85% is not particularly impressive. I would expect someone with a significant obstructive or ductal-dependent lesion to have significantly lower oxygen saturation. In addition, commonly in infants, particularly 2 or 3 day olds and infants with congenital heart disease, you cannot obtain a good pulse oximetry reading; it's almost like you're getting a pulse oximetry of the ambient air more than their fingers or their earlobes. So, sometimes, there is a discrepancy between how the patient looks, or how cyanotic he is, and how low his oxygen level is.

PR: What would make one suspect a ductal-dependent congenital heart lesion? Is the clue the age of the child, as this child is still in the first week of life, which is when physiologic changes normally occur? If the child was a month or 2 old with the same presentation, would we need to worry about be a different kind of heart lesion? Are we clued in to the possible use of prostaglandins because it's the first week of life?

CT: Normally the ductus will close in the first 24–48 hours after birth. If you have a ductal-dependent cardiac lesion, sometimes closure will be a little bit delayed. Those kids will sometimes stay open a little bit longer, which is why occasionally they are discharged from the hospital before the ductus closes. If this child were 1 or 2 months old, presenting with an initial presentation of congenital heart disease, that would make me think of one of two problems. Particularly if the presentation was less dramatic, I would rule out a ductal-dependent lesion, because that should have presented earlier. Additionally, a baby with a ventricular septal defect can present in heart failure. These infants tend to be a little bit older (1–3 months), and as the right-sided and left-sided pressures equal out, they will develop congestive heart failure.

PR: Right-heart predominance is often seen in pediatric EKGs. Is there anything on this EKG description that would point you towards a congenital heart disease?

SG: Although the right-heart strain can be a normal variant, right-heart strain would be expected in a disease process with a cyanotic child, and any of those diseases that impair flow out of the right ventricle would give you right-heart strain. This could include a transposition, tetralogy of Fallot, or even hypoplastic left-heart syndrome.

PR: If we saw an adult with this degree of cyanosis, our immediate reaction would be to intubate the patient. Intubation of children, however, is not such an easy technical task, and is fraught with some difficulties in management once the tube is in place, as you shouldn't use a cuffed tube in a child this size and age. One might have also some difficulty finding the

appropriate equipment with which to bag ventilate the child. Would an oxygen tent, rather than intubation, be a better initial choice?

KB: This is one of the settings where you will want to intubate the child as early as you can regardless of the oxygen saturations. The prostaglandin infusions will likely be life-saving for this child. The most concerning problem with prostaglandin infusion is that it causes apnea. The apnea appears, to some degree, to be dose-dependent, but is also related to the length of time that the patient is receiving the infusion. Usually one can intubate the patient faster than starting the prostaglandin infusion, although they are both equally important.

PR: Do you have any technical tricks for intubating a child this age?

KB: The greatest difficulty in intubating patients this age is that we haven't the experience of intubating a large number of 3, 4, and 5 kilogram infants. Many people don't use rapid sequence intubation (RSI), often intubating in the delivery room without medications. I would advocate using RSI, gathering all of your equipment as quickly as possible. This scenario is not a crash intubation, so you have a few minutes. One must remember how much smaller your equipment will need to be, and how much more precise you need to be with your intubation skills. You'll need an uncuffed tube, a Miller or straight blade, and you'd want to have slightly smaller endotracheal tubes available. Most of us usually use a 4.0 tube for infants, but in this case, you should have a 3.5 and maybe even a 3.0 tube styletted and ready to be used.

PR: Do you need a special ambu bag?

KB: No, you will probably be better off using the pediatric ambu bag than searching and trying something new. Most of the time, if there are newborn resuscitations that are happening regularly in your hospital, they'll have the smaller pediatric bag readily available.

PR: How useful is fingerstick glucose in this child?

CT: Any child, as with adults, presenting with an altered mental status should have a glucose checked as soon as possible, as severe symptomatic hypoglycemia could be the etiology. As the child becomes sicker and sicker and more hypoperfused, they could also become hypoglycemic. Hypoglycemia is one of the few easily corrected presentations of altered mental status.

KB: Although it is difficult to remember all of the congenital metabolic abnormalities that children can have, all of them have the potential to result in hypoglycemia. Without having to remember the individual genetic problem, one may be able to fix all of these patients simply by keeping the glucose at a proper level.

PR: What diagnostic tests would you want to utilize before giving any therapy to this child or while you are giving the therapy, as in this age group one should probably intubate and start a prostaglandin infusion as soon as possible; you can then try to figure out which particular disease is the culprit? Is there an age constraint for an echocardiogram (ECHO), or is there any other initial diagnostic maneuver that might help?

SG: Checking a hemoglobin would be very useful, as anemia could cause this presentation. With a normal oxygen saturation, we might worry about peripheral cyanosis-type diseases, such as methemoglobinemia. There are no constraints to obtaining an echocardiogram. Not only are there no constraints, this test will likely be diagnostic, and should be done as expeditiously as possible.

CT: After intubating this patient, it will be useful to look at the infant's response to oxygenation and intubation. If the baby's oxygenation improves to 100%, this is probably sepsis, but if the oxygenation is still 80% post-intubation, then one begins to think that this is not a new pneumonia or sepsis; some other disease process is preventing the child from oxygenating the blood.

PR: How do you choose a prostaglandin to infuse?

KB: Prostaglandin-E1 is the only one we routinely use for infant infusion in the ED. The dose is between 0.05 mcg/kg/min and 0.1 mcg/kg/min. As we mentioned, there seems to be a relationship between the strength of the infusion and the side effects. I would plan on the patient becoming apneic.

PR: Once you've started your prostaglandin infusion, intubated the child, ordered an ECHO, and spoken with the pediatric intensive care unit physician and hopefully a pediatric cardiologist, what else do you need to do in the ED for this child?

CT: This child will also probably benefit from a 20 cc/kg bolus of normal saline to help support the blood pressure. If the patient remains in shock after you've given the saline boluses, you might start a peripheral pressor for support while waiting for the prostaglandins to kick in.

PR: One of my technical nightmares is the thought of starting an IV on a 3-day-old infant. Would you start with an intraosseous line (IO) initially? Can prostaglandins be given through an intraosseous line?

KB: I wouldn't spend too much time trying to get an IV; while we are doing our initial evaluation, I would expect the nurse to try to get an IV. I wouldn't hesitate about putting an IO in an infant. Prostaglandins can be given through the IO as well. The newer IO access devices, particularly the intraosseous lines that are more like a hand drill, have markedly changed our threshold for using intraosseous lines. They are easier and faster than getting an IV in the best of hands.

PR: Do you see any need for putting in a femoral line for central access?

CT: As long as you are able to give the prostaglandins, and the baby is responding and able to maintain some degree of hemodynamic stability, I would not waste time putting a femoral line in at this point.

SG: Until when can one cannulate an umbilical vein, and would that be feasible in this case?

KB: My understanding is that it is feasible until about day seven of life, particularly if you still have the umbilical stump present, and you can slice down to nondesiccated stump material. The biggest problem with the umbilical vein catheterization is that the vast majority of emergency physicians haven't done one, or may have never even seen one done, so practically this may not be useful.

PR: I haven't done one since before the implementation of the intraosseous route; the problem we had with umbilical vein catheterization was not the technical difficulty, but picking the vessel, since there are two arteries and one vein and it's hard to remember which is which. I think that many of the umbilical cut downs ended up being intraarterial instead of intravenous. I'm not sure that it makes that much of a difference, but it probably reflects the fact that we don't do these procedures very often.

PR: If the baby's pulse rate did not slow down with a fluid and prostaglandin infusion, what would be your next step? Would you have any concern that you are dealing with a dysrhythmia that needs cardioversion?

SG: Unless there was electrocardiographic evidence of a dysrhythmia, I would not worry about one. If the heart rate doesn't slow down, then I would try and obtain an ECHO sooner rather than later, because perhaps you are dealing with something that you are not going to be able to fix in an ED and need an operative intervention.

PR: Can you summarize the most common ductal-dependent congenital lesions?

CT: More important than the specific diagnoses is to remember the two-way communication between your left-sided circulation and your right-sided circulation. I think of ductal-dependent lesions as either blood flow being obstructed and not flowing to the lungs, or not flowing to the systemic circulation. If you can keep the communication open, then you can distribute the blood where it needs to go. For example, in left-sided obstructive lesions, if you have a coarctation of the aorta or a hypoplastic left ventricle, then by maintaining patency of the ductus arteriosus, you can move the blood that is congesting the pulmonary system into the circulation. With gray or cyanotic babies who are in shock or with congenital heart abnormalities like tricuspid atresia, tetralogy of Fallot, or transposition obstructing blood flow to the lungs, you want to open the ductus so the systemic circulation can infuse the lungs and oxygenate the blood.

PR: After the first life-saving surgery, what complications will bring the child back to the ED: sepsis, failure of the shunt, or congestive heart failure?

CT: With a hypoplastic left heart, congestive failure is possible in that ventricle, as the right ventricle needs to supply the systemic circulation. The lungs are supplied by first a synthetic shunt, and second from an anastamosis of the superior vena cava and inferior vena cava to the pulmonary arteries, and they can have heart failure if the ventricle fails. These patients are very preload dependent as the blood supplied to the lungs is a passive system, and they need an adequate intravascular volume. More commonly, when

this child has a respiratory infection, particularly RSV, or anything that raises intrathoracic pressure, even dehydration for any reason, he may present with low oxygen saturation.

PR: Are they more prone to bacterial infections like endocarditis?

KB: Surprisingly, endocarditis seems to be quite rare in these children, despite all of their artificial hardware and the underdeveloped immune system of an infant. Their biggest problems are the result of simple viral infections causing them to stop or limit feeding. As tenuous as they are to begin with, they very quickly decompensate if they don't have enough intravascular volume to keep their blood pressure in a reasonable range, and often present in shock.

SG: What do you need to worry about when this patient becomes an adult? What kinds of things would you need to keep in mind when a patient presents to the ED with a history of having had congenital heart disease?

KB: The greatest challenge I experience with these patients is finding them a physician. Adults with a history of congenital heart disease tend to have extraordinarily complex anatomical alterations, and will often fall through the cracks, unless they are well set up with a pediatric cardiologist. They are similar to 40-year-old patients with cystic fibrosis. They often don't have a medical home or a physician following them, and this is why enlisting a pediatric cardiologist is very important. Moreover, the adult cardiologists don't usually take care of these problems.

PR: These cases can be very scary to the emergency physician, particularly one who doesn't see critical infants very often. To summarize, check the blood sugar, check the oxygen, and see if the child responds to oxygenation. Don't be afraid to put an intraosseous line in quickly, be sure to look at the age of the child, and administer your prostaglandins promptly to keep the shunt open.

Case resolution

The physician intubated the patient, and administered prostaglandin at a rate of 0.05 mcg/kg/min.

The child was subsequently transferred to a tertiary referral center where he was admitted to the ICU. The patient had an echocardiogram demonstrating a hypoplastic left-heart syndrome, and he underwent surgery the next day. After a weeklong stay in the ICU, he was transferred to the floor for an additional 5 weeks prior to discharge home with his parents. The patient will require close cardiology follow up for examination and echocardiography as an outpatient.

Section III: Concepts

Background/epidemiology

Congenital heart disease occurs in 4–12 per 1000 live births.[1-3] Increasingly, congenital heart disease can be detected in utero.[4] Despite this progress in early detection, some studies indicate up to 25% of patients with congenital heart disease are discharged home after birth undiagnosed.[5] Many infants are asymptomatic at birth, but deteriorate rapidly as the amount of blood flow through the pulmonary circulation increases and the foramen ovale and ductus arteriosus close over the first days to weeks of life. In cyanotic congenital heart disease, the patient has a right to left shunt, allowing the deoxygenated blood to bypass the lungs and pass directly through the circulation. These infants are dependent on the presence of a patent ductus arteriosus to allow deoxygenated blood to flow back into the pulmonary arteries from the aorta.[6] To obtain an oxygen saturation of 85%, at least 3–5 g/dL of deoxygenated hemoglobin is needed in the neonatal circulation.[7] Infants with lesions such as hypoplastic left-heart syndrome and aortic coarctation, which obstruct blood flow from the heart to the rest of the body, require a patent ductus to maintain their systemic circulation, and will present in profound shock when the ductus closes. Furthermore, neonates do not have the same ability to increase their stroke volume, and thus rely on tachycardia to increase their cardiac output in response to stressors. Therefore, changes in volume status, such as dehydration or a relative bradycardia, can have disastrous effects on the cardiac output. This helps to explain why neonates will compensate by increasing the systemic vascular resistance to maintain blood pressure, and will clinically have cool, pale extremities.[8]

Initial workup, history and physical

As these infants are typically critically ill, initial resuscitation efforts should begin immediately. The infant should be placed on supplemental oxygen if in respiratory distress. Intravenous access should be established rapidly; if unable to place a peripheral line quickly, an umbilical line or intraosseous access should be performed. An umbilical line can be placed until the stump has desiccated, between 7–14 days after birth. The physician should obtain a brief pediatric history, focusing on events surrounding birth for both the neonate and mother, and a description of the onset of the current symptoms. If the patient is febrile, this may point toward an infectious etiology and a septic infant. Questioning about diaphoresis, tachypnea, or fatigue, or difficulties during feeding is often helpful.[9] Feeding is often the most stressful activity for an infant.

The history can guide the physical examination. If congenital heart disease is suspected, blood pressure readings and oxygen saturations in both the arms and the legs should be obtained. A general guideline is any number less than 70 plus the age in years for the systolic blood pressure indicates a pediatric patient is hypotensive. The general appearance of the neonate should be noted, looking for signs of dehydration or signs of fluid overload, which may suggest heart failure. If the infant is crying, determine if this improves or worsens the cyanosis, as improvement in color with crying suggests a pulmonary etiology. On cardiac auscultation, a third heart sound can be physiologic, but the presence of a fourth heart sound is almost always pathologic. The chest should be auscultated and percussed for evidence of fluid. Central and peripheral cyanosis can be distinguished by evaluating the mucus membranes, lips, and nail beds. The extremities should be evaluated for capillary refill, clubbing, temperature and moisture of skin, as well as the quality of pulses.[3,10]

A crucial aspect of the evaluation centers on discriminating between noncardiac etiologies and cardiac etiologies. In this case, a hyperoxia test is very helpful. In a standard hyperoxia test, the infant is placed on 100% oxygen for 10 minutes. If the arterial oxygenation is greater than 150 mmHg as measured on an arterial blood gas, a respiratory cause is more likely. If the oxygenation is less than 100 mmHg, congenital heart disease is more likely.[3,10,11] Since an arterial blood gas may not be feasible in all situations, it is more straightforward to place the infant on 100% oxygen and note the response. If the saturation fails to improve, cardiac disease is the more likely explanation.

Etiologies/differential diagnosis

The differential diagnosis of a critically-ill infant is broad, but a basic evaluation can generally guide the initial resuscitation. Sepsis is one of the most common causes of critical illness in newborns. The infectious etiologies include pneumonia, bronchiolitis, and meningitis.[12] Central nervous system abnormalities include shallow breathing from a perinatal asphyxia and encephalopathy.[13] Less common congenital malformations include diaphragmatic hernias or tracheoesophageal fistulas. One would expect an improvement of the cyanosis with oxygen administration with a diaphragmatic hernia, and a tracheoesophageal fistula may be distinguished by exacerbations during periods of feeding. Other pulmonary etiologies include a pneumothorax or pleural effusions; these can be identified on physical examination and further testing. Infantile botulism or muscular dystrophy should also be considered with a floppy infant.

Lastly, the differential diagnosis of cyanotic congenital heart diseases (CHD) includes the causes of right to left shunts: tetralogy of Fallot, transposition of the great arteries, tricuspid atresia, total anomalous pulmonary venous return, truncus arteriosis, pulmonary atresia, Ebstein's anomaly, and single ventricle states such as the hypoplastic left-heart syndrome. Fortunately, the initial resuscitation is similar for each of these lesions, so it is not necessary to determine the likely etiology to begin effectively stabilizing the infant.

Testing

Patients who present with altered consciousness should have a blood glucose obtained as soon as possible. Thereafter, all patients should have a baseline chemistry panel to evaluate for a metabolic acidosis. A complete blood count should also be obtained, looking at the white blood cell count as a marker for possible infection, as well as for erythrocytosis, a marker of chronic cyanosis. The I/T ratio, or immature to total ratio, for white blood cells is also frequently requested. An umbilical artery line should be placed to obtain a baseline arterial blood gas on room air. A second sample should be taken after administration of 100% oxygen for 10 minutes (hyperoxia test). A chest radiograph is helpful to determine if there is a pulmonary cause of the cyanosis; this also allows one to assess if the pulmonary blood flow is increased or decreased, as well as note the presence of a pneumothorax or a pleural effusion and the appearance of the cardiac silhouette. In many instances, the chest radiograph will be unremarkable. An EKG can evaluate dysrhythmias, axis deviation, hypertrophy, strain, and metabolic abnormalities, but may appear normal despite life-threatening pathology.[14]

Management

It is common to witness oxygen saturations of less than 70% in patients with ductal-dependent lesions. To maintain patency of the ductus arteriosus, administer prostaglandin-E1 as a continuous infusion; the initial dose is 0.05–0.1 mcg/kg/min.[6,15,16] This dosage may also be given via the IO route. Patients with ductal-dependent lesions should not be left on a 100% nonrebreather mask, as the high level of oxygen actually triggers closure of the ductus arteriosus. Depending on the stability of the patient, the child may need to be intubated for airway protection and as protection against apnea, one of the more serious side effects of prostaglandin administration. There often is time to utilize rapid sequence intubation, preparing a spectrum of styletted endotracheal tubes ranging from 2.5–4.0, depending on the age of the infant. Recent evidence, however, suggests that in the stable patient, intubation prior to transfer may actually produce more complications in the infant, and therefore should be deferred until the tertiary care destination is reached.[17] Regardless, the FiO_2 of the oxygen should remain as close to 40% as possible. If dehydration is also a concern, small fluid boluses should be administered at 10–20 mL/kg. Attempts should also be made to get the patient to a tertiary referral center as soon as possible to obtain a pediatric ECHO, and for evaluation by pediatric cardiologists. In recent years, telemedicine has come to the aid of smaller hospitals to facilitate and expedite care.[18]

Disposition

Most of these patients presenting with newly diagnosed CHD, should be admitted to the pediatric

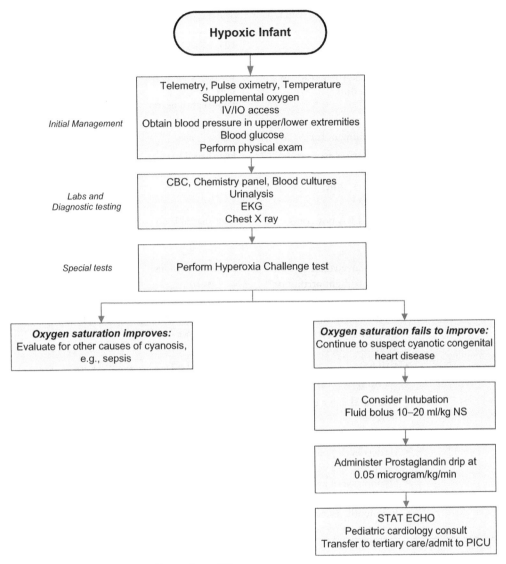

Figure 27.1 Cyanotic congenital heart disease[6,20].

intensive care unit. It is often prudent to administer broad spectrum antibiotics, as sepsis is typically still on the differential diagnosis list.

If the child deteriorates into pulseless electrical activity or cardiac dysrhythmia while still in the ED, standard pediatric advance life support pathways should be followed.[19] Inotropic agents, such as dopamine at 5–20 mcg/kg/min or dobutamine at 5–20 mcg/kg/min, can be added for pressure support.

Section IV: Decision making

- A targeted history and physical examination can help distinguish between cardiac and noncardiac etiologies in the cyanotic infant.
- Initial resuscitation involves rapid intravenous or intraosseous access, oxygen administration, and prostaglandin administration as indicated (Figure 27-1).
- See Table 27-1 for specific characteristics of cyanotic congenital heart disease.

Table 27-1. Rate control medications for atrial fibrillation with rapid ventricular response.

Etiology	Percentage of CHD*	Anatomy	Chest X-ray Findings	EKG Findings
Tetrology of Fallot	10%	• Right ventricle outflow obstruction • RVH • VSD • Overriding aorta	Decreased pulmonary flow Boot-shaped heart	RVH Right axis deviation
Transposition of the great arteries	5%	• Aorta arises from right ventricle • Requires either PDA or VSD	Egg-shaped heart	RVH, LVH Right axis deviation
Tricuspid atresia	1–2%	• RV and RA not connected	Boot-shaped heart	RVH, Right axis deviation LVH in severe cases
Total anomalous pulmonary venous return	1%	• Pulmonary venous blood drains to right atrium or systemic circulation	Pulmonary venous congestion	RVH, Right axis deviation
Truncus arteriosus	<1%	• Single artery supplies pulmonary, coronary, and systemic blood	Right aortic arch +/− evidence of CHF	RVH, LVH
Pulmonary atresia	<1%	• RVH • Blood flows through PFO	Right atrial enlargement	RVH, Right axis deviation
Ebsteins's anomaly	<1%	• Tricuspid valve develops in RV • Smaller functioning RV	Cardiomegaly (sometimes described as box or funnel shaped)	
Hypoplastic left-heart syndrome	<1%	• Underdeveloped mitral/aortic valve and left ventricle • Hypoplasia of ascending aorta • Blood supply via PDA • Frequently associated with coarctation of aorta	Increased pulmonary flow Cardiomegaly	RVH, Right axis deviation

*The majority of congenital heart disease can be attributed to acyanotic heart disease presentations.
Abbreviations: RVH–Right Ventricle Hypertrophy, VSD–Ventricular Septal Defect, PFO–Patent Foramen Ovale, PDA–Patent Ductus Arteriosus, RV–Right Ventricle, RA–Right Atrium, and LVH–Left Ventricular Hypertrophy.

Adapted from: Yee L. Cardiac emergencies in the first year of life. *Emerg Med Clin North Am.* 2007;25(4):981–1008, vi. And Samánek M, Slavík Z, Zborilová B, Hrobonová V, Vorísková M, Skovránek J. Prevalence, treatment, and outcome of heart disease in live-born children: A prospective analysis of 91,823 live-born children. *Pediatr Cardiol.* 1989;10(4):205–211.

References

1 Sissman NJ, Willerson JT, Lefkowit RJ. Incidence of congenital heart disease. *JAMA*. 2001:285(20):2579–2580.

2 Sadowski SL. Congenital cardiac disease in the newborn infant: past, present, and future. *Crit Care Nurs Clin North Am*. 2009;21(1):37–48, vi.

3 Tanner K, Sabrine N, Wren C. Cardiovascular malformations among preterm infants. *Pediatrics*. 2005;116(6): e833–838.

4 Lee W, Comstock C. Prenatal diagnosis of congenital heart disease: where are we now? *Ultrasound Clin*. 2006;1(2):273–291.

5 Wren C, Reinhardt Z, Khawaja K. Twenty-year trends in diagnosis of life-threatening neonatal cardiovascular malformations. *Arch Dis Child Fetal Neonatal Ed*. 2008;93(1):F33–F35.

6 Yee L. Cardiac emergencies in the first year of life. *Emerg Med Clin North Am*. 2007;25(4):981–1008, vi.

7 Woolridge DP, Love JC. Congenital heart disease in the pediatric emergency department. Part I: Pathophyisiolgy and clinical characteristics. *Pediatr Emerg Med Rep*. 2002;7:69–75.

8 Inaba A. Cardiac Disorders. In: Marx, JA, Hockberger R, Walls R, eds. *Rosen's Emergency Medicine: Concepts and Clinical Practice*. 6th ed. Philadelphia: Elsevier; 2006;2567–2601.

9 Sharieff GQ, Wylie TW. Pediatric cardiac disorders. *J Emerg Med*. 2004;26(1):65–79.

10 Woods WA, McCulloch MA. Cardiovascular emergencies in the pediatric patient. *Emerg Med Clin North Am*. 2005;23(4):1233–1249.

11 Yabek SM. Neonatal cyanosis: reappraisal of the response to 100% oxygen breathing. *Am J Dis Child*. 1984;138:880–884.

12 Brousseau, T, Kisson N. Common neonatal problems. In: Tintinalli, J, Kelen GD, Stapczynski JS, eds. *ACEP. Emergency Medicine: A Comprehensive Study Guide*. 6th ed. New York: McGraw-Hill; 2003; 593–594.

13 Park MK. Cyanotic congenital heart defects. In: *Pediatric Cardiology for Practioners*. 5th ed. Philadelphia: Mosby; 2008:176–231.

14 O'Connor M, McDaniel N, Brady WJ. The pediatric electrocardiogram part III: Congenital heart disease and other cardiac syndromes. *Am J Emerg Med*. 2008;26(4):497–503.

15 Barst RJ, Gersony WM. The pharmacological treatment of patent ductus arteriosus. A review of the evidence. *Drugs*. 1989;38(2):249–266.

16 Woolard R. Congenital heart disease, cyanotic. In: Schaider J, Barkin R, Hayden S, Rosen P, Wolfe R, eds. *Rosen and Barkin's 5 Minute Emergency Medicine Consult*. 2nd ed. Philadelphia: Lippincott, Williams, Wilkins; 2003:252–253.

17 Meckler GD, Lowe C. To intubate or not to intubate? Transporting infants on prostaglandin E1. *Pediatrics*. 2009;123(1):e25–e30.

18 Sable CA, Cummings SD, Pearson GD, et al. Impact of telemedicine on the practice of pediatric cardiology in community hospitals. *Pediatrics*. 2002;109(1):E3.

19 American Heart Association. 2005 American Heart Association (AHA) guidelines for cardiopulmonary resuscitation (CPR) and emergency cardiovascular care (ECC) of pediatric and neonatal patients: pediatric basic life support. *Circulation*. 2005;112 (24 Suppl):IV1–203.

Index

Cardiovascular Problems in Emergency Medicine: A discussion-based review, First Edition.
Edited by Shamai A. Grossman and Peter Rosen.
© 2011 John Wiley & Sons, Ltd. Published 2011 by John Wiley & Sons, Ltd.

Printed and bound by CPI Group (UK) Ltd, Croydon, CR0 4YY

09/06/2025

14686002-0004